KU-467-500

Practical Transfusion Medicine

Practical Transfusion Medicine

EDITED BY

Michael F. Murphy MD, FRCP, FrcPath

Professor of Blood Transfusion Medicine
University of Oxford;
Consultant Haematologist
NHS Blood and Transplant and Department of Haematology
John Radcliffe Hospital
Oxford, UK

Derwood H. Pamphilon MD, MRCPCH, FRCP, FrcPath

Formerly, Consultant Haematologist
NHS Blood and Transplant
Bristol, UK;
Honorary Clinical Reader
Department of Cellular and Molecular Medicine
University of Bristol
Bristol, UK

Nancy M. Heddle MSc, FCSMLS(D)

Director, MTRP
Professor, Department of Medicine
McMaster University
Canadian Blood Services
Hamilton, ON, Canada

FOURTH EDITION

WILEY-BLACKWELL

A John Wiley & Sons, Ltd., Publication

This edition first published 2013 © 2001, 2005, 2009, 2013 by John Wiley & Sons Ltd.

Wiley-Blackwell is an imprint of John Wiley & Sons, formed by the merger of Wiley's global Scientific, Technical and Medical business with Blackwell Publishing.

Registered office: John Wiley & Sons, Ltd, The Atrium, Southern Gate, Chichester, West Sussex, PO19 8SQ, UK

Editorial offices: 9600 Garsington Road, Oxford, OX4 2DQ, UK
The Atrium, Southern Gate, Chichester, West Sussex, PO19 8SQ, UK
111 River Street, Hoboken, NJ 07030-5774, USA

For details of our global editorial offices, for customer services and for information about how to apply for permission to reuse the copyright material in this book please see our website at www.wiley.com/wiley-blackwell

The right of the author to be identified as the author of this work has been asserted in accordance with the UK Copyright, Designs and Patents Act 1988.

All rights reserved. No part of this publication may be reproduced, stored in a retrieval system, or transmitted, in any form or by any means, electronic, mechanical, photocopying, recording or otherwise, except as permitted by the UK Copyright, Designs and Patents Act 1988, without the prior permission of the publisher.

Designations used by companies to distinguish their products are often claimed as trademarks. All brand names and product names used in this book are trade names, service marks, trademarks or registered trademarks of their respective owners. The publisher is not associated with any product or vendor mentioned in this book. This publication is designed to provide accurate and authoritative information in regard to the subject matter covered. It is sold on the understanding that the publisher is not engaged in rendering professional services. If professional advice or other expert assistance is required, the services of a competent professional should be sought.

The contents of this work are intended to further general scientific research, understanding, and discussion only and are not intended and should not be relied upon as recommending or promoting a specific method, diagnosis, or treatment by physicians for any particular patient. The publisher and the author make no representations or warranties with respect to the accuracy or completeness of the contents of this work and specifically disclaim all warranties, including without limitation any implied warranties of fitness for a particular purpose. In view of ongoing research, equipment modifications, changes in governmental regulations, and the constant flow of information relating to the use of medicines, equipment, and devices, the reader is urged to review and evaluate the information provided in the package insert or instructions for each medicine, equipment, or device for, among other things, any changes in the instructions or indication of usage and for added warnings and precautions. Readers should consult with a specialist where appropriate. The fact that an organization or Website is referred to in this work as a citation and/or a potential source of further information does not mean that the author or the publisher endorses the information the organization or Website may provide or recommendations it may make. Further, readers should be aware that Internet Websites listed in this work may have changed or disappeared between when this work was written and when it is read. No warranty may be created or extended by any promotional statements for this work. Neither the publisher nor the author shall be liable for any damages arising herefrom.

Library of Congress Cataloging-in-Publication Data

Practical transfusion medicine / edited by Michael F. Murphy, Derwood H. Pamphilon, Nancy M. Heddle. – 4th ed.
      p. ; cm.
   Includes bibliographical references and index.
   ISBN 978-0-470-67051-4 (hardback : alk. paper)
   I. Murphy, Michael F. (Michael Furber) II. Pamphilon, Derwood H. III. Heddle, Nancy M.
   [DNLM: 1. Blood Transfusion.   2. Blood Grouping and Crossmatching.
3. Blood Preservation.   4. Cross Infection–prevention & control.
5. Hematopoietic Stem Cell Transplantation.   WB 356]
615.3′9–dc23

                                                                                    2012037179

A catalogue record for this book is available from the British Library.

Wiley also publishes its books in a variety of electronic formats. Some content that appears in print may not be available in electronic books.

Cover image: Cover image from left to right: © drliwa/iStockphoto; withgod/iStockphoto; luchshen/iStockphoto; Michelle Del Guercio/Science Photo Library
Cover design by Steve Thompson

Set in 9/11.5pt Sabon by Aptara® Inc., New Delhi, India
Printed and bound in Singapore by Markono Print Media Pte Ltd

1   2013

Contents

List of contributors

Jean-Pierre Allain MD, PhD, FrcPath, FMedSc
NHS Blood and Transplant Cambridge;
Division of Transfusion Medicine
Department of Haematology
University of Cambridge
Cambridge, UK

David L. Allen FIBMS
Clinical Scientist
NHS Blood and Transplant;
Research Scientist
University of Oxford
John Radcliffe Hospital
Oxford, UK

Donald M. Arnold MD, MSc
Associate Professor
Department of Medicine
McMaster University;
Canadian Blood Services
Hamilton, ON, Canada

James P. AuBuchon MD, FCAP, FRCP(Edin)
President & CEO
Puget Sound Blood Center and University of
    Washington Seattle
Seattle, WA, USA

Imelda Bates FRCP, FrcPath
Senior Clinical Lecturer in Tropical Haematology
Liverpool School of Tropical Medicine
Liverpool, UK

Susan J. Brunskill MSc
Senior Scientist
NHS Blood and Transplant
Systematic Review Initiative
Oxford, UK

Rebecca Cardigan BSc, PhD, FrcPath
Consultant Clinical Scientist
National Head of Components Development
NHS Blood and Transplant
Cambridge, UK

Akila Chandrasekar MB BS, FrcPath
Consultant in Transfusion Medicine
NHS Blood and Transplant Tissue Services
Liverpool, UK

Nicola Curry RA, MA, MB Bchir, MRCP,
    FrcPath
Haematology Research Fellow
John Radcliffe Hospital
Oxford, UK

Geoff Daniels PhD, FrcPath
Consultant Clinical Scientist
Bristol Institute for Transfusion Sciences
NHS Blood and Transplant
Bristol, UK

Robertson D. Davenport MD
Associate Professor
Department of Pathology
University of Michigan Health System
Ann Arbor, MI, USA

Dana V. Devine PhD
Vice President, Medical, Scientific & Research Affairs
Canadian Blood Services
Ottawa, ON, Canada;
Professor of Pathology and Laboratory Medicine
Centre for Blood Research
University of British Columbia
Vancouver, BC, Canada

Roger Y. Dodd PhD
Vice President, Research and Development
American Red Cross
Holland Laboratory for the Biomedical Sciences
Rockville, MD, USA

Carolyn Doree PhD
Information Scientist
NHS Blood and Transplant
Systematic Review Initiative
Oxford, UK

Katharine A. Downes MD
Assistant Professor
University Hospitals Case Medical Center and
    Case Western Reserve University
Cleveland, OH, USA

Walter H. Dzik MD
Blood Transfusion Service
Massachusetts General Hospital;
Associate Professor
Harvard Medical School
Boston, MA, USA

Khaled El-Ghariani MA, FRCP, FrcPath
Consultant in Haematology and Transfusion
    Medicine
NHS Blood and Transplant and Sheffield Teaching
    Hospitals NHS Trust;
Honorary Senior Lecturer
University of Sheffield
Sheffield, UK

Lise J. Estcourt MB BChir, MA, MA(MEL), MRCP,
    FrcPath
Research Registrar
NHS Blood and Transplant
John Radcliffe Hospital
Oxford, UK

Dean Fergusson MHA, PhD
Senior Scientist
University of Ottawa Center for Transfusion
    Research
Clinical Epidemiology Program

The Ottawa Health Research Institute
Ottawa, ON, Canada

Stephen Field FrcPath (SA), MMed, MBChB
Medical Director
Welsh Blood Service
Cardiff, Wales, UK

Peter Flanagan FRCP, FrcPath, FRCPA
National Medical Director
New Zealand Blood Service
Auckland, New Zealand

Ronan Foley MD, FRCPC
Associate Professor of Pathology and Molecular
    Medicine
Department of Pathology and Molecular
    Medicine
McMaster University
Hamilton, ON, Canada

J. J. Francis PhD
Health Services Research Unit
University of Aberdeen
Aberdeen, Scotland, UK

Richard O. Francis MD, PhD
New York Blood Center
New York, NY;
Department of Pathology and Cell Biology
Columbia University Medical Center
New York, NY, USA

Ian M. Franklin PhD, FRCP, FrcPath
Medical & Scientific Director
Consultant Haematologist
Irish Blood Transfusion Service
National Blood Centre
Dublin, Republic of Ireland

Mark K. Fung MD, PhD
Associate Professor of Pathology and Laboratory
    Medicine
University of Vermont;
Fletcher Allen Health Care
Burlington, VT, USA

Mindy Goldman MD
Executive Medical Director
Donor and Transplantation Services
Canadian Blood Services
Ottawa, ON, Canada

Lawrence Tim Goodnough MD
Professor of Pathology and Medicine
Departments of Pathology and Medicine
Stanford University
Stanford, CA, USA

Andreas Greinacher MD
Professor of Transfusion Medicine and Haemostasis
Department of Immunology and Transfusion
   Medicine
Universitätsmedizin Greifswald
Greifswald, Germany

Paul C. Hébert MD, FRCPC, MHSc(Epid)
Professor
University of Ottawa Center for Transfusion
   Research
Clinical Epidemiology Program
The Ottawa Health Research Institute
Ottawa, ON, Canada

Nancy M. Heddle MSc, FCSMLS(D)
Director, MTRP
Professor, Department of Medicine
McMaster University;
Canadian Blood Services
Hamilton, ON, Canada

John R. Hess MD, MPH, FACP, FAAAS
Departments of Pathology and Medicine
University of Maryland School of Medicine
Baltimore, MD, USA

Patricia E. Hewitt FRCP, FrcPath
Consultant in Transfusion Medicine/Clinical
   Transfusion Microbiology
NHS Blood and Transplant
London, UK

Christopher D. Hillyer MD
President & CEO
New York Blood Center
New York, NY, USA;
Professor
Department of Medicine
Weill Cornell Medical College
New York, NY, USA

Sally Hopewell MSc, DPhil
UK Cochrane Centre
Oxford, UK

Rachael Hough BmedSci, BMBS, MD, FRCP,
   FrcPath
Consultant Haematologist and Clinical Lead of the
   Children and Young People's Cancer Service
University College Hospital's NHS Foundation Trust
London, UK

Beverley J. Hunt MD, FRCP, FrcPath
Professor of Thrombosis and Haemostasis
Kings College, London;
Consultant
Departments of Haematology, Pathology and
   Rheumatology
Guy's and St Thomas' NHS Foundation Trust
London, UK

Ram Kakaiya MD
Medical Director
Life Source Blood Services
Rosemont, IL, USA

Louis M. Katz MD
Executive Vice President, Medical Affairs
America's Blood Centers
Washington, DC, USA

Richard M. Kaufman MD
Medical Director, BWH Adult Transfusion Service
Assistant Professor of Pathology, Harvard Medical
   School
Blood Bank
Brigham and Women's Hospital
Boston, MA, USA

John Kearney BSc, PhD, CBiol, MIBiol, SRCS
Head of Tissue Services/Lead Scientist/PI for
  Research
Tissue Services
NHS Blood and Transplant
Liverpool, UK

Alan D. Kitchen PhD
Head, National Transfusion Microbiology Reference
  Laboratory;
NHS Blood and Transplant
Colindale, London, UK

Steven H. Kleinman MD
Clinical Professor of Pathology
University of British Columbia
Victoria, BC, Canada

Mark W. Lowdell BSc, MSc, PhD, FrcPath
Senior Lecturer in Haematology
Royal Free and University College Medical School
Royal Free Hospital
London, UK

Naomi Luban BA, MD
Professor of Paediatrics and Pathology
George Washington University School of Medicine
  and Health Sciences
Washington, DC, USA

Geoffrey F. Lucas PhD, FIBMS, DMS
Principal Clinical Scientist
NHS Blood and Transplant
Bristol, UK

Samuel J. Machin MD, FRCP, FrcPath
Professor of Haematology
Haemostasis Research Unit
Department of Haematology
University College London
London, UK

Edwin J. Massey MB ChB, FRCP, FrcPath
Associate Medical Director, Patient Services
NHS Blood and Transplant;
Consultant Haematologist
University Hospitals Bristol NHS Foundation Trust
Bristol, UK

Vickie McDonald MA, PhD, MRCP, FrcPath
Consultant Haematologist
University College London Hospitals NHS
  Foundation Trust
London, UK

I. Grant McQuaker DM, MRCP, FrcPath
Consultant Haematologist
BMT Unit
Beatson West of Scotland Cancer Centre
Glasgow, Scotland, UK

Ellen McSweeney MB, MRCP(UK), FrcPath
Consultant Haematologist
Irish Blood Transfusion Service
National Blood Centre
Dublin, Republic of Ireland

Siraj A. Misbah MSc, FRCP, FrcPath
Consultant Clinical Immunologist
Lead for Clinical Immunology
Oxford University Hospitals, University of Oxford
Oxford, UK

Emma Morris MA, PhD, MRCP, MRCPath
Reader in Immunotherapy
Department of Immunology and Molecular
  Pathology
Royal Free and University College Medical School
  London;
Honorary Consultant Haematologist (BMT)
Department of Haematology
University College London Hospitals
  NHS Trust
London, UK

William G. Murphy MD, FRCPEdin, FrcPath
Clinical Lead, Blood Transfusion Programme,
  Health Service Executive, Clinical Strategies and
  Programmes
Dublin;
Clinical Senior Lecturer
School of Medicine and Medical Science
University College Dublin
Dublin, Republic of Ireland

Gavin J. Murphy MBChB, MD, FRCS
British Heart Foundation Professor of Cardiac
  Surgery
School of Cardiovascular Sciences
University of Leicester
Leicester, UK

Michael F. Murphy MD, FRCP, FrcPath
Professor of Blood Transfusion Medicine
University of Oxford;
Consultant Haematologist
NHS Blood and Transplant and Department of
  Haematology
John Radcliffe Hospital
Oxford, UK

Cristina V. Navarrete PhD, FrcPath
Consultant Clinical Scientist
Director of Histocompatibility & Immunogenetics
  Services
NHS Blood and Transplant
Colindale Centre;
Honorary Reader in Immunology
University College London
London, UK

Paul M. Ness MD
Director, Transfusion Medicine Division
Johns Hopkins Medical Institutions;
Professor, Pathology, Medicine, and Oncology
Johns Hopkins University School of Medicine
Baltimore, MD, USA

Helen V. New PhD, MRCP, FrcPath
Honorary Senior Lecturer
Consultant in Paediatric Haematology and
  Transfusion Medicine
Department of Paediatrics
Imperial College Healthcare NHS Trust/NHS Blood
  and Transplant
London, UK

Pamela O'Hoski ART
Department of Pathology and Molecular Medicine
McMaster University
Hamilton, ON, Canada

Derwood H. Pamphilon MD, MRCPCH,
  FRCP, FrcPath
Formerly, Consultant Haematologist
NHS Blood and Transplant
Bristol;
Honorary Clinical Reader
Department of Cellular and Molecular Medicine
University of Bristol
Bristol, UK

Nishith Patel MBBS, MRCS
Clinical Research Fellow in Cardiac Surgery
School of Clinical Sciences
University of Bristol
Bristol, UK

Chris V. Prowse MA, DPhil, FrcPath
Retired, Professor of Transfusion Science
Edinburgh University,
Edinburgh, Scotland, UK

Sandra Ramírez-Arcos MSc, PhD, ARMCCM
Development Scientist and Adjunct Professor
Canadian Blood Services
Ottawa, ON, Canada

David Rees MA, FRCP, FrcPath
Senior Lecturer and Honorary Consultant in
  Paediatric Haematology
Department of Haematological Medicine
NHS Foundation Trust
King's College Hospital
London, UK

Biddy Ridler Mb, ChB, DObst, RCOG, AHEA
Blood Conservation Specialty Doctor
Honorary University Fellow
Peninsula College of Medicine and Dentistry
Royal Devon and Exeter Hospitals
Exeter, UK

David J. Roberts DPhil, MRCP, FrcPath
Professor of Haematology
University of Oxford;
Consultant Haematologist

NHS Blood and Transplant and Department of
  Haematology
John Radcliffe Hospital
Oxford, UK

Irene Roberts MD, FRCP, FrcPath, FRCPCH,
  DRCOG
Professor of Paediatric Haematology and Honorary
  Consultant Paediatric Haematologist
Departments of Haematology and Paediatrics
Imperial College London
London, UK

Paul Rooney BSc, PhD
Research and Development Manager for Tissue
  Services
NHS Blood and Transplant Tissue Services
Liverpool, UK

Marion Scott BSc, PhD
National Research and Development Manager
NHS Blood and Transplant
Bristol, UK

Aryeh Shander MD, FCCM, FCCP
Chief, Department of Anesthesiology, Critical Care
  and Hyperbaric Medicine
Englewood Hospital and Medical Center
Englewood, NJ;
Professor of Anesthesiology, Medicine and Surgery
Mount Sinai School of Medicine
New York, NY, USA

Beth H. Shaz MD
Chief Medical Officer
New York Blood Center
New York, NY;
Clinical Associate Professor
Department of Pathology and Laboratory
  Medicine
Emory University School of Medicine
Atlanta, GA, USA

Simon J. Stanworth MRCP (Paeds), DPhil,
  FrcPath
Consultant Haematologist
University of Oxford;

NHS Blood and Transplant and Department of
  Haematology
John Radcliffe Hospital
Oxford, UK

Susan L. Stramer MS, PhD
Executive Scientific Officer
American Red Cross
Scientific Support Office
Gaithersburg, MD, USA

Zbigniew 'Ziggy' M. Szczepiorkowski
  MD, PhD, FCAP
Section Chief, Clinical Pathology
Medical Director, Transfusion Medicine Service
Director, Cellular Therapy Center
Medical Director, Center for Transfusion Medicine
  Research
Dartmouth-Hitchcock Medical Center;
Lebanon, NH;
Associate Professor of Pathology and of
  Medicine
Geisel School of Medicine at Dartmouth
Hanover, NH, USA

Richard Tedder BA, MA Cantab, MB BChir
  Cantab, FRCP, FrcPath
NHSBT/HPA Epidemiology Unit
NHS Blood and Transplant
Colindale, London, UK

Dafydd Thomas MBChB, FRCA
Consultant in Intensive Care Medicine
Morriston Hospital
Swansea, Wales, UK

Stephen Thomas BSc, PhD
Manager, Component Development Laboratory
NHS Blood and Transplant
Brentwood, UK

John Thompson MS, FRCSed, FRCS
Consultant Surgeon
Peninsula College of Medicine and Dentistry
Royal Devon and Exeter Hospitals
Exeter, UK

Alan T. Tinmouth MD, MSc (Clin Epi), FRCPC
Head, General Hematology and Transfusion
  Medicine
Division of Hematology, Department of Medicine,
  Ottawa Hospital;
Scientist, University of Ottawa Centre for
  Transfusion Research
Clinical Epidemiology Program
The Ottawa Health Research Institute
Ottawa, ON, Canada

Marc L. Turner MB, ChB, MBA, PhD, FRCP,
  FrcPath
Professor of Cellular Therapy
Medical Director
Scottish National Blood Transfusion Service
Edinburgh, Scotland, UK

Eleftherios C. Vamvakas MD, PhD, MPH
Rita & Taft Schreiber Chair in Transfusion Medicine
Professor and Vice-Chair, Clinical Pathology
Department of Pathology and Laboratory Medicine
Cedars-Sinai Medical Center
Los Angeles, CA, USA

S. Marieke van Ham PhD
Professor of Biological Immunology
Head, Department of Immunopathology
Sanquin Research and Landsteiner Laboratory
Academic Medical Center, University of Amsterdam
Amsterdam, The Netherlands

Timothy S. Walsh BSc(Hons), MBChB(Hons)
  FRCP, FRCA, MD, MRes(PHS)
Professor of Critical Care, Clinical and
  Surgical Sciences
Edinburgh University;
Consultant in Anaesthetics and Intensive Care
Edinburgh Royal Infirmary
Edinburgh, Scotland, UK

Theodore E. Warkentin MD, FRCPC, FACP
Professor, Department of Pathology and Molecular
  Medicine and Department of Medicine
Michael G. DeGroote School of Medicine,
  McMaster University;
Regional Director, Transfusion Medicine
Hamilton Regional Laboratory Medicine Program;
Hematologist, Service of Clinical Hematology
Hamilton Health Sciences
Hamilton, ON, Canada

Kathryn E. Webert MD, MSc, FRCPC
Associate Professor
Department of Medicine and Department of
  Molecular Medicine and Pathology
McMaster University;
Canadian Blood Services
Hamilton, ON, Canada

Erica M. Wood MBBS, FRACP, FRCPA
Consultant Haematologist, Monash Medical Centre;
Clinical Associate Professor
Departments of Clinical Haematology and
  Epidemiology and Preventive Medicine
Monash University;
Melbourne, VIC, Australia

Mark H. Yazer MD
The Institute for Transfusion Medicine, Pittsburgh;
Associate Professor of Pathology
Department of Pathology
University of Pittsburgh
Pittsburgh, PA, USA

Jaap J. Zwaginga MD, PhD
Senior Lecturer
Jon J. van Rood Center for Clinical Transfusion
  Research
Sanquin, Leiden and The Department of
  Immunohematology and Blood Transfusion
Leiden University Medical Center
Leiden, The Netherlands

Preface to the Fourth Edition

The pace of change in transfusion medicine is relentless with new scientific and technological developments, and continuing efforts to improve clinical transfusion practice and avoid the use of blood wherever possible. This fourth edition has become necessary because of rapid changes in transfusion medicine since the third edition was published in 2009.

The primary aim of the fourth edition remains the same as the first, that is to provide a comprehensive guide to transfusion medicine. The book aims to include information in more depth than contained within handbooks of transfusion medicine and to present that information in a more concise and 'user-friendly' manner than standard reference texts. The feedback we receive from reviews and colleagues is that this objective continues to be achieved and that the book has a consistent style and format. We have again strived to maintain this in the fourth edition to provide a text that will be useful to the many clinical and scientific staff, both established practitioners and trainees, who are involved in some aspect of transfusion medicine and require an accessible text.

We considered that the book had become big enough for its purpose, and the number of chapters has been reduced by one from 49 to 48. It is divided into seven sections, which systematically take the reader through the principles of transfusion medicine, the complications of transfusion, practice in blood centres and hospitals, clinical transfusion practice, alternatives to transfusion, cellular and tissue therapy and organ transplantation and the development of the evidence base for transfusion. The final chapter on 'Scanning the future of transfusion medicine' has generated much interest, and it has been updated for this edition.

We wish to continue to develop the international readership and are very pleased to welcome Professor Nancy Heddle as a co-editor. The authorship likewise has become more international with each successive edition to provide a broad perspective. We are very grateful to the colleagues who have contributed to this book at a time of continuing challenges and change. Once again, we acknowledge the enormous support we have received from our publishers, particularly Jennifer Seward and Maria Khan.

1 Introduction: recent evolution of transfusion medicine

Paul M. Ness

Transfusion Medicine Division, Johns Hopkins Medical Institutions, Baltimore, Maryland, USA

Introduction to the introduction

'May you live in interesting times' (attributed to an ancient Chinese proverb).

This quotation, sometimes referred to as the Chinese curse, seems to be an appropriate statement to introduce the fourth edition of *Practical Transfusion Medicine*. Although it has been attributed to an unknown ancient Chinese proverb, its origin has not been determined, its attribution remains unclear and several of my Chinese colleagues suggest that it does not sound like a saying that emanated from China. One theory suggests that an original proverb translated to say 'It's better to be a dog in a peaceful time than be a man in a chaotic period' may be the origin and additional Wikipedia information suggests sources from the *American Society of International Law Proceedings* in 1939, or attributions to Polish or Jewish roots.

Regardless of its source, this curse has become a blessing readily demonstrated by the growth of transfusion medicine as witnessed by the evolution of *Practical Transfusion Medicine* into this fourth edition. The transfusion medicine world has used transformational problems such as the HIV epidemic and growing concerns of patients and physicians about blood safety to address and anticipate transfusion-related problems. Physicians now seek evidence that our current and evolving practices are based upon a solid foundation. This current volume has evolved from its humble original purpose to provide transfusion medicine educational material for haematology trainees in the United Kingdom (the first edition in 2001 through subsequent editions in 2005 and 2009) to become a comprehensive text with a distinguished international cast of authors. Former editions of the text have described the developing and broadening field of transfusion medicine for a multidisciplinary group of primary transfusion medicine practitioners to an increasingly diverse group of clinicians and supporting personnel dependent upon our services. This fourth edition continues the documentation of this movement to enhance blood safety and evaluates a growing armamentarium of options for blood and cellular therapies, based upon a foundation of evidence that continues to look forward but also has looked backward to substantiate or refute practices of the past. The transitions documented in the past ten years of the book's history have not always been easy or straightforward, but readers of the text will understand that the transfusion medicine community has addressed the challenges of the curse of 'interesting times' and turned them into enhanced patient care opportunities.

Modern transfusion therapy would not be possible without the discoveries of the heterogeneity of blood group antigens by pioneers such as Landsteiner, Levine and Wiener, the development of anticoagulant preservative solutions for red cells stimulated

Practical Transfusion Medicine, Fourth Edition. Edited by Michael F. Murphy, Derwood H. Pamphilon and Nancy M. Heddle.
© 2013 John Wiley & Sons, Ltd. Published 2013 by John Wiley & Sons, Ltd.

by military requirements, evolving blood separation and storage systems that have permitted collection of platelets and haemopoietic stem cells, and laboratory systems that permit matching of blood components from donors to recipients, after other laboratory systems have been utilized to maximize the likelihood that donor blood is free of transmissible pathogens. Much of this development has been documented in other venues. It is highly unlikely that any attempt that I might make to highlight these developments would add value to this introduction, so I will avoid any attempt to recapitulate this history so well documented in other transfusion texts.

Drs Michael Murphy and Derwood Pamphilon, now joined in this fourth edition by Nancy Heddle, have provided an excellent matrix for this introduction, emphasizing the recent evolution of transfusion medicine by their selection of seven sections of transfusion medicine activity in the current text. Although I have only seen the outline of the carefully selected list of authors, I will attempt to highlight some of the areas that have evolved recently in the last ten years that will be fully discussed in the text. You will have to wait like me to see what is ultimately written in the book, but I have no doubt that you and I will enjoy and benefit from this fourth edition of *Practical Transfusion Medicine*.

Basic principles of immunohaematology

In the lifetime of this book, there has been an explosion of development in molecular testing of blood groups on red cells and other blood and cellular components that are beginning to be applied in donor screening and pretransfusion testing. Although the serological tests that are used to identify blood donor antigens and recipient blood groups and antibodies are still widely applied in hospital and donor centre settings, the capability of these testing systems has been enhanced by automated methodology that reduces human testing errors and enhances turnaround time in transfusion services.

Many blood centres and transfusion services are starting to use molecular red cell antigen detection methods to screen blood donor inventories and to resolve difficult patient problems where recent transfusions, autoantibodies or complicated transfusion histories make these testing systems a valuable adjunct

to routine methods. With these methodologies, blood centres have the capability of performing routine red cell phenotype analysis that could permit more specific donor–patient matching of transfusion therapies. While this capability has clear-cut advantages for problem patients, the value of moving to more comprehensive transfusion matching remains unproven. Similar systems may enhance platelet transfusion therapy as well. Although prospective matching has not been shown to reduce alloimmunization for red cells or platelets in the past, even for high risk patient groups, future studies are likely to continue to explore the utility of prospective matching; if shown to have value for patients, it can then be determined if the clinical advantages justify the costs of these developments. Enhanced antigen screening capability for cellular antigen systems such as HLA may prove to be particularly important for cellular therapies that are expected to grow rapidly in the future. Broader application to platelet therapies will probably be seen in coming years. Leucocyte reduction was shown to be important in reducing platelet alloimmunization by the trial to reduce alloimmunization to platelet (TRAP) study in the 1990s, but the problems of platelet alloimmunization and specific platelet donor matching have not vanished, remaining a persistent problem for referral centres treating alloimmunized patients.

As one who studied alloimmunization to red cells and other transfusion components in the past, it is encouraging that a number of investigators are applying immunological methods in animal systems to determine how the process of alloimmunization occurs and whether there are therapies that could be applied to prevent alloimmunization or reverse clinically significant alloantibodies in affected patients. Our future transfusion therapies may be enhanced by learning which patients are at risk for alloimmunization and the pathophysiological underpinnings of alloimmunization as they apply to transfusion therapy. Leucocyte reduction can reduce platelet alloimmunization, suggesting that more extensive reduction of white cells or white cell function via pathogen reduction systems could become critical components for transfusion therapy. Prevention or reversal of alloimmunization to HLA would enhance solid organ transplant programmes, where previously immunized recipients are currently denied transplant options or required to undergo dangerous and expensive treatments to permit an incompatible solid organ or haemopoietic cell transplant. The growing capability to manoeuvre around previously impenetrable ABO barriers shown in the last ten years provides some encouragement that we will become equally successful in dealing with HLA barriers or xenotropic antigens that prevent transplants of solid organs from donor animals.

Our increased understanding of immunohaematological principles has improved our capability to reduce adverse transfusion complications. The past ten years featured the recognition and attack of TRALI, identifying and mitigating these reactions for some but not all blood recipients. Other persistent transfusion problems such as delayed haemolytic transfusion reactions, TRALI not caused by donor antibodies and allergic transfusion reactions should be amenable to detection and prevention by better use of our evolving knowledge of immunohaematology. It may also be possible to gain better quantification and understanding of the adverse effects due to immunomodulation, such that we can reduce this transfusion complication for patients.

Complications of transfusion

Having been the director of a large community blood centre and a major academic transfusion service during the chaotic era of HIV awareness and prevention from 1980 onward, it is refreshing that the overwhelming concerns about blood safety that affect patients and their physicians have lessened dramatically during the lifespan of this book. The HIV era followed by identification of HCV and its detection were clearly an episode of 'life in interesting times'. When providing transfusion medicine education to medical students or clinical updates to practitioners nowadays, however, they seem unconcerned with the current risk of HIV from a blood transfusion, a topic that dominated our interactions ten years ago. Although this state of relief is apparent in the developed world, blood safety concerns still remain high in developing countries, where donor screening and testing capabilities are still being developed. In a similar vein, the media in developed countries still remains eager to find the next transfusion pestilence, as shown by our recent flirtation with XMRV and SARS. Over the past ten years, with little public recognition, we enhanced testing for HCV, identified and prevented a major epidemic of

West Nile Virus infections from blood donors and made initial steps to reduce the risk of septic transfusions from platelets.

As we take pride in this collective record of accomplishment and recent track record in mitigating transfusion-transmitted infections, complacency is not an option; diligence towards reducing and eliminating transfusion risks must remain a primary transfusion medicine objective. In the United States, there is growing evidence that babesia transmission and dengue infection should remain high on a surveillance list of emerging concerns. These infections and how we address them will continue to raise conflicting points of view, however. Although we initiated routine screening for Chagas' disease, the limited detection rates and minimal evidence of transmission from previously infected donors using lookback studies has led to modifications of testing algorithms. These steps were justified to reduce costs to the blood centres and hospitals, but test kit providers have lost expected revenue, which may lessen their enthusiasm to develop new testing methods for infections that are not widespread or remain geographically constrained. As new candidate pathogens are identified and we continue to investigate these potential transfusion threats in keeping with the precautionary principle, these recent events may limit our ability to respond rapidly without expensive studies and unrewarded investments by test providers. In many cases, our concern for blood safety and mitigating transfusion risks from emerging infections gets ahead of regulatory guidance, so that the process by which we prioritize our activities in the blood safety arena remains difficult in the developed world. In the developing world and perhaps with increased frequency in developed countries, these processes will be affected by cost constraints and concerns about cost effectiveness in an era where reimbursement concerns loom large. As a discipline, we have also been ineffective in getting input from clinicians who order blood about these evolving blood safety concerns.

A number of blood safety concerns could be reduced by adoption of pathogen reduction systems. There is widespread use of pathogen reduction for plasma fractions from donor pools and increased use in blood components such as platelets and plasma in Europe and other developed countries outside the USA. In the USA, licensure and adoption have been delayed by regulatory concerns about adverse reactions in clinical trials and the lack of significant emerging infections on the horizon that would make favourable risk/benefit calculations. Pathogen reduction for red cells is still under development and may be slow to achieve licensed status due to antibody development with early formulations. Even if licensure is achieved, adoption may be stymied by cost considerations if pathogen reduction is advantageous for disease transmission issues alone. If these systems can be shown to reduce or eliminate some donor loss through travel history exclusions or elimination of unnecessary tests, or demonstrate other advantages for patients such as reduction of alloimmunization or prevention of graft versus host disease, the case for adoption by transfusion services will be enhanced.

Although most sections of transfusion complications focus upon infectious problems, the remaining chapters of this section provide extensive discussions of noninfectious transfusion complications. Progress in reducing these often ignored transfusion complications has been enhanced by the stable state of transfusion infections and our attempts to document the occurrence of all adverse effects through haemovigilance systems which began in the UK and have now spread to other countries throughout the world. The UK Serious Hazards of Transfusion (SHOT) programme highlighted TRALI cases as an important issue in its early versions, prompting actions of donor screening, consensus building, case reporting and product manipulations, which have lowered the rates of these reactions. It is hoped that these systems will become more widespread, move towards active rather than passive reporting and provide prioritized problem lists for further blood safety activities. A recent review reminds us that 'blood still kills', so attacks on common adverse transfusion effects such as immunomodulation, bacterial sepsis and the persistent problems with haemolytic reactions will move higher on the action list of transfusion medicine. The recent past has featured more discussion and action on these persistent problems affecting transfusion recipients, and the discussions of the status of these issues in the fourth edition of *Practical Transfusion Medicine* will provide an update of recent progress and opportunities for improvement.

The chapters of this section will also provide perspective on another issue of growing importance, the controversial debate of whether older blood has deleterious effects on transfused patients that could potentially be reduced by using fresher red cells. The medical literature is replete with retrospective studies from surgical cohorts that purport to show that older blood is harmful. These studies have stimulated the appropriate response from our community to initiate prospective clinical trials now underway in cardiac surgery and intensive care unit patients to address these issues. Basic and applied research studies on red cell storage, an area where we may have been inappropriately complacent, have been funded and are being reported in the literature and lay press. Ongoing research will determine whether the suggested culprits of nitric oxide, microparticles, nontransferrin bound iron or other biologic modifiers can be manipulated by storage systems to reduce adverse effects for patients if the prospective trials prove that there is a problem with older blood.

Practice in blood centres and hospitals

This section of the text provides the background and status report for transfusion-related activities in hospitals and blood centres. The shifting breadth in the new edition highlights international activities more broadly than previous editions, which were more Europe focused. Although recent editions were strong and comprehensive, multiauthored chapters from international authorities will address the challenge of describing current systems throughout the world, with the goal of broadening the experience base of all readers. As examples, the UK-based hospital chapter is now written by authors from Australia, the USA and the UK, and regulatory aspects that emphasized UK issues now include the perspective of authors from the USA, Canada and New Zealand as well as the UK. Increased emphasis is placed upon the global context of transfusion.

One of the triumphs of the last ten years has been advances made in developing countries through local initiatives, stimulated and enhanced by support from developed countries. The US President's Emergency Plan for AIDS Relief (PEPFAR) aided the development of national blood programmes in sub-Saharan Africa with funding by the CDC, which were implemented by experts from the USA including AABB and Europe from Sanquin. The National Institutes of Health in the US funded international epidemiological research programmes in Brazil and China through the Retrovirus

Epidemiology Donor Study (REDS) programme and other national blood service organizations provided financial support and expertise for blood programmes in the developing world. While the progress has been substantial, it remains an uphill climb to bring transfusion safety and an adequate supply of safe volunteer donor blood throughout the world, but we can take pride that we are collectively pursuing the challenge with documented results.

Although much of the text is aimed at educating clinicians about blood services, there have been major developments in blood centres and hospital transfusion services to apply standardized procedures to improve patient care. The activities in blood centres in the developed world to bring standardized blood components from a heterogeneous group of blood donors to enhance blood safety have reduced transfusion complications; the parallel development of quality-based laboratory systems for testing, storage and distribution of blood components to patients upon the request of an educated physician base has also addressed these objectives. The chapters in this section prove to be of more utility to committed transfusion medicine practitioners but will be helpful to clinicians who advise on transfusion programmes through medical staff committees and provide transfusion consultation and support to less knowledgeable clinical colleagues.

Clinical transfusion practice

One of the positive outcomes from blood safety initiatives has been our response to regulatory pressures to standardize blood collection and preparation processes. Although there are clear benefits in terms of blood safety from standardized procedures, we have become increasingly aware that modifications in the components we transfuse are required to meet the unique needs of different patient populations. Neonatal and paediatric transfusions have required hospital transfusion services to modify their practices to administer effective therapies in reduced volumes to these patients. Fresher blood components may be required for subsets of these patients and blood components with reduced potassium loads for massively transfused children are more commonly provided. The availability of recombinant coagulation factors has revolutionized the care of haemophilia. In a similar

manner, new factors such as VIIa have been introduced for broader patient groups with acute haemorrhage, raising concerns about efficacy, toxicity and costs for these agents. Reducing the plasma load in platelet recipients, a process initiated in Europe to save plasma for the production of fractionation products, is becoming more common as a means to reduce ABO haemolytic reactions or allergic transfusion reactions in platelet recipients who receive the platelets for haemostasis but do not really benefit from the accompanying plasma.

We have begun to recognize that our approaches to patients with massive blood loss require rethinking. Data from the military suggest that early resuscitation using large volumes of plasma can save lives, leading to the development of massive transfusion protocols in hospitals with red cells, plasma and platelets being administered in a 1:1:1 ratio. These practices are now being extended to other patients with major haemorrhage who clearly require red cell support, but the documentation that they would benefit from 1:1:1 support is not available. Meeting the needs of trauma patients, but avoiding overtransfusion for patients who might not benefit has become an ongoing challenge. At the same time, as frozen plasma use is increasing dramatically in trauma, we recognize that frozen plasma is our most inappropriately ordered blood component, commonly used to correct trivial elevations of coagulation tests or prevent bleeding in procedures where evolving evidence has shown no medical value from this risky transfusion intervention. Complicating these issues are the many problems with plasma administration: ABO antibodies that make products unavailable as a universal therapy, large volumes that put patients at risk when acute care is needed, slow processing times due to thawing requirements and inadequate potency for acute haemorrhage or reversal of anticoagulation.

These evolving medical transfusion issues suggest that the transfusion service may become more important as a source of product modifications, becoming more of a wet pharmacy for blood components. Since the pretransfusion testing functions are becoming more automated in hospitals and centralized in some communities, these laboratory functions will probably decrease in importance in the coming years. As a parallel development, transfusion services and their leadership will need to emphasize their critical role as transfusion consultants for clinicians, who will be faced with a growing menu of product modifications and new offerings from donor blood or the recombinant engineers. If laboratory functions are reduced by testing automation, product manipulations such as antigen stripping and reduced alloimmunization from product manipulations or treatment options, the traditional hospital blood bank could have its role diminished. On the other hand, if we embrace the growing heterogeneity of products we can offer from donor blood, recombinant proteins, cellular engineering and bone and tissue banking, and continue to offer these services with emphasis upon our critical consultative role, the transfusion medicine discipline will continue to grow and flourish with benefits to patients and their supporting clinicians.

Alternatives to transfusion

The progress in another area of growing activity is documented in the chapter on patient blood management. Although the risks of infectious complications have been dramatically reduced in recent times, given their choice, many patients continue to search for transfusion options that would drive these risks even lower. The continuing perception of unnecessary transfusion risks led some hospitals to develop programmes to provide medical care to patients who refuse to receive transfusion support for religious reasons; in many cases, other concerned patients reluctant to receive blood were made aware that they might avoid transfusion support by taking advantage of the practices developed to address the needs of religious objectors. These programmes have emphasized the development of impeccable surgical techniques, the recruitment of physicians willing to care for these patients understanding this therapeutic limitation, the use of transfusion alternatives, the restriction of transfusions to lower triggers based upon evolving clinical evidence and the need for presurgical assessments and informed consent discussions with patients well in advance of surgical procedures.

Although the evidence base for these practices remains somewhat anecdotal and is derived at best from heterogeneous cohorts, the practices that have been developed for bloodless medicine have formed the basis for patient blood management programmes where the lack of supporting evidence for many transfusion interventions is driving the performance of clinical trials to provide evidence going forward. Patient blood management offers transfusion medicine a growing opportunity to provide better care through evidenced guided transfusion support, develop new products to reduce the risk of documented adverse transfusion effects and reduce the costs of unnecessary and potentially harmful transfusions for patients and hospitals.

Our enthusiasm for transfusion alternatives has been somewhat squashed by recent developments in the field. The advantages of pharmacological alternatives to blood (sterility, dose standardization, lack of immunogenicity) led to enthusiastic use of erythropoietin to stimulate red cell production, aprotinin to reduce intraoperative blood loss and VIIa to promote rapid haemostasis. Ensuing reports of adverse effects with these agents has led to more cautious use of these products for more limited indications and removal of aprotinin from the market. The long search for a haemoglobin-based oxygen carrier (HBOC) to replace blood in trauma was impaired by clinical trial evidence from a major trial in trauma showing limited efficacy and a meta-analysis demonstrating that the HBOC class has adverse effects of increased myocardial infarctions and mortality compared to controls as a result of nitric oxide effects. While a continuing clinical need for patients with severe anaemia who cannot be transfused due to auto-antibodies, alloantibodies or religious objection remains unmet, recent developments lead to the pessimistic conclusion that blood substitutes will not be available in the foreseeable future.

Cellular and tissue therapy and organ transplantation

The hospital transfusion service has expanded its limited, traditional portfolio (blood components and associated services) to provide support for developing cellular therapy needs in many hospitals. Moving beyond routine transfusion support and expanded HLA and blood grouping activities to support complicated transplant recipients, many transfusion services now provide graft engineering support, collection support for peripheral blood haemopoietic stem cells and tissue and bone banking services. In many cases, these activities originated in haematology–oncology laboratories; as these activities have expanded their scope and providers have addressed the needs to augment their regulatory compliance, providing services to patients outside of the oncology realm, the hospital transfusion service has taken on these clinical laboratory responsibilities on its own or in conjunction with oncology-based laboratories. As cellular therapy services become more broadly required in disciplines such as cardiology, neurology and orthopaedics, this transition from separate discipline managed services to a centralized facility managed by transfusion medicine professionals has become an increasingly wise approach. In areas of the country or the world where hospitals may lack these capabilities, these functions can also be assumed and managed by a blood centre or national transfusion programme.

As transfusion medicine continues the transition to include cellular therapy, it is encouraging to note the increased attention and involvement by our discipline in therapeutic apheresis. Extending our services to offer direct patient care throughout the hospital provides an important clinical outreach activity for transfusion physicians, enabling us to be better recognized as clinicians by our colleagues and making our consultative activities in traditional transfusion support more likely to be sought and tolerated. It moves us beyond the role of the telephone police, rejecting unnecessary requests for transfusion support, to a role where we can readily demonstrate our primary concern for patients and not hospital expenses. Involvement in therapeutic apheresis also provides an important bridge to our provision of cellular therapy support to other clinical disciplines.

Development of the evidence base for transfusion

One of the most encouraging developments of the recent past is the recognition of our lack of robust evidence to support transfusion therapy decisions and some initial success in designing and implementing studies to fill this mounting void. These gaps have become more apparent as transfusion authorities and clinical transfusion prescribers have attempted to develop transfusion guidelines to improve transfusion practice and remove the burden of unnecessary transfusions, which are wasteful of resources and potentially harmful to blood recipients. As these groups have strived for consensus, it has become apparent that the strength of these guidelines is constrained by the level of evidence that supports the recommendations. We can thank a growing number of epidemiologists and transfusion authorities who have become converts to the epidemiology cause for moving us on the path to correct these deficiencies.

A major challenge for transfusion medicine is reconciling the differing levels of evidence we must consider for provision of blood components and recommending clinical transfusion practices. In the blood safety arena, it has been deemed inappropriate for us to wait for substantial evidence to change our practices if we believe that patients may be at risk, a concept deemed as the precautionary principle. In many cases, we have implemented changes in donor screening and testing based upon unproven assumptions that were clearly not cost effective or based upon statistically significant data collections. These actions are now taken more commonly because of the medicolegal and political risks of waiting for definitive proof of efficacy before taking action on blood safety issues.

Our decision making can be more rational in clinical practice where we can look at the available evidence for practice and design controlled clinical intervention trials to determine the best course for subsequent actions. In some cases the results of well-designed trials have been counterintuitive, such as the Transfusion Requirements in Critical Care (TRICC), which showed that less may be more when applied to transfusions in the ICU. In other cases, carefully performed studies implemented by transfusion practitioners have become available to prove that lower platelet transfusion triggers are acceptable for patients with haematologic malignancies. Based upon these trials, practice guidelines carry more weight. We need to be careful, however, not to overextend the interpretation of clinical trial data beyond the scope of the study populations; as an example, we understand that low platelet counts are acceptable in oncology but we have not performed clinically robust studies to determine the appropriate platelet thresholds in trauma or whether platelets stored at room temperature to maximize *in vivo* survival provide sufficiently rapid haemostatic correction in trauma situations.

The editors of *Practical Transfusion Medicine* clearly anticipated the importance of this area in earlier editions of the book and their prescient wisdom has rewarded readers with discussions of the mechanisms of trial design, how to evaluate evidence from trials and other data collections, and how to apply these findings to clinical practice. The fourth edition continues on this path, with evidence-enriched early chapters on specific practice issues and modified discussions of taking the next logical steps.

Afterthoughts

I appreciate the editors' invitation to provide this rambling retrospective view of the evolution of transfusion medicine. I came into the field at a time when transfusion practices were rarely questioned, cost pressures were minimal and the overriding concern was the development of a sufficient donor base to meet the growing demands for red cells and platelets. HIV and viral hepatitis brought this quiet era to an abrupt end, generating a revolution to embrace blood safety as a pre-eminent cause and generating incisive questions from patients and the physicians about whether they really need the blood we could provide and what they might do to avoid the risks. Our track record to enhance blood safety has been remarkable, but new infections, haemovigilance systems that demonstrate persistent noninfectious problems for patients and conflicting clinical data that suggests that blood transfusions are a two-edged sword continue to perplex us. We are addressing these concerns with clinical trials, innovations in blood component design and expansion of transfusion services beyond our traditional boundaries. *Practical Transfusion Medicine* reviews much of the recent history, provides an update of where we are in this expanding field and reminds us of the continuing challenges that we must address. The 'interesting times' are clearly not over.

Further reading

Blumberg N, Sime PJ & Phipps RP. The mystery of transfusion-related acute lung injury. *Transfusion* 2011; 51: 2055–2057.

Glynn SA. The red blood cell storage lesion: a method to the madness. *Transfusion* 2010; 50: 1164–1169.

Josephson CD, Glynn SA, Kleinman ST & Blajchman MA for the State of the Science Symposium Transfusion Medicine Committee. A multidisciplinary 'think tank': the top 10 clinical trial opportunities in transfusion medicine from the National Heart, Lung, and Blood Institute-sponsored 2009 State of the Science Symposium. *Transfusion* 2011; 51: 828–841.

Klein HG, Anderson D, Bernardi MJ, Cable R, Carey W, Hoch JS, Robitaille N, Sivlotti ML & Smaill F. Pathogen inactivation: making decisions about new technologies. Report of a consensus conference. *Transfusion* 2007: 47: 2338–2347.

McLeod BC. Therapeutic apheresis: history, clinical application, and lingering uncertainties. *Transfusion* 2010; 50: 1413–1426.

Moulds JM, Ness PM & Sloan SR (eds). *Bead Chip Molecular Immunohematology*. New York: Springer; 2011.

Natanson C, Kern SJ, Luire P, Banks SM & Wolfe SM. Cell-free hemoglobin-based blood substitutes and risk of myocardial infarction and death. *J Am Med Assoc* 2009: 299; 2304–2312.

Ness PM. Pharmacologic alternatives to transfusion. *Vox Sanguinis* 2002; 83 (Suppl. 1); 3–6.

Perkins HA & Busch MP. Transfusion-associated infections: 50 years of relentless challenges and remarkable progress. *Transfusion* 2010; 50: 2080–2089.

Snyder E & Choate J. The emergence of cellular therapy: impact on transfusion medicine. *Transfusion* 2010; 50: 2301–2309.

Vamvakas EC, Blajchman MA. Blood still kills: six strategies to further reduce allogeneic blood transfusion-related mortality. *Trans Med Rev* 2010; 24: 257.

Wilkinson KL, Brunskill SJ, Doree C, Hopewell S, Stanworth S, Murphy MF & Hyde C. The clinical effects of red blood cell transfusions. *Trans Med Rev* 2011; 25: 145.

Young PP, Colton BA & Goodnough LT. Massive transfusion protocols for patients with substantial hemorrhage. *Trans Med Rev* 2011; 25: 293.

PART ONE

Basic Principles of Immunohaematology

2

Essential immunology for transfusion medicine

Jaap Jan Zwaginga[1] *& S. Marieke van Ham*[2]

[1] Jon J. van Rood Center for Clinical Transfusion Research, Sanquin, Leiden and the Department of Immunohematology and Bloodtransfusion, Leiden University Medical Center, Leiden, The Netherlands
[2] Department of Immunopathology, Sanquin Research and Landsteiner Laboratory, Academic Medical Center, University of Amsterdam, Amsterdam, The Netherlands

Cellular basis of the immune response

Leucocytes from the myeloid and lymphoid lineage are the key effector cells of both the innate and adaptive immune system, and are differentiated from haemopoietic stem cells (HSC) in the bone marrow.

Innate immune cells

Phagocytes and antigen presenting cells (APCs)
Cells of the myeloid lineage include monocyte-derived macrophages, neutrophils (polymorphonuclear neutrophils, PMNs) and dendritic cells (DCs). All three function as phagocytes that remove dead cells and cell debris or immune complexes. Foremost, these cells act as the first line of innate defence, ingesting and clearing pathogens. Very important in this is their activation via specific receptors, termed PRR (pattern recognition receptors) by danger signals derived from pathogens or inflamed tissue. This triggers their differentiation and their expression and/or secretion of signalling proteins, which lead to further activation of the immune response. Some of these proteins (like IL-1, IL-6 and TNF) increase acute phase proteins that activate complement, while others (chemokines) attract circulating immune cells to the site of infection. DCs, and also macrophages, additionally serve as APCs that process and present digested proteins as antigen to specific T cells of the lymphoid lineage. PRR ligation in this setting induces maturation of APCs with acquisition of chemokine receptors, which allow their migration to the lymph nodes where the resting T cells reside. Simultaneously, mature APCs acquire costimulatory molecules and secrete cytokines. All are needed for T-cell activation and differentiation and eventually the immune response to the specific pathogen. The type of PRR ligation determines the formation of defined cytokines and with it an optimal pathogen class-specific immune answer, with minimal tissue damage.

NK lymphocytes
Natural killer (NK) cells are capable of killing virus-infected cells either specifically targeted by the presence of antibody on the cell's surface (antibody-dependent cell-mediated cytotoxicity – ADCC) or through the recognition of changes in the infected cell surfaces. Moreover, NK cells are normally kept from killing by expression of inhibiting receptors that recognize the presence of self-MHC molecules (see below) on autologous cells. Allogeneic cells with non-compatible MHC but also aberrant autologous cells (e.g. tumour cells) with lowered MHC expression lack sufficient of these NK inhibiting structures and trigger the default killing potential of NK cells.

Adaptive immune cells

T-lymphocytes
After migration of progenitor T cells to the thymus epithelium, billions of T cells are formed with billions of antigen receptor variants. Each lymphocyte

Practical Transfusion Medicine, Fourth Edition. Edited by Michael F. Murphy, Derwood H. Pamphilon and Nancy M. Heddle.
© 2013 John Wiley & Sons, Ltd. Published 2013 by John Wiley & Sons, Ltd.

expresses only one kind of heterodimeric T-cell receptor (TCR). For the large majority of T cells this is an alpha and a beta chain, which form a structure that is similar to the specific antigen binding site of immunoglobulin molecules. Immature T cells initially express a TCR receptor in complex with CD4 and CD8 molecules, which respectively interact with major histocompatibility complex class II and class I molecules. The presentation of self-antigens within such MHC molecules on thymic stromal cells determines the fate of the immature T cells. First of all, these interactions induce T-cell maturation into T cells that express only CD4 or CD8. Most important, however, is that these interactions are responsible for the removal of T cells that have a TCR with high binding affinity for the MHC complexes that express the self-antigen. The cells that survive this so-called 'negative selection' process migrate to the secondary lymphoid organs. There TCR specific binding to complexes of MHC can activate them with non-self (e.g. pathogen-derived) antigens on matured APCs. Interactions between the costimulatory molecules CD80 and CD86 on the APC with CD28 on the T cell subsequently drives the activated T cells into proliferation. Without this costimulation (e.g. by not fully differentiated APCs by insufficient or absent PRR ligation), T cells can become nonfunctional (anergized). The requirement of PRR-induced danger signals thus forms a second checkpoint of T-cell activation to prevent reactivity to self-antigens. Additionally, APC-released cytokines direct T-cell differentiation.

While immunoglobulins bind to amino acids in the context of the tertiary structure of the antigen, the TCR recognizes amino acids on small digested antigen fragments in the context of an MHC molecule. As indicated, there are two classes of MHC (called human leucocyte antigens of HLA in humans) molecules that are similar in their two polypeptide structure with an antigen binding groove (see Chapter 4). The MHC is polygenic determined, resulting in different sets of peptide binding specificities. Moreover, MHC genes are polymorphic, with many allelic variations in the population. Both MHC characteristics ensure endless protein/antigen binding capacities and thus adaptation of the immune response to new/rapidly evolving pathogens. MHC class I is expressed on all nucleated cells and presents so called 'endogenous' antigen constituting self-antigens, but also antigens from

viruses and other pathogens that use the replication machinery of eukaryotic cells for their propagation. To be loaded on to MHC I, proteins need to be processed in smaller antigen parts by the proteasome. Subsequently, processed proteins are shuttled into the endocytoplasmatic reticulum for loading on to newly synthesized MHC class I molecules. Finally, this complex is cell surface expressed. CD8+ cytotoxic T cells (CTLs) recognize the MHC class I/antigen complex on the cells. Although viruses and parasites (like *Plasmodium falciparum*) can hide in red blood cells because the latter lack MHC, red cells also lack the DNA replication machinery for such pathogens.

MHC class II molecules of APCs present antigenic proteins that are ingested or endocytosed from the extracellular milieu. Upon cell activation these proteins are protease digested in acidified endocytic vesicles yielding smaller antigen fragments. Again after fusion with the MHC class II containing compartments, the antigen is loaded on to the MHC class II molecule and routed to the plasma membrane.

The described antigen expression routes, however, are not absolute. Specialized DC in this respect can also express viral and other extracellular-derived proteins on MHC class I to CD8+ CTLs while, vice versa, primarily cytosolic proteins via so-called autophagy can become localized in the endocytic system and become expressed in MHC class II. This so-called antigen cross-presentation adds flexibility to the adaptive immune response.

Paradoxically, having described the fact that T cells become activated only when the specific TCR recognizes antigen in the context of its own MHC (termed MHC restriction) seems to refute the condition that MHC/HLA mismatched tissue transplants are rejected. Many acceptor T cells, however, can be activated because their TCR perceives donor-specific MHC as foreign in itself. A large circulating pool of T cells reacting with non-self MHC is usually present and explains the acute CD8-dependent rejection of non-self MHC in transplant rejection that occurs without previous immunization.

T helper (Th) cells

Differentiation into T helper cells is dependent on signals (cytokines and/or plasma membrane molecules) derived from the APC. Different Th subsets can be characterized by their cytokine release and their extralymphatic action in infected tissues. Th1 cells release

IFN gamma and IL-2 and bind and help macrophages to kill intracellular pathogens. In addition, Th1 cells support CTL function and are required for optimal CTL memory formation. Th17 cells releasing IL-17 and IL-6 probably enhance the early innate response by activating granulocytes and seem most needed for antifungal immunity. Both Th1 and Th17 are drivers from strong proinflammatory immune responses, which might explain why they are also associated with auto-immunity. Classically, Th2 cells are thought to be the main Th subsets to support B-cell differentiation and the formation of antibodies. The IL-4, -5 and -13 releasing Th2 cells, furthermore, help to kill parasites by inducing IgE production, which activates mast cells, basophils and eosinophils. Th2, however, is also associated with aberrant immunity, as observed in allergies. Finally, the recently defined follicular Thelper cells (Tfh) seem to be required for long-lived immunity and to induce antibody formation upon primary immunization and upon reactivation of memory B cells in the case of a re-encounter with an antigen.

Regulatory T cells (T regs)
These form a specialized CD4+ T-cell subset, which limits T-cell activation and autoimmunity. While naturally occurring T regs are already formed in the thymus, induced T regs are likely to be induced by APC that show suboptimal costimulation and that release anti-inflammatory cytokines (IL-10 and TGF-beta). These inhibit proinflammatory T-cell differentiation as well as many innate cell functions like DC differentiation.

B lymphocytes
In the bone marrow, progenitor B cells upon local cues from stromal cells, divide and are directed towards acquisition of their antigen-specific B-cell receptor (BCR). With initially millions of different binding affinities of this surface expressed immunoglobulin, immature B-cell clones that show self-antigen binding affinity are eliminated by premature stimulation. B cells mature in the peripheral lymphoid tissues where they respond to foreign antigens via activation of the BCR. Upon receipt of additional survival signals, they proliferate and differentiate into plasma cells that in their turn secrete immunoglobulins with identical binding specificities as the activated B cells they are derived from. Depending on their differentiation pathway, plasma cells secrete specific classes of effector antibodies (i.e. IgM, IgD, IgG, IgA and IgE). Long-lived IgG producing plasma cells migrate to the bone marrow where they can survive for many years. In addition to plasma cells, memory B cells are formed during the first antigen encounter, awaiting reactivation in a following infection.

B-cell activation and T-cell-dependent antibody formation

The binding of antigens by the BCR also leads to intracellular signalling and activation of the B cells upon antigen (re-)challenge. The antigen-BCR complex is internalized and processed into fragments, which can be re-expressed on MHC class II molecules at the B-cell surface. This APC function of B cells is first of all designed to recruit T helper cells that are activated by DCs that have presented the same antigen. This process ensures that T helper cells only support B-cell differentiation of those B cells that have become activated by the same pathogen, thus minimizing the risk of activation of autoreactive B cells. Activated B cells and activated T cells have an enhanced change to meet as both cells are induced to migrate to the border of the B–T cell zones in the secondary lymphoid organs upon activation. Activated Th cells express CD40L, which provides costimulation to the B cells. Ligation of the B cell via the CD40 costimulatory molecule together with cytokines secreted by the Th cells modulate the direction of B-cell differentiation. For example, Th1 support differentiation into IgG1 producing plasma cells and Th2 support formation of IgE producing plasma cells. Some pathogens that have a repetitive structure (called thymus-independent antigens) can activate B cells to produce IgM antibodies against mostly extracellular pathogens without T-cell help. This offers a fast response mechanism, but of low affinity. Higher affinity antibody formation requires T-cell helper interactions.

Humoral immune response

Immunoglobulins (Igs) are in fact the secreted form of the B-cell receptor. This specific effector molecule is secreted by plasma cells. The Ig's basic structure is a roughly Y-shaped molecule made up of two identical heavy chains with four domains and two identical (kappa or lambda) light chains with two domains. These heavy and light chains are interlinked by non-covalent and disulfide bonds. Two identical highly specific antigen binding sites (the arms of the Y) are formed by the amino terminus domains of the heavy and light chains and form the variable (Fab) domain of the Igs. The specificity and variability of these antigen binding sites is a result of two extra beta strands in these variable domains. Connected to the normal seven beta strands found in the 'constant' domains, these additional amino acid sequences form tertiary protein structures with an almost unending repertoire of different three-dimensional 'binding locks' for antigens (Figure 2.1). Both heavy chains combine via their carboxy terminal domains to the so-called constant (Fc) region (the trunk of the Y) of the Ig, which is more or less flexibly attached to the antigen binding part by a so-called hinge area in the heavy chains. The Fc region determines the Ig class and consequently the Ig effector function, which is different for each Ig class. Some effector Igs form higher order structures, with secreted IgA being a dimer and IgM a pentamer.

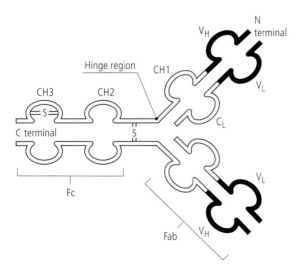

Fig 2.1 Basic structure of an immunoglobulin molecule. Domains are held in shape by disulfide bonds, though only one is shown. CH1–3, constant domain of an H chain; C$_L$, constant domain of a light chain; V$_H$, variable domain of an H chain; V$_L$, variable domain of a light chain.

Basis of antibody variability

The BCR/antibody variability via the variable region originates from random DNA recombination of two or three of many variable region gene segments. The endless recombinations are the pretranscriptional basis of the extremely variable tertiary structures of the immunoglobulin molecule (Figure 2.1) and the enormous B-cell repertoire in the bone marrow. Of these cells, each having one single antigen specificity, cells with self-reactive BCRs will be destroyed. From the remainder, clones are selected on the basis of their specific pathogen antigen binding abilities and these mature and expand into antibody producing plasma cells. This secondary diversification of the antibody repertoire takes place in extrafollicular tissues or in the germinal centres of the lymphoid organs and consists of:

• Several sequential enzyme-driven steps leading to point mutations or so-called *somatic hypermutations* of the variable regions of both the heavy and light chains.

• A process called *affinity maturation* leads to selection of B cells with a BCR type that has the highest affinity for the antigen. Random mutations are thus eventually directed towards plasma cells that secrete Igs with optimized antigen affinity.

• *Immunoglobulin (sub)class switching* by helper T-cell-released cytokines that induce transcription of so-called switch regions. This process enables the first produced IgM by naïve B cells to evolve into IgG or IgE class antibodies. There are five immunoglobulin classes (isotypes) based on different genes that are used for the C domains of the H chain and an additional four and two immunoglobulin subclasses for IgG and IgA. These subclasses determine the effector functions of the Ig, as well as their serum half-life and their ability for placental transfer (Table 2.1).

• The combination of somatic hypermutation/affinity maturation and class switching explains why during immune responses the first formed IgM Igs generally show low binding affinity to the antigen, while the later formed IgGs have undergone affinity maturation and indeed show enhanced antigen binding.

Antibody effector functions

The class (isotype) of an Ig is determined by coupling variable domains with identical binding specificities

Table 2.1 Immunoglobulin classes and their functions.

	Structure			Function		
Isotype	Heavy chain	Light chain	Configuration	Complement fixation*	Cells reacting with FcR	Placental passage
IgM	μ	κ, λ	Pentamer	+++	L	–
IgG1	γ1	κ, λ	Monomer	++	M, N, P, L, E	+++
IgG2	γ2	κ, λ	Monomer	+	P, L	+
IgG3	γ3	κ, λ	Monomer	+++	M, N, P, L, E	++
IgG4	γ4	κ, λ	Monomer	–	N, L, P	+/–
IgA1	α1	κ, λ	Monomer	+	–	–
IgA2	α2	κ, λ	Dimer in secretion	–	–	–
IgD	δ	κ, λ	Monomer	–	–	–
IgE	ε	κ, λ	Monomer	–	B, E, L	–

*Classical pathway.
B, basophils/mast cells; E, eosinophils; L, lymphocytes; M, macrophages; N, neutrophils; P, platelets.

to different constant regions of the heavy (H) chain. While IgM only functions in circulation, other classes also function in other body compartments. IgA in this respect is mostly localized in epithelial tissues like the gut. As a dimer, IgA can be excreted into the intestines and into exocrine (e.g. milk, saliva and tear producing) glands and act there as an early defence to pathogen invasion of these tissues and of the newborn via transfer in mother's milk. Although antibodies can neutralize toxins and pathogens, e.g. by blocking their adhesion to cell surfaces, definite clearing them from the body is achieved by the following processes.

• For pathogens, mostly by phagocytes, which are triggered to ingest and destroy antibody-coated structures by their Fc receptors crosslinking Fc tails of antigen-bound Igs. This IgG-mediated process is responsible for the clearance of antigen–Ig complexes from circulation in the spleen and liver.

• For parasites, by exocytosis of stored mediators, e.g. from mast cells that are triggered by their Fcε receptor recognizing the Fc region of IgE.

• Activation of the complement cascade (see Figure 2.2). The system is part of innate immunity but is also vital to the effector functions of complement-fixing immunoglobulin isotypes. Central to the complement's function is the activation of C3 by three routes:

(a) The classical pathway: this pathway can be powerfully activated by IgM but in decreasing order by IgG3, 1 and 2 as well and consists of four numbered components (C1–C4) and two regulatory proteins (C1 inhibitor, C4 binding protein). The first component (C1) consists of three subcomponents, C1q, C1r and C1s. It is the interaction between C1q and aggregated IgG or IgM bound to antigen that initiates activation of the classical complement sequence. The fixation of C1q activates C1r and C1s. C1s cleaves C4 and C2, whose active fragments C4b and C2a form the classical pathway C3 convertase.

(b) The alternative pathway, consisting of C3b, factor B and factor D, and the regulatory proteins, properdin, factors H and I. Factor B binds to a cleavage fragment of C3, C3b, to form C3bB. Factor D cleaves the bound factor B to form the alternative pathway C3 convertase (C3bBb). It activates C3 in a fashion similar to the C3 convertase of the classical pathway, C4b2a. Properdin acts to stabilize this alternative pathway C3 convertase, as do carbohydrate-rich cell surfaces, by partially shielding the convertase from inhibitors. The alternative pathway is inhibited by default and always shows some activation.

(c) The lectin pathway is initiated by soluble proteins like mannose binding lectin and ficolins that are structurally related to C1q and that recognize and bind carbohydrates on the surface of microorganisms. Serine proteases associated with these recognition proteins activate C4, which, similar to C1r and C1s, leads to the same outcome, namely generation of C3 convertase.

The fate of antibody-coated cells (e.g. red blood cells in auto- or alloimmune haemolysis) is dependent

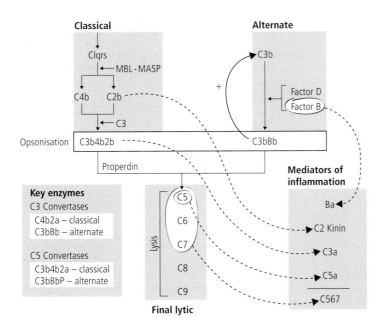

Fig 2.2 The different pathways for complement activation. MBL, mannan-binding lectin; MASP, MBL-associated serine protease.

on whether there is partial or total activation downstream from C3. Total activation in this respect generates the membrane attack complex with the formation of the trimolecular complex of C4b2a3b or C5 convertase. This complex cleaves C5 into two fragments, C5a and C5b. C5b forms a complex with C6, C7 and C8, which facilitates the insertion of a number of C9 molecules in the membrane. This so-called membrane attack complex (MAC) creates lytic pores in the membrane that destroys the target cell. IgM mediates this process especially well. MAC can also be transferred to cells close by and leads to so-called bystander lysis.

Partially activated complement, in contrast, recruits and activates phagocytes to sites of infection, but moreover it can mediate homing and clearance of complement-coated cells in macrophage areas of the spleen or liver, which next to Fc receptors also carry complement receptors.

Red blood cell antibodies illustrating the above principles

Several hundreds of red cell transfusion-related antigens have been identified. Blood group antigens are inherited polymorphic structures located on proteins, glycoproteins and glycolipids (Chapter 3).

Alloimmunization can happen after contact with non-self blood antigens by transfusion or during pregnancy and delivery. The responsible cellular mechanisms are still largely unclear but powerful animal models will generate definite knowledge in this respect [1]. The humoral response, however, is much easier to investigate. IgM class antibodies are formed first but are usually shortly present after immunization, as T-cell-independent B-cell activation and IgM production does not generate memory B cells and IgM producing plasma cells are often short lived. As so called *naturally occurring* antibodies, IgM, however, can also be present permanently. The binding affinity of antibodies increases in germinal centre reactions, coinciding with the switch from IgM to IgG. The chemical nature of the antigen itself also determines the elicited humoral response. Blood cell antibodies against carbohydrate antigens are generally IgM or IgG2 and IgG4, or a combination of these. Antibodies against protein blood group antigens are typically of the IgG class with predominantly IgG1 and IgG3.

Best known of the so-called *naturally occurring* IgM antibodies are those directed against the A or B blood group antigens. Some antigens, mostly bacterial polysaccharides A or B, can stimulate subsets of mature B cells directly due to the ability of these molecules to crosslink several BCRs and, concomitantly, FcR and complement receptors if antigen is opsonized. It is in this respect supposed that gastrointestinal bacteria trigger this so-called anti-A, B isoagglutinin production. This explains their presence from the first months of life. They are of the IgM class because T cells – as a necessary trigger of isotype switching – are not involved. Although some IgM to IgG switching does occur for A and B antigens, the T-cell-independent antibody formation for these carbohydrate antigens, however, has to be discerned from the T-cell-dependent high affinity IgG forming mechanisms for the polypeptide blood groups. Immunization and antibody formation can occur after allogeneic blood contact, e.g. by transfusion, transplantation or associated with pregnancy. This can cause direct or later haemolysis of subsequent transfused mismatched red blood cells but also haemolytic disease of a (next) child with incompatible fatherly antigens. While IgM cannot pass the placenta, motherly IgG directed against antigens on the fetus' blood cells can. Fortunately A and B antigens are only expressed at low levels on fetal red blood cells. Therefore, the anti-A or -B IgG transferred from the mother's blood usually does not lead to haemolysis in the fetus. On the other hand, organ transplants from donors that are AB incompatible can be acutely rejected by recipient anti-A or -B directed to A or B expression on the organ vasculature.

The mechanisms responsible for gradually increasing antibody specificities and subclass changes can also be witnessed by studies on the molecular structure of the V domains (like the predominant use of IGHV3 superspecies genes) of monoclonal antibodies against the protein antigen RhD on the red cell membrane. This selective use of V genes in antibody production against a certain antigen was found in pregnancy-induced RhD immunized females who volunteered for further immunization with RhD [2]. These hyperimmunization programmes are of great importance in the acquisition of therapeutic quantities of anti-D antibodies.

Antibody and complement-mediated blood cell destruction

A transfusion into a recipient with circulating antibodies against transfused antigens can cause an acute (within 24 hours posttransfusion) haemolytic

syndrome (Chapter 7). This clinical picture can be life threatening, especially when intravascular haemolysis is induced. The delayed form of haemolysis occurs between 1 and 7 days after an antigen-incompatible transfusion and is typically less severe. The latter namely depends on boosting of a previous, but at the moment of transfusion, undetectable memory immunization [3].

Most red blood group allo- and autoantibodies of the IgG isotype bring about lysis via the interaction of the IgG constant domain with Fcγ receptors on cells of the mononuclear phagocytic system. Several receptor types are described.

• FcγRI is the most important receptor that causes blood cell destruction. This is a high-affinity receptor found predominantly on monocytes. The consequence of adherence of IgG-coated red cells to FcγRI-positive cells is phagocytosis and lysis. This is usually extravascular and takes place in the spleen. The lysis can be demonstrated in vitro as ADCC.

• FcγRII is a lower affinity receptor found on monocytes, neutrophils, eosinophils, platelets and B cells.

• FcγRIII is also of relatively low affinity and found on macrophages, neutrophils, eosinophils and NK cells. It is responsible for the ADCC demonstrable in vitro with NK cells.

• There is also an FcRn (neonatal) on the placenta and other tissues of a different molecular family, which mediates the transfer of IgG into the fetus and is involved in the control of IgG concentrations.

The severity of haemolysis by IgG antibodies is determined by the concentration of antibody, its affinity for the antigen, antigen density, the IgG subclass and their complement activating capacity (see below). IgG2 antibodies generally do not reduce red cell survival, whilst IgG1 and IgG3 do. There is ample evidence in patients with warm-type autoimmune haemolytic anaemia that IgG1 and IgG3 are more effective in causing red cell destruction than IgG2. The level of IgG1 coating of red cells needs to exceed a threshold of approximately 1000 molecules per red cell to cause cell destruction. For a long time, it has been speculated that polymorphisms in the genes of the family of FcγRs might be significant in causing differences of severity of blood cell destruction observed between patients with apparently similar levels of IgG coating. In line with this, a single amino acid polymorphism of the FcγRIIa receptor dramatically alters the affinity for human IgG2 and additional polymorphisms might have an effect on the interaction with IgG1 and IgG3.

The complement system, either working alone or in concert with an antibody, plays an important part in immune red cell destruction. In contrast to extravascular FcγR-mediated destruction, complement-mediated lysis occurs in the intravascular compartment. The ensuing release of anaphylatoxins such as C3a and C5a contributes to acute systemic effects. IgM antibodies against the A and B antigens are mostly known for this rapid complement-mediated destruction and intravascular haemolysis of incompatible red cells. These events are due to incorrectly typed transfusion units or misidentification of product or recipient and, although rarely happening, remain the most important cause of transfusion-related mortality and morbidity.

Apart from intravascular lysis, blood cells coated with C3b will bind to cells carrying receptors for C3b (CR1 or CD35). This leads to extravascular cell destruction mainly in the liver. If, however, the bound C3b degrades to its inactive components iC3b and C3dg before the cell is lysed, then the cell is protected from lysis. Membrane-bound molecules such as decay accelerating factor (DAF) and membrane inhibitor of reactive lysis (MIRL) also protect red cells from lysis in this way.

Clinical aspects related to alloimmunization against blood cell antigens

Although platelet-directed antibodies (both directed against HLA class I and human platelet antigen or HPA) can lead to refractoriness to platelet transfusions (see Chapters 4 and 5), the consequences of red cell antibodies in the case of incompatible transfusions are much more significant. The effects not only lead to direct (destruction of the allogeneic red cells) but also to indirect (haemolysis-dependent thrombosis, multiple organ damage) morbidity and sometimes mortality (see Chapter 7). The latter can and has to be prevented by determining and recording alloimmune antibody specificities and matching further transfusions for the absence of reactive antigens.

Red cell alloimmunization is reported with large variations between 2 and 21%, with a strong predominance for specific antigens. This reported variation is certainly influenced by the quantity of alloexposures (the number of transfusions) [4]. On the other hand, medication-suppressed immunity or an activated immune system by the presence of autoimmune disorders, infection [5] or pre-existing haemolysis priming APCs with danger signals are all likely to influence auto- and alloimmunization efficacy. Such factors might protect and also be critical as additional triggers of red cell alloimmunization because most peptide red cell antigens only differ by single amino acid substitutions. In contrast, the much more immunogenic red cell antigens like the A, B and the RhD antigens, which are present or absent, are routinely matched for and therefore of less importance for transfusion-mediated alloimmunization. Finally, alloimmunization efficacy is influenced by factors involving the compatibility between donor and patient, e.g. the extent of their genetic or ethnic differences. The latter is not only the case for red cell blood groups themselves but also for HLA differences between donor and recipient. Certain HLA types are associated with a higher red blood cell alloimmunization risk, suggesting specific HLA restriction for the presentation of some red cell antigens [6, 7]. Interestingly, a first alloimmunization increases the risk of further antibody formation. This again might indicate a subgroup of so-called *responder* patients that have an intrinsic higher risk for alloimmunization [8]. On the other hand, the observation that preventative matching of donor blood for highly immunogenic antigens like Rh E and Kell prevents alloimmunization against other antigens might alternatively indicate that a first immunization itself changes the susceptibility for subsequent events [9]. Better identification of clinical or genetic patient factors and possibly also product (like storage) risk factors for red cell antigen alloimmunization will be of great importance; this might enable a cost-effective matching in specific high-risk conditions. This would prevent antibody formation that is especially important in later acute conditions when only low level matching is possible.

Although alloimmunization against red cell antigens – because of the many patients who undergo repetitive exposure to obligatory more or less mismatched blood – is important enough, (co-)transfused platelets and leucocytes, respectively expressing MHC class I and both class I and II, are more effective in inducing alloimmunization. This is first clear from the formation of non-self-directed transfusion-dependent

HPA and HLA and other leucocyte-directed antibodies. Leucocyte reduction in this respect, first introduced in the late 1990s to prevent the merely theoretical transmission of variant Creutzfeldt–Jacob disease by leucocytes in blood components, did decrease transfusion-associated primary HLA antibody formation. Antigens of the human leucocyte antigen (HLA) system can be recognized directly or indirectly by the cells of the immune system. The direct pathway involves the direct recognition of non-self HLA molecules on the donor antigen presenting cells (APC) in blood or in the transplanted tissues and involves activation of immunologically naive T cells. The indirect pathway involves processing and presentation of donor-derived HLA peptides by the host APC. Interesting, alloimmunization, e.g. against red cells, is associated with the additional presence of HLA antibodies [10, 11]. Again, it is unclear if this observation involves the so-called (more easily immunized) responder patients or that it merely indicates a general non-self antigen exposure, which is inherent to allogeneic blood exposure.

HLA and HPA antibodies are associated with various subsequent effects. First of all, recipient HLA antibodies can cause refractoriness to platelet transfusions because donor platelets express (although varying amounts of) incompatible HLA class I molecules. The same can happen on the basis of alloimmunization against inherited polymorphisms in platelet-specific antigens (HPA variants). These HPA antibodies can cause platelet transfusion refractoriness, but in contrast to HLA antibodies also neonatal alloimmune thrombocytopenia (NAITP) and sometimes fatal bleeding complications (see Chapter 5). HLA antibodies in this respect do not seem able to cross the placental barrier as can HPA antibodies. Second, donor HLA (but also other leucocyte binding) antibodies are instrumental in at least part of transfusion-related acute lung injury (TRALI) cases (see Chapter 9). Third, HLA antibodies in the recipient itself can cause cytokine-induced febrile nonhaemolytic transfusion reactions (FNHTR) when reacting with and destroying donor leucocytes in transfusion products (see Chapter 8).

Finally, hyperhaemolysis and posttransfusion purpura are associated with antibodies acting against transfused blood components. Posttransfusion purpura is a rare bleeding complication typically 5–10 days after transfusion [12] (see Chapter 12).

Hyperhaemolysis is a similar event but then lowering the haemoglobin below pretransfusion levels due to destruction of transfused and autologous red blood cells. Hyperhaemolysis is most seen in transfused haemoglobinopathy patients with a background of active haemolysis [13] (see Chapter 7).

Next to the alloimmunization against red blood groups, HPA, HLA and other leucocyte antigens, it seems only logical that transfusion of various amounts and degrees of functional and viable leucocytes can have additional effects on the immune system of the recipient. This transfusion-related immunomodulation (TRIM) (see Chapter 10) is mostly studied by comparing outcomes of leucocyte-rich and leucocyte-reduced transfusion products [14]. Patients with cancer and infections – disorders that for their outcome are determined by immune competence – are most likely to be affected by possible TRIM effects.

Key points

1 Transplants and allogeneic blood are intrinsically non-self and capable of eliciting an immune response; additional danger signals (as in inflammatory conditions) are needed to prime and activate the blood cells that are most important for alloantibody formation.
2 The ability of antibodies to bring about erythrocyte or platelet destruction varies according to their isotype and their antigenic, Fc receptor and complement binding and activating capacities.
3 Most clinical problems encountered in transfusion medicine are antibody-based; also the responsible and modulating cellular mechanisms, still need more elucidation [15].
4 Better identification of high risk patients (responders) and conditions together with increasing possibilities to perform extensive (genotypic) typing for RBC and platelet antigens will enable selective preventative and cost-effective donor–recipient matching [15].
5 High alloimmunization risk patients and conditions might additionally benefit from immunomodulatory therapies that aim at the prevention of allo-specific B-cell activation and plasma cell differentiation.

References

1 Gilson CR & Zimring JC. Alloimmunisation to transfused platelets requires priming of CD4+ T cells in the

splenic microenvironment in a murine model. *Transfusion* 2011; 52: 849–859.

2 Dohmen SE, Verhagen OJHM, Muit J, Ligthart PC & van der Schoot CE. The restricted use of IGHV3 super-species genes in anti-Rh is not limited to hyperimmunized anti-D donors. *Transfusion* 2006; 46: 2162–2168.

3 Vamvakas EC, Pineda AA, Reisner R, Santrach PJ & Moore SB. The differentiation of delayed hemolytic and delayed serologic transfusion reactions: incidence and predictors of hemolysis. *Transfusion* 1995; 35: 26–32.

4 Zalpuri S, Zwaginga JJ, le Cessie S, Elshuis J, Schonewille H & van der Bom JG. Red-blood-cell alloimmunisation and number of red-blood-cell transfusions. *Vox Sanguinis* 2011, July: 6.

5 Hendrickson JE, Desmarets M, Deshpande SS, Chadwick TE, Hillyer CD, Roback JD & Zimring JC. Recipient inflammation affects the frequency and magnitude of immunization to transfused red blood cells. *Transfusion* 2006; 46: 1526–1536.

6 Hoppe C, Klitz W, Vichinsky E & Styles L. HLA type and risk of alloimmunisation in sickle cell disease. *Am J Hematol* 2009; 84: 462–464.

7 Noizat-Pirenne F, Tournamille C, Bierling P, Roudot-Thoraval F, Le Pennec PY, Rouger P & Ansart-Pirenne H. Relative immunogenicity of Fya and K antigens in a Caucasian population, based on HLA class II restriction analysis. *Transfusion* 2006; 46: 1328–1333.

8 Higgins JM & Sloan SR. Stochastic modelling of human RBC alloimmunisation: evidence for a distinct population of immunologic responders. *Blood* 2008; 112: 2546–2553.

9 Schonewille H, Rene RP, de Vries RRP & Brand A. Alloimmune response after additional red blood cell antigen challenge in immunized hemato-oncology patients. *Transfusion* 2009; 49: 453–457.

10 Buetens O, Shirey RS, Goble-Lee M, Houp J, Zachary A, King KE & Ness PM. Prevalence of HLA antibodies in transfused patients with, without red cell antibodies. *Transfusion* 2006; 46: 754–756.

11 Sanz C, Ghita G, Franquet C, Martínez I & Pereira A. Red-blood-cell alloimmunisation and female sex predict the presence of HLA antibodies in patients undergoing liver transplant. *Vox Sanguinis* 2010; 99: 261–266.

12 Hendrickson JE & Hillyer CD. Noninfectious serious hazards of transfusion. *Anesth Analg* 2009; 108: 759–769.

13 Win N. Hyperhemolysis syndrome in sickle cell disease. *Expert Rev Hematol* 2009; 2: 111–115.

14 Hebert PC, Fergusson D, Blajchman MA, Wells GA, Kmetic A, Coyle D, Heddle N, Germain M, Goldman M, Toye B, Schweitzer I, van Walraven C, Devine D & Sher GD. Leukoreduction Study Investigators: clinical outcomes following institution of the Canadian universal leukoreduction program for red blood cell transfusions. *J Am Med Assoc* 2003; 289: 1941–1949.

15 Zimring JC, Welniak L, Semple JW, Ness PM, Slichter SJ & Spitalnik SL, for the NHLBI Alloimmunisation Working Group. Current problems and future directions of transfusion-induced alloimmunisation: summary of an NHLBI working group. *Transfusion* 2011; 51: 435–441.

Further reading

Murphy K. *Janeway's Immunobiology*, 8th edn. London and New York: Garland Science; 2011.

3

Human blood group systems

Geoff Daniels

Bristol Institute for Transfusion Sciences, NHS Blood and Transplant, Bristol, UK

Introduction

A blood group may be defined as an inherited character of the red cell surface detected by a specific alloantibody. This definition would not receive universal acceptance as cell surface antigens on platelets and leucocytes might also be considered blood groups, as might uninherited characters on red cells defined by autoantibodies or xenoantibodies. The definition is suitable, however, for the purposes of this chapter.

Most blood groups are organized into blood group systems. Each system represents a single gene or a cluster of two or more closely linked homologous genes. Of the 339 blood group specificities recognized by the International Society for Blood Transfusion, 297 belong to one of 33 systems (Table 3.1). All these systems represent a single gene, apart from Rh, Xg and Chido/Rodgers, which have two closely linked homologous genes, and MNS with three genes [1, 2].

Most blood group antigens are proteins or glycoproteins, with the blood group specificity determined primarily by the amino acid sequence, and most of the blood group polymorphisms result from single amino acid substitutions, though there are many exceptions. Some of these proteins cross the membrane once, with either the N-terminal or C-terminal outside the membrane, some cross the membrane several times and some are outside the membrane to which they are attached by a glycosylphosphatidylinositol anchor. Some blood group antigens, including

those of the ABO, P1PK, Lewis, H and I systems, are carbohydrate structures on glycoproteins and glycolipids. These antigens are not produced directly by the genes controlling their polymorphisms, but by genes encoding transferase enzymes that catalyse the final biosynthetic stage of an oligosaccharide chain.

The two most important blood group systems from the clinical point of view are ABO and Rh. They also provide good models for contrasting carbohydrate- and protein-based blood group systems.

The ABO system

ABO is often referred to as a histo-blood group system because, in addition to being expressed on red cells, ABO antigens are present on most tissues and in soluble form in secretions. At its most basic level, the ABO system consists of two antigens, A and B, indirectly encoded by two alleles, *A* and *B*, of the *ABO* gene. A third allele, *O*, produces neither A nor B. These three alleles combine to effect four phenotypes: A, B, AB and O (Table 3.2).

Clinical significance

Two key factors make ABO the most important blood group system in transfusion medicine. First, almost without exception, the blood of adults contains antibodies to those ABO antigens lacking from their red

Practical Transfusion Medicine, Fourth Edition. Edited by Michael F. Murphy, Derwood H. Pamphilon and Nancy M. Heddle.
© 2013 John Wiley & Sons, Ltd. Published 2013 by John Wiley & Sons, Ltd.

Table 3.1 Human blood group systems.

Number	Name	Symbol	Number of antigens	Gene symbol(s)	Chromosome
001	ABO	ABO	4	*ABO*	9
002	MNS	MNS	46	*GYPA, GYPB, GYPE*	4
003	P1PK	P1PK	3	*A4GALT*	22
004	Rh	RH	54	*RHD, RHCE*	1
005	Lutheran	LU	20	*BCAM*	19
006	Kell	KEL	35	*KEL*	7
007	Lewis	LE	6	*FUT3*	19
008	Duffy	FY	5	*DARC*	1
009	Kidd	JK	3	*SLC14A1*	18
010	Diego	DI	22	*SLC4A1*	17
011	Yt	YT	2	*ACHE*	7
012	Xg	XG	2	*XG, CD99*	X/Y
013	Scianna	SC	7	*ERMAP*	1
014	Dombrock	DO	8	*ART4*	12
015	Colton	CO	4	*AQP1*	7
016	Landsteiner–Wiener	LW	3	*ICAM4*	19
017	Chido/Rodgers	CH/RG	9	*C4A, C4B*	6
018	H	H	1	*FUT1*	19
019	Kx	XK	1	*XK*	X
020	Gerbich	GE	11	*GYPC*	2
021	Cromer	CROM	18	*CD55*	1
022	Knops	KN	9	*CR1*	1
023	Indian	IN	4	*CD44*	11
024	Ok	OK	3	*BSG*	19
025	Raph	RAPH	1	*CD151*	11
026	John Milton Hagen	JMH	6	*SEMA7A*	15
027	I	I	1	*GCNT2*	6
028	Globoside	GLOB	1	*B3GALT3*	3
029	Gill	GIL	1	*AQP3*	9
030	RHAG	RHAG	4	*RHAG*	6
031	Forssman	FORS	1	*GBGT1*	9
032	Junior	JR	1	*ABCG2*	4
033	Lan	LAN	1	*ABCB6*	2

Table 3.2 The ABO system.

Phenotype	Genotypes	Frequency Europeans*	Africans†	Indians‡	Antibodies present
O	O/O	43%	51%	31%	Anti-A, -B, -A,B
A_1	A^1/A^1, A^1/O, A^1/A^2	35%	18%	26%	Anti-B
A_2	A^2/A^2, A^2/O	10%	5%	3%	Sometimes anti-A_1
B	B/B, B/O	9%	21%	30%	Anti-A
A_1B	A^1/B	3%	2%	9%	None
A_2B	A^2/B	1%	1%	1%	Sometimes anti-A_1

*English donors.
†Donors from Kinshasa, Congo.
‡Makar from Mumbai.

cells (Table 3.2). In addition to anti-A and anti-B, group O individuals have anti-A,B, an antibody to a determinant common to A and B. Second, ABO antibodies are IgM, though they may also have an IgG component, have thermal activity at 37°C, activate complement and cause immediate intravascular red cell destruction, which can give rise to severe and often fatal haemolytic transfusion reactions (HTRs) (see Chapter 7). Major ABO incompatibility (i.e. donor red cells with an ABO antigen not possessed by the recipient) must be avoided in transfusion and, ideally, ABO-matched blood (i.e. of the same ABO group) would be provided.

ABO antibodies seldom cause haemolytic disease of the fetus and newborn (HDFN) but when they do it is usually mild. The prime reasons for this are (1) that IgM antibodies do not cross the placenta, (2) IgG ABO antibodies are often IgG2, which do not activate complement or facilitate phagocytosis and (3) ABO antigens are present on many fetal tissues and in body fluids, so the haemolytic potential of the antibody is greatly reduced.

A and B subgroups

The A (and AB) phenotype can be subdivided into A_1 and A_2 (and A_1B and A_2B). In a European population, about 80% of group A individuals are A_1 and 20% A_2 (Table 3.2). A_1 and A_2 differ quantitatively and qualitatively. A_1 red cells react more strongly with anti-A than A_2 cells. In addition, A_2 red cells lack a component of the A antigen present on A_1 cells and some individuals with the A_2 or A_2B phenotype produce anti-A_1, an antibody that agglutinates A_1 and A_1B cells, but not A_2 or A_2B cells. Anti-A_1 is seldom reactive at 37°C and is generally considered clinically insignificant.

There are numerous other ABO variants, involving weakened expression of A or B antigens, but all are rare. They are often subdivided into categories (A_3, A_x, A_m, A_{el}, B_3, B_x, B_m and B_{el}) based on serological characteristics, but molecular analyses have shown that most of the subgroups are genetically heterogeneous.

Biosynthesis and molecular genetics

Red cell A and B antigens are expressed predominantly on oligosaccharide structures on integral membrane glycoproteins, mainly the anion transporter band 3

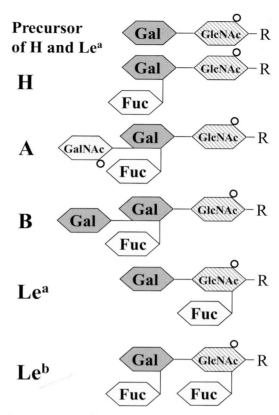

Fig 3.1 Diagram of the oligosaccharides representing H, A, B, Le^a and Le^b antigens, and the biosynthetic precursor of H and Le^a. R, remainder of molecule.

and the glucose transporter GLUT1, but are also on glycosphingolipids embedded in the membrane. The tetrasaccharides that represent the predominant form of A and B antigens on red cells are shown in Figure 3.1, together with their biosynthetic precursor, the H antigen, which is abundant on group O red cells. The product of the *A* allele is a glycosyltransferase that catalyses the transfer of N-acetylgalactosamine (GalNAc) from a nucleotide donor substrate, UDP-GalNAc, to the fucosylated galactose (Gal) residue of the H antigen, the acceptor substrate. The product of the *B* allele catalyses the transfer of Gal from UDP-Gal to the fucosylated Gal residue of the H antigen. GalNAc and Gal are the immunodominant sugars of A and B antigens, respectively. The O allele produces no transferase, so the H antigen remains unmodified.

The *ABO* gene on chromosome 9 consists of seven exons. The *A¹* and *B* alleles differ by seven nucleotides in exons 6 and 7, four of which, in exon 7, encode amino acid substitutions in their glycosyltransferase products: Arg176, Gly235, Leu266 and Gly268 in A; Gly176, Ser235, Met266 and Ala268 in B [3]. It is primarily the amino acids at positions 266 and 268 that determine whether the gene product is a GalNAc-transferase (A) or Gal-transferase (B). The most common *O* allele (*O¹*) has an identical sequence to *A¹*, apart from a single nucleotide deletion in exon 6, which shifts the reading frame and introduces a translation stop codon before the region of the catalytic site, so that any protein produced would be truncated and have no enzyme activity. Another common *O* allele, called *O¹ᵛ*, differs from *O¹* by at least nine nucleotides, but has the same single nucleotide deletion as that in *O¹* and so cannot produce any functional enzyme. *O²*, which represents about 3% of *O* alleles in a European population, does not have the nucleotide deletion characteristic of most *O* alleles and encodes a complete protein product, but with a charged arginine residue instead of a neutral glycine (A) or alanine (B) at position 268, which completely blocks the donor GalNAc-binding site and prevents any enzyme activity. The *A²* allele has a sequence almost identical to *A¹*, but has a single nucleotide deletion immediately before the translation stop codon. The resultant frame shift abolishes the stop codon, so the protein product has 21 extra amino acids at its C-terminal, which reduces the efficiency of its GalNAc-transferase activity and might alter its acceptor substrate specificity [4].

Biochemically related blood group systems – H, Lewis and I

H antigen is the biochemical precursor of A and B (Figure 3.1). It is synthesized by an α1,2-fucosyltransferase, which catalyses the transfer of fucose from its donor substrate to the terminal Gal residue of its acceptor substrate. Without this fucosylation neither A nor B antigens can be made. Two genes, active in different tissues, produce α1,2-fucosyltransferases: *FUT1*, active in mesodermally derived tissues and responsible for H on red cells, and *FUT2*, active in endodermally derived tissues and responsible for H in many other tissues and in secretions. Homozygosity for inactivating mutations in *FUT1* leads to an absence of H from red cells and,

therefore, an absence of red cell A or B, regardless of *ABO* genotype. Such mutations are rare, as are red cell H-deficient phenotypes. In contrast, inactivating mutations in *FUT2* are relatively common and about 20% of White Europeans (nonsecretors) lack H, A and B from body secretions despite expressing those antigens on their red cells. Very rare individuals who have H-deficient red cells and are also H nonsecretors (Bombay phenotype) produce anti-H together with anti-A and -B and can cause a severe transfusion problem.

Antigens of the Lewis system are not produced by erythroid cells, but become incorporated into the red cell membrane from the plasma. Their corresponding antibodies are not usually active at 37°C and are not generally considered clinically significant. Leᵃ and Leᵇ are not the products of alleles. The Lewis gene (*FUT3*) product is an α1,3/4-fucosyltransferase that transfers fucose to the GlcNAc residue of the secreted precursor of H in nonsecretors to produce Leᵃ and to secreted H in secretors to produce Leᵇ (Figure 3.1). Consequently, H secretors are Le(a–b+) or Le(a+b+), H nonsecretors are Le(a+b–) and individuals homozygous for *FUT3* inactivating mutations (secretors or nonsecretors) are Le(a–b–).

I antigen represents branched *N*-acetyllactosamine (Galβ1–4GlcNAc) structures in the complex carbohydrates that also express H, A and B antigens. The I gene (*GCNT2*) encodes a branching enzyme, which only becomes active during the first months of life. Consequently, red cells of neonates are I-negative. Rare individuals are homozygous for inactivating mutations in *GCNT2* and never form I on their red cells [5]. This phenotype, called adult i, is associated with production of anti-I, which is usually only active below 37°C, but may occasionally be haemolytic at body temperature.

The Rh system

Rh is the most complex of the blood group systems, with 54 specificities. The most important of these is D (RH1).

Rh genes and proteins

The antigens of the Rh system are encoded by two genes, *RHD* and *RHCE*, which produce D and CcEe

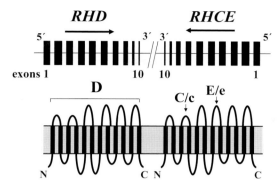

Fig 3.2 Diagrammatic representation of the Rh genes, *RHD* and *RHCE*, shown in opposite orientations as they appear on the chromosome, and of the two Rh proteins in their probable membrane conformation, with 12 membrane-spanning domains and 6 extracellular loops expressing D, C/c and E/e antigens.

antigens, respectively. The genes are highly homologous, each consisting of 10 exons. They are closely linked, but in opposite orientations, on chromosome 1 [6] (Figure 3.2). Each gene encodes a 417 amino acid polypeptide that differs by only 31–35 amino acids, according to Rh genotype. The Rh proteins are palmitoylated, but not glycosylated, and span the red cell membrane 12 times, with both termini inside the cytosol and with six external loops, the potential sites of antigenic activity (Figure 3.2).

D antigen

The most significant Rh antigen from the clinical point of view is D. About 85% of White people are D+ (Rh-positive) and 15% are D– (Rh-negative). In Africans, only about 3–5% are D– and in the East Asia D– is rare.

The D– phenotype is usually associated with the absence of the whole D protein from the red cell membrane. This explains why D is so immunogenic, as the D antigen comprises numerous epitopes on the external domains of the D protein. In White people, the D– phenotype almost always results from homozygosity for a complete deletion of *RHD*. D-positives are either homozygous or heterozygous for the presence of *RHD*. In Africans, in addition to the deletion of *RHD*, D– often results from an inactive *RHD* (called *RHD*Ψ) containing translation stop codons within the reading frame. Other genes containing inactivating mutations are also found in D– Africans and Asians.

Numerous variants of D are known, though most are rare [7]. They are often split into two types, partial D and weak D, though this dichotomy is not adequately defined and of little value for making clinical decisions. Partial D antigens lack some or most of the D epitopes. If an individual with a partial D phenotype is immunized by red cells with a complete D antigen, they might make antibodies to those epitopes they lack. The D epitopes comprising partial D may be expressed weakly or may be of normal or even enhanced strength. Weak D antigens appear to express all epitopes of D, but at a lower site density than normal D. D variants result from amino acid substitutions in the D protein occurring either as a result of one or more mis-sense mutations in *RHD* or from one or more exons of *RHD* being exchanged for the equivalent exons of *RHCE* in a process called gene conversion.

Anti-D

Anti-D is almost never produced in D– individuals without immunization by D+ red cells. However, D is highly immunogenic and at least 30% of D– recipients of transfused D+ red cells make anti-D. Anti-D can cause severe immediate or delayed HTRs and D+ blood must never be transfused to a patient with anti-D.

Anti-D is the most common cause of severe HDFN. The effects of HDFN caused by anti-D are, at its most severe, fetal death at about the seventeenth week of pregnancy. If the infant is born alive, the disease can result in hydrops and jaundice. If the jaundice leads to kernicterus, this usually results in infant death or permanent cerebral damage. The prevalence of HDFN resulting from anti-D has been substantially reduced by anti-D immunoglobulin prophylaxis. In 1970, at the beginning of the anti-D prophylaxis programme, there were 1.2 deaths per thousand births in England and Wales due to HDFN caused by anti-D; by 1989, this figure had been reduced to 0.02.

Prediction of fetal Rh genotype by molecular methods

Knowledge of the molecular bases for D– phenotypes has made it possible to devise tests for predicting fetal

D type from fetal DNA. This is a valuable tool in assessing whether the fetus of a woman with anti-D is at risk from HDFN [8]. Most methods involve PCR tests that detect the presence or absence of *RHD*. It is important that the tests are devised so that *RHD*Ψ and other variant *RHD* genes do not give false phenotype predictions. Initially, the usual source of fetal DNA was amniocytes obtained by amniocentesis, which has an inherent risk of fetal loss and of feto-maternal haemorrhage. A far superior source of fetal DNA, avoiding invasive procedures, is the small quantity of free fetal DNA present in maternal plasma. This non-invasive form of fetal D typing is now provided as a reference service in some countries for alloimmunized D– women. In addition, in a few European countries noninvasive fetal *RHD* genotyping is offered to all D– pregnant women, so that only those with a D+ fetus receive routine antenatal anti-D prophylaxis (see Chapter 32).

C and c, E and e

C/c and E/e are two pairs of antigens representing alleles of *RHCE*. The fundamental difference between C and c is a serine–proline substitution at position 103 in the second external loop of the CcEe protein (Figure 3.2), though the situation is more complex than that [9]. E and e represent a proline–alanine substitution at position 226 in the fourth external loop. Taking into account the presence and absence of D and of the C/c and E/e polymorphisms, eight different haplotypes can be recognized. The frequencies of these haplotypes and the shorthand symbols often used to describe them are shown in Table 3.3.

Anti-c is clinically the most important Rh antibody after anti-D and may cause severe HDFN. On the other hand, anti-C, -E and -e rarely cause HDFN and when they do the disease is generally mild, though all have the potential to cause severe disease.

Other Rh antigens

Of the 54 Rh antigens, 20 are polymorphic, i.e. have a frequency between 1 and 99% in at least one major ethnic group, 22 are rare antigens and 12 are very common antigens. Antibodies to many of these antigens have proved to be clinically important and it is prudent to treat all Rh antibodies as being potentially clinically significant [10].

Other blood group systems

Of the remaining blood group systems (Table 3.1), the most important clinically are Kell, Duffy, Kidd, Diego and MNS, and these are described below.

The Kell system

The original Kell antigen, K (KEL1) (Met193), has a frequency of about 9% in Caucasians, but is rare in other ethnic groups. Its antithetical (allelic) antigen, k (KEL2) (Thr193), is common in all populations. The remainder of the Kell system consists of one triplet and five pairs of allelic antigens – Kpa, Kpb and Kpc; Jsa and Jsb; K11 and K17; K14 and K24; VLAN and VONG; KYO and KYOR – plus 17 high frequency and 3 low frequency antigens. Almost all represent single amino acid substitutions in the Kell glycoprotein.

Anti-K can cause severe HTRs and HDFN. About 10% of K– patients who are given one unit of K+ blood produce anti-K, making K the next most immunogenic antigen after D. In most cases of HDFN caused by anti-K, the mother will have had previous blood transfusions. HDFN caused by anti-K differs from Rh HDFN in that anti-K appears to cause fetal anaemia by suppression of erythropoiesis, rather than immune destruction of mature fetal erythrocytes. Anti-k is a very rare antibody. It is always immune and has been incriminated in some cases of mild HDFN [10]. Most other Kell system antibodies are rare and best detected by an antiglobulin test.

The Kell antigens are located on a large glycoprotein, which crosses the cell membrane once and has a glycosylated, C-terminal extracellular domain, maintained in a folded conformation by multiple disulfide bonds. The Kell glycoprotein belongs to a family of endopeptidases, which process biologically important peptides, and is able to cleave the biologically inactive peptide big endothelin-3 to produce endothelin-3, an active vasoconstrictor.

The Duffy system

Fya and Fyb represent a single amino acid substitution (Gly42Asp) in the extracellular N-terminal domain of the Duffy glycoprotein. Their incidence in Caucasians is Fya 68%, Fyb 80%. About 70% of African Americans and close to 100% of West Africans are

Table 3.3 Rh phenotypes and the genotypes that produce them (presented in DCE and shorthand terminology).

Phenotype					Frequency (%)				
D	C	c	E	e	Europeans*	Africans[†]	Asians[‡]	Genotypes	
+	+	−	−	+	18.5	0.7	56.0	DCe/Dce	R^1/R^1
								DCe/dCe	R^1r'
+	−	+	+	−	2.3	1.3	3.5	DcE/DcE	R^2R^2
								DcE/dcE	R^2r''
+	−	+	−	+	2.1	58.9	0.2	Dce/dce	$R^\circ r$
								Dce/Dce	$R^\circ R^\circ$
+	+	−	+	−	Rare	Rare	Rare	DCE/DCE	R^zR^z
								DCE/dCE	R^zr^y
+	+	+	−	+	34.9	13.2	8.4	DCe/dce	R^1r
								DCe/Dce	R^1R°
								Dce/dCe	$R^\circ r'$
+	−	+	+	+	11.8	18.3	2.1	DcE/dce	R^2r
								DcE/Dce	R^2R°
								Dce/dcE	$R^\circ r''$
+	+	−	+	+	0.2	Rare	1.1	DCe/DCE	R^1R^z
								DCE/dCe	R^zr'
								DCe/dCE	R^1r^y
+	+	+	+	−	0.1	Rare	0.3	DcE/DCE	R^2R^z
								DCE/dcE	R^zr''
								DcE/dCE	R^2r^y
+	+	+	+	+	13.4	2.1	28.1	DCe/DcE	R^1R^2
								DCe/dcE	R^1r''
								DcE/dCe	R^2r'
								DCE/dce	R^zr
								Dce/DCE	$R^\circ R^z$
								Dce/dCE	$R^\circ r^y$
−	+	−	−	+	Rare	0.1	Rare	dCe/dCe	$r'r'$
−	−	+	+	−	Rare	Rare	Rare	dcE/dcE	$r''r''$
−	−	+	−	+	15.1	4.1	0.1	dce/dce	rr
−	+	−	+	−	Rare	Rare	Rare	dCE/dCE	r^yr^y
−	+	+	−	+	0.1	1.3	0.1	dCe/dce	$r'r$
−	−	+	+	+	0.1	Rare	Rare	dcE/dce	$r''r$
−	+	−	+	+	Rare	Rare	Rare	dCe/dCE	$r'r^y$
−	+	+	+	−	Rare	Rare	Rare	dcE/dCE	$r''r^y$
−	+	+	+	+	Rare	Rare	Rare	dcE/dCe	$r''r'$
								dCE/dce	r^yr

*English donors.
[†]Yoruba of Nigeria.
[‡]Cantonese of Hong Kong.

Fy(a−b−) (Table 3.4). They are homozygous for an *FY*B* allele containing a mutation in a binding site for the erythroid-specific GATA-1 transcription factor, which means that Duffy glycoprotein is not expressed in red cells, though it is present in other tissues [11]

(Table 3.5). The Duffy glycoprotein is the receptor exploited by *Plasmodium vivax* merozoites for penetration of erythroid cells. Consequently, the Fy(a−b−) phenotype confers resistance to *P. vivax* malaria. The Duffy glycoprotein (also called Duffy antigen

27

Table 3.4 The Duffy system: phenotypes and genotypes.

Phenotype	Genotype	Frequency (%)	
		Europeans	Africans
Fy(a+b–)	FY*A/A or FY*A/Null[†]	20	10
Fy(a+b+)	FY*A/B	48	3
Fy(a–b+)	FY*B/B or FY*B/Null	32	20
Fy(a–b–)	FY*Null/Null	0	67

*Null represents the allele that produces no Duffy antigens on red cells.

chemokine receptor, DACR) is a red cell receptor for a variety of chemokines, including interleukin-8.

Anti-Fy[a] is not infrequent and is found in previously transfused patients who have usually made other antibodies. Anti-Fy[b] is very rare. Both may cause acute or delayed HTRs and HDFN varying from mild to severe [10].

The Kidd system

Kidd has two common alleles, *JK*A* and *JK*B*, which represent a single amino acid change (Asp280Asn) in the Kidd glycoprotein. Both Jk[a] and Jk[b] antigens have frequencies of about 75% in Caucasian populations. A Kidd-null phenotype, Jk(a–b–), results from homozygosity for inactivating mutations in the Kidd gene, *SLC14A1*. It is very rare in most populations, but reaches an incidence of greater than 1% in

Table 3.5 Nucleotide polymorphisms in the promoter region and in exon 2 of the three common alleles of the Duffy gene.

Allele	GATA box sequence –64 to –69 (promoter)	Codon 42 (exon 2)	Antigen
FY*A	TTATCT	GGT (Gly)	Fy[a]
FY*B	TTATCT	GAT (Asp)	Fy[b]
FY*Null	TTACCT	GAT (Asp)	Red cells – none Other tissues – probably Fy[b]

Polynesians. The Kidd glycoprotein is a urea transporter in red cells and in renal endothelial cells.

Anti-Jk[a] is uncommon and anti-Jk[b] is very rare, but they both cause severe transfusion reactions and, to a lesser extent, HDFN [10]. Kidd antibodies have often been implicated in delayed HTRs. They are often difficult to detect serologically and tend to disappear rapidly after stimulation.

The Diego system

Diego is a large system of 22 antigens: three pairs of allelic antigens – Di[a] and Di[b] (Leu854Pro), Wr[a] and Wr[b] (Lys658Glu), Wu and DISK (Gly565Ala) – plus 16 antigens of very low frequency. All represent single amino acid substitutions in band 3, the red cell anion exchanger. The original Diego antigen, Di[a], is very rare in Caucasians and Black people, but relatively common in Mongoloid people, with frequencies varying between 1% in Japanese and 50% in some native South Americans. Anti-Di[a] and -Di[b] are immune and rare, and can cause severe HDFN [10]. Wr[a] has a frequency of about 0.1%. Its high frequency allelic antigen, Wr[b], is dependent on an interaction of band 3 with glycophorin A for expression. Naturally occurring anti-Wr[a] is present in approximately 1% of blood donors and can cause severe HTRs. Very rarely, anti-Wr[a] causes HDFN. Autoanti-Wr[b] is a relatively common autoantibody and may be implicated in autoimmune haemolytic anaemia.

The MNS system

MNS, with a total of 46 antigens, is second only to Rh in complexity. These antigens are present on one or both of two red cell membrane glycoproteins, glycophorin A (GPA) and glycophorin B (GPB). They are encoded by two homologous genes, *GYPA* and *GYPB*, on chromosome 4.

The M and N antigens, both with frequencies of about 75%, differ by amino acids at positions 1 and 5 of the external N-terminus of GPA (Ser1Leu, Gly5Glu). S and s have frequencies of about 55% and 90%, respectively, in a Caucasian population and represent an amino acid substitution in GPB (Met29Thr). About 2% of Black West Africans and 1.5% of African Americans are S– s–, a phenotype virtually unknown in other ethnic groups, and most of these lack the U antigen, which is present when either S or s is expressed. The numerous MNS variants mostly result from amino acid substitutions in GPA or GPB and from hybrid GPA–GPB molecules, formed by intergenic recombination between *GYPA* and *GYPB*. The phenotypes resulting from these hybrid proteins are rare in Europeans and Africans, but the GP.Mur (previously Mi.III) phenotype occurs in up to 10% of East Asians. GPA and GPB are exploited as receptors by the malaria parasite *Plasmodium falciparum*.

Anti-M and -N are not generally clinically significant, though anti-M is occasionally haemolytic [10]. Anti-S, the rarer anti-s and anti-U can cause HDFN and have been implicated in HTRs. Although rare elsewhere, anti-Mur, which detects red cells of the GP.Mur phenotype, is common in East Asia and Oceanic regions and causes severe HTRs and HDFN.

The biological significance of blood group antigens

The functions of several red cell membrane protein structures bearing blood group antigenic determinants are known, or can be deduced from their structure. Some are membrane transporters, facilitating the transport of biologically important molecules through the lipid bilayer: band 3 membrane glycoprotein, the Diego antigen, provides an anion exchange channel for HCO_3^- and Cl^- ions; the Kidd glycoprotein is a urea transporter; the Colton glycoprotein is aquaporin 1, a water channel; the GIL antigen is aquaporin 3, a glycerol transporter; the Junior and Lan antigens are possibly porphyrin transporters. The Lutheran, LW and Indian (CD44) glycoproteins are adhesion molecules, possibly serving their primary functions during erythropoiesis. The MER2 antigen is located on the tetraspanin CD151, which associates with integrins within basement membranes, but its function on red cells is not known. The Duffy glycoprotein is a chemokine receptor and could function as a 'sink' or scavenger for unwanted chemokines. The Cromer and Knops antigens are markers for the decay accelerating factor (CD55) and complement receptor 1 (CD35), respectively, which protect the cells from destruction by autologous complement. Some blood group glycoproteins appear to be enzymes, though their functions on red cells are not known: the Yt antigen is acetylcholinesterase, the Kell antigen is an endopeptidase and the sequence of the Dombrock

glycoprotein suggests that it belongs to a family of adenosine diphosphate (ADP)-ribosyltransferases. The C-terminal domains of the Gerbich antigens, GPC and GPD, and the N-terminal domain of the Diego glycoprotein, band 3, are attached to components of the cytoskeleton and function to anchor it to the external membrane. The carbohydrate moieties of the membrane glycoproteins and glycolipids, especially those of the most abundant glycoproteins, band 3 and GPA, constitute the glycocalyx, an extracellular coat that protects the cell from mechanical damage and microbial attack [12, 13].

The Rh proteins are associated as heterotrimers with the glycoprotein RhAG in the red cell membrane, and these trimers are part of a macrocomplex of red cell surface proteins that include tetramers of band 3 plus LW, GPA, GPB and CD47, and are linked to the red cell cytoskeleton through protein 4.2 and ankyrin. There is probably another protein complex containing Rh proteins and dimers of band 3, plus Kell, Kx and Duffy blood group proteins, and is linked to the cytoskeleton through glycophorin C (Gerbich blood group), MMP1, and protein 4.1R. It is likely that RhAG forms a carbon dioxide and, possibly, oxygen channel, and could function as an ammonia/ammonium transporter [13, 14]. The function of the Rh proteins is not known, but they may play a role in facilitating the assembly of the band 3 macrocomplex.

The structural differences between antithetical red cell antigens (e.g. A and B, K and k, Fy^a and Fy^b) are small, often being just one monosaccharide or one amino acid. The biological importance of these differences is unknown and there is little evidence to suggest that the product of one allele confers any significant advantage over the other. Some blood group antigens are exploited by pathological microorganisms as receptors for attaching and entering cells, so in some cases absence or changes in these antigens could be beneficial. It is likely that interaction between cell surface molecules and pathological microorganisms has been a major factor in the evolution of blood group polymorphism.

Key points

1 The International Society of Blood Transfusion recognizes 339 blood group specificities, 297 of which belong to one of 33 blood group systems.

2 The most important blood group systems clinically are ABO, Rh, Kell, Duffy, Kidd and MNS.

3 ABO antibodies are almost always present in adults lacking the corresponding antigens and can cause fatal intravascular HTRs.

4 ABO antigens are carbohydrate structures on glycoproteins and glycosphingolipids.

5 Anti-RhD is the most common cause of HDFN.

6 Red cell surface proteins serve a variety of functions, though many of their functions are still not known.

References

1 Red Cell Immunogenetics and Blood Group Terminology Working Party of the International Society of Blood Transfusion. http://www.isbtweb.org/working-parties/red-cell-immunogenetics-and-blood-group-terminology.

2 Storry JR, Castilho L, Daniels G, *et al.* International Society of Blood Transfusion Working Party on red cell immunogenetics and blood group terminology: Berlin Report. *Vox Sanguinis* 2011; 101: 77–82.

3 Yamamoto F, Clausen H, White T, Marken J & Hakomori S. Molecular genetic basis of the histo-blood group ABO system. *Nature* 1990; 345: 229–233.

4 Chester AM & Olsson ML. The ABO blood group gene: a locus of considerable genetic diversity. *Transfus Med Rev* 2001; 15: 177–200.

5 Yu L-C, Twu Y-C, Chou M-L, *et al.* The molecular genetics of the human I locus and molecular background explaining the partial association of the adult I phenotype with congenital cataracts. *Blood* 2003; 101: 2081–2088.

6 Wagner FF & Flegel WA. *RHD* gene deletion occurred in the *Rhesus box*. *Blood* 2000; 95: 3662–3668.

7 Rhesus base website. http://www.uni-ulm.de/~fwagner/RH/RB.

8 Daniels G, Finning K, Martin P & Massey E. Non-invasive prenatal diagnosis of fetal blood group phenotypes: current practice and future prospects. *Prenat Diagn* 2009; 29: 101–107.

9 Mouro I, Colin Y, Chérif-Zahar B, Cartron J-P & Le Van Kim C. Molecular genetic basis of the human Rhesus blood group system. *Nature Genet* 1993; 5: 62–65.

10 Poole J & Daniels G. Blood group antibodies and their significance in transfusion medicine. *Transfus Med Rev* 2007; 21: 58–71.

11 Tournamille C, Colin Y, Cartron JP & Le Van Kim C. Disruption of a GATA motif in the *Duffy* gene promoter abolishes erythroid gene expression in Duffy-negative individuals. *Nature Genet* 1995; 10: 224–228.

12 Daniels G. Functions of red cell surface proteins. *Vox Sanguinis* 2007; 93: 331–340.

13 Anstee DJ. The functional importance of blood group-active molecules in human red blood cells. *Vox Sanguinis* 2011; 100: 140–149.

14 Mohandas N & Gallagher PG. Red cell membrane: past, present, and future. *Blood* 2008; 112: 3939–3948.

Further reading

Anstee DJ. Red cell genotyping and the future of pretransfusion testing. *Blood* 2009; 114: 248–256.

Anstee DJ. The relationship between blood groups and disease. *Blood* 2010; 115: 4635–4643.

Avent ND & Reid ME. The Rh blood group system: a review. *Blood* 2000; 95: 375–387.

Daniels G. *Human Blood Groups*, 3rd edn. Oxford: Wiley-Blackwell 2013.

Daniels G. The molecular genetics of blood group polymorphism. *Hum Genet* 2009; 126: 729–742.

Daniels G & Bromilow I. *Essential Guide to Blood Groups*, 2nd edn. Oxford: Blackwell Publishing; 2010.

Daniels G & Reid ME. Blood groups: the past 50 years. *Transfusion* 2010; 50: 3–11.

Reid ME & Lomas-Francis C. *The Blood Group Antigen Facts Book*, 2nd edn. New York: Academic Press; 2004.

Roback JD, Combs MR, Grossman BJ & Hillyer CD. *AABB Technical Manual*, 17th edn. Bethesda, MD: AABB; 2011.

Watkins WM. (ed.) Commemoration of the centenary of the discovery of the ABO blood group system. *Transfus Med* 2001; 11: 239–351.

4

Human leucocyte antigens

Cristina V. Navarrete

NHS Blood and Transplant, Colindale Centre and University College London, London, UK

Introduction

The genes coding for human leucocyte antigens (HLAs) are located on the short arm of chromosome 6, spanning a distance of approximately 4 Mb. This genomic region is divided into three subregions [1, 2].
• Class I subregion contains genes coding for the heavy (α) chain of the classical (*HLA-A, -B* and *-C*) and nonclassical (*HLA-E, -F* and *-G*) class I molecules. The nonclassical major histocompatibility complex class I chain-related gene *A* and gene *B* (*MICA* and *MICB*) have also been mapped to this subregion, centromeric to the *HLA-B* gene (Figure 4.1).
• Class II subregion contains the classical *HLA-DR*, *-DQ* and *-DP* genes and the nonclassical *HLA-DMA*, *-DMB*, *-DOA* and *-DOB* genes. The low-molecular-mass polypeptide genes *LMP2* and *LMP7*, *TAP1* and *TAP2* transporters and the Tapasin (*Tpn*) genes involved in the processing, transport and loading of HLA class I antigenic peptides are also located in this subregion (see Figure 4.1).
• Class III subregion lies between the other two subregions and contains genes coding for a diverse group of proteins, including complement components (C4Bf), tumour necrosis factor (TNF) and heat-shock proteins (HSPs).

The nonclassical class I-like gene *HFE* has been mapped to a locus located 4 Mb telomeric to *HLA-F*. Single point mutations in this gene are associated with the development of hereditary haemochromatosis (HH).

HLA class I genes

The HLA class I genes are classified according to their structure, expression and function as classical (*HLA-A, -B* and *-C*) and nonclassical (*HLA-E, -F* and *-G*). Both classical and nonclassical HLA class I genes code for a heavy (α) chain, of approximately 43 kDa, non-covalently linked to a nonpolymorphic light chain, the β_2-microglobulin of 12 kDa, which is coded for by a gene on chromosome 15. The extracellular portion of the heavy chain has three domains (α1, α2 and α3) of approximately 90 amino acids long. These domains are encoded by exons 2, 3 and 4 of the class I gene, respectively. The α1 and α2 domains are the most polymorphic domains of the molecule and they form a peptide-binding groove that can accommodate antigenic peptides approximately eight to nine amino acids long.

The exon/intron organization of the nonclassical HLA class I genes (*E, F* and *G*) is very similar to the classical class I genes, but they have a more restricted polymorphism. The *MICA* and *MICB* gene products, however, do not bind β_2-microglobulin and do not present antigenic peptides.

A schematic representation of the classical HLA class I gene and molecule is shown in Figure 4.2.

HLA class II genes

The classical HLA class II DR, DQ and DP *A* and *B* genes code for heterodimers formed by noncovalently

Practical Transfusion Medicine, Fourth Edition. Edited by Michael F. Murphy, Derwood H. Pamphilon and Nancy M. Heddle.
© 2013 John Wiley & Sons, Ltd. Published 2013 by John Wiley & Sons, Ltd.

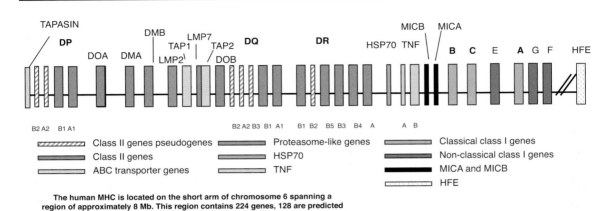

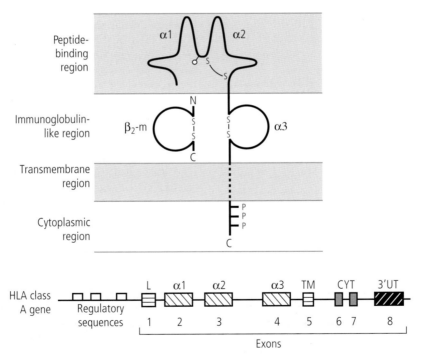

Fig 4.1 Map of the human leucocyte antigen complex. HSP, heat-shock protein; TNF, tumour necrosis factor. Based on Trowsdale and Campbell, 1997, in Dominique Charron (ed.), *HLA Genetic Diversity of HLA Functional and Medical Implication*, Vol. 1, pp. 499–504.

Fig 4.2 HLA class I molecule. β₂-m, β₂-microglobulin.

associated α and β chains of approximately 34 and 28 kDa, respectively. The expressed α and β chains consist of two extracellular domains and a transmembrane and cytoplasmic domains. The α1/β1 and α2/β2 domains are encoded by exon 2 and exon 3 of the class II gene, respectively. The majority of the polymorphism is located in the β1 domain of the DR molecules and in the α1 and β1 domains of the DQ and DP molecules. Similarly to the class I molecules, these domains also form a peptide-binding groove. However, in the case of the class II molecules (DR), the groove is open at both sides and it can accommodate antigenic peptides of varying size, although most of them are approximately 13–25 amino acids long. A schematic representation of the HLA class II gene and molecule is shown in Figure 4.3.

The nonclassical HLA class I DMA, DMB, DOA and DOB genes have a similar structure to the classical class II genes, but show limited polymorphism.

Genetic organization and expression of HLA class II genes

There is one DRA gene of limited polymorphism and nine DRB genes, of which B1, B3, B4 and B5 are highly polymorphic and B2, B6 and B9 are pseudogenes. The main serologically defined DR specificities (DR1–DR18) are determined by the polymorphic DRB1* gene. The number of DRB genes expressed in each individual varies according to the DRB1 allele expressed (Figure 4.4). There are a few exceptions to this pattern of gene expression, e.g. a DRB5 gene has been found to be expressed with some DR1 alleles. Some nonexpressed or null DRB5 and DRB4 genes have also been identified. In contrast to the DRB genes, there are two DQA and three DQB genes, but only the DQA1 and DQB1 are expressed and both are polymorphic. Similarly, there are two DPA and two DPB genes, but only the DPA1 and DPB1 are expressed and both are polymorphic.

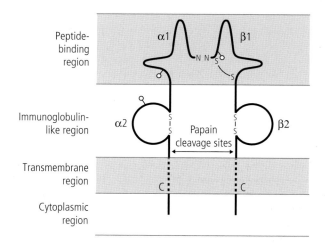

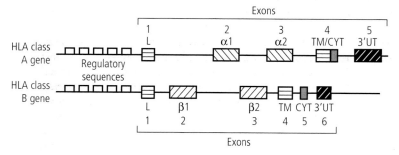

Fig 4.3 HLA class II molecule.

Specifications

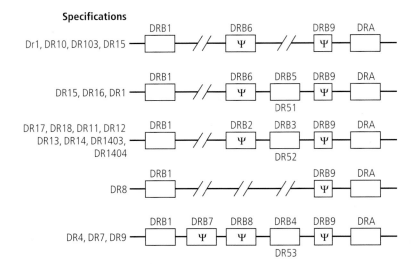

Fig 4.4 Expression of *HLA-DRB* genes.

Expression of HLA molecules

The classical HLA class I molecules (A, B, C) are expressed on the majority of tissues and blood cells, including T and B lymphocytes, granulocytes and platelets. Low levels of expression have been detected in endocrine tissue, skeletal muscle and cells of the central nervous system. HLA-E and -F are also expressed on most tissues tested, but HLA-G shows a more restricted tissue distribution and to date HLA-G products have only been found on extravillous cytotrophoblasts of the placenta and mononuclear phagocytes. MICA and MICB molecules are expressed on fibroblasts, endothelial, intestinal and tumour epithelial cells.

The HLA class II molecules are constitutively expressed on B lymphocytes, monocytes and dendritic cells, but can also be detected on activated T lymphocytes and activated granulocytes. It is not clear whether they are also present on activated platelets. HLA class II expression can be induced on a number of cells such as fibroblasts and endothelial cells as the result of activation and/or the effect of certain inflammatory cytokines, such as interferon (IFN)-γ, TNF and interleukin (IL)-10.

Both classical and nonclassical HLA molecules can also be found in soluble forms and it has been suggested that they may play a role in the induction of peripheral tolerance.

Genetics

HLA genes are codominantly expressed and are inherited in a Mendelian fashion. One of the main features of the HLA genes is their high degree of polymorphism and the strong linkage disequilibrium (LD) in which they segregate. LD is a phenomenon where the observed frequency of alleles of different loci segregating together is greater than the frequency expected by random association. Whereas some of the polymorphism and the patterns of LD are expressed with similar frequencies in all populations, others are unique to some population groups. For example, HLA-A2 is expressed at a relatively high frequency in most population groups studied so far, whereas B53 is found predominantly in Black people.

The genetic region containing all HLA genes on each chromosome is termed the haplotype. Some HLA haplotypes are also found across different ethnic groups, e.g. HLA-B44-DR7, whereas others are unique to a particular population, e.g. HLA-B42-DR18 in Black Africans. This characteristic is particularly relevant for the selection of HLA-compatible family donors for patients requiring solid organ or haemopoietic stem cell (HSC) transplantation.

Function of HLA molecules

The main function of HLA molecules is to present antigenic peptides to T cells and this requires a fine interaction between the HLA molecules, the antigenic peptide and the T-cell receptor. A number of costimulatory molecules (e.g. CD80 and CD86) and adhesion molecules such as ICAM-1 (CD54) and LFA-3 (CD58) also contribute to these interactions.

The HLA class I molecules are primarily, but not exclusively, involved in the presentation of endogenous antigenic peptides to CD8 cytotoxic T cells. Both the classical and nonclassical HLA class I molecules also interact with a new family of receptors present on natural killer (NK) cells [3]. Some of these receptors, which are polymorphic and differentially expressed, have an inhibitory role whereas others are activating. The killer-activating and killer-inhibitory receptors belong to two distinct families: the immunoglobulin superfamily called killer immunglobulin receptors (KIRs) and the C-type lectin superfamily CD94-NKG2. The interaction between the inhibitory receptors and the relevant HLA ligand results in the prevention of NK lysis of the target cell. Thus, NK cells from any given individual will be alloreactive towards cells lacking their corresponding inhibitory KIR ligands, e.g. tumour or allogeneic cells. In contrast, NK cells will be tolerant to cells from individuals who express the corresponding KIR ligands. The MICA and MICB molecules, which are induced by stress, are polymorphic but do not have a peptide binding groove and nor do they bind β2m. These molecules also interact with the NK activatory receptor NKG2D and with $\gamma\delta$T cells.

The *LMP2* and *LMP7* genes are thought to improve the capacity of the proteosomes to generate peptides of the appropriate size and specificity to associate with the class I molecules whereas *TAP1* and *TAP2* are primarily involved in the transport of the proteosome-generated peptides to the endoplasmic reticulum, where they associate with the class I molecules.

Classical HLA class II molecules are mostly involved in the presentation of exogenous antigenic peptides to CD4 helper T cells. Once activated, these CD4 cells can initiate and regulate a variety of processes leading to the maturation and differentiation of cellular (CD8 cytotoxic T cells) and humoral effectors (such as antibody production by plasma cells). Activated effectors also secrete proinflammatory cytokines (IL-2, IFN-γ, TNF-α) and regulatory cytokines (IL-4, IL-10 and transforming growth factor-β).

The main function of HLA-DM molecules is to facilitate the release of the class II-associated invariant chain (Ii) peptide from the peptide-binding groove of the HLA-DR molecules so that the groove can be loaded with the relevant antigenic peptide and this function is modulated by the DO molecules [4].

Identification of HLA gene polymorphism

The HLA polymorphisms were initially defined using serological and cellular techniques. With the development of gene cloning and DNA sequencing, it is now possible to perform a detailed analysis of these genes at the single nucleotide level. This analysis has shown the existence of certain locus-specific nucleotide sequences in both coding (exons) and noncoding (introns) regions of the genes and also the existence of regions of nucleotide sequences that are common to several alleles of the same and/or different loci. The DNA sequencing of a number of HLA alleles of various loci has also demonstrated that the majority of the variation is located in the α1 and α2 domain of the class I molecules and in the α1 and β1 domain of the class II molecules. These are called hypervariable regions.

Based on this information, a number of techniques have been developed to characterize these polymorphisms. Most of the described techniques make use of the polymerase chain reaction (PCR) to amplify the specific genes or region to be analysed. These techniques include PCR-SSP (PCR sequence-specific priming), PCR-SSOP (PCR sequence-specific oligonucleotide probing) and DNA sequencing-based typing (SBT).

The number of recognized serologically defined antigens and DNA-identified HLA alleles is shown in Table 4.1 and can be accessed from http://hla.alleles .org/nomenclature/stats.html.

Due to the complexity of the HLA polymorphism and to the vast number of new alleles defined each year, a revised nomenclature has now been implemented [5, 6] (see Figure 4.5). In this revised version optional suffixes may be added to an allele to indicate its expression status. Alleles that have been shown not to be expressed, 'Null' alleles, have been given the suffix 'N'. An allele with 'Low' cell surface expression when compared with normal levels is

Table 4.1 Number of recognized HLA antigens/alleles. Adapted from Marsh *et al.* [5]. Taken from http://hla.alleles.org/nomenclature/stats.html. Accession date 07/12/11.

Gene	Alleles	Protein	Antigens[†]
HLA class I			
HLA-A	1729	1264	24
HLA-B	2329	1766	50
HLA-C	1291	938	9
HLA-E	10	3	
HLA-F	22	4	
HLA-G	47	15	
HLA class II			
HLA-DRB1	1051	729	17
HLA-DRA1	7	2	—
HLA-DRB3	57	46	1
HLA-DRB4	15	8	1
HLA-DRB5	19	16	1
HLA-DQB1	160	111	6
HLA-DQA1	45	29	—
HLA-DPB1	150	130	6*
HLA-DPA1	33	16	—

*Cellularly defined.
[†]Serologically defined.

indicated by the suffix 'L'. Suffix 'S' is used to describe an allele specifying a protein that is expressed as a soluble 'secreted' molecule but is not present on the cell surface. A 'C' suffix describes an allele product that is present in the 'Cytoplasm' but not on the cell surface. An 'A' suffix indicates an 'Aberrant' expression and a 'Q' suffix is used when the expression of an allele is 'Questionable'.

PCR sequence-specific priming

This technique involves the use of primers designed to anneal with DNA sequences unique to each allele and locus. The detection of the PCR-amplified product is then carried out by running the amplified product on an agarose gel. This technique allows the rapid identification of the HLA alleles in individual samples since the readout of this method is the presence or absence of the product for which specific primers were used. However, although this is a very rapid procedure, many PCR reactions have to be set up per sample in order to detect most of the defined alleles,

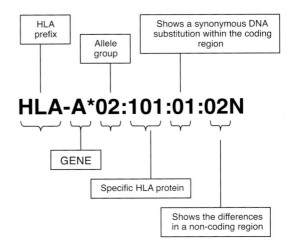

A synonymous substitution (also called a *silent* substitution) is the evolutionary substitution of one base for another in an exon of a gene coding for a protein, such that the produced amino acid sequence is not modified. Synonymous substitutions and mutations affecting noncoding DNA are collectively known as silent mutations. A nonsynonymous substitution results in a change in amino acid that may be arbitrarily further classified as conservative (change to an amino acid with similar physiochemical properties), semi-conservative (e.g. negative to positively charged amino acid) or radical (vastly different amino acid).

Fig 4.5 An example for a current HLA nomenclature. Taken from Nunes E, Heslop H, Fernandez-Vina M *et al.* Definitions of histocompatibility typing term. *Blood* 2011; 118: e180–e183 [6].

e.g. at least 24 reactions for low resolution DR typing. Furthermore, for PCR-SSP typing the DNA sequence of the alleles must be known since novel unknown sequences may not always be detected.

PCR sequence-specific oligonucleotide probing

In this technique, the gene of interest is amplified using primers designed to anneal with DNA sequences common to all alleles of the loci of interest. The amplified PCR product is then immobilized on to support (e.g. nylon) membranes and the specificity of the products analysed by reacting the membranes with labelled allele-specific oligonucleotides. By scoring the probes that bind to specific regions, it is possible to assign the HLA type.

A modification of this technique, called reverse blot, involves the binding of the PCR-amplified product to labelled probes immobilized on membranes (strips) or plates. More recently, Luminex analysers are used to read the binding of the DNA to beads coated with an oligonucleotide probe. Reverse SSOP is useful when large numbers of samples need to be HLA-typed, e.g. bone marrow or cord blood donors.

DNA sequencing-based typing

DNA sequencing involves the denaturation of the DNA to be analysed to provide a single-strand template. Sequencing primers, exon- or locus-specific, are then added and the DNA extension is performed by the addition of Taq polymerase in the presence of excess nucleotides. The sequencing mixture is divided into four tubes, each of which contains specific dideoxyribonucleoside triphosphate (ddATP). When these are incorporated into the DNA synthesis, elongation is interrupted with chain-terminating inhibitors. In each reaction, there is random incorporation of the chain terminators and therefore products of all sizes are generated. The sequencing products are detected by labelling the nucleotide chain inhibitors with radioisotopes and, more recently, with fluorescent dyes. The products of the four reactions are then analysed by electrophoresis in parallel lanes of a polyacrylamide–urea gel and the sequence is read by combining the results of each lane using an automated DNA sequencer. In HLA SBT, some ambiguous results can be obtained with heterozygous samples and these may need to be retested by using PCR-SSP or reverse PCR-SSOP. SBT permits high resolution HLA typing, which is known to be important in the selection of HLA-matched HSC unrelated donors.

A major advantage of all DNA-based techniques is that no viable cells are required to perform HLA class I and II typing. Furthermore, since all the probes and primers are synthesized to order, there is a consistency of reagents used, allowing the comparison of HLA types from different laboratories. However, although serological typing is being rapidly replaced by DNA-based typing techniques, serological reagents may still be required for antigen expression studies.

The advantages and disadvantages of the various techniques described above are given in Table 4.2.

Table 4.2 Advantages and disadvantages of DNA-based techniques.

Technique	Advantages	Disadvantages
Sequence-specific oligonucleotide probing (SSOP)	Needs only one pair of genetic primers; fewer reactions to set up	Different temperatures required for each probe
	Larger number of samples can be processed simultaneously	Probes can cross-react with different alleles
	Requires small amount of DNA cheap	Large numbers of probes required to identify specificity
		Difficult to interpret pattern of reactions
Sequence-specific priming (SSP)	Provides rapid typing with higher resolution than SSOP	Too many sets of primers are needed to fulfil HLA type
	All PCR amplifications are carried out at same time, temperature and conditions	Requires a two-stage amplification to provide HR typing
	Fast and simple to read and interpret	
Sequencing-based typing (SBT)	Provides the highest level of resolution	Not easy to perform
	Able to identify new alleles	Requires expensive reagents and equipments
	Does not require previous sequence data to identify new allele	
Difficult to interpret		Requires DNA sequence data to compare results
		Slower than rSSOP and SSP
		Limited throughput analyses
		High cost

More recently a new approach to perform high resolution and high throughput HLA typing involving massive parallel clonal sequencing strategies and next-generation sequencing (NGS) platforms has been described. These NGSs are able to produce a large volume of HR HLA data.

Formation of HLA antibodies

HLA-specific antibodies are induced by pregnancy, transplantation, blood transfusions and planned immunizations. The affinity, avidity and class of the antibodies produced depend on various factors, including the route of immunization, the persistence and type of immunological challenge and the immune status of the host. Cytotoxic HLA antibodies can be identified in approximately 20% of human pregnancies. The antibodies produced are normally multispecific, high titre, high affinity and of the IgG class. Although these HLA IgG antibodies can cross the placenta, they are not harmful to the fetus. Antibodies produced following transplantation are mostly IgG, although rarely HLA IgM antibodies have been identified. In contrast, the majority of HLA antibodies found in multitransfused patients are multispecific IgM and IgG and are mostly directed at public epitopes. The introduction of leucocyte-reduced blood components (see Chapter 21) may lead to a reduction in alloimmunization in naive recipients, but it may not be very effective in preventing alloimmunization in already sensitized recipients, i.e. women who have become immunized as a result of pregnancy.

The deliberate immunization of healthy individuals to produce HLA-specific reagents is nowadays difficult to justify ethically. However, planned HLA immunization is still carried out in some countries to treat women with a history of recurrent miscarriages. These women are immunized with white cells from their partners or a third party to attempt to induce an immunomodulatory response that results in the maintenance of the pregnancy.

Detection of HLA antibodies

HLA antibodies are responsible for some of the serious immunological reactions to the transfusion of blood and blood components and play a pivotal role in the rejection of solid organ transplants.

A number of techniques to detect HLA antibodies have been developed. These include the complement-dependent lymphocytotoxicity (LCT) test, enzyme-linked immunosorbent assay (ELISA) and flow cytometry and, more recently, a Luminex-based technique [7, 8].

Complement-dependent cytotoxicity test

The complement-dependent cytotoxicity (CDC) test, developed by Terasaki and McClelland (1964) [9], involves mixing equal volumes of serum and cells to allow the binding of the specific antibody to the target cell followed by the addition of rabbit complement. Complement-fixing antibodies reacting with the HLA antigen present on the cell surface lead to the activation of complement via the classical pathway and result in the disruption of the cell membrane. The lysed cells are then detected by adding ethidium bromide (EB) and the live cells are identified by adding acridine orange (AO) at the end of the incubation period. Live cells stained with AO when exposed to ultraviolet (UV) light appear green, whereas lysed cells allow the entry of EB, which binds to DNA, and they appear red under UV light. The reactions are scored by estimation of the percentage of dead cells in each well after establishing baseline values in the negative and positive as follows: 0–10% (one background cell death, negative), 11–20% (two doubtful negative), 21–50% (four weak positive), 51–80% (six positive) and 81–100% (eight strong positive).

The CDC assay, however, does not discriminate between HLA and non-HLA cytotoxic lymphocyte-reactive antibodies including autoantibodies. However, the majority of lymphocytotoxic autoantibodies are IgM and can be identified by screening the serum with and without dithiothreitol (DTT). The addition of DTT to the serum results in the breakdown of the intersubunit disulfide bonds in the IgM molecule, leading to the loss of cytotoxicity due to IgM. Prolonged exposure or excess DTT can lead to the breakdown of intramolecular disulfide bonds in the IgG molecules and also inactivate complement, but this can be inhibited by the addition of cystine.

The presence of lymphocytotoxic autoreactive antibodies in itself is not thought to be of clinical significance in solid organ transplant recipients or in patients immunologically refractory to random donor platelet transfusions.

Since the CDC test only detects cytotoxic HLA-specific antibodies, other techniques such as the ELISA or flow cytometry are needed to detect noncytotoxic HLA-specific antibodies.

Enzyme-linked immunosorbent assay

ELISA-based methods have often been the technique of choice for antibody detection, particularly where there has been a requirement for testing large numbers of samples. In this technique, a pool of purified HLA antigens is immobilized on a microwell plate, directly or via an antibody directed against a non-polymorphic region of the HLA antigen or against the β2-microglobulin. Antibodies directed against the nonpolymorphic region of the HLA class I molecule, i.e. the α3 domain, are used to immobilize the specific HLA antigen to the microwell, ensuring that the more polymorphic α1 and α2 domains are available for antibody binding. HLA-specific antibodies bound to the immobilized antigens are then detected with an enzyme-linked secondary antibody which, upon addition of specific substrate, catalyses a colour change reaction that is detected in an ELISA reader.

In order to detect HLA specificity, each specific HLA antigen is isolated from an individual cell or cell line. Large panels of cells are cell lines used to purify these antigens in order to cover all the major HLA specificities at least once. A number of commercial kits are now available to screen for HLA antibodies and to define their specificities.

One of the main advantages of this ELISA technique is that they detect HLA-specific antibodies since it relies on the binding of the antibodies to wells coated with pools of solubilized or purified HLA antigens.

Flow cytometry

In this technique, cells and serum are incubated to allow the binding of the antibody to the target antigen. The bound antibody is then detected by using an antibody against human immunoglobulin labelled with a fluorescent marker such as fluorescein isothiocyanate or R-phycoerythrin. At the end of the incubation period, the cells are passed through the laser beam of the flow cytometer to identify the different cell populations based on their morphology/granularity and on the fluorescence. Normally, test sera with median fluorescence values greater than the mean + 3SD of the negative controls are considered positive, but each laboratory needs to establish its own positive and negative cut-off point values. By using a second antibody against cell-specific markers such as CD3 or CD19, it is possible to identify T- or B-cell reactivity.

The main advantages of flow cytometric techniques are the increased sensitivity when compared with LCT- and ELISA-based techniques and the detection of non-complement-fixing antibodies, allowing early detection of sensitization. However, one of the disadvantages is that it also detects non-HLA lymphocyte-reactive antibodies that are of unclear clinical relevance.

The use of flow cytometric techniques was initially investigated as an alternative cross-match technique and was shown to be more sensitive than previously described techniques. The increased sensitivity may be due to the fact that it detects both cytotoxic and noncytotoxic antibodies, some of which may be HLA specific.

Luminex

This technique uses fluorochrome-dyed polystyrene beads coated with specific HLA antigens. The precise ratio of these fluorochromes creates 100 distinctly coloured beads, each of which is coated with a different antigen. The beads are then incubated with the patient's serum and the reaction is developed using a PE-conjugated antihuman IgG (Fc-specific) antibody. The positive or negative reactions are then read using a Luminex analyser, which can distinguish between up to 100 different beads sets in a single tube. Luminex is the most sensitive technique currently available for the detection of HLA antibodies. Most recently, this technology has been further improved by the introduction of beads coated with single antigens, which improve the identification of antibody specificities that were not previously detected. In this technique, the beads can be coated with either HLA antigens for antibody screening or HLA oligonucleotide probes for HLA typing.

The CDC test and flow cytometry are the two main techniques used to perform antibody cross-matching between the patient's serum and the potential donor's cells in the solid organ transplant setting.

Clinical relevance of HLA antigens and antibodies

Although the main role of the HLA molecules is to present antigenic peptides to T cells, HLA molecules can themselves be recognized as foreign by the host T cells by a mechanism known as allorecognition. Two pathways of allorecognition have been identified, direct and indirect.

In the direct pathway, the host's T cells recognize HLA molecules (primarily class II) expressed on donor tissues, e.g. tissue dendritic cells and endothelial cells. Indirect allorecognition involves the recognition by the host T cells of donor-derived HLA class I and II antigenic peptides presented by the host's own antigen-presenting cells. Because of this mechanism, HLA antigen incompatibility is one of the main barriers to success of solid organ or HSC transplantation and also results in the strong alloimmunization seen in patients following transplantation or blood transfusion [10].

Solid organ transplantation

Matching for HLA-A, -B and -DR antigens is an important factor influencing the outcome of solid organ transplantation and particularly renal transplants. The application of the PCR-based techniques has allowed the identification of molecular differences between otherwise serologically identical HLA types of donor and recipient pairs, particularly in the HLA-DRβ1 chain. Correlation of these results with graft survival has shown a higher kidney graft survival rate when recipients and donors are HLA-DR identical by serological and molecular techniques than when they were HLA-DR identical by serological but not molecular methods (87% versus 69%) [11].

The presence of circulating HLA-specific antibodies directed against donor antigens in renal and cardiac recipients has been associated with hyperacute rejection of the graft. It is therefore important that these antibodies are detected and identified as soon as the patient is registered on the transplant waiting list to ensure that incompatible donors are not considered for transplantation [12]. Antibodies against the MICA

and HLA DP antigens also seem to influence graft outcome, suggesting the possible need to screen for these antibodies in patients awaiting transplantation.

Furthermore, the appearance of donor-specific antibodies after transplantation has been associated with graft rejection, indicating the importance of post-transplant antibody monitoring for some groups of patients.

HLA and haemopoietic stem cell transplantation

HLA-DR incompatibility is one of the main factors associated with the development of acute graft-versus-host disease (aGVHD) but mismatches at the HLA-A and -B alleles, and to lesser extent HLA-C alleles, are also independent risk factors, particularly when using matched unrelated donors. Although HSC transplantation between HLA-identical siblings ensures matching for all HLA-A, -B, -C, -DR and -DQ genes, acute GVHD still develops in about 20–30% of these patients. This is probably due to the effect of untested HLA antigens, such as DP, or minor histocompatibility antigens in the activation of donor T cells. However, patients receiving grafts from HLA-matched unrelated donors have a higher risk of developing GVHD than those transplanted using an HLA-identical sibling [13].

The use of DNA-based methods has provided a unique opportunity to improve the HLA matching of patients and unrelated donors and to reduce the development of GVHD. However, it has been shown that the increased GVHD seen as a result of HLA mismatch is also associated with lower relapse rates, probably due to a graft-versus-leukaemia (GVL) response associated with the graft-versus-host response. On the other hand, the use of T-cell-depleted marrow, which has successfully decreased the incidence of GVHD, has resulted in an increased incidence of leukaemia relapse. Thus, it appears that mature T cells in the marrow, which may be responsible for GVHD, may also be involved in the elimination of residual leukaemic cells. Conversely, the rate of graft rejection is significantly higher in recipients of an HLA-mismatched transplant than in those receiving a transplant from an HLA-identical sibling (12.3 versus 2.0%) [13, 14].

HSC transplantation using cord blood from HLA-matched and HLA-mismatched donors has now been associated with a reduced risk and severity of GVHD and with no increase in relapse rates. It is possible that the immaturity of the immunological effectors present in cord blood may contribute to the reduced GVHD without impairment of the GVL effect.

Graft failure, which is thought to be mediated by residual recipient T and/or NK cells reacting with major or minor histocompatibility antigens present in the donor marrow cells, has been shown to be associated also with antibodies reacting with donor's HLA antigens. Thus, rejection is particularly high in HLA-alloimmunized patients. However, in spite of these reports, HLA antibodies are more relevant in the post-transplant period, where highly immunized patients can develop immunological refractoriness to random platelet transfusions due to the presence of HLA antibodies. These patients require transfusions of HLA-matched platelets (see Chapter 27).

Blood transfusion

White cells and platelets present in transfused products express antigens that, if not identical to those present in the recipient, are able to activate T cells and lead to the development of antibodies and/or effector cells responsible for some of the serious complications of blood transfusion. Also, antibodies (and T cells) present in the transfused product may react directly with the relevant antigens in the recipient and lead to the development of a transfusion reaction. Amongst the transfusion reactions due to the presence of antibodies in the recipient are a febrile nonhaemolytic transfusion reaction (FNHTR) and immunological refractoriness to random platelet transfusions [15, 16].

Although the occurrence of FNHTR has been commonly associated with the presence of HLA (and to a lesser extent HPA (human platelet antigen) or HNA (human neutrophil antigen)) antibodies in the recipient reacting with white blood cells or platelets present in the transfused product, it has recently been described that FNHTR may also be triggered by the direct action of cytokines such as IL-1β, TNF-α, IL-6 and/or by chemokines such as IL-8, which are found in transfused products.

Immunological refractoriness to random platelet transfusions is primarily due to the presence of HLA and, to a lesser extent, HPA and high titre ABO alloantibodies in the patient and reaction with the transfused incompatible platelets leading to the lack of

platelet increments after the transfusion. Following the introduction of universal leucodepletion, the proportion of multitransfused patients with HLA antibodies seems to have decreased to approximately 10–20% and these patients are, in general, previously sensitized transplanted or transfused recipients and multiparous women.

The development of transfusion-related acute lung injury (TRALI) has been associated with the transfusion of blood components containing HLA and HNA antibodies able to recognize the relevant antigen(s) on recipient white cells and triggering an immunological reaction leading to the accumulation of neutrophils in the lungs and oedema. TRALI has sometimes been associated with the presence of HLA or HNA antibodies in recipients reacting with transfused leucocytes and/or to interdonor antigen–antibody reactions in pooled platelets.

Transfusion-associated (TA) GVHD, which is a rare but often severe and fatal transfusion reaction, is the result of immunocompetent HLA-matched T lymphocytes present in blood or blood components reacting with HLA and/or minor histocompatibility antigens present on the recipient cells. TA-GVHD occurs primarily in immunosuppressed individuals, although it can also occur in immunocompetent recipients. The diagnosis of TA-GVHD depends on finding evidence of donor-derived cells, chromosomes or DNA in the blood and/or affected tissues of the recipient.

HLA and disease

HLA genes are known to be associated with a number of autoimmune and infectious diseases [17, 18] and different mechanisms to explain these associations have been postulated, including linkage disequilibrium with the relevant disease susceptibility gene, the preferential presentation of the pathogenic peptide by certain HLA molecules and molecular mimicry between certain pathogenic peptides and host-derived peptides. A number of diseases associated with both HLA class I and II have been described in Table 4.3. More recently genome-wide association studies (GWAS) [19] using over a thousand single nucleotide polymorphisms (SNPs) located in the MHC have identified a number of these SNP in strong linkage disequilibrium with some of the HLA associated diseases such as RA and SLE.

Table 4.3 HLA-associated diseases.

HLA class I genes
  Birdshot chorioretinopathy: *HLA-A29*
  Behçet's disease: *HLA-B51*
  Ankylosing spondylitis: *HLA-B27*
  Psoriasis: *HLA-Cw6*
  Malaria: *HLA-B53*
HLA class II genes
  Rheumatoid arthritis
    *HLA-DRB1*0401*
    *HLA-DRB1*0404*
    *HLA-DRB1*0405*
    *HLA-DRB1*0408*
    *HLA-DRB1*0101/0102*
    *HLA-DRB1*1402*
    *HLA-DRB1*1001*
  Narcolepsy: *HLA-DQB1*0602/DQA1*0102*
  Coeliac disease: *HLA-DQB1*0201/DQA1*0501*
  Neonatal allo-immune thrombocytopenia:
    *HLA-DRB3*0101*
  Malaria: *HLA-DRB1*1302/DQB1*0501*
  Insulin-dependent diabetes mellitus:
    *HLA-DQB1*0302/DQA1*0301*
HLA-linked diseases
  Haemochromatosis: (*HLA-A3*) HFE gene *C282Y, H63D*
    and *S65C*
  21-OH deficiency: (*HLA-B47*) 21-OH gene
  Abacavir hypersensititvy: *B*5701*

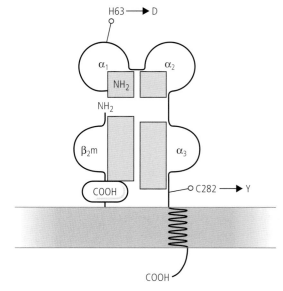

Fig 4.6 HFE molecule. β_2-m, β_2-microglobulin.

Hereditary haemochromatosis

Hereditary haemochromatosis (HH) is a clinical condition of iron overload caused by an inherited disorder in the genes involved in the metabolism of iron. HH is a common genetic disorder in Northern Europe, where between 1 in 200 and 1 in 400 individuals suffer from the disease, with an estimated carrier frequency of between 1 in 8 and 1 in 10. Clinical manifestations of HH include cirrhosis of the liver, diabetes and cardiomyopathy. Detection of asymptomatic iron overload is important since removal of excess iron by phlebotomy can prevent organ damage [20, 21].

HH was originally described associated to HLA-A3, although this was not very specific since the majority of HLA-A3-positive individuals do not have HH. It was later found that mutations in the HFE gene located 3 Mb telomeric from the HLA-F gene was partly responsible for this condition. A number of mutations have now been identified and clinical data indicate that at least three of these mutations (C282Y, H63D and S65C) may predispose to and affect the clinical outcome of this condition. Over 90% of HH patients in the UK are homozygous for the mutation that replaces a cysteine (C) with a tyrosine (Y) at codon 282 in the *HFE* gene. The second and third mutations (H63D and S65C) are thought to be less important, although it may have an additive effect if inherited with the first mutation (Figure 4.6). Recent studies on blood donors have shown that approximately 1 in 280 donors is homozygous for the mutations.

A DNA-based technique to detect these three mutations simultaneously has now been developed and provides a simple, rapid and unambiguous definition of these mutations.

Neonatal alloimmune thrombocytopenia

Neonatal alloimmune thrombocytopenia (NAIT) is a serious condition in the newborn and is due to feto-maternal incompatibility for HPAs (see also Chapters 5 and 26). More than 80% of cases occur in women who are homozygous for the *HPA-1b* allele. Although the majority of cases are associated with the presence of HPA-1a antibodies, about 15% of cases are due to anti-HPA-5b. The production of HPA-1a antibodies is strongly associated with the *HLA-DRB3*0101* allele. However, only approximately 35% of HPA-1a-negative, DRB3*0101-positive women develop antibodies upon exposure to the antigen, suggesting that other genes or factors may be involved in the development of alloimmunization against HPA-1a.

Other diseases

Diseases in which the molecular mimicry mechanism has been postulated include ankylosing spondylitis and *Klebsiella* infection. However, the precise pathogenic mechanisms involved remain unknown. More recently, it has been shown that HLA genes are also involved in the response to certain drugs, such as the association of HLAB-57 and abacavir, a drug used in the treatment of HIV [22].

Key points

1 HLA molecules are crucial in the induction and regulation of immune responses and in the outcome of transplantation using allogeneic-related and -unrelated donors and are also responsible for some of the serious immunological complications of blood transfusion.
2 The main feature of HLA genes is their high degree of polymorphism and linkage disequilibrium and, depending on their molecular structure, expression and function, they are classified as classical or nonclassical.
3 The detection of HLA polymorphisms is currently performed using DNA-based techniques at various degrees of resolution depending on the clinical needs and relevance.
4 The techniques currently used to screen and define the specificity of HLA antibodies allow the discrimination of HLA and non-HLA cytotoxic and noncytotoxic antibodies.
5 HLA antibodies produced following transfusion, transplantation or pregnancy are responsible for some of the most serious complications of blood transfusion.
6 HLA matching and cold ischaemia time are the two most important factors influencing the outcome of renal transplantation.

7 In the HSC transplantation setting, HLA matching for HLA class I and II genes is essential to minimize the development of a GVHD.
8 HLA genes are involved in the pathogenesis of a variety of diseases either directly through the presentation of pathogenic peptides or indirectly through their linkage disequilibrium with the relevant disease susceptibility gene(s).

References

1 Campbell RD. The human major histocompatibility complex: a 4000-kb segment of the human genome replete with genes. In: KE Davies & SM Tilghman (eds), *Genome Analysis*, Vol. 5: *Regional Physical Mapping*. New York: Cold Spring Harbor Laboratory Press; 1993, pp. 1–33.
2 Horton R, Wilming L, Rand V *et al*. Gene map of the extended human MHC. *Nat Rev* 2004; 5: 889–899.
3 Parham P & McQueen KL. Alloreactive killer cells: hindrance and help for haematopoietic transplants. *Nat Rev Immunol* 2003; 3: 108–121.
4 Traherne JA. Human MHC architecture and evolution: implications for disease association studies. *J Immunogenet* 2008; 35: 179–192.
5 Marsh SG, Albert ED, Bodmer WF *et al*. Nomenclature for factors of the HLA system. *Tissue Antigens* 2010; 75: 291–455.
6 Nunes E, Heslop H, Fernandez-Vina M *et al*. Definitions of histocompatibility typing term. *Blood* 2011; 118: e180–e183.
7 Brown C & Navarrete C. HLA antibody screening by LCT, LIFT and ELISA. In: J Bidwell & C. Navarrete (eds), *Histocompatibility Testing*. London: Imperial College Press; 2000, pp. 65–98.
8 Howell WM, Carter V & Clark B. The HLA system: immunobiology, HLA typing, antibody screening and crossmatching techniques. *J Clin Pathol* 2010, 63: 387–390.
9 Terasaki PL & McClelland JD. Microdroplet assay of human serum cytokines. *Nature* 2000; 204: 998–1000.
10 Choo SY. *Yonsei Med J*. 2007; 48(1): 11–23.
11 Opelz G & Döhler B. Effects of human leucocyte antigen compatibility of kidney graft survival: comparative analysis of two decades. *Transplantation* 2007; 84: 137–143.
12 Dyer PA & Claas FHJ. A future for HLA matching in clinical transplantation. *Eur J Immunogenet* 1997; 24: 17–28.
13 Madrigal JA, Arguello R, Scott I & Avakian H. Molecular histocompatibility typing in unrelated donor bone marrow transplantation. *Blood Rev* 1997; 11: 105–117.

14 Petersdorf EW, Malkki M, Gooley TA *et al*. MHC haplotype matching for unrelated hematopoietic cell transplantation. *PloS Med* 2007; 4: 59–68.

15 Harrison J & Navarrete C. Selection of platelet donors and provision of HLA matched platelets. In: J Bidwell & C. Navarrete (eds), *Histocompatibility Testing*. London: Imperial College Press; 2000, pp. 379–390.

16 Brown CJ and Navarette CV. Clinical relevance of the HLA system in blood transfusion. *Vox Sanguinis* 2011; 101: 93–105.

17 Caillat-Zucman S. Molecular mechanisms of HLA association with autoimmune diseases. *Tissue Antigens* 2009; 73(1): 1–8.

18 Gambaro G, Anglani F & D'Angelo A. Association studies of genetic polymorphisms and complex disease. *The Lancet* 2000; 355: 308–311.

19 Metzker ML. Sequencing technologies – the next generation. *Nature Rev Genet* 2010; 11: 31–46.

20 Mura C, Raguenes O & Ferec C. HFE mutations analysis in 711 haemochromatosis probands: evidence for S65C implication in mild form of hemochromatosis. *Blood* 1999; 93: 2502–2505.

21 Bomford A. Genetics of haemochromatosis. *The Lancet* 2002; 360: 1673–1681.

22 Profaizer T & Eckels D. HLA alleles and drug hypersensitivity reactions. *Int J Immunogenet* 2011; 39: 99–105.

Further reading

Brown CJ & Navarette CV. Clinical relevance of the HLA system in blood transfusion. *Vox Sanguinis* 2011; 101: 93–105.

Contreras M & Navarrete C. Immunological complications of blood transfusion. In: M Contreras (ed.), *ABC of Transfusion*, 4th edn. Wiley-Blackwell; 2009, pp. 61–68.

Navarrete C. Human leucocyte antigens. In: MF Murphy & DH Pamphilon (eds), *Practical Transfusion Medicine*, 3rd edn. Wiley-Blackwell; 2009, pp. 30–43.

Ouwehand H & Navarrete C. The molecular basis of blood cell alloantigens. In: D Proven & J Gribben (eds), *Molecular Hematology*, 3rd edn. Blackwell Publishing; 2010, pp. 259–275.

Platelet and neutrophil antigens

David L. Allen[1], Geoffrey F. Lucas[2] & Michael F. Murphy[3]

[1]NHS Blood and Transplant, John Radcliffe Hospital, Oxford, UK
[2]NHS Blood and Transplant, Bristol, UK
[3]University of Oxford and NHS Blood and Transplant and Department of Haematology, John Radcliffe Hospital, Oxford, UK

Antigens on platelets and granulocytes

Antigens on human platelets and granulocytes can be categorized according to their biochemical nature into:

- carbohydrate antigens on glycolipids and glycoproteins:
    (a) A, B and O,
    (b) P and Le on platelets, I on granulocytes;
- protein antigens:
    (a) human leucocyte antigen (HLA) class I (A, B and C),
    (b) glycoprotein (GP)IIb/IIIa, GPIa/IIa, GPIb/IX/V, etc., on platelets,
    (c) FcγRIIIb (CD16), CD177, etc., on granulocytes;
- hapten-induced antigens:
    (a) quinine, quinidine,
    (b) some antibiotics, e.g. penicillins and cephalosporins,
    (c) heparin.

These antigens can be targeted by some or all of the following types of antibodies:

- autoantibodies,
- alloantibodies,
- isoantibodies and
- drug-dependent antibodies.

Many platelet and granulocyte antigens, e.g. ABO and HLA class I, are shared with other cells (Table 5.1); others, however, are restricted to single lineages. This chapter is divided into two sections: the first focuses on proteins expressed predominantly on platelets, and in particular the human platelet antigens (HPAs), whilst the second section focuses on the equivalent proteins and alloantigens expressed predominantly on neutrophils (human neutrophil antigens, HNAs).

Human platelet antigens

Twenty-one polymorphisms have been described (Table 5.2); most were first discovered during investigation of cases of neonatal alloimmune thrombocytopenia (NAIT). The majority of these antigens are located on the GPIIIa subunit of the GPIIb/IIIa integrin (CD41/CD61), which is present at high density on the platelet membrane and seems to be particularly polymorphic and immunogenic. Others are located on the GPIIb subunit, on GPIa/IIa (CD49b), GPIb/IX/V and CD109.

These receptor complexes are critical to platelet function and are responsible for the stepwise process of platelet attachment to the damaged vessel wall. GPIb/IX/V is the receptor for the von Willebrand factor (vWF) and is implicated in the initial tethering of platelets to damaged endothelium. The GPIbα-bound vWF interacts with collagen, facilitating the interaction of collagen with its signalling (GPVI) and attachment receptors (GPIa/IIa). Outside-in signalling via GPVI leads to conformational changes in integrins

Practical Transfusion Medicine, Fourth Edition. Edited by Michael F. Murphy, Derwood H. Pamphilon and Nancy M. Heddle.
© 2013 John Wiley & Sons, Ltd. Published 2013 by John Wiley & Sons, Ltd.

Table 5.1 Antigen expression on peripheral blood cells.

Antigen	Erythrocytes	Platelets	Neutrophils	B-lymphocytes	T-lymphocytes	Monocytes
A, B, H	+++	++/(+)	–	–	–	–
I	+++	++	++	–	–	–
Rh*	+++	–	–	–	–	–
K	+++	–	–	–	–	–
HLA class I	–/(+)	+++	+++	+++	+++	+++
HLA class II	–	–	–/+ + +†	+++	–/+++†	+++
GPIIb/IIIa	–	+++	(+)‡	–	–	–
GPIa/IIa	–	+++	–	–	++	–
GPIb/IX/V	–	+++	–	–	–	–
CD109	–	(+)/++†	–	–	–/++†	(+)
FcγRIIIb (CD16b)	–	–	+++	–	–	–
CD177	–	–	+++§	–	–	–
CTL-2	–	+	+++	++ (B- and T-lymphocytes not separated)		?
CD11b/18	–	–	++	–	–	++¶
CD11a/18	–	–	++	++	++	++

+++, ++, + indicates level of antigen expression in decreasing order. (+) indicates weak expression, ? indicates not known.
*Nonglycosylated.
†On activated cells.
‡GPIIIa in association with an alternative α chain (α_v).
§Expressed on a subpopulation of neutrophils.
¶Also expressed on natural killer cells.

GPIIb/IIIa and GPIa/IIa from 'locked' to 'open' configurations, exposing the high affinity binding sites for collagen and fibrinogen, respectively. GPIIb/IIIa is the main platelet fibrinogen receptor and is critical to the final phase of platelet aggregation, but it also binds fibronectin, vitronectin and vWF. The function of CD109 has not been fully elucidated although recent studies suggest a role in regulation of transforming growth factor beta (TGF-β)-mediated signalling. Glanzmanns thrombasthenia and Bernard–Soulier syndrome are rare and severe, autosomal recessive, platelet bleeding disorders caused by deletions or mutations in the genes encoding GPIIb and GPIIIa, or GPIbα, GPIbβ and GPIX, respectively.

Inheritance and nomenclature

Most HPAs have been shown to be bi-allelic, with each allele being codominant, although recently the HPA-1, -5 and -7 systems have been shown to have third alleles. Historically, platelet-specific antigens were named using an abbreviation of the name of the propositus in which the alloantibody was first detected. Some systems were described simultaneously by different investigators and, confusingly, several names were assigned to the same polymorphism, e.g. Zw and Pl^A and Zav, Br and Hc. In 1990, an International Society of Blood Transfusion working group agreed a new nomenclature for platelet-specific alloantigens, the HPA nomenclature, and subsequently guidelines for naming of newly discovered platelet-specific alloantigens [1]. Each system is now numbered consecutively (HPA-1, -2, -3 and so on) (Table 5.2) according to its date of discovery, with the major allele in each system designated 'a' and the minor allele 'b'. Antigens are only included in a system if antibodies against the alloantigen encoded by both the major and minor alleles have been reported; if an antibody against only one system antigen has been reported, a 'w' (for workshop) is added after the antigen name, e.g. HPA-10bw.

Table 5.2 HPA systems.

HPA system	Antigen	Alternative names	Phenotype frequency* (%)	Glycoprotein	SNP	SNP rs number	Amino acid change
1	1a	Zw^a, Pl^{A1}	97.9	GPIIIa	T^{196}	rs5918	Leucine^{33}
	1b	Zw^b, Pl^{A2}	28.8		C^{196}		Proline^{33}
2	2a	Ko^b	>99.9	GPIbα	C^{524}	rs6065	Threonine^{145}
	2b	Ko^a, Sib^a	13.2		T^{524}		Methionine^{145}
3	3a	Bak^a, Lek^a	80.95	GPIIb	T^{2622}	rs5911	Isoleucine^{843}
	3b	Bak^b			G^{2622}		Serine^{843}
4	4a	Yuk^b, Pen^a	>99.9	GPIIIa	G^{526}	rs5917	Arginine^{143}
	4b	Yuk^a, Pen^b	<0.1		A^{526}		Glutamine^{143}
5	5a	Br^b, Zav^b	99.0	GPIa	G^{1648}	rs10471371	Glutamic acid^{505}
	5b	Br^a, Zav^a, Hc^a	19.7		A^{1648}		Lysine^{505}
6				GPIIIa	G^{1564}	rs13306487	Arginine^{489}
	6bw	Ca^a, Tu^a	0.7		A^{1564}		Glutamine^{489}
7				GPIIIa	C^{1267}	rs121918448	Proline^{407}
	7bw	Mo^a	0.2		G^{1267}		Alanine^{407}
8				GPIIIa	T^{2004}		Arginine^{636}
	8bw	Sr^a	<0.01		C^{2004}		Cysteine^{636}
9				GPIIb	G^{2603}		Valine^{837}
	9bw	Max^a	0.6		A^{2603}		Methionine^{837}
10				GPIIIa	G^{281}		Arginine^{62}
	10bw	La^a	<1.6		A^{281}		Glutamine^{62}
11				GPIIIa	G^{1996}		Arginine^{633}
	11bw	Gro^a	<0.25		A^{1996}		Histidine^{633}
12				GPIbβ	G^{141}		Glycine^{15}
	12bw	Iy^a	0.4		A^{141}		Glutamic acid^{15}
13				GPIa	C^{2531}		Threonine^{799}
	13bw	Sit^a	0.25		T^{2531}		Methionine^{799}
14				GPIIIa			
	14bw	Oe^a	<0.17	Δ AAG$^{1929-1931}$			Δ Lysine^{611}
15	15a	Gov^b	74	CD109	C^{2108}	rs10455097	Serine^{703}
	15b	Gov^a	81		A^{2108}		Tyrosine^{703}
16					C^{517}		Threonine^{140}
	16bw	Duv^a	<1	GPIIIa	T^{517}		Isoleucine^{140}
17					C^{622}		Threonine^{195}
	17bw	Va^a	<0.4	GPIIIa	T^{622}		Methionine^{195}
18					G^{2235}		Glutamine^{716}
	18bw	Cab^a	<1	GPIa	T^{2235}		Histidine^{716}
19					A^{487}	ss120032848	Lysine^{137}
	19bw	Sta	<1	GPIIIa	C^{487}		Glutamine^{137}
20					C^{1949}	ss120032852	Threonine^{619}
	20bw	Kno	<1	GPIIb	T^{1949}		Methionine^{619}
21					G^{1960}	ss120032849	Glutamic acid^{628}
	21bw	Nos	<1	GPIIIa	A^{1960}		Lysine^{628}

*Based on studies of Caucasians.

SNP, single nucleotide polymorphism; rs, the international SNP reference number in dbSNP database.

With the advent of techniques such as immunopre-cipitation of radioactive-labelled platelet membrane proteins, the monoclonal antibody-specific immobilization of platelet antigen (MAIPA) assay (Figure 5.1) and the polymerase chain reaction (PCR), the genetic and molecular basis of all HPAs has been elucidated (Figure 5.2 and Table 5.2). For all but one of the 21 HPAs, the difference between the two alleles is a single nucleotide polymorphism (SNP), which changes the amino acid in the corresponding protein (Figure 5.2). Twelve of the HPAs are grouped into six HPA systems (HPA-1 to -5 and HPA-15) and for all of these, except HPA-3 and HPA-15, the minor allele frequency is ≤ 0.2. Homozygosity for the minor allele is therefore relatively rare so providing compatible blood components for patients with antibodies against high frequency HPA antigens can be difficult. Some SNPs are population-specific, e.g. SNP rs5918 (HPA-1 system) is absent in populations of the Far East; conversely, SNP rs5917 (HPA-4) is not present in Caucasians but is present in Far Eastern populations. It is therefore important to take ethnicity into account when investigating clinical cases of suspected HPA alloimmunization.

Typing for HPAs

Until the early 1990s, HPA typing was performed by serological assays ('phenotyping'). This required the use of monospecific antisera, which were relatively uncommon as the majority of immunized individuals produced HLA class I antibodies in addition to HPA antibodies. The development of more advanced assays, e.g. the MAIPA assay (Figure 5.1) that were able to elucidate complex mixtures of antibodies against different GPs, permitted more extensive phenotyping, but some antisera were simply not available.

Many DNA-based typing techniques have been developed; these have largely replaced phenotyping in the majority of platelet immunology laboratories. One such assay is the polymerase chain reaction using sequence-specific primers (PCR-SSP). This is a fast and reliable technique and has become one of the cornerstone techniques in platelet immunology laboratories (see Figure 5.3). High throughput HPA SNP typing techniques with automated readout, such as Taqman assays, are now also in routine use and allow typing at reduced cost. Novel techniques for the simultaneous detection of numerous SNPs are emerging and these may become the routine method for donor typing in blood centres.

Genotyping of fetal DNA from amniocytes or from chorionic villus biopsy samples is of clinical value in cases of HPA alloimmunization in pregnancies where there is a history of severe NAIT and the father is heterozygous for the implicated HPA SNP. Noninvasive HPA genotyping assays based on the presence of trace amounts of fetal DNA in maternal plasma have been described and reduce the risk to the fetus from invasive sampling procedures.

Platelet isoantigens, autoantigens and hapten-induced antigens

GPIV is absent from the platelet membrane in 4% of African Blacks and 3–10% of Japanese. If these individuals are exposed to GPIV-positive blood through pregnancy or transfusion, they may produce GPIV isoantibodies. These antibodies may cause NAIT or platelet refractoriness and may be responsible for febrile nonhaemolytic transfusion reactions (FNHTRs). Similarly, formation of isoantibodies can complicate both the pregnancies and transfusion support of patients with Glanzmanns' thrombasthenia or Bernard–Soulier syndrome.

The GPs carrying the HPAs are the target of autoantibodies in autoimmune thrombocytopenia (AITP); these autoantibodies bind to the platelets of all individuals, regardless of their HPA type. Platelet autoimmunity is frequently associated with B-cell malignancies and during immune cell re-engraftment following haemopoietic stem cell transplantation. In both situations, the presence of autoantibodies may contribute to the refractoriness to donor platelets.

Some drugs too small to elicit an immune response in their own right may bind to platelet GPs *in vivo* and act as a hapten [2]. In some patients, the haptenized platelet GP can trigger the formation of antibodies that only bind to the GP in the presence of hapten; a classic example is quinine. Typically, quinine-dependent antibodies bind to GPIIb/IIIa and/or GPIb/IX/V although other GPs are sometimes the target. Many other drugs, including several antibiotics, have been associated with hapten-mediated thrombocytopenia. In haemato-oncology patients, who often receive a

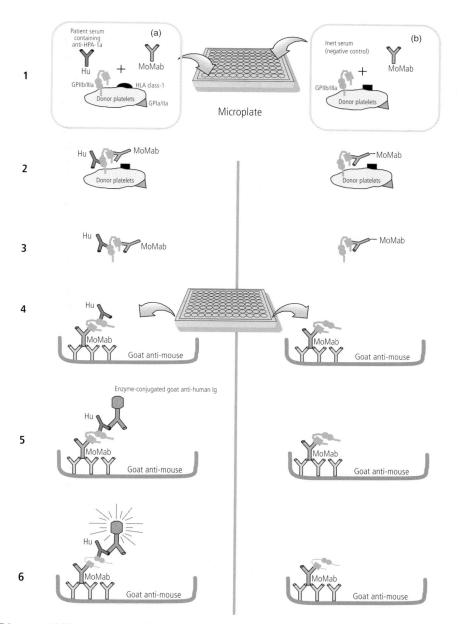

Fig 5.1 MAIPA assay. (1) Human serum and murine monoclonal antibody (MoMab) directed against glycoprotein being studied; e.g. GPIIb/IIIa are sequentially incubated with target platelets: in (a) the test serum contains anti-HPA-1a and in (b) no platelet antibodies are present. (2) After incubation a trimeric (a) or dimeric (b) complex is formed. Excess serum antibody and MoMab is removed by washing. (3) The platelet membrane is solubilized in nonionic detergent, releasing the complexes into the fluid phase; particulate matter is removed by centrifugation. (4) The lysates containing the glycoprotein/antibody complexes are added to wells of a microtitre plate previously coated with goat antimouse antibody. (5) Unbound lysate is removed by washing and enzyme-conjugated goat antihuman antibody is added. (6) Excess conjugate is removed by washing and substrate solution is added. Cleavage of substrate, i.e. a colour reaction, indicates binding of human antibody to target platelets.

49

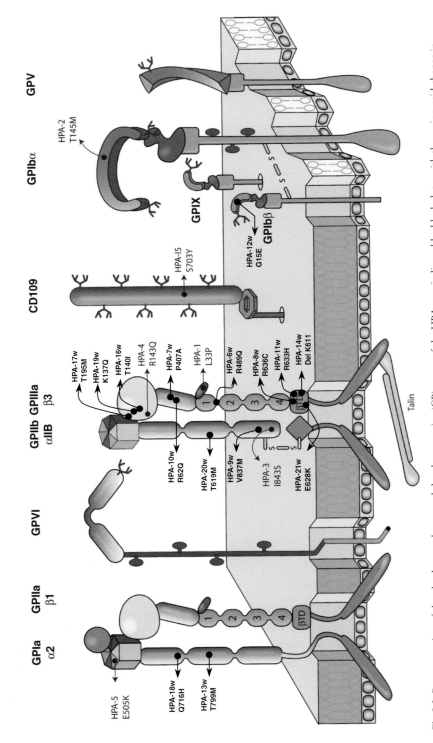

Fig 5.2 Representation of the platelet membrane and the glycoproteins (GP) on which the human platelet antigens (HPA) are localized. From left to right are depicted GPIa/IIa, GPIIb/IIIa, CD109 and GPIb/IX/V. The molecular basis of the HPAs are indicated by black dots, with the amino acid change in single-letter code and by residue number in the mature protein.

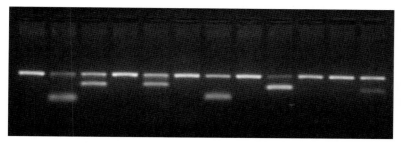

Fig 5.3 PCR-SSP determination of HPA-1, -2, -3, -4, -5 and -15 genotypes. The upper band present in all lanes is the 429-bp product of human growth hormone; lower bands are the products of sequence-specific primers. The results are read from left to right, i.e. lane 1 HPA-1a, lane 2 HPA-1b, etc. The HPA genotype in this case is 1b/1b, 2a/2a, 3a/3a, 4a/4a, 5a/5a, 15b/15b. Courtesy of Dr Paul Metcalfe (NIBSC).

spectrum of drugs, unravelling the causes of persistent thrombocytopenia or poor responses to platelet transfusions can be complex because of the many possible causes of thrombocytopenia. If the thrombocytopenia is hapten-mediated, withdrawal of the drug will result in rapid recovery of the platelet count.

Another form of drug-dependent thrombocytopenia may be observed in coronary artery disease patients treated with ReoPro (Abciximab). This function-blocking chimeric human–mouse F(Ab) fragment against GPIIb/IIIa causes precipitous thrombocytopenia in approximately 1% of patients due to the presence of pre-existing antibodies against ReoPro-induced neoepitopes.

The interaction of heparin with platelet factor 4 induces epitope formation that can cause antibody production and lead to heparin-induced thrombocytopenia (HIT) (see Chapter 30), but the reduction in platelet count is less profound than in classic examples of hapten-mediated immune thrombocytopenia. The risk of thrombotic complications is the main concern in patients with HIT who show a mild but significant reduction in their platelet count after heparin administration.

Detection of HPA alloantibodies

Over the last five decades, techniques for the detection of HPA antibodies have evolved significantly. Early assays, e.g. the platelet agglutination test, were both insensitive and nonspecific. The platelet immunofluorescence test (PIFT) improved sensitivity but is still classified as a nonspecific assay as it is unable to distinguish between HPA and HLA class I antibodies. Despite this limitation, the PIFT with a flow cytometric endpoint remains widely used since it is a whole cell assay capable of detecting a wide range of antibody specificities and is especially useful in detecting both autoantibodies and alloantibodies against HPA-2 and -3. The principles of the PIFT are shown in Plate 5.1 (see the plate section). Later assays that use purified or captured GPs, e.g. the MAIPA assay and solid-phase ELISA assays, were developed; these are both sensitive and specific and have become cornerstone techniques for the detection and identification of HPA antibodies. The widely used MAIPA assay captures specific GPs using monoclonal antibodies and can be used to analyse complex mixtures of platelet antibodies in patient sera [3]. The principle of this assay is shown in Figure 5.1. The MAIPA assay requires considerable operator expertise in order to ensure maximum sensitivity and specificity and selection of appropriate screening cells is critical. The use of platelets heterozygous for the relevant HPA or from donors who have a low expression of particular antigens, e.g. HPA-15, may result in the failure to detect clinically significant alloantibodies. Furthermore, recent evidence suggests that integrin conformation is an important factor in assay sensitivity. A disadvantage of assays that use purified GPs, rather than captured GPs as in the MAIPA assay, is that not all clinically important GPs are available, e.g. CD109. It can thus be seen that the detection and characterization of platelet antibodies can be problematic. More recently the use of biotinylated recombinant GPIIIa proteins coupled to microbeads suitable for use in high throughput assays has been described, with the potential to multiplex and streamline laboratory investigations of platelet alloimmunization.

Clinical significance of HPA alloantibodies

HPA alloantibodies are responsible for the following clinical conditions:
• NAIT: this condition is described in detail below (but also see Chapter 32);
• refractoriness to platelet transfusions (described in detail in Chapter 28); and
• posttransfusion purpura (PTP) (described in detail in Chapter 12).

Neonatal alloimmune thrombocytopenia

History

The first case of NAIT was described by van Loghem in 1959. The existence of the platelet equivalent of haemolytic disease of the fetus and newborn (HDFN) had long been suspected, but laboratory confirmation was delayed because the detection of platelet antibodies was extremely technically demanding.

NAIT is now a well-recognized clinical entity with an estimated incidence of severe thrombocytopenia due to maternal HPA antibodies of 1 per 1000–1200 live births. Unlike HDFN, about 30% of cases of NAIT occur in first pregnancies.

Definition and pathophysiology

NAIT is due to maternal HPA alloimmunization caused by feto-maternal incompatibility for a fetal HPA inherited from the father and which is absent in the mother. Maternal IgG alloantibodies against the fetal HPA cross the placenta and bind to fetal platelets and, depending on a number of factors, may reduce platelet survival. Severe thrombocytopenia in the term neonate, accompanied by haemorrhage, is generally caused by HPA-1a antibodies if the mother is Caucasian or Black African. Antibodies against HPA-2 and HPA-4 antigens are generally implicated in cases of Far Eastern ethnicity. In the latter and in Black Africans, GPIV deficiency should also be considered.

Anti-HPA-5b tends to cause much less severe NAIT than anti-HPA-1a.

NAIT due to alloantibodies against other HPAs is infrequent and HLA class I antibodies, present in 15–25% of multiparous women, are not thought to cause NAIT. Destruction of IgG-coated fetal platelets takes place predominantly in the spleen through interaction with mononuclear cells bearing $Fc\gamma$ receptors for the constant domain of IgG.

HPA-1a is known to be expressed on fetal platelets from 16 weeks' gestation and placental transfer of IgG antibodies can occur from 14 weeks, so thrombocytopenia can occur early in pregnancy and ICH has been reported as early as 16 weeks' gestation.

Incidence

Prospective screening of pregnant Caucasian women has shown that about 1 in 1200 neonates has severe thrombocytopenia ($<50 \times 10^9$/L) because of alloimmunization against HPA-1a. However, the authors' experience and other studies, where prospective screening was not carried out, indicate that the number of samples referred for investigation of suspected NAIT is considerably less, which suggests that many cases are undiagnosed [4]. HPA-5b antibodies are often found in pregnant women, but they cause clinically significant platelet destruction much less frequently than anti-HPA-1a, possibly due to the low copy number of the GPIa/IIa complex (<2000/platelet compared to 50 000/platelet for GPIIb/IIIa).

Clinical features

A typical case of NAIT presents with skin bleeding (purpura, petechiae and/or ecchymoses) or more serious haemorrhage, such as intracranial haemorrhage (ICH), in a full-term and otherwise healthy newborn with a normal coagulation screen and isolated thrombocytopenia. There are less common presentations *in utero*, including ventriculomegaly, cerebral cysts and hydrocephalus, which may be discovered by routine ultrasound. Although rare, hydrops fetalis has been reported in association with NAIT and this diagnosis should be considered if there are no other obvious reasons for the hydrops.

The precise incidence of ICH due to NAIT is unknown, but conservative estimates suggest that it is as low as 1 in 20 000 live births, which equates to approximately 35 cases per annum in the UK. Nearly 50% of severe ICHs occur *in utero*, usually between 30 and 35 weeks' gestation, but sometimes before 20 weeks. At the other end of the clinical spectrum, NAIT can be discovered incidentally when a blood count is performed for other reasons.

Severe NAIT in a neonate is a serious condition and requires correction of the platelet count. Appropriate management (see below) is essential to prevent ICH and the possibility of a lifelong disability.

Differential diagnosis

Other causes of neonatal thrombocytopenia are infection, prematurity, intrauterine growth retardation, inherited chromosomal abnormalities (particularly trisomy 21), maternal AITP and, very rarely, inherited forms of inadequate megakaryopoiesis. Precise figures on the incidence of neonatal thrombocytopenia caused by viral infection are not available. Maternal platelet autoimmunity is rarely associated with severe thrombocytopenia in the neonate, but should be considered in women with a history of AITP.

Platelet-type von Willebrand's disease, in which mutations in the GPIbα gene are associated with a propensity for *in vitro* platelet aggregation, can lead to falsely low platelet counts.

Laboratory investigations

Only antibodies against HPAs or isoantibodies against GPIIb/IIIa, GPIb/IX, CD109 and GPIV are thought to cause alloimmune thrombocytopenia in the fetus and neonate, although there are reports of platelet autoantibodies from patients with AITP crossing the placenta and causing neonatal thrombocytopenia.

For appropriate clinical management, the cause of severe thrombocytopenia in an otherwise healthy neonate should be urgently investigated. Screening for maternal HPA antibodies must be carried out, using techniques with appropriate sensitivity and specificity. The combination of two techniques such as the indirect PIFT and MAIPA assays, using a panel of group O, HPA-typed platelets, remains the preferred option in many reference laboratories and is an approach supported by results of quality assessment exercises.

HPA antibodies are detected in approximately 15% of referrals of suspected NAIT referred to the National Platelet Immunology Reference Laboratory in England. The most frequently detected antibody specificities are HPA-1a and HPA-5b, which are implicated in about 85% and 10% of clinically diagnosed cases of NAIT, respectively. The ability of an HPA-1a-negative mother to form anti-HPA-1a is partly controlled by the HLA *DRB3*01:01* allele. This allele is present in approximately 30% of Caucasoid women and the chance of HPA-1a antibody formation is greatly enhanced in HPA-1a-negative women who are HLA *DRB3*01:01*-positive compared to *DRB3*01:01*-negative women (odds ratio of 140). This high level association between HLA class II type and the formation of alloantibodies has not been observed for any other blood group antigen. The absence of HLA *DRB3*01:01* has a negative predictive value of >90% for HPA-1a alloimmunization but its positive predictive value is only 35%, limiting its potential usefulness as part of an antenatal screening programme. However, it remains of clinical use when counselling female siblings from index cases who have formed HPA-1a antibodies in pregnancy. About 15% of HPA-1a-negative pregnant women develop anti-HPA-1a in pregnancy, and of these about 30% will deliver a neonate with a platelet count $<50 \times 10^9$/L. The HPA-15 system was described a decade ago, but its clinical relevance has only recently been demonstrated, with a number of studies having shown that it is the third most commonly encountered HPA antibody specificity and that its effects may be as severe as in anti-HPA-1a-mediated NAIT.

Molecular typing of the parents and neonate for HPA-1, -2, -3, -5 and -15 should be performed because the results will be informative when interpreting antibody investigation results. For patients from the Far East, HPA-4 must also be included and the platelets should be investigated for GPIV expression status.

Alloimmunization against low frequency HPAs, e.g. HPA-9bw, explain some NAIT referrals that have a negative antibody screen for the common HPA antibody specificities [5]. A practical approach to detecting antibodies against low frequency antigens that are absent from cells used in antibody screening panels is to perform a cross-match against paternal platelets, although it is necessary to exclude positive findings due to ABO or HLA class I antibodies.

Genotyping of the maternal, paternal and affected infants' DNA samples for HPA-bw SNPs is also a cost-effective approach in this clinical setting.

Neonatal management

A cord platelet count of $<100 \times 10^9$/L should be repeated using a venous sample and a blood film examined. The neonate should be examined for skin or mucosal bleeding if a low platelet count is confirmed. If the platelet count is $<30 \times 10^9$/L or if there are signs of bleeding with a low count, it is strongly recommended that the neonate is transfused with donor platelets that are HPA-1a and -5b-negative, as these will be compatible with the maternal HPA alloantibody in $\geq 95\%$ of NAIT cases. The authors have shown that the transfusion of such platelets to infants affected by HPA-1a or -5b mediated NAIT results in a higher increment and more prolonged platelet survival than transfusion of random donor (HPA-1a-positive) platelets. However, if HPA-1a- and -5b-negative platelets are not immediately available and there is an urgent clinical need for transfusion then random, ABO and RhD compatible, donor platelets should be used in the first instance. A platelet count should be performed approximately 1 hour after completion of the platelet transfusion, and subsequently at least daily until the platelet count has been demonstrated not to be falling.

The results of laboratory investigations should not delay immediate platelet transfusion, as full investigation may be time-consuming and the risk of cerebral bleeds is highest in the first 48 hours post-delivery. In a typical case, the platelet count should recover to normal within a week, although a more protracted recovery can occur. Intravenous immunoglobulin (IvIgG) is not recommended as a first-line treatment as it is only effective in about 75% of cases and there is a delay of 24–48 hours before a satisfactory count is achieved; this is in contrast to the immediate effect of transfusion of HPA-compatible donor platelets. A cerebral ultrasound scan of the baby within the first week of life should be considered if the platelet count is $<50 \times 10^9$/L, and is recommended when the platelet count is 30×10^9/L.

Antenatal management

In a subsequent pregnancy of a mother with a known history of NAIT, the clinical management needs to be planned by a team experienced in the management of the risks of this condition. Treatment during the subsequent pregnancy is based on the history of haemorrhage and fetal/neonatal thrombocytopenia in previous pregnancies.

The mother should be advised to avoid nonsteroidal anti-inflammatory drugs as well as aspirin. There are two main treatment options: high dose IvIgG to the mother, or in utero platelet transfusion. Over the last decade, it has become increasingly clear that the former is the safest and most effective intervention to reduce the risk of ICH in the fetus [6]. The dose is 1 g/kg body weight at weekly intervals, usually from 20 weeks' gestation onwards; some fetal medicine specialists use a lower dose (0.5 g/kg/week) and may start between 12 and 20 weeks' gestation, depending on the history of NAIT in previous pregnancies. Early commencement of treatment is indicated where there is a history of antenatal ICH in previous pregnancies, because the earliest reports of ICH are at 16 weeks. A beneficial effect of IvIgG on the fetal platelet count occurs in approximately 70% of cases. There is a debate about the need to perform fetal blood sampling (FBS) to ascertain the platelet count and many centres do this at 28 weeks (usually after 8 weeks' treatment with IvIgG). If FBS reveals IvIgG to be ineffective in achieving a safe fetal platelet count, doubling the dose of IvIgG and/or adding corticosteroids (prednisolone, 0.5 mg/kg body weight) should be considered. If the increased intensity of treatment is ineffective, it may be necessary to switch to weekly fetal platelet transfusions. In utero platelet transfusions, carried out with FBS, carry a significant risk of fetal morbidity and mortality and should not be chosen as the first-line treatment but as a rescue therapy or in the management of pregnancies with a history of treatment failure on IvIgG. The transfusion of platelets has more complications compared to red cell transfusions for HDFN, e.g. bradycardia, post-needle withdrawal cord bleeds. Once commenced, the technically demanding procedure of in utero platelet transfusions is generally repeated at weekly intervals (Figure 5.4) or as indicated by the fetal platelet count.

The delivery needs careful planning between obstetric, paediatric and haematology teams to ensure an appropriate mode of delivery, and close liaison with blood transfusion services for timely provision of HPA-compatible platelets for the neonate. For neonates that have been transfused in utero, irradiation of cellular blood components is recommended.

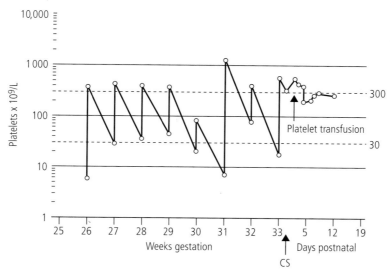

Fig 5.4 Seventh pregnancy of a patient who has had five miscarriages. The last of these was shown to have hydrops and hydrocephalus and a platelet count of only 17×10^9/L, and the serological findings supported a diagnosis of anti-HPA-1a mediated NAIT. The fetal platelet count was $<10 \times 10^9$/L at 25 weeks' gestation in the sixth pregnancy, and a cord haematoma developed during FBS resulting in fetal death. In the seventh pregnancy, prednisolone 20 mg/day and IvIgG 1 g/kg/week were administered to the mother from 16 weeks until delivery. The figure shows pre- and posttransfusion platelet counts following serial FBS and platelet transfusions. The fetal platelet count was $<10 \times 10^9$/L at 26 weeks. The aim was to maintain the fetal platelet count above 30×10^9/L by raising the immediate posttransfusion platelet count to above 300×10^9/L after each transfusion. The fetal platelet count fell below 10×10^9/L on one occasion when there were problems in preparing the fetal platelet concentrate and the dose of platelets was inadequate. CS, caesarean section.

Counselling

Counselling of couples with an index case about the risks of severe fetal/neonatal thrombocytopenia in a subsequent pregnancy needs to be based on disease severity in the infant(s) and outcome of immunological investigations. The following should be taken into account:

• thrombocytopenia in subsequent cases is as severe or, generally, more severe;
• the best predictors of severe fetal thrombocytopenia in a future pregnancy are antenatal ICH and severe thrombocytopenia (platelet count $<30 \times 10^9$/L) in a previous pregnancy;
• antibody specificity;
• antibody titre and bioactivity have been investigated to determine if these parameters have a predictive role in determining the severity of NAIT and contradictory data have been obtained [7–9], and currently are probably of no value in informing clinical management;
• HPA zygosity of the partner.

HPA-typed donor panels

Establishing donor panels for fetal and neonatal platelet transfusion requires a major commitment from blood services and identification of suitable donors requires the use of high throughput typing techniques. Although the frequency of HPA-1a-negative individuals amongst Caucasians is 2.5%, potential donors for fetal/neonatal transfusions must also be negative for the mandatory microbiological tests, negative for antibodies against red cells, platelets and leucocytes, and be cytomegalovirus (CMV) seronegative. The donors should also ideally be HPA-5b-negative to ensure that the panel

55

is of potential benefit to the maximum number of cases of suspected NAIT. In order to recruit a single HPA-1a-negative donor satisfying the above criteria, approximately 1500–2000 donors have to be typed for HPA-1a. In addition, therapeutic platelets should be RhD matched, as small amounts of red cells present in platelet concentrates may immunize RhD-negative recipients and be negative for high titre anti-A and anti-B antibodies. To recruit a single RhD-negative HPA-1a-negative donor whose platelets will be suitable for a first fetal or neonatal platelet transfusion, where the fetal/neonatal blood group is unknown, approximately 6000–7000 donors need to be typed.

Human neutrophil antigens

Antigens on the membrane of human neutrophils can, as with platelets, be divided into different categories. There are common antigens that have a wider distribution on other blood cells and tissues, e.g. I and P blood group systems and HLA class I. There are 'shared' antigens that have a limited distribution amongst other cell types, e.g. HNA-4a and HNA-5a polymorphisms associated with CD11/18. There are also a limited number of truly neutrophil-specific antigens, e.g. HNA-1a, HNA-1b, HNA-1c polymorphisms on FcγRIII or CD16. The current nomenclature for the HNA systems includes polymorphisms that are both cell-specific and 'shared' (see Table 5.3) [10].

HNA-1 system

The three antigens that comprise the HNA-1 system are localized on neutrophil FcγRIIIb (CD16), one of two low affinity receptors (R) for the constant domain (Fc) of human IgG(γ) that are found on neutrophils. There are normally 100 000–200 000 copies of FcγRIIIb per neutrophil. Four amino acid differences with arginine/serine, asparagine/serine, aspartic acid/asparagine and valine/isoleucine substitutions at positions 36, 65, 82 and 106, respectively, define the difference between HNA-1a and -1b, while a single amino acid substitution (alanine 78 > asparagine) defines the HNA-1c polymorphism (see Figure 5.5). The expression of HNA-1c is frequently associated with the presence of an additional FcγRIIIb gene and increased expression of FcγRIIIb. The expression of HNA-1 antigens varies with ethnicity, with HNA-1a

being more common in Chinese and Japanese populations than in Caucasians.

Two other FcγRIIIb-associated high frequency alloantigens, LAN and SAR, have been reported. The FcγRIIIb 'Null' phenotype is rare and is based on a double deletion or mutation of the *FcγRIIIb* gene and is, in some cases, associated with a deletion of the *FcγRIIc* gene. A maternal deficiency of FcγRIIIb can cause immune neutropenia in the newborn due to maternal FcγRIIIb isoantibodies. The FcγRIIIb molecule (but not necessarily the HNA-1 sites) can also be the antigenic target in autoimmune neutropenias.

HNA-2

HNA-2, formerly known as HNA-2a or NB1, is localized on a 58–64 kDa glycoprotein (CD177), expressed as a glycosylphosphatidylinositol-anchored membrane GP found both on the neutrophil surface membrane and on secondary granules. The term HNA-2a should no longer be used since it is now known that there is no antithetical antigen.

The percentage of neutrophils expressing HNA-2 varies between individuals and HNA-2 alloantibodies typically give a bimodal fluorescence profile with granulocytes from HNA-2-positive donors in immunofluorescence tests with a flow cytometric endpoint. HNA-2 antigen status can be determined by phenotyping with polyclonal or monoclonal antibodies. The HNA-2-negative phenotype is associated with particular sequence haplotypes from which nonproductive HNA-2 transcripts are generated, thereby causing a failure to express HNA-2.

HNA-3 system

HNA-3a (previously known as 5^{b}) and HNA-3b (previously known as 5^{a}) were originally described using antisera obtained from women immunized during pregnancy and were reported as being present on granulocytes, platelets, lymphocytes, kidney, spleen and lymph node tissue. Biochemical studies localized the HNA-3a antigen to a granulocyte glycoprotein with a molecular weight of 70–95 kDa. The polymorphism has been further localized to choline transporter-like protein 2 (CTL2) and a single point mutation at amino acid 154 (HNA-3a is encoded by Arginine and HNA-3b by Glutamine). The gene frequency of HNA-3a

Table 5.3 HNA systems.

HNA system	Antigen	Original acronym for antigen	Phenotype frequency* (%)	Glycoprotein	Nucleotide change	Amino acid change
1	1a	NA1	46	FcγRIIIb	G^{108}	Arginine[36]
						None
					A^{197}	Asparagine[65]
					G^{247}	Aspartic acid[82]
					G^{319}	Valine[106]
	1b	NA2	88	FcγRIIIb	C^{108}	Serine[36]
					T^{114}	None
					G^{197}	Serine[65]
					A^{247}	Asparagine[82]
					A^{319}	Isoleucine[106]
	1c	SH+	5	FcγRIIIb	A^{266}	Aspartic acid[78]
		SH–			C^{266}	Alanine[78]
2	2	NB1	97	CD177	nk	nk
3a	Five	5b	94.5	CTL2	G^{461}	Arginine[154]
3b	Five	5a	35.9	CTL2	A^{461}	Glutamine[154]
4a	Mart	Mart[a](+)	99.1	CD11b	G^{302}	Arginine[61]
		Mart[a](–)		CD11b	A^{302}	Histidine[61]
5a	Ond	Ond[a](+)	>99	CD11a	G^{2466}	Arginine[766]
		Ond[a](–)		CD11a	C^{2466}	Threonine[766]
—		NB2	32	nk	nk	nk
—	ND	ND1	98.5	nk	nk	nk
—	NE	NE1	23	nk	nk	nk
—	LAN	LAN[a]	>99	FcγRIIIb	nk	nk
—	SAR	SAR[a]	>99	FcγRIIIb	nk	nk

*Frequencies based on studies of Caucasians.
nk, not known.

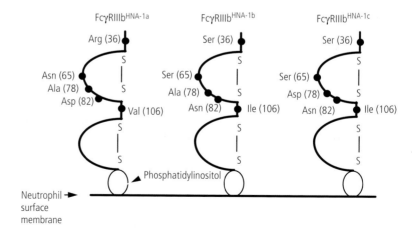

Fig 5.5 Representation of the amino acid substitutions resulting in the HNA-1a, -1b, -1c forms of *FcγRIIIb*. The positions of the amino acid substitutions arising from the allelic variation of the *FcγRIIIb* gene are depicted by black dots. Amino acids are given in three-letter acronyms. The intrachain disulfide bonds create two domains, which are closely related to the C-terminal heavy chain domains of IgG.

and HNA-3b has been reported as 0.792 and 0.207, respectively, in the German population. HNA-3a antibodies have been implicated in transfusion-related acute lung injury (TRALI) and neonatal alloimmune neutropenia (NAIN). HNA-3b antibodies have also been described but the clinical significance of these antibodies is not known.

Alloantigens on CD11a and CD11b

The genes encoding the α_M and α_L subunits of the β_2 integrin or CD11b and CD11a are polymorphic and are associated with HNA-4a and HNA-5a, respectively. Alloantibody formation against these two polymorphisms has been observed in transfusion recipients, and recently cases of NAIN due to HNA-4a and HNA-5a antibodies have been described. The low incidence of neonatal neutropenia associated with these antibodies is probably explained by the wide distribution of these proteins on granulocytes, monocytes and lymphocytes.

Detection of neutrophil antibodies

The reliable detection and identification of neutrophil antibodies can be technically difficult. The main problems are the abundant expression of the two low affinity receptors (FcγRII and FcγRIIIb) for the constant domain of human IgG, which results in increased and variable binding of circulating immunoglobulins in normal sera and the requirement for fresh and typed donor neutrophils as panel cells, since neutrophils cannot be stored. The incidence of antibody-mediated neutropenias is comparatively rare and, therefore, the best strategy for investigation of clinical cases is a national reference laboratory where adequate technical expertise and reagents are available.

Many techniques for neutrophil/granulocyte antibody detection have been evaluated over the years. Early assays such as the granulocyte cytotoxicity and agglutination tests had a very low specificity. The granulocyte immunofluorescence and granulocyte chemiluminescence tests have the advantage of good sensitivity but are not specific, i.e. they cannot readily distinguish between granulocyte-specific

and HLA class I antibodies without further investigations. For some HNA systems, e.g. antigens expressed on CD16, CD177 and CD11/18, the monoclonal antibody immobilization of granulocyte antigens (MAIGA) assay can be applied but, otherwise, immunoprecipitation of membrane-labelled neutrophil proteins remains the only reliable technique to determine the nature of the antigen. The principles of the granulocyte immunofluorescence test and the MAIGA assays are analogous to the equivalent platelet tests (Plate 5.1 and Figure 5.1, respectively). Increased understanding of the molecular nature of HNAs has opened up the potential to develop recombinant HNAs and both cell lines expressing recombinant proteins (rHNA) and soluble rHNA coupled to a solid phase have been described. These new assays have shown promise but, currently, generally lack the sensitivity and specificity of established techniques. The introduction of such techniques does, however, have the potential to transform the serological investigation of granulocyte alloantibodies and the high throughput capability of assays using beads coupled to rHNA proteins would be particularly beneficial for blood donor screening in TRALI-reduction programmes [11].

HNA typing has historically been based on the use of monospecific alloantisera derived from immunized patients or blood donors, but monoclonal antibodies against HNA-1a, -1b and -2 are now available. Recent advances in the understanding of the molecular basis of the HNA systems means that it is now possible to type for HNA-1a, -1b, -1c, -3a, -3b, -4a, -4b, -5a and -5b using PCR-SSP or sequence-based typing techniques.

Clinical significance of HNA antibodies

Neutrophil-specific antibodies are implicated in:
• neonatal alloimmune neutropenia (NAIN);
• febrile nonhaemolytic transfusion reactions (see Chapter 8);
• transfusion-related acute lung injury (TRALI) (see Chapter 9);
• transfusion-related alloimmune neutropenia (TRAIN);
• autoimmune neutropenia; and
• persistent post-bone marrow transplant neutropenia.

Neonatal alloimmune neutropenia

Maternal alloimmunization against neutrophil-specific alloantigens on fetal/neonatal neutrophils is a condition analogous to NAIT in terms of pathophysiology but, with an estimated incidence of 0.1–0.2% of live births, is comparatively rare as a clinically significant entity although there are no reliable figures. Clinical presentation is mainly one of bacterial infections with isolated neutropenia being the only haematological abnormality. The neutropenia may be severe but is reversible and newborn infants may require treatment with antibiotics and/or GCSF to control bacterial infections and hasten recovery to a normal neutrophil count. The neutropenia in some cases caused by HNA-1a and -1b antibodies has been reported to extend for up to 28 weeks. HNA-1a and -2 are the most commonly implicated antibody specificities.

FNHTR and TRALI (see Chapters 8 and 9)

FNHTRs have a number of different causes. They can occasionally be associated with the presence of leucocyte (HLA and HNA) alloantibodies in the recipient. In the UK, where there is universal leucocyte reduction of blood components, investigations for other causes of high fever associated with transfusion are carried out, e.g. tests for bacterial contamination and IgA-deficiency. Serological investigations for platelet, HLA and granulocyte antibodies are of limited clinical value as the diagnostic specificity of these tests for FNHTRs is low. Nonetheless, testing for HNA antibodies may be required in rare cases in which a severe FNHTR cannot be otherwise explained and washed components have proved ineffective. The management of FNHTRs is described in detail in Chapter 8.

TRALI is a severe and sometimes life-threatening transfusion reaction. The majority of cases are caused by donor leucocyte alloantibodies against alloantigens present on the patient's leucocytes, although patient alloantibodies may be involved in some cases. In most TRALI cases, HLA class I- and II-specific antibodies are implicated but HNA antibodies have also been implicated as causal agents with HNA-1a and HNA-3a antibody specificities being found most commonly [12]. TRALI investigations are logistically complex because of the need to contact all of the implicated donors to obtain fresh blood samples. Investigations are usually stratified to include only female donors initially. The donor samples are screened for both HLA and HNA alloantibodies. If antibodies are found it is necessary to type the patient to determine whether they have the cognate antigen and to type the donor to establish that they lack the antigen. In some cases, it may be necessary to screen a recipient's serum for antibodies or to perform a cross-match between donor sera and the patient's granulocytes and lymphocytes.

Many blood transfusion services have taken steps to reduce the incidence of TRALI, e.g. by reducing the proportion of female donors for plasma and platelet components, and more recently by screening female donors for HLA and HNA antibodies. The success of these strategies has been demonstrated by the reduced incidence of TRALI in haemovigilance schemes.

Transfusion-related alloimmune neutropenia (TRAIN)

The first documented case of TRAIN occurred following the infusion of 80 mL of plasma-reduced blood after cardiac surgery on a 4-week-old infant [13]. The plasma from the blood donor was found to contain HNA-1b alloantibodies that resulted in an absolute neutropenia in the infant, who typed as HNA-1a(+), -1b(+). The neutropenia resolved after 7 days after treating the infant with GCSF. The condition is of interest since it demonstrates that, in some circumstances, passively infused HNA antibodies can trigger neutropenia rather than TRALI. This clinical entity has recently been confirmed by an additional report.

Autoimmune neutropenia

Autoimmune neutropenia is a rare condition that can occur as a transient, self-limiting autoimmunity in young children [14] or a chronic form in adults [15]. The autoantibodies tend to target the FcγRIIIb (CD16), CD177 or CD11/18 molecules but can also be HNA-specific, e.g. HNA-1a antibodies are found in autoimmune neutropenia of childhood.

The most sensitive method for the detection of autoantibodies is to test the patient's neutrophils using the direct immunofluorescence test. However, the combination of severe neutropenia, high blood sample volume requirements to recover sufficient granulocytes and the need for a fresh sample limits the applicability of this test, especially in children. Screening of a patient's serum with a panel of typed neutrophils in the indirect granulocyte immunofluorescence and granulocyte chemiluminescence or granulocyte agglutination tests provides a suitable alternative and, in some studies, this approach has been found to be only slightly less sensitive than performing a direct test.

Persistent post-bone marrow transplant neutropenia

Antibody-mediated neutropenia may be a serious complication of bone marrow transplantation. In this context, as the neutrophil antibodies may be autoimmune and/or alloimmune in nature, laboratory investigation requires serological and typing studies to elucidate the nature of the antibodies involved.

Key points

1 Allo-, auto-, iso- and drug-induced antigens may be found on platelets and neutrophils and are implicated in a range of immune cytopenias.
2 Alloantigens on platelets are known as HPAs; alloantigens on neutrophils are known as HNAs.
3 Reliable detection and identification of HPA- and HNA-specific antibodies requires the use of both whole-cell type assays such as the PIFT/GIFT and antigen-capture type assays such as the MAIPA/MAIGA assays.
4 HPA and HNA types can mostly be determined using PCR-based methodologies.
5 NAIT is a common disorder and HPA-1a or HPA-5b antibodies are responsible for approximately 95% of cases.
6 Optimal postnatal treatment of NAIT is the transfusion of HPA-1a/5b-negative donor platelets.
7 Optimal antenatal treatment of NAIT is yet to be determined but maternal treatment with IvIgG is the recommended initial treatment.
8 HNA antibodies can be associated both with alloimmune and autoimmune neutropenia.
9 TRALI can be a life-threatening condition, especially if HNA-3a antibodies are involved.
10 The incidence of antibody-mediated TRALI has been reduced by implementation of a number of different strategies.

References

1 Metcalfe P, Watkins NA, Ouwehand WH, Kaplan C, Newman P, Kekomaki R et al. Nomenclature of human platelet antigens. Vox Sanguinis 2003 October; 85(3): 240–245.
2 Aster RH, Curtis BR, McFarland JG & Bougie DW. Drug-induced immune thrombocytopenia: pathogenesis, diagnosis, and management. J Thromb Haemost 2009 June; 7(6): 911–918.
3 Kiefel V, Santoso S, Weisheit M & Mueller-Eckhardt C. Monoclonal antibody-specific immobilization of platelet antigens (MAIPA): a new tool for the identification of platelet-reactive antibodies. Blood 1987 December; 70(6): 1722–1726.
4 Tiller H, Killie M, Skogen B, Oian P & Husebekk A. Neonatal alloimmune thrombocytopenia in Norway: poor detection rate with nonscreening versus a general screening programme. BJOG 2009 March; 116(4): 594–598.
5 Ghevaert C, Rankin A, Huiskes E, Porcelijn L, Javela K, Kekomaki R et al. Alloantibodies against low-frequency human platelet antigens do not account for a significant proportion of cases of fetomaternal alloimmune thrombocytopenia: evidence from 1054 cases. Transfusion 2009 October; 49(10): 2084–2089.
6 Kamphuis MM & Oepkes D. Fetal and neonatal alloimmune thrombocytopenia: prenatal interventions. Prenat Diagn 2011 July; 31(7): 712–719.
7 Bertrand G, Drame M, Martageix C & Kaplan C. Prediction of the fetal status in noninvasive management of alloimmune thrombocytopenia. Blood 2011 March 17; 117(11): 3209–3213.
8 Killie MK, Husebekk A, Kjeldsen-Kragh J & Skogen B. A prospective study of maternal anti-HPA 1a antibody level as a potential predictor of alloimmune thrombocytopenia in the newborn. Haematologica 2008 April 28; 93(6): 870–877.
9 Ghevaert C, Campbell K, Stafford P, Metcalfe P, Casbard A, Smith GA et al. HPA-1a antibody potency and bioactivity do not predict severity of fetomaternal alloimmune thrombocytopenia. Transfusion 2007 July; 47(7): 1296–1305.
10 Bux J. Nomenclature of granulocyte alloantigens. ISBT Working Party on Platelet and Granulocyte Serology, Granulocyte Antigen Working Party. International Society of Blood Transfusion. Transfusion 1999 June; 39(6): 662–663.
11 Lucas G, Win N, Calvert A, Green A, Griffin E, Bendukidze N et al. Reducing the incidence of TRALI in the UK: the results of screening for donor leucocyte antibodies and the development of national guidelines. Vox Sanguinis 2012 July; 103(1): 10–17.

12 Bux J & Sachs UJ. The pathogenesis of transfusion-related acute lung injury (TRALI). *Br J Haematol* 2007 March; 136(6): 788–799.

13 Wallis JP, Haynes S, Stark G, Green FA, Lucas GF & Chapman CE. Transfusion-related alloimmune neutropenia: an undescribed complication of blood transfusion. *The Lancet* 2002 October 5; 360(9339): 1073–1074.

14 Bruin M, Dassen A, Pajkrt D, Buddelmeyer L, Kuijpers T & de Haas M. Primary autoimmune neutropenia in children: a study of neutrophil antibodies and clinical course. *Vox Sanguinis* 2005 January; 88(1): 52–59.

15 Shastri KA & Logue GL. Autoimmune neutropenia. *Blood* 1993 April 15; 81(8): 1984–1995.

Further reading

Bassler D, Greinacher A, Okascharoen C *et al*. A systematic review and survey of the management of unexpected neonatal alloimmune thrombocytopenia. *Transfusion* 2008; 48: 92–98.

Bux J. Human neutrophil alloantigens. *Vox Sanguinis* 2008; 94: 277–285.

Capsoni F, Sarzi-Puttini P & Zanella A. Primary and secondary autoimmune neutropenia. *Arthritis Res Therapy* 2005; 7: 208–214.

Fung YL, Minchinton RM & Fraser JF. Neutrophil antibody diagnostics and screening: review of the classical versus the emerging. *Vox Sanguinis* 2011; 101: 282–290.

Lucas GF & Metcalfe P. Platelet and granulocyte glycoprotein polymorphisms. *Transfus Med* 2000; 10: 157–174.

Murphy MF & Bussel JB. Advances in the management of alloimmune thrombocytopenia. *Br J Haematol* 2007; 136: 366–378.

Ouwehand WH, Stafford P, Ghevaert C *et al*. Platelet immunology, present and future. *ISBT Sci Ser* 2006; 1: 96–102.

Warkentin TE & Smith JW. The alloimmune thrombocytopenic syndromes. *Transfus Med Rev* 1997; 11: 296–307.

PART TWO
Complications of Transfusions

6 Investigation of acute transfusion reactions

Kathryn E. Webert[1] & Nancy M. Heddle[2]

[1]Department of Medicine and Department of Pathology and Molecular Medicine, McMaster University and Canadian Blood Services, Hamilton, Ontario, Canada

[2]Department of Medicine, McMaster University and Canadian Blood Services, Hamilton, Canada

The investigation of suspected acute reactions to blood components and plasma derivatives cannot be summarized in a single simple algorithm for several reasons:
- signs and symptoms are not specific for one type of reaction;
- the frequency and type of reactions vary with different blood components, e.g. leucocyte-reduced or not;
- risks are variable with different patient populations;
- the severity and risk of reactions must be taken into account to ensure a balance between the safety, availability and costs due to wastage.

In this chapter, an algorithmic approach is provided for the clinical management and laboratory investigation of transfusion reactions.

Understanding the clinical presentation and differential diagnosis

Acute reactions are defined as adverse events occurring during or within four to six hours of transfusion. They can usually be placed into the following categories [1, 2]:
- acute haemolysis (AHTR);
- allergic;
- anaphylactic;
- transfusion-related acute lung injury (TRALI);
- febrile nonhaemolytic reactions (FNHTR);
- bacterial sepsis;
- hypotension;
- transfusion-associated circulatory overload (TACO);
- acute pain reaction
- metabolic complications (hyperkalemia, hypokalemia, hypocalcemia, hypothermia).

There are other types of reactions that can occur following the acute period including delayed haemolytic reactions, transfusion-associated graft-versus-host disease, posttransfusion purpura, alloimmune thrombocytopenia and alloimmune neutropenia. These reactions are discussed in other chapters.

The diagnosis of an acute transfusion reaction can be challenging as signs and symptoms are not specific for each type of reaction, all possible signs and symptoms do not present with every reaction and different types of reactions can occur simultaneously. In Table 6.1, signs and symptoms have been grouped into nine categories. The information summarized in this table illustrates how similar signs and symptoms can occur in different reactions (e.g. bacterial sepsis, allergic and analyphylactic reactions can all present with cutaneous symptoms).

To ensure management strategies and investigations that minimize risks to patients, healthcare professionals need to understand the aetiology and pathophysiology of each type of acute reaction (Table 6.2). It is also essential to understand the typical clinical presentation for each type of reaction so that a differential diagnosis can be formulated as part of the investigative process. Some considerations to assist in the

Practical Transfusion Medicine, Fourth Edition. Edited by Michael F. Murphy, Derwood H. Pamphilon and Nancy M. Heddle.
© 2013 John Wiley & Sons, Ltd. Published 2013 by John Wiley & Sons, Ltd.

Table 6.1 Summary of the signs/symptoms typically observed with different types of acute transfusion reactions.

Reaction type	Cutaneous	Pain	Inflammatory	Respiratory	Hypo-tension	Hyper-tension	Other cardio-vascular	GI	Neuro-muscular	CNS	DIC	Haemo-globinuria	Renal failure
AHTR		✓		✓	✓		✓				✓	✓	✓
Allergic	✓			✓									
Anaphylactic	✓		✓*	✓	✓	✓	✓	✓					
TRALI			✓	✓	✓		✓	✓					
FNHTR		✓	✓	✓				✓					
Bacterial sepsis	✓	✓	✓	✓	✓	✓	✓	✓		✓	✓	✓	
Hypotensive		✓	✓	✓	✓		✓	✓					
TACO		✓	✓	✓		✓	✓						
Acute pain		✓	✓	✓		✓	✓						
Hyperkalemia							✓	✓	✓				
Hypokalemia							✓	✓	✓	✓			
Hypocalcemia		✓	✓				✓	✓	✓				
Hypothermia				✓									
Hypotensive		✓	✓	✓	✓								

*Flushing only.

AHTR, acute haemolytic transfusion reaction; TRALI, transfusion-related acute lung injury; FNHTR, febrile nonhaemolytic transfusion reaction; TACO, transfusion-associated circulatory overload; GI, gastrointestinal; CNS, central nervous system; DIC, disseminated intravascular coagulation.

Table 6.2 Summary of acute transfusion reactions [3, 4].

Reaction	Frequency	Mechanism	Clinical presentation	Differential diagnosis	Laboratory investigations	Management
AHTR	1:25 000 (fatal 1:600 000)	Result from the destruction of donor red cells by preformed recipient antibodies	Fever, flank pain and red/brown urine	FNHTR bacterial contamination TRALI Nonimmune causes of haemolysis	Positive DAT free haemoglobin in plasma and urine Positive cross-match	Stop the transfusion immediately Begin infusion of normal saline
		Antibodies fix complement and cause rapid intravascular haemolysis	Hypotension, shock, death			Alert the blood transfusion laboratory, check for clerical error, send entire transfusion setup to blood transfusion laboratory for testing
		Usually due to ABO incompatibility which is most often the result of clerical error				Obtain bloodwork: DAT, plasma for free haemoglobin, antibody screen Obtain urine sample: haemoglobinuria
Allergic transfusion reaction	1:100–300 transfusions	Soluble allergenic substances in the plasma of the donated blood product react with pre-existing IgE antibodies in the recipient	Hives Urticaria Flushing	Anaphylactic transfusion reaction TRALI TACO	Rule out anaphylactic reaction	Stop the transfusion until a more serious reaction is ruled out
		Causes mast cells and basophils to release histamine, leading to hives or urticaria				Antihistamine may improve symptoms
						If no evidence of dyspnea or anaphylaxis, the transfusion may be continued with close observation
Anaphylactic transfusion reaction	1:20 000–50 000 transfusions	Usually due to the presence of anti-IgA antibodies in recipients who are IgA deficient	Rapid onset of shock, hypotension, angioedema and respiratory distress (2° to bronchospasm and laryngeal oedema)	Allergic transfusion reaction TRALI TACO	IgA level Testing for anti-IgA (if IgA deficient)	Stop the transfusion Adrenaline Airway maintenance, oxygenation Maintain haemodynamic status (IV fluids, vasopressor medications)

(continued)

Table 6.2 (*Continued*)

Reaction	Frequency	Mechanism	Clinical presentation	Differential diagnosis	Laboratory investigations	Management
TRALI	2–8 cases per 10 000 allogeneic transfusion (0.014–0.08%) 0.5–2 cases per 1000 patients transfused (0.04–0.16%)	Antibodies or neutrophil-priming agents in the infused blood product likely interact with the recipient's leucocyte antigens Activation of the WBC results in the production of inflammatory mediators that increase vascular permeability Leads to capillary leak and pulmonary tissue damage	Shortness of breath Fever Hypotension or hypertension Acute noncardiogenic pulmonary oedema (elevated JVP, bilateral lung crackles)	Bacterial contamination TACO Anaphylactic transfusion reaction Cardiogenic pulmonary oedema ARDS Pneumonia	Antigranulocyte or anti-HLA antibodies in the donor CXR (bilateral pulmonary infiltrates) BNP (possibly useful)	Stop the transfusion Respiratory support as required (supplemental oxygen, mechanical ventilation) Maintain haemodynamic status (IV fluids, vasopressor medications)
FNHTR	Commonly occur during transfusions of red cells, platelets or plasma 1:100 RBC transfusions; 1:5 platelet transfusions	Likely caused by cytokines that are generated and accumulate during the storage of blood components Less frequently caused by leukocyte antigen/antibody interactions between recipient and blood product	Fever, rigors, chills Other: nausea, vomiting, dyspnea, hypotension Typically occur during or within 2 hours of transfusion but may present up to 6 hours after transfusion	AHTR Bacterial contamination TRALI Comorbid conditions causing fever (i.e. infection, haematologic malignancies, solid tumour) Drugs causing fever	No specific tests Rule out other transfusion reactions	Stop the transfusion until a more serious reaction is ruled out Antipyretics to decrease fever and meperidine may help patients with severe chills and rigors

Bacterial contamination	Previously estimated as 1:10 000 for symptomatic reactions (platelets), 1:>1 million (RBC) Likely lower if pre-transfusion bacterial detection is in place	Bacteria in the blood product from: donor skin (venipuncture site); donor with bacteremia; contamination during collection/storage	High fever, rigors Hypotension	AHTR FNHTR Allergic transfusion reaction	Gram stain and culture of remaining blood component Gram stain and culture of patient's blood	Stop the transfusion IV fluids Broad spectrum antibiotics
Hypotensive transfusion reaction	Unknown but thought to be rare	Unknown May be related to generation of bradykinin and/or its active metabolite Majority of reactions occur during transfusion of blood components administered through a negatively charged filter or to patients receiving an angiotensin-converting enzyme (ACE) inhibitor	Hypotension Dyspnea, urticaria, flushing, pruritis, GI symptoms Most reactions occur within minutes of the beginning of the transfusion and resolve rapidly with cessation of the transfusion and supportive care	AHTR Bacterial contamination TRALI Anaphylactic transfusion reaction Unrelated to blood transfusion (i.e. due to blood loss)	No specific tests Rule out other transfusion reactions	Stop the transfusion
TACO	May be as high as 1:100 transfusions	Increase in central venous pressure, increase in pulmonary blood volume and decrease in pulmonary compliance with resultant secondary congestive heart failure and pulmonary oedema	Elevated JVP Bilateral crackles on auscultation Hypertension Dry cough Orthopnoea Pedal oedema	TRALI Anaphylactic transfusion reaction	Chest X-ray Clinical examination BNP (possibly useful)	Stop the transfusion Supplemental oxygen Diuretics

(continued)

Table 6.2 (*Continued*)

Reaction	Frequency	Mechanism	Clinical presentation	Differential diagnosis	Laboratory investigations	Management
Acute pain reaction	Unknown Data suggest it may occur with 0.02% of blood products transfused	Unknown	Acute pain during transfusion (chest, abdominal, back or flank) Other symptoms include: dyspnea, hypertension, chills, tachycardia, restlessness, flushing, headache	AHTR TRALI TACO Allergic	No specific tests	Temporarily stop transfusion Rule out other causes of reaction Pain management
Hyperkalemia	Unknown Likely more common in infants and children and individuals receiving massive transfusion	During storage of red blood cells, increasing potassium concentration of the supernatant occurs	Muscle weakness Cardiac effects: ECG changes (e.g. peaked T waves, loss of P wave amplitude, prolonged PR interval and QRS duration), arrhythmias, cardiac arrest Death		Electrolytes ECG	May possibly be prevented by such modalities as: slow rate of infusion, the use of fresher blood, washing of red cells, use of in-line potassium filters (in development)
Hypokalemia	Rare May occur in association with massive transfusion (especially large amounts of FFP)	Unknown Possibly caused by metabolic alkalosis secondary to citrate metabolism, release of catecholamines, aldosterone and/or antidiuretic hormone	ECG changes (flattened or inverted T waves, U wave, ST depression, wide PR interval) Muscle weakness Cardiac arrhythmias	Rapid infusion of other solutions low in potassium	Electrolytes ECG	Consider replacement of potassium

Hypocalcemia	Rare May occur in association with massive transfusion	May occur in massive transfusion recipients with liver failure. Liver normally rapidly metabolized transfused citrate. If rate of citrate delivery exceeds liver's ability to clear citrate, citrate may be able to bind to calcium, resulting in hypocalcemia	ECG changes (prolongation of QT interval), depressed left ventricular function, increased neuromuscular excitability, hypotension	Calcium level Magnesium level (also bound by citrate)	Consider calcium replacement when ionized calcium concentration is less than 50% of normal value with symptoms of hypocalcemia
Hypothermia	Unknown Most commonly seen with rapid massive transfusion of red cells (stored between 1 and 6 °C)	Occurs with rapid transfusion of large volumes of cold blood (red cells)	Decreased core body temperature Hypothermia may be associated with metabolic derangements (hyperkalemia, increased lactate, increased oxygen affinity of haemoglobin), abnormalities in hemostasis and cardiac disturbances	Other causes associated with massive transfusion and trauma include infusion of cold fluids, opening of body cavities due to injuries, impaired thermoregulatory control	May be prevented by use of blood warmers when rapid massive transfusion is required

AHTR, acute haemolytic transfusion reaction; FNHTR, febrile nonhaemolytic transfusion reaction; TRALI, transfusion-related acute lung injury; DAT, direct antiglobulin test; TACO, transfusion-associated circulatory overload; IV, intravenous; HLA, human leucocyte antigen; CXR, chest X-ray; JVP, jugular venous pressure; ARDS, adult respiratory distress syndrome; GI, gastrointestinal; BNP, brain natriuretic peptide; ECG, electrocardiogram; WBC, white blood cell; RBC, red blood cell; FFP, fresh frozen plasma.

decision-making process and investigation are summarized below [3, 4].

Patient history

• The reason for the patient's admission and current diagnosis may give some indication as to the type of reaction. For example, if the patient is being transfused because of anaemia but is also in congestive heart failure, TACO could be the cause of the reaction.

• Consider whether the patient has been previously transfused or pregnant as this can lead to alloimmunization to red cell and leucocyte antigens, which are known to be associated with certain types of reactions (acute haemolytic, FNHTR).

• What blood components have been transfused and what is the transfusion timeline? If plasma-containing products have been recently transfused, consider whether the reaction could be caused by passive infusion of antibody or soluble allergens that may now be reacting with the product being transfused.

• Has the patient had a history of reactions when blood components are transfused? Some patients are prone to developing recurrent FNHTR and/or allergic reactions when transfused.

• Is the patient known to be IgA deficient? Some patients with IgA deficiency develop anti-IgA antibodies, which may cause anaphylactic transfusion reactions when an IgA-containing blood component is transfused.

Medications

• Determine what medications the patient is receiving or has received in the time period leading up to the transfusion. Considerations should include:
  ◦ the use of premedications given to prevent acute reactions such as allergic (antihistamines) or FNHTR (antipyretics);
  ◦ antimicrobial medication;
  ◦ pyrogenic agents that are known to cause fever such as amphotericin or monoclonal antibodies;
  ◦ ACE inhibitors, which have been associated with hypotensive reactions; and
  ◦ pruritogenic agents such as vancomycin, narcotics, etc.

Type of blood component being transfused

• Does the component contain significant volumes of plasma? Infusion of plasma is associated with a variety of reactions including allergic, anaphylactic, TRALI and acute haemolysis caused by passive antibody incompatibility with the patient's red cells [3, 4].

• Does the component contain a significant number of red cells? If greater than 50 mL of red cells are present in the component, acute haemolysis needs to be considered as a possible cause of the adverse reaction.

• Was the component stored at room temperature or in a refrigerator? Platelets have a higher risk of bacterial contamination as they are stored at room temperature. However, products stored at colder temperatures can also be contaminated with bacteria, especially those strains that are known to grow at cold temperatures [3].

• Is the component leucocyte-reduced and if so was leucocyte reduction performed pre- or post-storage? Non-leucocyte-reduced blood components (especially platelets) are associated with a higher frequency of FNHTR. Post-storage leucocyte reduction also has limited effectiveness in preventing FNHTR to platelets whereas pre-storage leucocyte reduction is highly effective. In contrast, both post- and pre-storage leucocyte reduction are effective in preventing most FNHTR to red cells [5].

Was fever present?

• Fever is a common finding in most types of reactions. However, it does not occur in allergic transfusion reactions or with anaphylaxis. Therefore, fever can be useful to help differentiate between severe hypotension caused by bacterial contamination, acute haemolysis or TRALI (fever may be present) versus hypotension caused by anaphylactic shock (fever is absent).

• Was the rise in temperature $\geq 2°C$? Significant temperature increases are typically seen with bacterial contamination, especially if the patient has not been premedicated with an antipyretic or is not receiving antibiotic therapy. Increases in temperature greater than 2°C are not usually seen with other types of reactions [6].

Volume of component transfused

The volume of the component transfused can also be an important consideration for a differential diagnosis.

• Some types of reactions are dose-dependent; hence, they tend to occur towards the end of the transfusion after most of the component has been given. Such reactions include allergic reactions, FNHTR and TRALI. This observation becomes less useful when symptoms occur during the transfusion of multiple blood components. In this situation, it is difficult to determine if the reaction is caused by the first unit transfused or the current unit that is being administered.

• Anaphylactic reactions can present after a small amount of component is transfused (1–10 mL) [7].

• Acute haemolytic reactions usually require at least 50–100 mL of red cells to be transfused before symptoms appear.

Other considerations

• Always remember that the patient's clinical comorbidities and therapies could also be causing many of the symptoms typical of acute transfusion reactions. Hence, these always need to be considered as part of the differential diagnosis.

• Although most reactions are relatively infrequent, it is possible for a patient to have more than one type of reaction concurrently. This possibility should always be considered when the patient presents with atypical findings.

• For many reaction types, there is a spectrum of severity, ranging from mild to severe, depending on such factors as characteristics of the patient and blood component, and amount of blood transfused. For example, bacterial contamination of a blood component may result in an acute septic reaction with high fever and hypotension. Alternately, such a component may cause no or only mild symptoms.

• Consider how well you know the patient and their previous response to blood component transfusions. Less concern may be appropriate for a patient who develops hives every time they are transfused, whereas action would be appropriate for the sudden development of moderate respiratory symptoms in the multi-transfused patient who has previously had no adverse events.

General approach for investigation and treatment of acute transfusion reactions

Using all of the information noted above, the clinician must make a decision whether to stop the administration of the blood component temporarily or discontinue the transfusion and must decide the extent of the investigations to be performed. Stopping and investigating every transfusion reaction is often assumed to provide the highest level of safety for the patient, but in reality may contribute to other morbidities such as bleeding or respiratory/cardiovascular morbidity if an essential transfusion is delayed. Hence, some clinical judgement is required to ensure a balance between risk and benefit. The following approach should be used if there is any concern about patient safety and an investigation is required.

Action to be taken on the clinical unit

• Stop the transfusion immediately. The severity of some reactions is dose-dependent. For example, the risk of severe morbidity and mortality with acute haemolysis is generally proportional to the volume of component transfused.

• Keep the IV line open with saline (or other appropriate IV solution) in the event that a decision is made to continue the transfusion or if the patient requires other IV therapy.

• Support the patient's clinical symptoms with appropriate medical therapy.

• Perform a bedside clerical check to ensure that the name on the blood component and requisition matches the patient's armband/identifier.

• Look carefully at the remaining blood component to determine if there is any evidence of haemolysis or particulate matter. A contaminated unit of red cells may have discoloration either in the primary bag or in the first few segments closest to the blood bag.

• Complete a transfusion reaction form and notify the blood transfusion laboratory that a reaction has occurred. The transfusion laboratory will perform relevant investigations, notify the blood supplier if applicable so appropriate actions can be taken and ensure that relevant reactions are reported to the country's haemovigilance system (see Chapter 18). This reporting provides cumulative statistics about reactions that may be the first clue of a new emerging threat to the blood supply or a problem with component manufacturing.

• If a decision is made to perform a more extensive investigation to rule out problems with a donor unit (e.g. serological incompatibility causing haemolysis,

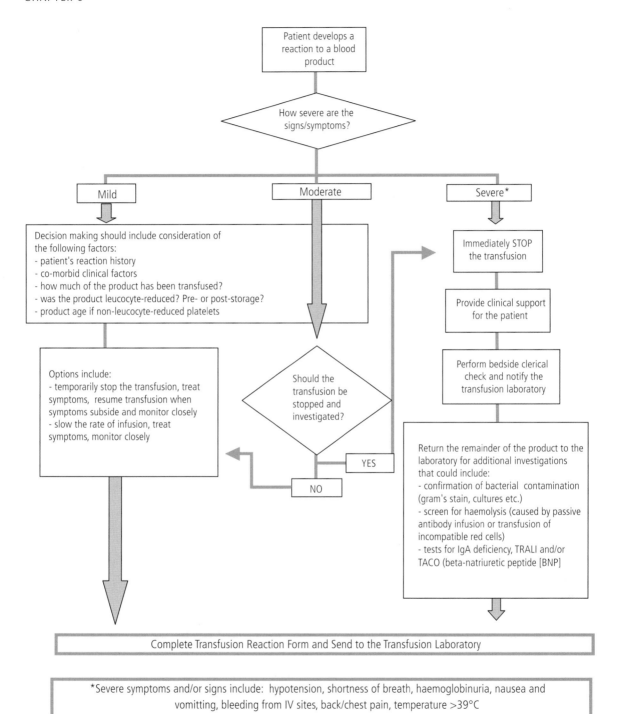

Fig 6.1 Flow diagram illustrating a possible approach for the management and investigation of an acute transfusion reaction.

bacterial contamination, TRALI), the remainder of the blood bag should be returned to the blood transfusion laboratory and/or blood service for further testing. Local policies should be followed for additional patient samples to be collected for specialized testing.

Action to be taken in the laboratory

When a reaction is reported to the blood transfusion laboratory, there should always be a clerical check performed to verify that the paperwork is accurate and that the correct component was issued for transfusion. To rule out haemolysis from the differential diagnosis, the following screening tests should be performed:
- clerical check as mentioned above;
- centrifuge a posttransfusion sample of the patient's blood and observe the plasma for visual evidence of haemolysis; and
- perform a direct antiglobulin test on a posttransfusion EDTA sample taken from the patient.

If the clerical check does not indicate any problems and the two screening tests are negative, acute haemolysis as the cause of the reaction can usually be eliminated. However, if the patient's symptoms are severe and consistent with a haemolytic reaction, a complete serological work-up may be indicated, including repeating the compatibility test on both the pre- and posttransfusion patient samples and specific tests for haemolysis (i.e. lactate dehydrogenase, haptoglobin, methaemalbumin, etc.).

All blood transfusion laboratories should have specific protocols for the investigation of other types of reactions. The Public Health Agency of Canada has developed guidelines for the investigation of suspected reactions caused by bacterial contamination, which can be accessed from the website (http://www.phac-aspc.gc.ca) [8]. Similar documents may be present in other countries. Investigation of TRALI, anaphylaxis and TACO requires specialized testing, which may be available only from a reference centre or specialized laboratory [9–11]. However, each facility should have policies and procedures in place to direct and facilitate these investigations. Results from these specialized tests are not usually available in a timely manner. Hence, treatment and prevention strategies must be made based on clinical findings and test results available on site.

Algorithm

As mentioned previously, some clinical judgement is required when deciding what reactions to investigate more fully and the management strategies required. Aggressive investigation of mild reactions can burden resources within the healthcare setting and may cause unnecessary delays in transfusion therapy for a patient in critical need of blood components. In contrast, patient safety should always be paramount. The algorithm in Figure 6.1 can be used as a guide to develop a safe but logical approach to managing acute transfusion reactions.

Key points

1 Decisions related to the investigation of acute transfusion reactions require some clinical judgement based on the severity of the reactions (Figure 6.1).
2 Effective management decision making requires that healthcare professionals understand the types of acute transfusion reactions that can occur and their pathophysiology (Tables 6.1 and 6.2).
3 Patient factors to consider when formulating the differential diagnosis include the history of transfusion, pregnancy, medications, previous reactions, types of symptoms and diagnosis and clinical morbidities.
4 Component factors to consider when formulating the differential diagnosis include the type of component, leucocyte reduction status, volume transfused and component age.
5 Each institution must have policies and procedures for the investigation of acute reactions.

References

1 Braendstrup P, Bjerrum OW, Nielsen OJ, Jensen BA, Clausen NT, Hansen PB et al. Rituximab chimeric anti-CD20 monoclonal antibody treatment for adult refractory idiopathic thrombocytopenic purpura. Am J Hematol 2005; 78: 275–280.
2 Hendrickson JE & Hillyer CD. Noninfectious serious hazards of transfusion. Anesth Analg 2009; 108: 759–769.
3 Callum J, Lin Y, Pinkerton PH, Karkouti K, Pendergrast JM, Robitaille N et al. Bloody Easy 3, Blood Transfusions, Blood Alternatives and Transfusion Reactions: A

Guide to Transfusion Medicine [Internet], 2011 [cited 16 November 2011]. Available from: http://www.transfusionontario.org/media/BE_Mds/HOPE-SUN-BloodyEasy-EN_FINAL-LoRes.pdf.

4 Popovsky, M (ed.). *Transfusion Reactions*. Bethesda, MD: AABB Press; 2007.

5 Heddle N. Febrile nonhemolytic transfusion reactions. In: M Popovsky (ed.), *Transfusion Reactions*, 3rd edn. Bethesda, MD: AABB Press; 2007, pp. 57–103.

6 Ramirez-Arcos S, Goldman M & Blajchman M. Bacterial contamination. In: M Popovsky (ed.), *Transfusion Reactions*, 3rd edn. Bethesda, MD: AABB Press; 2007, pp. 163–206.

7 Vamvakas E. Allergic and anaphylactic reactions. In: M Popovsky (ed.), *Transfusion Reactions*, 3rd edn. Bethesda, MD: AABB Press; 2007, pp. 105–156.

8 Public Health Agency of Canada. *Guidelines for the Investigation of Suspected Transfusion Transmitted Bacterial Contamination* [Internet], 2007 [updated January 2008; cited 16 November 2011]. Available from: URL: http://www.phac-aspc.gc.ca/hcai-iamss/tti-it.

9 Stroncek DF, Fadeyi E & Adams S. Leukocyte antigen and antibody detection assays: tools for assessing and preventing pulmonary transfusion reactions. *Transfus Med Rev* 2007; 21: 273–286.

10 Vassallo RR. Review: IgA anaphylactic transfusion reactions. Part I. Laboratory diagnosis, incidence, and supply of IgA-deficient products. *Immunohematology* 2004; 20: 226–233.

11 Zhou L, Giacherio D, Cooling L & Davenport RD. Use of B-natriuretic peptide as a diagnostic marker in the differential diagnosis of transfusion-associated circulatory overload. *Transfusion* 2005; 45: 1056–1063.

Further reading

Bakdash S & Yazer MH. What every physician should know about transfusion reactions. *Can Med Assoc J* 2007; 177: 141–147.

Bux J & Sachs UJH. Pulmonary transfusion reactions. *Transf Med Hemotherapy* 2008; 35: 337–345.

Eder AF & Benjamin RJ. TRALI risk reduction: donor and component management strategies. *J Clin Apher.* 2009; 24: 122–129.

Eder AF & Chambers LA. Noninfectious complications of blood transfusion. *Arch Pathol Lab Med* 2007; 131: 708–718.

Sandler SG. How I manage patients suspected of having had an IgA anaphylactic transfusion reaction. *Transfusion* 2006; 46: 10–13.

Vamvakas EC & Blajchman MA. Blood still kills: six strategies to further reduce allogeneic blood transfusion-related mortality. *Transfus Med Rev* 2010; 24: 77–124.

Haemolytic transfusion reactions

Edwin J. Massey[1], Robertson D. Davenport[2] &
Richard M. Kaufman[3]

[1]Department of Pathology, NHS Blood and Transplant, Bristol, UK
[2]University of Michigan Health System, Ann Arbor, Michigan, USA
[3]Brigham and Womens Hospital, Boston, Massachusetts, USA

Definition of a haemolytic transfusion reaction

A haemolytic transfusion reaction (HTR) is the occurrence of lysis or accelerated clearance of red cells in a recipient of a blood transfusion. With few exceptions, these reactions are caused by immunological incompatibility between the blood donor and the recipient [1].

HTRs are usually classified with respect to the time of their occurrence following the transfusion but may also be classified on the pathophysiological basis of the site of red cell destruction, intravascular or extravascular. The classification used by the Serious Hazards of Transfusion (SHOT) haemovigilance scheme in the UK is as follows [2]:
• *Acute HTRs* (AHTRs) occur during or within 24 hours of the transfusion.
• *Delayed HTRs* (DHTRs) occur more than 24 hours after a transfusion, typically 5–7 days later.

In general, with some exceptions, intravascular haemolysis is seen in AHTRs and extravascular haemolysis in DHTRs. During intravascular haemolysis, the destroyed red cells release free haemoglobin and other red cell contents directly into the intravascular space. These reactions are characterized by gross haemoglobinaemia and haemoglobinuria, which can potentially precipitate renal and other organ failure.

During extravascular haemolysis, red cells are removed from circulation primarily by the spleen.

In these reactions the only feature may be a fall in haemoglobin (Hb), but clinically significant DHTRs can occur, which may contribute to morbidity and even mortality in patients who are otherwise compromised by single or multiple organ failure prior to the reaction.

Pathophysiology of HTRs

There are three phases involved (Figure 7.1):
• antibody binding to red cell antigens, which may involve complement activation;
• opsonized red cells interacting with and activating phagocytes; and
• production of inflammatory mediators.

Antigen–antibody interactions

Where an immunological incompatibility is responsible, the course of the reaction depends upon:
• the class and the subclass (in the case of IgG) of the antibody;
• the blood group specificity of the antibody;
• the thermal range of the antibody;
• the number, density and spatial arrangement of the red cell antigen sites;
• the ability of the antibody to activate complement;
• the concentration of antibody in the plasma; and
• the amount of red cells transfused.

Practical Transfusion Medicine, Fourth Edition. Edited by Michael F. Murphy, Derwood H. Pamphilon and Nancy M. Heddle.
© 2013 John Wiley & Sons, Ltd. Published 2013 by John Wiley & Sons, Ltd.

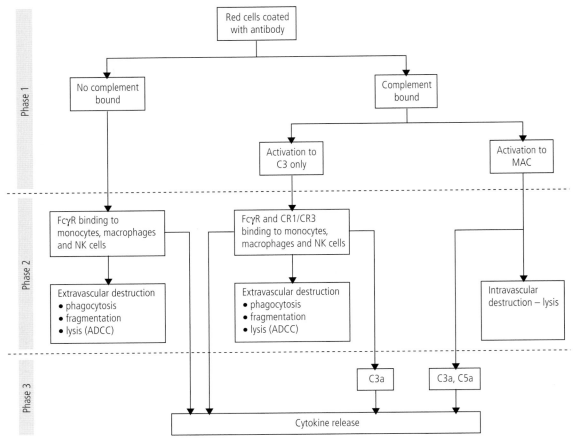

Fig 7.1 Pathophysiology of the haemolytic transfusion reaction (HTR). ADCC, antibody-dependent cell-mediated cytotoxicity; MAC, membrane attack complex; NK, natural killer.

The characteristics of the antibody and antigen

The characteristics of the antibody (such as immunoglobulin class, specificity and thermal range) and those of the antigen sites against which antibody activity is directed (such as site density and spatial arrangement) are interrelated. Antibodies of a certain specificity, from different individuals, are often found only within a particular immunoglobulin class and have similar thermal characteristics; in addition, red cells of a certain blood group phenotype, from different individuals, tend to be relatively homogeneous regarding the attributes of the relevant antigen. It is for this reason that knowledge of the specificity of an antibody can be highly informative in predicting its

clinical significance [3]. Three examples illustrate this concept.
• Anti-A, anti-B and anti-A,B antibodies are regularly present in moderate to high titre in the plasma of group O persons. These 'naturally occurring' antibodies are often both IgM and IgG, having a broad thermal range up to 37°C, and are often strongly complement-binding. The A and B antigens are often present in large numbers (e.g. up to 1.2×10^6 A_1 antigen sites per cell) and are strongly *immunogenic* (provoking an immune response in an individual lacking the antigen). If an individual who has anti-A, anti-B or anti-A,B in their plasma is transfused with donor red cells that express the cognate antigen (i.e. A and/or B), an AHTR is highly likely to occur, which may be

fatal. The infusion of group O donor plasma (200–300 ml in an adult pack of platelets or plasma) can similarly cause haemolysis of the recipient's red cells if they are A, AB or B; this will be discussed later in this chapter.

• Anti-Jk^a antibodies may be produced following immunization of a Jk(a–) person via pregnancy or transfusion. They are usually IgG (but may also have an IgM component), are active at 37°C and may be complement-binding. In Jk(a+b–) persons, there are about 1.4×10^4 Jk^a antigen sites per cell. Jk^a antigens are not particularly immunogenic; however, the antibody is sometimes difficult to detect in pretransfusion testing (because of the low titre of antibody); consequently, Jk(a+) blood may be inadvertently transfused to patients with pre-existing anti-Jk^a. These antibodies are frequently implicated in DHTRs.

• Anti-Lu^a antibodies may be produced following the immunization of an Lu(a–) person, or may be 'naturally occurring'. They are usually IgM (but often have IgA and IgG components), are only sometimes reactive at 37°C and are not usually complement-binding. The Lu^a antigens show variable distribution on the red cells of an individual and are poorly immunogenic. The antibody may not be detected in pretransfusion testing, because screening cells usually do not possess the Lu^a antigen and because antibody levels fall after immunization. Anti-Lu^a antibodies have not been implicated in AHTRs and have only rarely been implicated in DHTRs, which are usually mild.

Complement activation

Antibody-mediated intravascular haemolysis is caused by sequential binding of complement components (C1–C9) on the red cell membrane. IgM alloantibodies are more efficient activators of C1 than IgG antibodies, since the latter must be sufficiently close together on the red cell surface to be bridged by C1q in order to activate complement. Activation to the C5 stage leads to release of C5a into the plasma and assembly of the remaining components of the membrane attack complex (MAC) on the red cell surface, leading to lysis.

Extravascular haemolysis is caused by non-complement-binding IgG antibodies or those that bind sublytic amounts of complement. IgG subclasses differ in their ability to bind complement, with the following order of reactivity: IgG3>IgG1>IgG2>IgG4.

Activation of C3 leads to the release of C3a into the plasma and to C3b and iC3b deposition on red cells, promoting binding of the red cell to two complement receptors, CR1 (CD35) and CR3 (CD11b), which are both expressed on macrophages and monocytes. Hence, C3b and iC3b augment macrophage-mediated clearance of IgG-coated cells, and antibodies binding sublytic amounts of complement (e.g. Duffy and Kidd antibodies) often cause more rapid red cell clearance and more marked symptoms than non-complement-binding antibodies (e.g. Rh antibodies).

C3a and C5a are anaphylatoxins with potent proinflammatory effects including oxygen radical production, granule enzyme release from mast cells and granulocytes, nitric oxide production and cytokine production [4].

Fc receptor interactions

IgG alloantibodies bound to red cell antigens interact with phagocytes through Fc receptors. The affinity of Fc receptors for IgG subclasses varies, with most efficient binding to IgG1 and IgG3. After attachment to phagocytes, the red cells are either engulfed or lysed through antibody-dependent cell-mediated cytotoxicity (ADCC).

Cytokines

Cytokines are generated during an HTR as a consequence of both anaphylotoxin generation (C3a, C5a) and phagocyte Fc receptor interaction with red-cell-bound IgG. Some biological actions of cytokines implicated in HTRs are given in Table 7.1.

ABO incompatibility stimulates the release of high levels of tumour necrosis factor (TNF)-α into the plasma, within 2 hours, followed by CXCL-8 (interleukin (IL)-8) and CCL-2 (monocyte chemotactic protein (MCP)-1). In IgG-mediated haemolysis, TNF-α is produced at a lower level together with IL-1β and IL-6. CXCL-8 production follows a similar time course to that in ABO incompatibility.

IgG-mediated haemolysis, as opposed to ABO incompatibility, also results in the production of the IL-1 receptor antagonist, IL-1ra. The relative balance of IL-1 and IL-1ra may also, at least in part, account for some of the clinical differences between intravascular and extravascular haemolysis [5].

Table 7.1 Cytokines implicated in haemolytic transfusion reactions.

Terminology	Biological activity
Proinflammatory cytokines	
TNF, IL-1	Fever
	Hypotension, shock, death
	Mobilization of leucocytes from marrow
	Activation of T and B cells
	Induction of cytokines (IL-1, IL-6, CXCL-8, TNF-α, CCL-2)
	Induction of adhesion molecules
IL-6	Fever
	Acute-phase protein response
	B-cell antibody production
	T-cell activation
Chemokines	
CXCL-8	Chemotaxis of neutrophils
	Chemotaxis of lymphocytes
	Neutrophil activation
	Basophil histamine release
CCL-2	Chemotaxis of monocytes
	Induction of respiratory burst
	Induction of adhesion molecules
	Induction of IL-1
Anti-inflammatory cytokines	
IL-1ra	Competitive inhibition of IL-1 type I and II receptors

Table 7.2 Antibody specificities associated with haemolytic transfusion reactions.

Blood group system	Intravascular haemolysis	Extravascular haemolysis
ABO, H	A, B, H	
Rh		All
Kell	K	K, k, Kp^a, Kp^b, Js^a, Js^b
Kidd	Jk^a (Jk^b, Jk^3)	Jk^a, Jk^b, Jk^3
Duffy		Fy^a, Fy^b, Fy^3
MNS		M, S, s, U
Lutheran		Lu^b
Lewis	Le^a	
Cartwright		Yt^a
Vel	Vel	Vel
Colton		Co^a, Co^b
Dombrock		Do^a, Do^b

Antibody specificities associated with HTRs

These are given, together with the site of red cell destruction, in Table 7.2. A helpful review paper on the clinical significance of red cell antibodies has been written by Daniels *et al.* [3].

Acute HTRs

Aetiology and incidence

These reactions arise as a result of existing antibodies, in either the recipient or donor plasma, which are directed against red cell antigens of the other party. In the developed world, transfusion reactions resulting from incompatibility are more common as a cause of morbidity and mortality than transfusion-transmitted infection. This may not be the perception of patients, the public, politicians and even clinical staff. Incompatible transfusion can occur for the following reasons:

1 Clerical error. This can occur at the point of taking and labelling the sample, laboratory compatibility testing and blood allocation, collection of the blood component from the refrigerator, freezer or agitator and bedside checking at administration.

2 Undetected antibody. Kidd (Jk) antibodies are a typical example of antibodies that may be missed by sensitive testing systems.

3 Intentional provision of blood components as the best available, lowest risk choice when the 'perfect' blood component is not available (e.g. ORhD negative cde/cde in an emergency to a patient who subsequently proves to have anti-c).

The majority of AHTRs have historically been due to the transfusion of ABO-incompatible red cells, but can also be due to the administration of donor plasma containing high titres of ABO haemolysins when platelets or less commonly fresh frozen plasma of a different ABO blood group is transfused (classically group O donor plasma into a group A recipient). ABO-incompatible red cell transfusions are the result of the 'wrong' blood being given to the 'wrong' patient because of clerical or administrative errors, occurring at any stage during the transfusion process. ABO-incompatible platelet administration is unlikely to cause a reaction and such

Table 7.3 Errors resulting in 'wrong blood' incidents.

Prescription, sampling and request
  Failure to identify correct recipient at sampling
  Correct patient identity at sampling but incorrectly
    labelled sample
  Selection of incompatible products in an emergency
Transfusion laboratory
  Took a correctly identified sample and aliquoted it
    into an improperly labelled test tube for testing
  Took a wrongly identified sample through testing
  Tested the correct sample but misinterpreted the
    results
  Tested the correct sample but recorded the results on
    the wrong record
  Correctly tested the sample but labelled the wrong
    unit of blood as compatible for the patient
  Incorrect serological reasoning, e.g. O-positive FFP
    to non-O-positive recipient
Collection and delivery of the wrong component to the
  ward
  Failure to check recipient identity with unit identity
Bedside administration error
  Recipient identity checked through case notes or
    prescription chart and not wristband
  Wristband absent or incorrect

Table 7.4 Fatal acute haemolytic transfusion reactions reported to the FDA between 1976 and 1985.

Incompatibility	Number of deaths
O recipient and A red cells	80
O recipient and B/AB red cells	26
B recipient and A/AB red cells	12
A recipient and B red cells	6
O plasma to A/AB recipient	6
B plasma to AB recipient	1
Total ABO incompatibilities	131
Anti-K	5
Anti-EKP$_1$	1
Anti-Jk^b	1
Anti-Jk^{a}Jk^{b}Jk^3	1
Anti-Fy^a	1
Total non-ABO incompatibilities	9

transfusions are 'intentional' to utilize the short shelf-life platelet stock in an efficient manner (see below). More recently in the UK, serious errors in the transfusion process have become less frequent and morbidity and mortality following HTR is now more commonly due to antibodies other than ABO [2].

The Serious Hazards of Transfusion (SHOT) confidential reporting scheme has shown that in cases where the patient was transfused with a blood component or plasma product that did not meet the appropriate requirements or that was intended for another patient, the sites of primary error were clinical areas in 65% of cases, hospital laboratories in 34% of cases and blood establishments in 1% of cases. The reports have also highlighted that multiple errors contribute to incorrect blood component transfusion (IBCT). Examples of reported errors from several series are given in Table 7.3. Estimates of ABO-incompatible transfusions vary and may be underestimates, since some may be unrecognized or not reported, but two surveys have found a frequency of 1 in approximately 30 000 transfusions [6, 7].

Not all ABO-incompatible transfusions cause morbidity and mortality; mortality is dependent on the amount of incompatible red cells transfused and is reported to be 25% in recipients receiving 1–2 units of blood and reaches 44% with more than 2 units. However, as little as 30 mL group A cells given to a group O recipient can be fatal. Less frequently, Kell, Kidd and Duffy antibodies can be responsible and the acute reaction is due to a failure to detect, or take account of, the red cell alloantibody in either the antibody screen or cross-match.

Errors are a major cause of morbidity due to HTRs. In the UK the SHOT voluntary reporting scheme HTR has accounted for 501/8110 (6%) and IBCT 2837/8110 (35%) of errors reported. Nearly all deaths as a result of IBCT are due to ABO-incompatible transfusions and there have been 27 deaths in which IBCT was causal or contributory, between 1996 and 2010. Over the same period there have been 118 cases of major morbidity due to IBCT and 50 others attributable to acute and delayed HTR [2]. Similar findings have been noted in other countries; details of the incompatibilities resulting in deaths reported to the Food and Drug Administration between 1976 and 1985 are provided in Table 7.4 [8].

On a positive note, the SHOT voluntary reporting scheme has demonstrated an increase in overall reporting of errors and reactions but simultaneously the number of reported errors resulting in preventable major morbidity or mortality has fallen. HTR, in particular AHTR due to ABO incompatible transfusion, has decreased. There was also a 29% reduction of IBCT cases in 2010 [2]. This suggests that increased awareness of the hazards of transfusion has led to a lower threshold to report and an improvement in patient safety. This progress is probably due to a number of initiatives to improve hospital transfusion practice, including providing better training of the large number of staff involved at some stage of the transfusion process (see Chapter 23).

Symptoms and signs

These may become apparent within receiving as little as 20 mL of ABO-incompatible red cells. Initial clinical presentations include the following:
- fever, chills or both;
- pain at the infusion site or localized to the lower back/flanks, abdomen, chest or head;
- hypotension, tachycardia or both;
- agitation, distress and confusion, particularly in the elderly;
- nausea or vomiting;
- dyspnoea;
- flushing; and
- haemoglobinuria.

In anaesthetized patients, the only signs may be uncontrollable hypotension or excessive bleeding from the operative site, as a result of disseminated intravascular coagulation (DIC).

Some of these symptoms and signs can also be features of other transfusion reactions including bacterial contamination of the unit, allergic reactions, transfusion-related acute lung injury and febrile non-hemolytic reactions (see Chapters 8, 9 and 14).

Complications

Acute kidney injury develops in up to 36% of patients with AHTR as a result of acute tubular necrosis induced by both hypotension and DIC. Thrombus formation in renal arterioles may also cause cortical infarcts.

DIC develops in up to 10% of patients. TNF-α can induce tissue factor expression by endothelial cells and together with IL-1 can reduce the endothelial expression of thrombomodulin. Thromboplastic material is also liberated from leucocytes during the course of complement activation [5].

Immediate management of suspected AHTR (see Chapter 6)

Actions for nursing staff

In the presence of a fever of more than 1°C above the patient's pretransfusion temperature and/or any symptoms or signs mentioned above, the nursing staff should:
- stop the transfusion, leaving the infusion line ('giving set') attached to the blood pack;
- use a new giving set and keep an intravenous infusion running with normal saline;
- call a member of the medical staff;
- check that the patient identity as provided on the wristband corresponds with that given on the label on the blood pack and on the compatibility form;
- save any urine the patient passes for later examination for haemoglobinuria; and
- monitor the patient's pulse (P), blood pressure (BP) and temperature (T) at 15-minute intervals.

Actions for medical staff

The immediate actions depend upon the presenting symptoms and signs, and are summarized in Table 7.5.

Investigation of suspected AHTR

Blood samples should be taken from a site other than the infusion site for the investigations listed in Table 7.6.

Other reactions characterized by haemolysis

In patients with autoimmune haemolytic anaemia, transfusion may exacerbate the haemolysis and be associated with haemoglobinuria.

Donor units of red cells may also be haemolysed as a result of:
- bacterial contamination;
- excessive warming;
- erroneous freezing;
- addition of drugs or intravenous fluids;
- trauma from extracorporeal devices; or
- red cell enzyme deficiency.

Table 7.5 Immediate medical management of an acute transfusion reaction.

Symptoms/signs	Likely diagnosis	Actions
Isolated fever or fever and shivering, stable observations, correct unit given	Febrile nonhaemolytic transfusion reaction (FNHTR)	Paracetamol 1 g orally/per os (PO) (in the US acetaminophen 625 mg), continue transfusion slowly observations of P, BP and T every 15 min for 1 h, then hourly. If no improvement then call haematology medical staff
Pruritus and/or urticaria	Allergic transfusion reaction	Chlorpheniramine 10 mg IV (US: diphenhydramine 25–50 mg PO or IV) and other actions as for suspected FNHTR
Any other symptoms/signs, hypotension or incorrect unit	Assume to be an acute haemolytic transfusion reaction in first instance	Discontinue transfusion, normal/saline to maintain urine output >1 mL/kg/h. Full and continuous monitoring of vital signs. Call haematology medical and transfusion laboratory staff immediately for further advice/action. Send discontinued unit of blood with attached giving set and other empty packs, after clamping securely, to the transfusion laboratory

Table 7.6 Laboratory investigation of suspected acute haemolytic transfusion reaction.

Blood test	Rationale/findings
Full blood count	Baseline parameters, red cell agglutinates on film
Plasma/urinary haemoglobin	Evidence of intravascular haemolysis
Haptoglobin, bilirubin, LDH	Evidence of intravascular or extravascular haemolysis
Blood group	Comparison of posttransfusion and retested pretransfusion samples, to detect ABO error not apparent at bedside. Unexpected ABO antibodies posttransfusion may result from transfused incompatible plasma. The donor ABO group should be confirmed
Direct antiglobin test (DAT)	Positive in majority, pretransfusion sample should be tested for comparison. May be negative if all incompatible cells destroyed
Compatibility testing	An IAT antibody screen and IAT cross-match using the pre- and posttransfusion sample provide evidence for the presence of alloantibody. Elution of antibody from posttransfusion red cells may aid identification of antibody or confirm specificities identified in serum in cases of non-ABO incompatibility. Red cell phenotype should also be performed on recipient pretransfusion sample and unit in cases of non-ABO incompatibility, to confirm absence in patient and presence in unit of corresponding antigen
Urea/creatinine and electrolytes	Baseline renal function
Coagulation screen	Detection of incipient DIC
Blood cultures from the patient and implicated pack(s)	In event of septic reaction caused by bacterial contamination of unit, which may be suspected from inspection of pack for lysis, altered colour or clots

Management of a confirmed AHTR

The management of haemolytic transfusion reactions should be determined by the severity of the clinical manifestations.

- Maintain adequate renal perfusion while avoiding volume overload by:
    (a) maintenance of circulating volume with crystalloid and/or colloid infusions and,
    (b) if necessary, inotropic support.
- Transfer to a high dependency area where continuous monitoring can take place.
- Repeat coagulation and biochemistry screens 2- to 4-hourly.
- If urinary output cannot be maintained at 1 mL/kg/h, seek expert renal advice.
- Haemofiltration or dialysis may be required for the acute tubular necrosis.
- In the event of the development of DIC, blood component therapy may be required.
- Having ascertained the nature of the incompatibility causing the AHTR, transfusion of compatible blood may be required for life-threatening anaemia.

Prevention of AHTRs

Prevention of 'wrong blood' incidents

- Prevention of the multiplicity of errors that can contribute to the transfusion of ABO-incompatible red cells must depend upon the creation of an effective quality system for the entire process, which will involve:
    (a) adherence to national guidelines and standards;
    (b) local procedures that are agreed, documented and validated;
    (c) training and retraining of key staff;
    (d) regular error analysis and review;
    (e) reporting to local Risk Management/Assurance Committee; and
    (f) reporting to regulatory bodies such as the Medicines and Healthcare Products Regulatory Agency (MHRA) in the UK, the Food and Drug Administration in the USA and to national haemovigilance schemes to contribute to the understanding of the extent and underlying causes.
    These aspects are specifically covered in Chapter 23.
- Since the majority of errors leading to an ABO-incompatible transfusion are due to misidentification of the patient or patient's sample, due attention must be paid to the comprehensive use of unique patient identifiers throughout the hospital and automation within the laboratory [2, 9, 10].
- Access to previous transfusion records containing historical ABO groups should be available at all times.
- It is desirable that computerized systems are used to verify at the bedside the matches between the patient and the sample taken for compatibility testing, and at the time of transfusion between the patient and the unit of blood.

Prevention of non-ABO AHTRs

- In the case of recurrently transfused patients, due attention should be paid to the interval between sampling and transfusion, to optimize the detection of newly developing antibodies. In the UK for patients transfused within the previous 14 days, the pretransfusion sample should not be taken more than 3 days before the next transfusion [11, 12]. In the USA the pretransfusion sample must be obtained within 3 days (72 hours) if the patient has been transfused or pregnant within the past three months. Similar requirements exist in other countries.
- In the presence of multiple red cell alloantibodies, when it is not feasible to obtain compatible red cells in an emergency, intravenous immunoglobulin (1 g/kg/day for 3 days) and/or steroids (hydrocortisone 100 mg 6-hourly or methylprednisolone 1 g daily for 3 days) have been used with anecdotal reports of ameliorating a potential haemolytic or 'hyperhaemolytic' episode (see below).

Delayed HTRs

Aetiology and incidence

With few exceptions, DHTRs are due to secondary immune responses following re-exposure to a given red cell antigen. The recipient has been primarily sensitized to the antigen in pregnancy or as a result of a previous blood transfusion and a few days after a subsequent transfusion there is a rapid increase in the antibody concentration, resulting in the destruction of red cells.

- The antibodies most commonly implicated and reported to SHOT between 1996 and 2006 were those from the Kidd blood group system followed by those from the Rh, Duffy and Kell systems. One analysis showed that in approximately 10% of reported cases, more than one alloantibody was found in the serum [13].

• Frequently, there are no clinical signs of red cell destruction, but subsequent patient investigations reveal a positive direct antiglobulin test (DAT) and the emergence of a red cell antibody. This situation has been termed a delayed serological transfusion reaction (DSTR) [14].

• Kidd and Duffy antibodies are more likely to cause symptoms and be associated with a DHTR rather than a DSTR.

• Estimates of the frequency of DHTR and DSTR vary, but in a series reported from the Mayo Clinic, the frequency of DHTR was 1 in 5405 units and of DSTR was 1 in 2990 units, giving a combined frequency of 1 in 1899 units transfused [15].

• DHTRs are in themselves rarely fatal, although in association with the underlying disease can lead to mortality.

• Of transfusion fatalities reported to the United States Food and Drug Administration (FDA) between 1976 and 1985 10% were due to DHTR; in 75% of cases, more than one alloantibody was present in the serum and the same proportion involved non-Rh antibodies.

• Six deaths reported to SHOT between 1996 and 2006 have been due to DHTRs [13]. Tragically, in some instances there were delays in diagnosis, investigation and provision of compatible units, which led to marked anaemia and contributed to mortality.

Signs and symptoms

These usually appear within 5–10 days following the transfusion, but intervals as short as 24 hours and as late as 41 days have been recorded. The exact onset may be difficult to define since haemolysis can be initially insidious and may only be appreciated from results of posttransfusion samples. The commonest features are:

• fever;
• fall in haemoglobin concentration; and
• jaundice and hyperbilirubinemia.

Hypotension and kidney injury are uncommon (6% of cases). In the postoperative period in particular, the diagnosis may be overlooked and the symptoms and signs incorrectly attributed to continuing haemorrhage or sepsis. In the setting of sickle cell disease,

DHTR can be particularly severe with destruction of autologous red cells (hyperhaemolysis) (see below).

Management

The majority of DHTRs require no treatment because red cell destruction occurs gradually as antibody synthesis increases. Haemolysis may, however, contribute to the development of life-threatening anaemia, particularly in patients with ongoing bleeding, and urgent investigations are required to ensure the timely provision of antigen-negative units.

Expert medical advice may be required for treatment of the hypotension and renal failure. When accompanied by circulatory instability and renal insufficiency, a red cell exchange transfusion with antigen-negative units can curtail the haemolytic process. Future transfusions of red cells should also be negative for the antigen in question.

Investigation of suspected DHTR (see Chapter 6)

• The peripheral blood film is likely to show spherocytosis.

• Other evidence of haemolysis – namely hyperbilirubinaemia, elevated lactate dehydrogenase (LDH), reduced serum haptoglobin, haemoglobinaemia, haemoglobinuria and haemosiderinuria – is useful to confirm the nature of the reaction and to monitor progress.

• The DAT usually becomes positive within a few days of the transfusion until the incompatible cells have been eliminated.

• Further serological testing on pre- and posttransfusion samples should be undertaken in accordance with the schedule provided for AHTR.

• The antibody may not be initially apparent in the posttransfusion serum but can be eluted from the red cells. If the red cell eluate is inconclusive, then a repeat sample should be taken after 7–10 days, to allow for an increase in antibody titre. However, additional, more sensitive techniques may have to be employed to detect the antibody and it is advisable to seek the help of a reference laboratory.

• Since a significant proportion of cases have more than one alloantibody in the serum, it is important that the panels used for antibody identification have sufficient cells of appropriate phenotypes to exclude additional specificities.

Prevention

Access to previous transfusion records may disclose the presence of antibodies undetectable at the time of cross-matching, and all patients should be questioned regarding previous transfusions and pregnancies. Patients found to have developed a clinically significant red cell alloantibody should be provided with an antibody card. When the care of patients requiring transfusion support is shared between hospitals, there must be adequate communication between laboratories and clinical teams.

Laboratories should ensure that their antibody screen is effective in detecting weak red cell alloantibodies and that screening cells are taken from homozygotes where the corresponding antibodies show a dosage effect (i.e. they are less easy to detect when red cells with heterozygous expression of the relevant antigen are used rather than cells with homozygous expression). Pretransfusion testing is covered in detail in Chapter 23.

Haemolysis resulting from haemopoietic stem cell transplantation (see Chapter 41)

Major ABO incompatible transplants

Infusion of bone marrow during major ABO-incompatible transplants can result in an AHTR (the recipient has antibodies against the donor's red cells, e.g. group A donor, group O recipient). The risk is dependent on the antibody titre of the recipient and the volume of red cells in the marrow harvest. Peripheral blood stem cell products rarely have enough red cells to result in clinical AHTR even if there is ABO incompatibility.

Minor ABO incompatible transplants

Most patients transplanted with minor ABO-incompatible marrow (the donor has antibodies against the recipient's red cells, e.g. O donor, A recipient) develop a positive DAT, but only 10–15% of patients develop clinically significant haemolysis. Haemolysis in minor ABO incompatibility is short-lived and exchange transfusion is rarely required. Red cells and plasma-containing components (platelets, FFP and cryoprecipitate) should be compatible with both recipient and donor.

It has been suggested that the use of peripheral blood stem cells may increase the risk of significant haemolysis since the number of lymphocytes infused with the graft is increased, and three deaths due to an AHTR were reported between 1997 and 1999 in minor ABO-incompatible transplants. Several cases due to anti-D have been described, and antibody production has persisted for up to 1 year [16].

Delayed haemolysis following organ transplantation (passenger lymphocyte syndrome)

Donor-derived B lymphocytes within the transplanted organ may mount an anamnestic response against the recipient's red cell antigens. Donor-derived antibodies are usually directed against antigens within the ABO and Rh systems. If ABO mismatched organs are transplanted, the frequency of occurrence of donor-derived antibodies and haemolysis increases with the lymphoid content of the graft, from kidney to liver to heart–lung transplants. The figures for haemolysis are 9%, 29% and 70%, respectively. The frequency of haemolysis increases with an O donor and an A recipient. Pretransplant isohaemaglutinin titres do not appear to predict the incidence or severity of haemolysis. The ABO antibodies, which appear 7–10 days after transplant, last for approximately one month. Haemolysis is usually mild, although several cases of renal failure and one death have been reported. It can be prevented by switching to group O cells, either at the end of surgery or postoperatively if the DAT becomes positive.

Rh antibodies have been described following kidney, liver and heart–lung transplants. They can cause haemolysis for up to 6 months, which can be sufficiently severe to merit therapy.

Haemolysis occurs 7–10 days after transplantation, with an unpredictable and abrupt onset [17].

Hyperhaemolytic transfusion reactions and haemolytic transfusion reactions in sickle cell disease

The frequency of alloimmunization in sickle cell anaemia is dependent upon the nature and success of the extended red cell antigen-matching policy employed. Approximately, 40% of patients who are alloimmunized have experienced or will experience a DHTR.

Although DHTRs are characteristically mild in other groups of recipients, they can be responsible for major morbidity in sickle cell disease. The term 'sickle cell haemolytic transfusion reaction (SCHTR) syndrome' has been suggested to capture some of the distinctive features that can be seen to accompany a reaction. A similar syndrome has been described in other transfusion-dependent patients, so the term 'hyperhaemolytic transfusion reaction (HHTR)' may be more appropriate. These features are as follows:
• symptoms suggestive of a sickle cell pain crisis that develop or are intensified during the HTR;
• marked reticulocytopenia (relative to pretransfusion levels);
• development of a more severe anaemia after transfusion than was present before. This may be due to the suppression of erythropoiesis as a result of the transfusion but hyperhaemolysis of autologous red cells (bystander immune haemolysis) has also been suggested. There have been reports that bone marrow aspirates performed on patients suffering from this complication have shown evidence of active erythropoiesis during the reticulocytopenic phase and haemophagocytosis. This has led to the suggestion that erythroid precursors and reticulocytes are removed by adhesion to monocytes via other mechanisms, in addition to IgG and Fc receptors, such as the integrins $\alpha 4\beta 1$ and VCAM-1;
• subsequent transfusions may further exacerbate the anaemia and it may become fatal; and
• patients often have multiple red blood cell alloantibodies and may also have autoantibodies, which make it difficult or impossible to find compatible units of red blood cells.

However, in other patients the DAT may be negative, no alloantibodies are identified and serological studies may not provide an explanation for the HTR; even red cells that are phenotypically matched with multiple patient antigens may be haemolysed.

Management involves withholding further transfusion and treating with corticosteroids (hydrocortisone 100 mg 6-hourly or methylprednisolone 1 g daily for 3 days), while IVIG (1 g/kg/day) may have been beneficial in some cases [18].

It is recommended that patients with sickle cell disease are phenotyped prior to transfusion and that blood is matched for Rhc, C, D, e, E and K (see Chapter 28).

Acute haemolysis from ABO-incompatible platelet transfusions

Rarely, the passive transfusion of anti-A or anti-B present in a platelet pack will cause haemolysis in the recipient. This is most commonly seen in type A recipients of type O platelets. Clinically significant reactions are rare: passive anti-A/B becomes diluted in the recipient's plasma and it will also bind to A or B antigen, both soluble in the recipient's plasma and on endothelial cells. The typical anti-A/B titre in a platelet donor is on the order of 1:128, but occasionally donors will have very high titres exceeding 10 000. Severe and even fatal AHTRs have been reported, particularly in cases where a large amount of incompatible ABO antibody is transfused into a recipient with a small plasma volume (e.g. pediatric patient). In the UK, all platelet units are required to be screened for anti-A/B using a cut-off titre of 1:100. Packs from donors who have titres below this level are marked 'HT-negative' or high titre negative. Approximately 10% of platelet units will have titres above 1:100 and will not be marked 'HT-negative'; these are restricted to ABO-identical recipients. In the USA, no preventative strategy is currently mandated and local practices vary. AABB accredited transfusion services are simply required to have a policy concerning the transfusion of products having significant amounts of incompatible ABO antibodies.

Key points

1 HTRs are the second commonest cause in the UK and the USA of immediate morbidity and mortality following a transfusion (the most common cause is transfusion-related acute lung injury, TRALI).
2 The clinical presentations are diverse and they can be unrecognized or misdiagnosed.
3 Most fatal AHTRs have historically been due to the transfusion of ABO-incompatible red cells but there is evidence that increased transfusion safety awareness has reduced the frequency of ABO incompatible red cell transfusion. Other causes of AHTR are overtaking ABO in countries where haemovigilance schemes have been successful.

4 The transfusion of ABO-incompatible red cells is the result of an error occurring at any stage in the transfusion process. Patient identification errors are the most frequent culprit.

5 Devising and successfully implementing measures to overcome these preventable and fatal errors is a challenge but should be a priority for those involved in hospital transfusion.

References

1 Beauregard P & Blajchman MA. Haemolytic and pseudo-haemolytic transfusion reactions: an overview of the haemolytic transfusion reactions and the clinical conditions that mimic them. *Transfus Med Rev* 1994; 8: 184–199.

2 Serious Hazards of Transfusion. *Annual Report 2010*. Manchester: SHOT Office. ISBN 978-0-9558648-3-4. Available at: www.shotuk.org.

3 Daniels G, Poole J, de Silva M, Callaghan T, MacLennan S & Smith N. The clinical significance of blood group antibodies. *Transfusion Medicine* 2002; 12(5): 287–295.

4 Davenport RD. Hemolytic transfusion reactions. In: MA Popovsky (ed.), *Transfusion Reactions*, 2nd edn. Bethesda, MD: AABB Press; 2001, pp. 2–36.

5 Davenport RD. Pathophysiology of hemolytic transfusion reactions. *Seminars in Hematology* 2005 July; 42(3): 165–168.

6 Linden JV, Wagner K, Voytovich AE & Sheehan J. Transfusion errors in New York State: an analysis of 10 years experience. *Transfusion* 2000; 40(10): 1207–1213.

7 Stainsby D. ABO incompatible transfusions – experience from the UK Serious Hazards of Transfusion (SHOT) scheme. *Transfusion Clinique et Biologique* 2005; 12(5): 385–388.

8 Sazama K. Reports of 355 transfusion-associated deaths: 1976 through 1985. *Transfusion* 1990; 30: 583–590.

9 National Patient Safety Agency. *Right Patient, Right Blood*. Safer Practice Notice No. 14. London: NPSA; 2006. Available at: www.npsa.nhs.uk.

10 National Patient Safety Agency. *Standardising Patient Wristbands Improves Patient Safety*. Safer Practice Notice No. 24. London: NPSA; 2007. Available at: www.npsa.nhs.uk.

11 British Committee for Standards in Haematology. Guidelines for pre-transfusion compatibility procedures in blood transfusion laboratories. Available at http://www.bcshguidelines.com/documents/Compat_Guideline_for_submission_to_TTF_011012.pdf (accessed November 15, 2012).

12 Milkins CE, Berryman J, Cantwell C, Elliott C & Rowley M. Timing of sample collection in relation to previous transfusion: a proposal for changing the recommendations. British Blood Transfusion Society Annual Conference prize winning poster 2010. http://hospital.blood.co.uk/library/pdf/Bloodlines_Issue_98.pdf (p. 27).

13 Stainsby D, Jones H, Asher D, Atterbury C, Bonicelli A, Brant L, Chapman C, Davidson K, Gerrard R, Gray A, Knowles S, Love E, Milkins C, McClelland B, Norfolk D, Soldan K, Taylor C, Revill J, Williamson L & Cohen H. Serious hazards of transfusion: a decade of haemovigilance in the UK. *Transfus Med Reviews* 2006; 20(4): 273–282.

14 Vamvakas EC, Pineda AA, Reisner R, Santrach PJ & Moore SB. The differentiation of delayed haemolytic and delayed serologic transfusion reactions: incidence and predictors of haemolysis. *Transfusion* 1995; 35: 26–32.

15 Pineda AA, Vamvakas EC, Gorden LD, Winters JL & Moore SB. Trends in the incidence of delayed hemolytic and delayed serologic transfusion reactions. *Transfusion* 1999; 39(10): 1097–1103.

16 Daniel-Johnson J & Schwartz J. How do I approach ABO-incompatible hematopoietic progenitor cell transplantation? *Transfusion* 2011; 51(6): 1143–1149.

17 Petz LD. Immune hemolysis associated with transplantation. *Semin Hematol* 2005; 42: 145–155.

18 Win N, Sinha S, Lee E & Mills W. Treatment with intravenous immunoglobulin and steroids may correct severe anemia in hyperhemolytic transfusion reactions: case report and literature review. *Transfus Med Rev* 2010; 24 (1): 64–67.

Further reading

Daniels G. *Human Blood Groups*, 2nd edn. Oxford: Blackwell Science; 2002.

Food and Drug Administration. *Fatalities Reported to FDA Following Blood Collection and Transfusion: Annual Summary for Fiscal Year 2010*. Available at: http://www.fda.gov/BiologicsBloodVaccines/SafetyAvailability/ReportaProblem/TransfusionDonationFatalities/ucm254802.htm.

Klein H & Anstee D. Haemolytic transfusion reactions. In: HG Klein & D Anstee (eds), *Mollison's Blood Transfusion in Clinical Medicine*. Oxford: Backwell Science; 2006.

Popovsky MA. *Transfusion Reactions*, 3rd edn. Bethesda, MD: AABB Press; 2007.

Serious Hazards of Transfusion (SHOT) resources and reports. Available at: www.shotuk.org.

Win N. The clinical significance of blood group alloantibodies and the supply of blood for transfusion; 2007. Available at: http://hospital.blood.co.uk/library/clinical_guidelines_and_policies_from_nhsbt.

8

Febrile and allergic transfusion reactions

Mark K. Fung[1] *& Nancy M. Heddle*[2]

[1]Department of Pathology, University of Vermont and Fletcher Allen Health Care, Burlington, Vermont, USA
[2]Department of Medicine, McMaster University and Canadian Blood Services, Hamilton, Canada

Febrile and allergic reactions are the most common acute adverse events that occur during or following the transfusion of blood components. Signs and symptoms typical of these reactions can also be associated with other types of transfusion reactions and/or caused by treatments and medications that the patient may be receiving as well as comorbidities; hence, to establish causation and an appropriate management strategy can be challenging. In this chapter, febrile nonhaemolytic transfusion reactions (FNHTRs) and both mild and severe forms of allergic reactions will be discussed.

Febrile nonhaemolytic transfusion reactions

Clinical presentation

The classical definition of an FNHTR includes fever (usually defined as $\geq 1°C$ rise in temperature) during or within 2 hours of completing the transfusion, along with other symptoms that can include a cold feeling, chills and a generalized feeling of discomfort. Less frequently headache, nausea and vomiting may also occur and in severe reactions rigors can be present. Although this is the classical definition, in practice only 15% of patients develop a fever, with chills, cold and discomfort being the primary findings [1].

Differential diagnosis

Unfortunately, these symptoms are not specific for an FNHTR. The challenge for the transfusing physician is to consider the other possibilities as part of the differential diagnosis and to develop a systematic approach for establishing a definitive diagnosis. When a patient presents with fever, the differential diagnosis should include:
- FNHTR;
- acute haemolytic reactions;
- delayed haemolytic reactions;
- bacterial contamination;
- transfusion-related acute lung injury (TRALI);
- acute pain reactions;
- comorbid conditions; and
- medications.

Although all of these reactions can be associated with fever, it is especially important to rule out acute haemolysis, bacterial contamination and TRALI, as these conditions can frequently be associated with morbidity and mortality unless rapidly recognized and treated. Bacterial contamination and TRALI also have implications for donor management and handling of other components prepared from the implicated donation, emphasizing the importance of considering these types of reactions in the differential diagnosis (see Chapters 9 and 14). In contrast, FNHTRs cause discomfort and distress, although not long-term morbidity, for the patient and consume additional healthcare

Practical Transfusion Medicine, Fourth Edition. Edited by Michael F. Murphy, Derwood H. Pamphilon and Nancy M. Heddle.
© 2013 John Wiley & Sons, Ltd. Published 2013 by John Wiley & Sons, Ltd.

resources for their treatment and investigation. Preliminary data were recently published suggesting that patients who experience FNHTR may be more likely to develop red cell alloimmunization. The hypothesis to explain this observation is that cytokines involved in causing FNHTR may alter the immune system towards a Th2 response to foreign red cell antigens, resulting in an increased risk of alloimmunizations [2]. Although this hypothesis needs to be confirmed, it illustrates the potential for secondary sequelae to be associated with FNHTR, emphasizing the importance of preventing this adverse event.

To further complicate the investigative process in patient populations where transfusion-associated fever occurs frequently, e.g. in haematology/oncology patients, clinical judgement should be incorporated into the decision-making process.

Frequency

The frequency of FNHTRs varies with the:
- patient population;
- type of blood components being transfused;
- age of the blood component.

Reactions to platelets occur more frequently than reactions to red cells. However, precise estimates of FNHTR associated with platelet transfusions are difficult as milder reactions are likely to be underreported. In a general hospital population, FNHTRs to red cells occur with 0.04–0.44% of transfusions, while the frequency of reactions to platelets is higher, ranging from 0.06 to 2.2%. In specific patient populations such as adult haematology/oncology patients, reactions to platelets are even more common, occurring in up to 37% of transfusions if non-leucocyte-reduced platelets are used [1]. When pre-storage leucocyte-reduced platelets are transfused, the frequency of acute reactions decreases dramatically (<2% of transfusions) [3]. In paediatric ICU patients 1.6% of blood components transfused (40/2509) were associated with acute reactions, with FNHTR accounting for 60% (24/40) of these events [4]. FNHTRs to blood components other than red cells and platelets are rare and there are limited data to estimate their frequency.

Pathogenesis

The pathogenesis of FNHTRs is multifactorial and varies for red cells and platelets. Our current understanding of the mechanisms causing these reactions with red cells and platelets are summarized below.

- *Antibody mechanism.* Patients' plasma contains a leucocyte antibody that reacts with leucocytes present in the blood component. An antigen–antibody reaction occurs, resulting in the release of endogenous pyrogens/cytokines by the donor leucocytes. These biological response modifiers act on the hypothalamus to cause fever. This antigen–antibody hypothesis is believed to be the primary mechanism causing FNHTRs to red cells, but probably accounts for less than 10% of FNHTRs to platelets [1].

- *Leucocyte/platelet-derived biological response modifiers.* During storage of the blood component, proinflammatory cytokines (interleukin 1 (IL-1), interleukin 6 (IL-6) and tumour necrosis factor α (TNFα)) are released from leucocytes present in the blood component. This typically happens when the component is stored at room temperature. Cytokines accumulate to high levels by the end of the product storage period and, when infused, cause fever by stimulation of the hypothalamus. This is the primary mechanism responsible for FNHTRs to platelets. Platelets are stored at room temperature for a maximum of 5 days and have high cytokine concentrations at the end of the storage period if contaminating leucocytes are present [5]. Platelet-derived cytokines such as CD40 ligand (sCD40L) and RANTES also accumulate in stored platelets and may play a role in some reactions. When the receptor for CD40L is engaged, proinflammatory cytokines are synthesized (IL-6, IL-8, monocyte chemotactic protein-1 (MCP-1)). One study suggested an incremental effect where reactions were more frequent when high levels of multiple biological response mediators were present [6]. There are over 15 different cytokines that have been shown to accumulate in platelet products during storage.

- *Other biological response modifiers (BRMs).* Other BRMs such as complement and neutrophil priming lipids have been detected in some stored blood components and it is hypothetically possible that they may cause or contribute to FNHTRs in some patients. However, there are no clinical data linking these substances to an increased risk of an adverse event [1].

Patient susceptibility

Patient factors may also play a role in susceptibility to FNHTRs. Reactions caused by leucocyte antibodies may be more common in females due to leucocyte antibody formation during pregnancy. Patients whose disease or treatments result in an inflammatory response may also be more likely to have reactions as the additive effect of transfusion-related cytokines may be sufficient to cause the symptoms and signs of FNHTRs. Recent data also suggests that certain gene polymorphisms may result in an increase in inflammatory cytokine gene expression, resulting in an increased susceptibility to FNHTR. One genotype that has been shown to increase susceptibility for FNHTRs is *IL1RN*2.2* [7].

Management of FNHTRs

The management of FNHTRs includes the exclusion of other causes of fever. However, the management strategy requires clinical judgement and must balance the benefits and risks of their investigation and treatment. The following questions should be considered.

• *Is the blood component leucocyte reduced*? The risk of an FNHTR in a setting where all red cell and platelet components are universally pre-storage leucocyte reduced is low (see above). In this latter situation, stopping the transfusion and investigating every reaction not only consumes significant healthcare resources but may put patients at risk as they may not receive the required components in a timely manner.

• *Does the patient have a history of FNHTRs*? Some patients are susceptible to repeated FNHTRs when blood components are transfused, e.g. because of the presence of leucocyte antibodies; hence the patient's history of reaction should be considered.

• *If a temperature increase occurred, was it greater than or equal to 2°C*? It is very uncommon for the temperature to rise more than 2°C with an FNHTR. In this situation, bacterial contamination should be suspected, the transfusion should be stopped immediately and appropriate investigations initiated.

• *Would you describe the patient's signs and symptoms as mild, moderate or severe*? If the symptoms are mild, a less aggressive management approach may be initiated but careful observation of the patient is essential. If the symptoms are severe, the transfusion should be stopped immediately and supportive care given to the patient. Investigations to rule out other possible causes of the reaction should be initiated. If

the clinical findings are categorized as moderate, the questions above need to be considered and clinical judgement is required as to how patient management should proceed.

Finally, the management strategy for FNHTRs associated with red cell transfusions should include an approach to rule out an acute haemolytic transfusion reaction. Haemolysis following platelet transfusion is rare but can occur when the plasma of the platelet product contains a high titre ABO antibody that reacts with the patient's red cells.

The management approach should also aim to alleviate the signs and symptoms associated with an FNHTR. This may involve temporary discontinuation of the transfusion while antipyretic medication is administered to the patient. Medications should never be injected into the blood component. In most cases, the transfusion can be resumed once the signs and symptoms subside. There is some evidence that pethidine (or meperidine in North America) is effective treatment for alleviating rigors associated with transfusions.

A conservative strategy for minimizing the risk to patients while investigating reactions would include the following steps:

• Temporarily stop the transfusion but keep the line open with saline.

• Perform a bedside clerical check between the blood and the patient to ensure that the right blood has been transfused.

• Observe the blood component to determine if there is discoloration or particulate matter present.

• Notify the blood transfusion laboratory and send appropriate samples if laboratory investigations are deemed necessary to rule out other causes of acute reactions with fever.

Prevention of FNHTRs

As the pathogenesis of FNHTRs is different for red cells and platelet transfusions, the strategy for their prevention also depends on the blood component being transfused.

Red cells

Since most reactions are caused by the leucocyte antigen–antibody mechanism, the primary way to prevent these reactions is to reduce the number of leucocytes in the red cell component. Prevention can be accomplished for most patients by removing approximately one log of leucocytes to a level of less than or equal to 10^8 leucocytes/unit of red cells. This can be achieved by post-storage filtration, centrifugation with buffy coat removal (either during the manufacturing process or post-storage) or pre-storage filtration during the component preparation phase. Filtration (pre- or post-storage) using current leucocyte reduction filters results in red cell products with less than 10^6 leucocytes, which is well below the threshold needed to prevent most FNHTRs. If a patient still reacts to a leucocyte-reduced red cell product, other options for preventing future reactions include washing and/or selecting fresher blood for transfusion [1].

Platelets

Most platelet reactions (90%) are caused by leucocyte-derived cytokine accumulation during storage. Hence, post-storage leucocyte reduction is not an effective strategy for preventing these reactions. FNHTRs to platelets can be prevented by pre-storage leucocyte reduction by either filtration or centrifugation (buffy coat method of platelet preparation). If pre-storage leucocyte-reduced platelets are not available, the plasma supernatant on the stored platelets can be removed and replaced with a suitable platelet additive solution washing to remove the cytokine-rich plasma, or fresher platelets (≤ 3 days of storage) can be transfused [1].

Premedication

Premedication of the patient with an antipyretic drug, paracetamol in the UK and acetaminophen in North America, has become standard practice to prevent FNHTRs. Aspirin should not be used as a premedication in any patient requiring platelet transfusions as it affects platelet function. In some centres, it is routine practice to premedicate all patients prior to transfusion. However, there are no clinical data to justify this universal approach and when using leucocyte-reduced blood components such a practice is not warranted. However, patients with recurrent FNHTRs can be treated with an antipyretic approximately 30 minutes prior to starting the transfusion, which should help to alleviate or prevent symptoms [8, 9].

Allergic transfusion reactions

Clinical presentation

Allergic transfusion reactions can be either nonsystemic/localized or systemic/generalized and are classified as mild, moderate or severe.

• Nonsystemic reactions are usually mild, consisting of urticaria and occasionally focal angioedema. These are benign and self-limiting though still cause symptoms that are distressing to the patient. However, such mild reactions may progress to more severe and systemic reactions with repeated transfusions.

• Systemic reactions range from moderate (generalized urticaria) to severe and life-threatening. Although urticaria is considered a pathognomonic finding for an allergic reaction, cutaneous signs or symptoms may not always be present in severe allergic reactions. Severe reactions usually present with a combination of skin, respiratory or circulatory changes, and less commonly with gastrointestinal symptoms. However, approximately 14% of severe reactions present only with respiratory symptoms or only with hypotension [10].

• Anaphylactic and anaphylactoid reactions behave identically clinically and are managed in the same way. These reactions should be considered a medical emergency as failure to initiate prompt treatment can have fatal consequences. Anaphylaxis usually begins 1–45 minutes after starting the transfusion and, in addition to an urticarial rash, presents with hypotension/shock, upper or lower airway obstruction (hoarseness, wheezing, chest pain, stridor, dyspnoea, anxiety, feeling of impending doom), gastrointestinal symptoms and rarely death.

Differential diagnosis

To ensure that appropriate treatment is administered in a timely fashion, patients presenting with systemic symptoms should also be promptly evaluated for:

• other causes of respiratory distress including circulatory overload, TRALI or any other comorbid condition such as pulmonary embolism and exacerbations of chronic lung disease;

• other causes of shock such as acute haemolytic transfusion reactions, sepsis and other comorbid clinical conditions that can be associated with shock;

• hypotension with or without cutaneous flushing due to bradykinin (BK) or des-Arg9-BK generation with the use of negatively charged bedside leucocyte reduction filters, or its transient accumulation in platelets during storage. Such hypotensive reactions may occur in a subset of patients being treated with an angiotensin-converting enzyme (ACE) inhibitor or who have inherited decreased ability to metabolize BK or des-Arg9-BK [11].

Incidence (frequency)

It is estimated that about 1% of transfusions are adversely affected by allergic reactions and that allergic reactions comprise 13–33% of all transfusion reactions. Rates of allergic transfusion reactions vary widely between the studies depending on product type and preparation. In a review of the studies done between 1990 and 2005 [8]:

• allergic reactions associated with packed red cell transfusions were reported to range from 0.03 to 0.61% with a median of 0.15% (1 reaction per 667 transfusions);

• allergic reactions associated with platelet transfusions occurred at a higher rate, ranging from 0.09 to 21% with a median of 3.7% (1 reaction per 27 transfusions); and

• the frequency of allergic reactions associated with the transfusion of plasma was lower than platelets but more common than reactions to red cells.

True anaphylaxis is a systemic reaction caused by antigen-specific crosslinking of IgE molecules on the surface of tissue mast cells and peripheral blood basophils, with immediate release of potent mediators. In contrast, immediate systemic reactions that mimic anaphylaxis but are not caused by an IgE-mediated immune response are termed anaphylactoid reactions. Both anaphylactic or anaphylactoid reactions are severe and life-threatening, but fortunately they are rare and comprise only about 1.3% of all transfusion reactions, affecting 1/20 000–1/47 000 transfusions.

Pathogenesis

Generally, an allergic transfusion reaction is defined as a type I hypersensitivity response mediated by IgE antibodies binding to a soluble allergen and resulting in the activation of mast cells. In these reactions, the allergen is often not known and the actual mechanism continues to remain largely speculative. In contrast, severe reactions that involve anaphylaxis which are not mediated by IgE antibodies but involve IgG anti-IgA are classified as type III reactions. These reactions result in complement activation with subsequent amplified release of anaphylotoxins C3a and C5a leading to anaphylaxis. When the aetiology of an allergic reaction is identified, it usually falls into one of the following categories:

• recipient pre-existing antibodies to plasma proteins in the blood component;

• recipient antibodies against a substance in the blood component that either is lacking or has a distinctly different allelic expression in the patient (i.e. IgA, haptoglobulin, C_4); and

• extraneous substances in the component (i.e. passively transmitted donor IgE antibodies, drugs, other allergens).

For the vast majority of patients, the underly aetiology is believed to be a recipient pre-existing antibody to plasma proteins in the blood component that cannot be specifically identified (i.e. deficiencies in IgA, haptogloblin and C4 are not commonly encountered and represent a very small minority of allergic reactions). In some instances, an allergic reaction can be traced back to donor-specific factors, but with only a 5% chance of causing an allergic reaction in another recipient; therefore patient-specific factors are a predominant cause of allergic reactions [12].

Management

When there is a suspicion for any transfusion reaction, a general principle of treatment is to discontinue the transfusion immediately and until the patient is clinically assessed.

• Mild nonsystemic allergic transfusion reactions are usually treated with an antihistamine, commonly diphenhydramine 25–50 mg IM or IV in North America and chlorphenamine (Piriton) 10–20 mg IM or IV in the UK. The transfusion can often be restarted at a slower rate once symptoms have settled.

• Moderate reactions can additionally be treated with a dose of corticosteroids and the transfusion is usually discontinued indefinitely.

• In severe reactions, the transfusion is never restarted. Anaphylaxis is treated as with any other anaphylactic reaction.

• In addition to discontinuation of the current transfusion, other blood components collected simultaneously from the same donor should be identified and avoided for this patient, particularly apheresis platelets, where two or three doses may have been created from a single collection. However, the likelihood of donor-specific factors triggering an allergic reaction in a different recipient is low relative to patient-specific factors; therefore it would be considered safe to use other associated blood components from this donor for other patients [12].

The management strategy for anaphylaxis differs for adults and paediatric patients. For adults/adolescents, immediate administration of adrenaline (epinephrine in the USA) 500 μg (0.5 mL of 1:1000 solution) IM is key. Aggressive volume expansion with IV normal saline, oxygen supplementation and antihistamines are also required. If the hypotension is intractable, adrenaline 500 μg (5 mL 1:10 000 solution) IV can be given every 5–10 minutes and preparations should be made to transfer the patient to an intensive care unit where an IV drip of inotropic therapy can be maintained. Intubation may be necessary if the airway becomes compromised.

For paediatric patients, the treatment of anaphylaxis should include: adrenaline 10 μg/kg 1:1000 concentration IM (e.g. under 6 months: 50 μg or 0.05 mL of adrenaline 1 in 1000; 6 months to 6 years: 120 μg or 0.12 mL; 6–12 years, 250 μg or 0.25 mL) that can be repeated every 5 minutes (maximum dose 300 μg). A μg/kg dose should be used rather than an mL/kg dose as there are different concentrations of adrenaline. Administration of chlorphenamine (250 μg/kg IV for children 1 month to less than 1 year of age; 2.5–5 mg for 1–5 years; 5–10 mg for 6–12 years; 10 mg for over 12 years) or diphenhydramine 1 mg/kg IV/IM in the USA and ranitidine 1 mg/kg IV (maximum dose 50 mg) are also effective for supportive management.

While the above drugs are being prepared, the focus should be on resuscitation, including oxygen therapy, suctioning and positioning of the patient to open the airway, maintenance of the circulation, oxygen saturation monitoring, establishing an IV if possible and administering a fluid bolus with 20 mL/kg sodium chloride 0.9% if venous access is established. If signs and symptoms persist despite a single-dose IM of adrenaline then a paediatric intensive care specialist should be consulted to provide airway and further haemodynamic support.

Prevention

Premedication with antipyretics and/or antihistamines

It has been reported that 50–80% of transfusions in Canada and the USA are premedicated. A recent systematic review of the literature assessing the efficacy of premedication in FNHTRs including the results of three small prospective randomized controlled trials found no evidence that premedication prevented NHTRs including allergic or febrile reactions [13]. A retrospective review of 7900 transfusions in 385 paediatric oncology patients also found no statistically significant difference in allergic transfusion reactions between those who received premedication and those who did not [14]. This study also found that there was no difference in allergic reactions with or without premedication, even in those with a previous history of two or more allergic reactions. In addition, allergic reactions were not more common in those with a history of two or more allergic transfusion reactions. Although premedication does not appear to affect the incidence of allergic reactions, there have been no studies to date that have evaluated whether premedication has an effect on the severity of such reactions.

Leucocyte reduction

Unlike FNHTRs, there is no significant reduction in allergic transfusion reactions with the use of leucocyte-reduced blood components.

Washed components/plasma-reduced components

Red cells have minimal volumes of residual plasma and would require washing to further reduce the amount of plasma proteins transfused. Washing was associated with a decrease in allergic reaction rates of 2.7% to 0.3% for red cells [15]. For apheresis platelets, plasma reduction was associated with a lowering of allergic reactions from 5.5% to 1.7%, and was further reduced with washing to 0.5% [15]. Platelet recovery was better with plasma reduction (80.7%) than with washing (70.5%), which was not considered a significant difference. Platelet activation was significantly higher with washing (24.2% increase) versus with plasma reduction (10.3% increase). In contrast, plasma reduction only removed 51.1% of plasma proteins versus 96% with washing [16]. With the exclusion of severe or life-threatening allergic reactions, which would benefit from washing of cellular products, the use of plasma reduction was sufficient to decrease the number of allergic reactions in 67.4% of patients with clinically significant or multiple urticarial reactions.

IgA-deficient blood components

IgA deficiency is the most common primary immunodeficiency in the Western world, affecting up to 1 in 20 people. Severe IgA deficiency, defined as IgA <0.05 mg/L, can be associated with anaphylactic reactions to blood components that almost always contain IgA [17]. Patients with anaphylactic transfusion reactions should have further testing using a pretransfusion patient serum sample to quantify their serum IgA level as well as anti-IgA antibody titres. However, in actual experience, the vast majority of patients with anaphylactic transfusion reactions are not IgA deficient. Only a small proportion of those individuals who are IgA deficient have anti-IgA antibodies, and only a small subset of individuals with antibodies have been documented to have anaphylactic reactions with non-IgA deficient products [17]. Given the near ubiquitous presence of IgA in blood components, a patient with a recent transfusion within the past 24 hours with no reaction has essentially passed an antigen (IgA) stimulus test and therefore is unlikely to have IgA deficiency as their underlying cause of anaphylaxis. If serum IgA is detectable in the patient, anaphylaxis due to IgA deficiency is very unlikely, though not entirely excluded, with 0.7% of patients with low or normal IgA levels having detectable anti-IgA [17]. Due to the limited sensitivity of the IgA assay in most hospital laboratories (0.20–50 mg/dL with nephelometry or turbidometry), additional testing is usually required to identify patients with severe IgA deficiency (less than 0.05 mg/dL) and to test for anti-IgA antibodies. Such testing is performed in a limited number of reference laboratories. Due to the additional time necessary to perform these confirmatory assays, it is possible that requests for additional transfusions are made prior to availability of results. In such circumstances, IgA-deficient or washed blood components should be used whenever possible until severe IgA deficiency and anti-IgA antibodies are confirmed or excluded with the additional laboratory tests. In the event that IgA-deficient or washed blood components (such as IgA-deficient plasma) are not immediately available for

a patient in a life-threatening situation, and where confirmatory testing is not yet completed, withholding transfusions may cause greater harm than a slow transfusion with careful monitoring [18]. If allergic transfusion reactions secondary to IgA antibodies due to IgA deficiency is confirmed, IgA-deficient products should be given in any future transfusions. Even in such circumstances, when faced with a life-threatening need for transfusion prior to the availability of IgA-deficient products, a slow transfusion with intense monitoring and immediate access to supportive care in the event of a severe reaction may outweigh the risk of anaphylaxis as a recurrence of anaphylaxis due to IgA is not a given certainty [19]. Since anaphylactic transfusion reactions are rare and often not due to IgA deficiency, while transfusions are common and often urgent, it is both impractical and not cost effective to widely screen for IgA deficiency in the pretransfused population.

Key points

1 Allergic and FNHTRs are the most common transfusion reactions. Anaphylaxis is rare.
2 Mild allergic reactions usually only require antihistamine treatment and the transfusion can be continued unless systemic symptoms develop.
3 Mild FNHTRs usually respond to the administration of an antipyretic.
4 If a moderate to severe transfusion reaction is suspected, the transfusion must be stopped until the patient is assessed and possible causes of the reaction are investigated.
5 Systemic symptoms warrant prompt clinical assessment as treatment can vary widely between diagnoses and, in particular, failure to administer adrenaline (epinephrine) in anaphylactic reactions can be fatal.

References

1 Heddle NM. Febrile non hemolytic transfusion reactions. In: MA Popovsky (ed.), *Transfusion Reactions*, 3rd edn. Bethesda, MD: AABB Press; 2007, pp. 57–103.
2 Yazer MH, Triulzi DJ, Shaz B, Kraus T & Zimring JC. Does a febrile reaction to platelets predispose recipients to red blood cell alloimmunization? *Transfusion* 2009; 49: 1070–1075.

3 Paglino JC, Pomper GJ, Fisch GS, Champion MH & Snyder EL. Reduction of febrile but not allergic reactions to RBCs and platelets after conversion to universal prestorage leukoreduction. *Transfusion* 2004; 44: 16–24.

4 Gauvin F, Lacroix J, Robillard P, Lapointe H & Hume H. Acute transfusion reactions in the pediatric intensive care unit. *Transfusion* 2006; 46: 1899–1908.

5 Heddle NM, Klama L, Singer J *et al*. The role of the plasma from platelet concentrates in transfusion reactions. *N Engl J Med* 1994; 331: 625–628.

6 Blumberg N, Gettings KF, Turner C, Heal JM & Phipps RP. An association of soluble CD40 ligand (CD154) with adverse reactions to platelet transfusions. *Transfusion* 2006; 46: 1813–1821.

7 Addas-Carvalho M, Salles TS & Saad ST. The association of cytokine gene polymorphisms with febrile non-hemolytic transfusion reaction in multitransfused patients. *Transfus Med* 2006; 16: 184–191.

8 Geiger TL & Howard SC. Acetaminophen and diphenhydramine premedication for allergic and febrile nonhemolytic transfusion reactions: good prophylaxis or bad practice? *Transfus Med Rev* 2007; 21: 1–12.

9 Tobian AA, King KE & Ness PM. Transfusion premedications: a growing practice not based on evidence. *Transfusion* 2007; 47: 1089–1096.

10 Domen RE & Hoeltge GA. Allergic transfusion reactions. An evaluation of 273 consecutive patients. *Arch Pathol Lab Med* 2003; 127: 316–320.

11 Eastlund T. Vasoactive mediators and hypotensive transfusion reactions. *Transfusion* 2007; 47: 369–372.

12 Savage WJ, Tobian AA, Fuller AK, Wood RA, King KE & Ness PM. Allergic transfusion reactions to platelets are associated more with recipient and donor factors than with product attributes. *Transfusion* 2011; 51: 1716–1722.

13 Martí-Carvajal AJ, Solà I, González LE *et al*. Pharmacological interventions for the prevention of allergic and febrile non-haemolytic transfusion reactions. *Cochrane Database Syst Rev* 2010; (6): CD007539.

14 Sanders RP, Maddirala SD, Geiger TL, Pounds S, Sandlund JT, Ribeiro RC, Pui CH & Howard SC. Premedication with acetaminophen or diphenhydramine for transfusion with leucoreduced blood products in children. *Br J Haematol* 2005; 130: 781–787.

15 Tobian AA, Savage WJ, Tisch DJ, Thoman S, King KE & Ness PM. Prevention of allergic transfusion reactions to platelets and red blood cells through plasma reduction. *Transfusion* 2011; 51: 1676–1683.

16 Veeraputhiran M, Ware J, Dent J, Bornhorst J, Post G, Cottler-Fox M, Pesek G, Theus J & Nakagawa M. A comparison of washed and volume-reduced platelets with respect to platelet activation, aggregation, and plasma protein removal. *Transfusion* 2011; 51: 1030–1036.

17 Vassallo RR. Review: IgA anaphylactic transfusion reactions. Part I. Laboratory diagnosis, incidence, and supply of IgA-deficient products. *Immunohematology* 2004; 20: 226–233.

18 Sandler SG & Zantek ND. Review: IgA anaphylactic transfusion reactions. Part II. Clinical diagnosis and bedside management. *Immunohematology* 2004; 20: 234–239.

19 Sandler SG. How I manage patients suspected of having had an IgA anaphylactic transfusion reaction. *Transfusion* 2006; 46: 10–13.

Further reading

Heddle NM, Klama L, Meyer R *et al*. A randomized controlled trial comparing plasma removal with white cell reduction to prevent reactions to platelets. *Transfusion* 1999; 39: 231–238.

Heddle NM, Blajchman MA, Meyer RM *et al*. A randomized controlled trial comparing the frequency of acute reactions to plasma-removed platelets and prestorage WBC-reduced platelets. *Transfusion* 2002; 42: 556–566.

Acute lung injury after transfusion

Steven H. Kleinman[1] *& Ram Kakaiya*[2]

[1]University of British Columbia, Victoria, British Columbia, Canada
[2]Life Source Blood Services, Rosemont Illinois, USA

Definition

The clinical syndrome of transfusion-related acute lung injury (TRALI) is characterised by acute onset of respiratory distress during or within 6 hours of transfusion, associated with oxygen desaturation (hypoxemia) and bilateral lung infiltrates, without evidence for left atrial hypertension or circulatory overload. However, differentiation of TRALI from circulatory overload can be difficult, if not impossible. No specific treatment for TRALI exists; in 90% of the cases, the patient recovers completely within 96 hours but the remaining 10% of cases are fatal.

Incidence

Haemovigilance data establish that TRALI is the number one cause of acute mortality from transfusion. In the USA, reports of transfusion-related fatalities to the Food and Drug Administration (FDA) indicate that TRALI has been the number one cause of fatalities from 2005 to 2010 [1]. In the UK, the Serious Hazards of Transfusion (SHOT) reported 36 cases of TRALI in 2003. This annual number decreased in subsequent years, coincident with the introduction of risk mitigation strategies; the 2010 annual SHOT report indicates only 15 reported cases [2].

There is a consensus that TRALI is both under-recognized and underreported; thus, the precise incidence of fatal plus nonfatal TRALI is unknown.

An overall risk of approximately 1:5000 transfused units in the general hospital population was reported in 1985 and this incidence number is frequently cited in the literature [3]. In research settings, computer-generated automatic alerts for respiratory distress after transfusion may improve detection of TRALI cases [4]. In a case control study of 89 TRALI cases at UCSF and Mayo Clinic, the investigators identified the following independent patient risk factors for TRALI: chronic alcohol abuse, current cigarette use, pre-existing shock, positive fluid balance, peak airway pressure greater than 30 cm H_2O if mechanically ventilated before transfusion, liver surgery (mainly transplantation) and elevated pretransfusion levels of interleukim-8 [5]. Acute lung injury (ALI) due to other causes is common in critically ill medical patients whether or not they are transfused; however, its frequency is increased in transfused patients (up to 40–45% in some studies) and shows a dose–response relationship [6, 7]. This points out the difficulty in determining whether ALI in patients with predisposing ALI risk factors is indeed TRALI or is instead due to other etiologies.

Pulmonary dysfunction that is not severe enough to meet the definition of TRALI may also occur following transfusion. This is consistent with a threshold model of TRALI in which the strength of the mediators (antibodies, activated lipids) may determine the severity of symptoms [8]. Some of these cases are classified as transfusion-associated dyspnea (TAD).

Practical Transfusion Medicine, Fourth Edition. Edited by Michael F. Murphy, Derwood H. Pamphilon and Nancy M. Heddle.
© 2013 John Wiley & Sons, Ltd. Published 2013 by John Wiley & Sons, Ltd.

Clinical manifestations

Males and females are equally affected. Most cases occur in adults. Previous transfusion history is unremarkable and recurrent TRALI is extremely rare. At least one case of TRALI from an autologous transfusion has been recorded. A few cases have occurred in children. Directed donations from mother to child can cause TRALI due to maternal leucocyte antibodies against the child's leucocyte antigens.

The onset of TRALI is often quite dramatic, with symptoms occurring either during the transfusion or usually within 2 hours (but this can be up to 6 hours) of its completion. Some investigators have also reported that TRALI can rarely have a delayed onset (>6 hours after transfusion) [9]. The syndrome manifests as acute respiratory distress syndrome (ARDS) or as noncardiogenic pulmonary oedema, and is characterized by acute onset of respiratory distress with dyspnoea, tachypnea and oxygen desaturation. The patient may appear cyanotic and may develop hypotension or hypertension. Oxygen desaturation is often severe, requiring mechanical ventilation in 70% of cases. Mild cases of respiratory distress that are unaccompanied by hypoxia, do not require any oxygen administration or resolve quickly do not fit the diagnostic criteria for TRALI. Some patients with TRALI experience a low grade fever for several hours. Symptoms and signs may be muted in patients under general anaesthesia and the first indication of TRALI might be the appearance of copious amounts of yellow frothy sputum from the endotracheal tube.

Auscultation of the lungs will detect the presence of bilateral rales or crackles. Hypoxia, defined as PaO_2/FiO_2 <300, and the development of new bilateral lung infiltrates on chest X-ray are essential in making a diagnosis. Hypoxia may also manifest as cyanosis or oxygen saturation of <90% on room air by pulse oximetry.

New acute lung injury (ALI) is defined by the development of new bilateral lung infiltrates on the chest X-ray. The chest X-ray may show 'white out', a radiographic finding in which both lungs show uniform white opacities throughout. More commonly, pulmonary infiltrates are located peripherally, especially in both lower lung fields (Figure 9.1). Because some patients with TRALI have acute transient leucopenia (neutropenia) around the

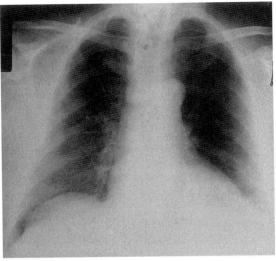

(a)

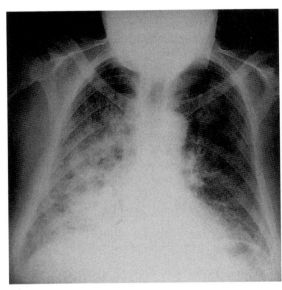

(b)

Fig 9.1 Chest X-rays of a patient with transfusion-related acute lung injury: (a) 1 day before a platelet transfusion and (b) shortly after transfusion showing diffuse bilateral shadowing of the lungs and a normal-sized heart. Reproduced with permission from AE Virchis, RK Patel, M Contreras, C Navarrete, RS Kaczmarski & R Jan-Mohamed. Lesson of the week: acute non-cardiogenic lung oedema after platelet transfusion. *British Medical Journal*, 1997; 314:880.

time of symptom onset, a complete blood count with a white cell count differential can be a useful adjunct test.

Types of blood components that can cause TRALI

TRALI has been caused by all types of blood components, including red cell concentrates, FFP, platelet concentrates, platelets collected by apheresis, cryoprecipitate and, rarely, intravenous immunoglobulin. Plasma-rich components, namely FFP, platelets collected by apheresis and platelet concentrates collected by the buffy coat method, which are resuspended in a large amount of plasma from one of the platelet donors, pose a greater per-unit risk than plasma-poor components (e.g. red cell concentrates) [10]. Plasma that has been treated by the solvent-detergent (SD) method that is currently in use in Europe, manufactured by pooling a large number of plasma units and thus diluting the leucocyte antibodies contained in donor blood, has not been shown to cause TRALI [11]. Leukocute-reduced cellular components can cause TRALI. It is unclear if the length of storage of cellular blood components influences the risk of TRALI occurrence.

Pathogenesis

Two different mechanisms – antibody-mediated and non-antibody-mediated – have been postulated as causes of TRALI [8]. It appears that cases caused by the antibody mechanism are of greater clinical severity and more often require mechanical ventilation. In some cases, TRALI may be due to the combined effects of both mechanisms.

• Leucocyte antibodies may bind to the recipient's neutrophils, which possess the corresponding cognate antigen/s, causing them to aggregate in the pulmonary vasculature, or may bind to endothelial cells, leading to neutrophil adherence and neutrophil activation. Activated neutrophils subsequently release cytotoxic enzymes, which lead to increased vascular permeability and intra-alveolar oedema. Antigen–antibody complex formation may also lead to increased vascular permeability through complement activation. A given threshold dose of antibody might be sufficient to cause

TRALI while a subthreshold dose may serve as the second 'hit' in a two-hit model of TRALI or cause a milder form of pulmonary injury that does not meet the definition of TRALI, a much more severe form of lung injury.

• Non-antibody-mediated TRALI results from transfusion of bioactive substances, which accumulate in cellular blood components during their storage. These bioactive substances include lipids (lysophosphatidylcholines), lipopolysaccharides, cytokines (IL-6 and IL-8), secretory phopholipase2 (sPLA2) and soluble CD40 ligand [12]. This mechanism of TRALI has been termed the two-hit hypothesis. The first hit is a patient stressor (e.g. surgery or sepsis) that causes the expression of endothelial cell adhesion molecules, leading to neutrophil adherence and activation in the pulmonary microvasculature. The second hit, consisting of passive administration of bioactive substances in stored blood components, leads to intravascular release of neutrophil enzymes, causing increased vascular permeability and resultant intra-alveolar oedema. Laboratory tests to measure bioactive substances are not widely available.

It is unclear what percentage of TRALI cases are due to each of these mechanisms. Most (but not all) series report that 80–85% of TRALI cases are caused by the antibody mechanism, with the large majority of these due to donor leucocyte antibodies directed at HLA or neutrophil-specific antigens present on the recipient's cells [13]. Some cases have been due to recipient antibody reacting with leucocytes in the transfused unit; however, this phenomenon is now very uncommon due to the widespread use of leucocyte-reduced blood components. The remaining 15–20% of cases are thought to be due to the non-antibody-mediated mechanism. Implicated antibodies include HLA class I antibodies directed against A, B and possibly C locus antigens, HLA class II antibodies directed mostly against DR antigens and neutrophil antibodies directed against human neutrophil antigens (HNAs). Involved donors can have multiple types of antibodies. The presence of a cognate antigen in the recipient that corresponds to the antibody specificity in the involved donor or a positive cross-match between the donor's serum and the recipient's leucocytes provide strong support for the serologic diagnosis of antibody-mediated TRALI. The presence of multiple antibodies in the involved donor that have the corresponding matching antigens in the recipient may be seen. It is possible that the presence of multiple donor antibodies corresponding to multiple cognate antigens poses a greater risk of TRALI than does a single congate antibody [14]. HNA-3a (formerly designated as 5b) antibodies are rare but are important to detect as these have been associated with several fatal cases of TRALI [15]. Currently, neutrophil antibody detection assays are not widely available and are just beginning to become automated. It has been reported that anti-HNA-3a may be missed unless a leucoaggultination assay or an enhanced immunofluorescense assay is used.

Lung histology

Fatal cases of TRALI show massive alveolar oedema on histological examination (Figure 9.2) [12]. Alveolar–capillary membrane disruption is widespread with hyaline membrane formation.

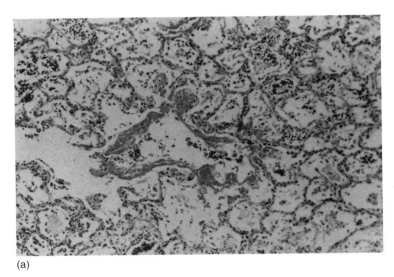

(a)

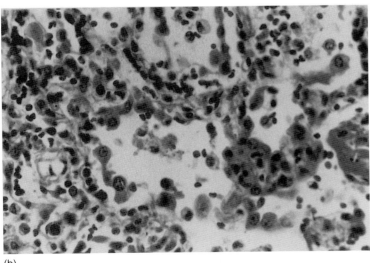

(b)

Fig 9.2 Thin sections of fixed lung from a patient with transfusion-related acute lung injury. There is acute diffuse alveolar damage with intra-alveolar oedema and haemorrhage. There was no histological evidence of infection and all post mortem cultures (bacterial, viral and fungal) were negative. Magnification: (a) ×40; (b) ×440. Reproduced with permission from C Silliman *et al*. The association of biologically active lipids with the development of transfusion-related acute lung injury: a retrospective study. *Transfusion*, 1997; 37: 719–726.

Interstitium and alveoli are infiltrated with inflammatory cells consisting of neutrophils and macrophages. The diffuse alveolar damage resembles findings seen in ARDS from other causes.

Differential diagnosis

Diagnosis of TRALI remains difficult because patients who experience severe respiratory distress during or after transfusion are often quite ill, have multiple other morbidities, may have cardiac or pulmonary compromise and could be suffering from conditions that are known to cause ALI or ARDS. Clinical evaluation should include investigation of other causes of ALI, which include sepsis syndrome (with or without septic shock), trauma, aspiration, smoke inhalation, near drowning, pneumonia, systemic inflammatory response syndrome, pancreatitis, postcardiopulmonary bypass and drug overdose. In any given patient, the presence of one or more of these other causes of ALI makes the diagnosis of TRALI quite difficult. A Consensus Conference has recommended that ALI occurring within 6 hours of transfusion in a patient with other ALI risk factors be designated as possible TRALI, as it is often extremely difficult to determine whether it was the transfusion or the alternate risk factor that caused the ALI [16]. The diagnosis of TRALI is difficult, if not impossible, to make in patients with pre-existing ALI.

The lack of certain clinical findings helps in the differential diagnosis between TRALI and transfusion-associated circulatory overload (TACO) [17]. This latter syndrome consists of cardiogenic pulmonary oedema, which may show one or more of the following features:
• positive fluid balance, weight gain, orthopnoea or paroxysmal nocturnal dyspnoea;
• peripheral oedema;
• hepatomegaly;
• hepatojugular reflux, heart murmur;
• new onset cardiac gallop rhythm (S3 and S4);
• an increased jugular venous pressure;
• elevated pulmonary artery wedge pressure (≥ 18 mm Hg) in invasively monitored patients;
• an enlarged heart with or without pleural effusion on the chest X-ray;
• radiographic appearance of pulmonary infiltrates that are more central with or without Kerley septal lines;
• echocardiograph findings of decreased systolic ejection fraction or diastolic dysfunction;
• a 50% elevation of B-type natriuretic peptide (BNP) in a posttransfusion-versus-a pretransfusion sample supports TACO whereas a BNP level of <250 pg/mL measured immediately after the onset of acute pulmonary oedema supports the diagnosis of TRALI. In critical care patients, BNP levels may be higher in patients who develop TACO compared to those who develop TRALI, yet may have a limited diagnostic value due to a large overlap among the observed values in these patient groups [18];
• some TRALI patients experience low grade fever and acute onset of leucopenia and these features, if present, suggest TRALI rather than TACO.

In addition to TACO, other conditions that can mimic TRALI include anaphylactic transfusion reactions and sepsis from transfusion of bacterially contaminated blood components. Respiratory stridor, localized or generalized skin rash, hypotension and/or shock favour a diagnosis of anaphylactic reaction. High fever, chills, rigor, shock, disseminated intravascular coagulation, a positive gram stain and culture from the transfused blood component and positive blood cultures from the recipient support a diagnosis of transfusion-transmitted bacterial sepsis. Finally, a low grade fever seen in TRALI must be differentiated from a haemolytic transfusion reaction. A clerical check of the transfusion episode showing the lack of any error, plus an absence of visual haemolysis in the posttransfusion serum or plasma and a negative direct antiglobulin test, suggest that a haemolytic transfusion reaction is unlikely.

More recently, the new term 'transfusion-associated dyspnoea' (TAD) has been coined for those cases of dyspnoea following transfusion that do not fit into any of the known transfusion reaction categories. A threshold model of TRALI can explain mild–moderate–severe symptoms as a consequence of the strength of the antibodies or other mediators combined with the predisposing 'activation state' of the patient's neutrophils and/or endothelium [8]. Further studies are needed to understand fully the entire clinical spectrum of posttransfusion lung injury.

Table 9.1 Clinical information that may assist in differential diagnosis of pulmonary transfusion reactions.

Clinical parameter	Interpretation
History	Underlying cardiac dysfunction and positive fluid balance may suggest TACO. Sepsis or aspiration in the previous 24 hours suggests ALI and the designation of 'possible TRALI'. IgA deficiency may suggest allergic reaction
Physical examination	Sudden elevation of blood pressure, jugular venous distension and wheezing suggest TACO. Hypotension suggests TRALI. Stridor, wheezing and urticaria suggest allergic reaction. Fever suggests febrile reaction, sepsis/bacterial contamination
Chest X-ray	Bilateral infiltrates indicate pulmonary oedema (TACO or TRALI). Cardiomegaly (cardiothoracic ratio >0.55) and increased vascular pedicle width (>65 mm) suggest TACO
Arterial blood gas analysis, arterial oxygen saturation (pulse oximetry)	$PaO_2/FIO_2 < 300$ (or O_2 saturation <90% on room air) meets the Consensus Conference definition of ALI (TRALI or possible TRALI)
Haemodynamic monitoring: central venous and pulmonary artery pressures	Increase in central venous (>12–15 mm Hg) or pulmonary artery wedge pressure (>18–20 mm Hg) at the time of reaction suggest TACO
Echocardiography	Systolic (ejection fraction <45%) or diastolic dysfunction suggest TACO or other cause of cardiogenic oedema
Pulmonary oedema fluid	The ratio of pulmonary oedema albumin over plasma albumin of >0.55 suggest ALI rather than hydrostatic (TACO) oedema
Beta-natriuretic peptide (BNP)	Low values of BNP (<250 pg/mL) suggest TRALI. Increase in BNP >1.5 of pretransfusion values may suggest TACO
Leucocyte and neutrophil count before and after the implicated transfusion	Sudden, transient drop in neutrophil or leucocyte count after the transfusion suggests TRALI
Response to diuretic therapy	Rapid (minutes to hours) resolution of pulmonary oedema after diuresis may suggest TACO
Timing of the reaction in relation to transfusion and other potential risk factors	Sudden onset during or shortly after the transfusion is suggestive of a transfusion reaction rather than a pulmonary complication related to another risk factor

Clinical information helpful in the differential diagnosis of TRALI is listed in Table 9.1.

Management

Patient management is supportive. Virtually all patients will require some sort of oxygen support with many requiring mechanical ventilation with or without intubation. There is no evidence to support the use of corticosteroids. Fluid management may include the use of intravenous fluids to correct profound hypotension. Diuretics may be indicated if blood pressure is stable and if an element of congestive heart failure or circulatory overload is present or cannot be excluded [9, 19].

Clinicians should obtain a chest X-ray, HLA phenotype and pre- and posttransfusion BNP levels in all suspected cases of TRALI. If the investigation of the involved donors fails to show the presence of and/or risk/s for leukocyte antibody, patient testing for leucocyte antibody may be considered. Patients with TRALI resulting from their leucocyte antibodies may benefit from transfusion of leucocyte-reduced blood components. Further transfusions, if needed, do not require any other special precautions since recurrent TRALI is extremely rare. The use of platelets that are stored for less than 4 days and red cell units less than

14 days have been advocated by some authors, but there are no clinical data to support the need for such products.

Outcome and morbidity

TRALI is often quite severe and patients require mechanical ventilation for adequate oxygenation in two-thirds or more of the cases. The remaining cases require oxygen therapy by nonmechanical modalities. Pulmonary infiltrates resolve in the vast majority of patients (≥80%) in 96 hours. Slow recovery of pulmonary functions occur in 10%. Mortality is approximately 6–10%. Recurrence is extremely rare. Those who recover do not have any chronic sequelae. TRALI may be associated with a decreased long-term survival in critically ill medical patients, but this may be due to an increased fatality rate during the initial hospitalization [20].

TRALI mitigation strategies

For non-antibody-mediated TRALI, no preventive steps have been recommended or undertaken. For antibody-mediated TRALI, there is general agreement that a donor who is clearly 'implicated' in a case of TRALI should be deferred. An 'implicated donor' is defined as one who is shown to possess leucocyte antibodies that correspond to the recipient's antigen/s or a donor whose serum is reactive against the recipient's leucocytes in a cross-match test. It remains uncertain if the donor should be deferred if he or she has leucocyte antibodies but cognate antigens are not present in the recipient or if the cross-match test is negative.

In the UK, steps were taken in late 2003 to reduce transfusing FFP units collected from female donors. With this intervention, the number of TRALI cases from FFP transfusion decreased from 14 cases in 2003 to 6 cases in 2004 to 1 case in 2005. In view of these and other data, in late 2006, the AABB (formerly, the American Association of Blood Banks) recommended that plasma for transfusions be prepared from donors who are less likely to be alloimmunized [10]. Therefore, plasma units for transfusion are now increasingly prepared predominantly from male donors. This strategy has now been demonstrated to have decreased the incidence of TRALI in several different countries, including the UK, USA, Germany and the Netherlands [1, 2, 9, 21]. In some European countries, SD plasma has been used as an alternative product to reduce the incidence of TRALI [11].

There are probably sufficient male donor plasma units available for blood groups O and A such that transfusion needs can be met almost exclusively by transfusion of male-only plasma. For blood groups B and AB plasma, some plasma from female donors may be necessary to meet the transfusion demand. In this regard, plasma from nulliparous female donors would be preferred to plasma from multiparous donors. Group B or AB plasma from multiparous donors can also be screened for HLA antibodies before release for transfusion. Prevention approaches for platelets require different measures as there are an insufficient number of male platelet apheresis donors to achieve a practice similar to the one described for plasma transfusion. Alternatively, deferral of females who have been pregnant at least once would still result in the loss of 40–60% of female platelet apheresis donors, and such a donor loss would likely create a critical shortage. Because of these considerations, screening blood donors, especially female donors with a history of pregnancy, for HLA antibodies and then deferring those who have them from plateletpheresis donations is a strategy that has been adopted in some jurisdictions [22]. At present, techniques for neutrophil antibody identification are cumbersome and cannot be applied for screening a large number of donors.

Key points

1 TRALI is a leading cause of death from transfusion.
2 It manifests as ARDS or noncardiogenic pulmonary oedema during or within 6 hours of transfusion.
3 Leucocyte antibodies (HLA and neutrophil-specific) and neutrophil priming agents in blood components are responsible for the syndrome.
4 Treatment is supportive, but fatality occurs in 10% of diagnosed cases.
5 Those who recover show no long-term lung injury.
6 TRALI is difficult to distinguish from transfusion-associated circulatory overload (TACO). Underlying cardiac dysfunction and positive fluid balance may suggest TACO.

7 Preventive measures include exclusion of blood donors implicated in TRALI cases and reduction of the number of transfusions of plasma-containing blood components from donors who are likely to possess leucocyte antibodies.

References

1 Fatalites reported to the FDA following blood collection and transfusion. Annual summary for fiscal year 2010. Available at: http://www.fda.gov/biologicsbloodvaccines/safetyavailability/reportaproblem/transfusiondonationfatalities/ucm254802.htm (accessed August 15, 2011).

2 Knowles S (ed.) & Cohen H, on behalf of the Serious Hazards of Transfusion (SHOT) Steering Group. The 2010 Annual SHOT Report (2011). Available at: http://www.shotuk.org/wp-content/uploads/2011/07/SHOT-2010-Report1.pdf (accessed August 15, 2011).

3 Popovsky MA & Moore SB. Diagnostic and pathogenetic considerations in transfusion-related acute lung injury. *Transfusion* 1985; 25: 573–577.

4 Finlay-Morreale HE, Louie C & Toy P. Computer-generated automatic alerts of respiratory distress after blood transfusion. *J Am Med Inform Assoc* 2008 May–June; 15(3): 383–385.

5 Toy P, Gajic O, Bacchetti P, Looney MR, Gropper MA, Hubmayr R & Clifford A. Transfusion related acute lung injury: incidence and risk factors. *Blood* 2012; 119: 1757–1767.

6 Khan H, Cartin-Ceba R & Gajic O. Transfusion and acute lung injury in the critically ill. In: S Kleinman & M Popovsky (eds), *TRALI: Mechanisms, Management, and Prevention*. Bethesda, MD: AABB Press; 2008, pp. 13–42.

7 Silverboard H, Aisiku I, Martin G et al. The role of acute blood transfusion in the development of acute respiratory distress syndrome among the critically ill: a cohort study. *J Trauma* 2005; 59: 717–723,

8 Bux J & Sachs UJH. The pathogenesis of transfusion-related acute lung injury (TRALI). *Br J Haematol* 2007; 136: 788–799.

9 Bux J. Antibody-mediated (immune) transfusion-related acute lung injury. *Vox Sanguinis* 2011; 100: 122–128.

10 Transfusion-related acute lung injury. Association Bulletin #05-09. Bethesda, MD: AABB; 2005. Available at: http://www.aabb.org/Content/Members-Area/.

11 Sachs UJH, Kauschat D & Bein G. White-blood cell reactive antibodies are undetectable in solvent/detergent plasma. *Transfusion* 2005; 45: 1628–1631.

12 Silliman CC, Paterson AJ, Dickey W et al. The association of biologically active lipids with the development of transfusion-related acute lung injury. *Transfusion* 1997; 37: 719–726.

13 Middelburg RA, van Stein D, Briet E, van der Bom JG. The role of donor antibodies in the pathogenesis of transfusion-related acute lung injury: a systematic review. *Transfusion* 2008; 48: 2167–2176.

14 Hashimoto S, Nakajima F, Kamada H, Kawamura K, Satake M, Tadokoro K & Okazaki H. Relationship of donor HLA antibody strength to the development of transfusion-related acute lung injury. *Transfusion* 2010; 50: 2582–2591.

15 Reil A, Keeler-Stanislawski B, Geuerney S et al. Specificities of leukocyte alloantibodies in transfusion-related acute lung injury and results of leukocyte antibody screening of blood donors. *Vox Sanguinis* 2008; 95: 313–317.

16 Kleinman S, Caufield T, Chan P et al. Toward an understanding of transfusion-related acute lung injury: statement of a consensus panel. *Transfusion* 2004; 44: 1774–1789.

17 Gajic O, Gropper MA & Hubmayr RD. Pulmonary edema after transfusion: how to differentiate transfusion-associated circulatory overload from transfusion-related acute lung injury. *Crit Care Med* 2006; 34: S109–S113.

18 Li G, Daniels CE, Kojicic T, Wilson GA, Winters JL, Moore SB & Gajic O. The accuracy of natriuretic peptides (brain natriuretic peptide and N-terminal pro-brain natriuretic) in the differentiation between transfusion-related acute lung injury and transfusion-related circulatory overload in the critically ill. *Transfusion* 2009; 49: 13–20.

19 Moore SB. Transfusion-related acute lung injury (TRALI); clinical presentation, treatment, and prognosis. *Crit Care Med* 2006; 34(Suppl.): S114–S117.

20 Li G, Kojicic M, Reriani MK, Fernandez Perez ER, Thakur L, Kashyap R, Van Buskirk CM & Gajic O. Long-term survival and quality of life after transfusion-associated pulmonary edema in critically ill medical patients. *Chest* 2010; 137: 783–789.

21 Wiersum-Osselton JC, Middelburg RA, Beckers EAM, vanTilborgh AJW, Zijliker-Jansen PY, Brand A, van der Bom JG & Schipperus MR. Male-only fresh-frozen plasma for transfusion-related acute lung injury prevention: before and after comparative cohort study. *Transfusion* 2011; 51: 1278–1283.

22 Kleinman S, Grossman B & Kopko P. A national survey of transfusion-related acute lung injury risk reduction policies for platelets and plasma in the United States. *Transfusion* 2010; 50: 1312–1321.

Further reading

Bux J. Transfusion-related acute lung injury (TRALI): a serious adverse event of blood transfusion. *Vox Sanguinis* 2005; 89: 1–10.

Goldman M, Webert KE, Arnold DM, Freedman J, Hannon J & Blajchman MA. Proceedings of a Consensus Conference: towards an understanding of TRALI. *Transfus Med Rev* 2005; 19: 2–31.

Kleinman S & Triulzi D. TRALI risk-reduction strategies. In S Kleinman and M Popovsky (eds), *TRALI: Mechanisms, Management, and Prevention.* Bethesda, MD: AABB Press; 2008, pp. 161–188.

Silliman CC, Ambruso DR & Boskov LK. Transfusion-related acute lung injury. *Blood* 2005; 105: 2266–2273.

Stroncek DF. Pulmonary transfusion reactions. *Semin Hematol* 2007; 44: 2–14.

10 Purported adverse effects of transfusion-related immunomodulation and of the transfusion of 'old blood'

Eleftherios C. Vamvakas

Department of Pathology and Laboratory Medicine, Cedars-Sinai Medical Center, Los Angeles, California, USA

Transfusion-related immunomodulation (TRIM) encompasses the documented laboratory immune alterations that follow allogeneic blood transfusion (ABT), as well as any established or purported, beneficial or deleterious, clinical effects that may be ascribed to immunosuppression resulting from ABT, including:

- enhanced survival of renal allografts;
- increased risk of recurrence of resected malignancies and of postoperative bacterial infections;
- increased short-term (up to 3-month posttransfusion) mortality from all causes; and
- activation of endogenous CMV or HIV infection in transfused compared with untransfused patients.

Any ABT-related increase in short-term posttransfusion mortality (perhaps secondary to an increased risk of multiple organ failure, MOF) would most likely be mediated by 'proinflammatory' rather than 'immunomodulatory' mechanisms; however, the term TRIM has recently been used more broadly, to encompass transfusion complications mediated via either immunomodulatory or proinflammatory pathways.

The only *established* clinical TRIM effect is beneficial, not deleterious. It is the enhanced survival of renal allografts after pretransplant ABT [1]. This effect has been confirmed by animal data and clinical experience worldwide. Before the advent of cyclosporine and potent immunosuppressive drugs, this ABT effect was exploited clinically, through the deliberate exposure of patients awaiting renal transplantation to transfusion of non-leucocyte-reduced red blood cells (RBCs).

The benefit from ABT is small in the current era, but a randomized controlled trial (RCT) documented that it is still evident. The existence of deleterious clinically relevant TRIM effects has not yet been established; neither do we know the mechanism(s) of TRIM or the specific blood constituent(s) that mediate(s) TRIM. TRIM may be mediated by one (or more) of the following (Figure 10.1):

- allogeneic mononuclear cells (AMCs) present in RBC units stored for less than 2 weeks;
- proinflammatory soluble mediators released from leucocyte granules or membranes and accumulating progressively in the supernatant of RBCs during storage; and/or
- soluble, class I HLA molecules circulating in allogeneic plasma.

Clinical studies of adverse TRIM effects

Some 200 observational studies and 22 RCTs reported before 2005 examined the purported adverse TRIM effects in humans. The RBC components transfused in these studies reflected the RBC components used in Europe and North America between the mid-1980s and the first few years of the 21st century. Sixteen RCTs assumed that the TRIM effect is mediated by allogeneic leucocytes and compared recipients of non-leucocyte-reduced versus leucocyte-reduced allogeneic RBCs or whole blood. Six RCTs assumed that the

Practical Transfusion Medicine, Fourth Edition. Edited by Michael F. Murphy, Derwood H. Pamphlon and Nancy M. Heddle.
© 2013 John Wiley & Sons, Ltd. Published 2013 by John Wiley & Sons, Ltd.

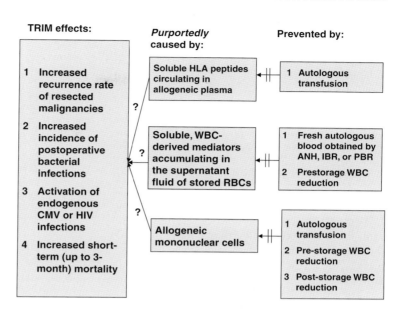

Fig 10.1 TRIM effects, postulated mediators of TRIM and preventive strategies that could be effective if the TRIM effects were mediated by each corresponding mediator. ANH, acute normovolemic hemodilution; IBR, intraoperative blood recovery; PBR, postoperative blood recovery. Modified with permission from Vamvakas EC. Deleterious effects of transfusion-related immunomodulation: fact or fiction? Update through 2005. *Am J Clin Pathol* 2006; 126 (Suppl 1): S71–S85.

TRIM effect is mediated by either allogeneic leucocytes or allogeneic plasma and compared recipients of non-leucocyte-reduced allogeneic versus autologous blood. Thus, the reported RCTs differed in ways that determined the conclusions to be drawn about mechanisms of TRIM. Patients randomized to receive non-leucocyte-reduced allogeneic RBCs received units that were either buffy-coat-reduced (in Europe) or buffy-coat-rich (in the USA). Buffy-coat-reduced RBCs are units from which approximately two-thirds of leucocytes are removed, without filtration, by the method used to separate blood into components. If leucocytes do indeed mediate TRIM, buffy-coat-rich RBCs should have more of a TRIM effect than buffy-coat-reduced RBCs.

Patients randomized to receive autologous or leucocyte-reduced allogeneic RBCs received units that were either replete with or devoid of leucocyte-derived soluble mediators. During storage of a non-leucocyte-reduced RBC unit, leucocytes deteriorate over 2 weeks, progressively releasing soluble mediators. RBCs leucocyte reduced by filtration after storage are full of leucocyte-derived mediators, because such mediators (as well as apoptotic or necrotic leucocytes) are not retained by leucocyte reduction filters. RBCs leucocyte reduced by filtration before storage are free of leucocyte-derived mediators, because their leucocytes are removed before they can release mediators

into the supernatant fluid. Stored autologous blood, obtained by preoperative donation, is full of mediators, because autologous leucocytes also deteriorate during storage, releasing mediators. Fresh autologous blood, obtained by acute normovolemic haemodilution (ANH), intraoperative blood recovery (IBR) or postoperative blood recovery (PBR), and transfused within hours of collection and processing, is free of leucocyte-derived soluble mediators.

Leucocyte reduction, performed either before or after storage, can prevent TRIM effects mediated by AMCs, but it cannot prevent TRIM effects mediated by soluble molecules circulating in allogeneic plasma (Figure 10.1). Only pre-storage, as opposed to post-storage, leucocyte reduction can prevent TRIM effects mediated by leucocyte-derived, soluble mediators. Autologous transfusion can prevent TRIM effects mediated by AMCs as well as by molecules circulating in allogeneic plasma. Only fresh, as opposed to stored, autologous blood can prevent TRIM effects mediated by leucocyte-derived, soluble mediators.

TRIM effects mediated by AMCs

The best argument that the adverse TRIM effects are mediated by AMCs is that the established beneficial TRIM effect in renal transplantation requires viable leucocytes. Also, immune suppression has been induced in mice receiving allogeneic leucocytes free of plasma and platelets. Viable allogeneic leucocytes in blood components can act as responder cells or as stimulator cells, inducing cellular immunity and antibody production in the recipient. After 10–14 days of storage, the capacity of donor antigen-presenting leucocytes to stimulate recipient T-helper cells is abrogated *in vitro* owing to a reduction in costimulatory molecules.

The only RCT to study the effect of AMCs has been the Viral Activation Transfusion Study, which studied transfusion-induced activation of endogenous CMV or HIV infection [2]. All RBCs transfused in this study had been stored for less than 2 weeks and could thus be presumed to contain immunologically competent AMCs. There was no difference between the arms of the RCT in the HIV–RNA level, the number of CD4-positive T cells or any other endpoint studied. Median survival was 13.0 months in recipients of pre-storage filtered, leucocyte-reduced allogeneic RBCs, as compared with 20.5 months in recipients of buffy-coat-rich, non-leucocyte-reduced allogeneic RBCs ($p = 0.12$). This difference was not significant in the intention-to-treat analysis but, after correction for various prognostic factors, transfusion of non-leucocyte-reduced RBCs was associated with a better outcome.

TRIM effects mediated by leucocyte-derived soluble mediators

Soluble immune response modifiers accumulating during storage of blood components include elastase, histamine, soluble HLA, soluble Fas ligand, transforming growth factor (TGF)-β1 and proinflammatory cytokines IL-1β, IL-6 and IL-8. *In vitro*, soluble leucocyte-derived factors from stored RBCs induce immediate upregulation of expression of inflammatory genes in third-party leucocytes [3]. Apoptosis of leucocytes begins immediately after the collection of donor blood. Gradual apoptosis and necrosis begins with granulocytes and continues with monocytes, while lymphocytes can remain viable for >25 days at 2–6°C. Apoptotic cells engage the phosphatidylserine/annexin-V receptor on macrophages, inducing release of prostaglandin E-2 and TGF-β – factors that suppress macrophages

and natural killer cells and impair antigen-presenting capacity.

However, the 12 RCTs that compared the risk of postoperative infection between patients randomized to receive non-leucocyte-reduced versus leucocyte-reduced ABT (in the event that they needed perioperative transfusion) have not supported the theory that attributes TRIM to leucocyte-derived soluble mediators. These RCTs are medically heterogeneous, having been conducted at various settings, having transfused various blood components and having diagnosed infection based on varying criteria. Thus, not all 12 RCTs targeted a TRIM effect that was *biologically* similar in all cases, making it inappropriate to combine the results of all 12 RCTs in a meta-analysis. However, if we were to integrate these findings despite the extreme heterogeneity of the studies, we would find no association between non-leucocyte-reduced ABT and an increased risk of infection across all the available RCTs, whether we relied on 'intention-to-treat' analyses (that retain all randomized subjects, whether transfused or not) or on 'as-treated' analyses (that remove the untransfused subjects) [4].

What has medical relevance, however, is the integration of medically homogeneous studies. Integration of such subsets of homogeneous studies produced results antithetical from those expected from theory. Across nine RCTs transfusing allogeneic RBCs filtered before storage to the leucocyte-reduced arm and enrolling approximately 5000 subjects, no TRIM effect was detected. If leucocyte-derived, soluble mediators did cause TRIM, pre-storage filtration should abrogate any increased infection risk associated with non-leucocyte-reduced ABT. Thus, a deleterious TRIM effect would be expected in this analysis, but no such effect was found (summary odds ratio (OR) = 1.06; 95% confidence interval (CI), 0.91–1.24; $p > 0.05$) (Figure 10.2a).

In contrast, across the four RCTs transfusing allogeneic RBCs or whole blood filtered after storage to the non-leucocyte-reduced arm, there was a 2.25-fold increase in the risk of infection in association with non-leucocyte-reduced ABT (summary OR = 2.25; 95% CI, 1.12–4.25; $p < 0.05$) (Figure 10.2b). Thus, the TRIM effect appeared to be prevented by post-storage filtration, contradicting the theory that attributes TRIM to leucocyte-derived, soluble mediators. Such mediators would have been present equally in both the non-leucocyte-reduced and leucocyte-reduced RBCs, because they would not have been removed by post-storage filtration.

TRIM effects mediated by soluble molecules circulating in allogeneic plasma

Only one RCT has been specifically designed to study the effects of soluble HLA molecules circulating in allogeneic plasma as mediators of TRIM. Wallis *et al.* [5] randomized patients undergoing open-heart surgery to receive plasma-reduced, buffy-coat-reduced or leucocyte-reduced RBCs. The highest risk of infection was observed in the plasma-reduced arm, although the difference between the three arms was not significant. This finding suggested that plasma removal does not prevent TRIM or, by extension, that allogeneic plasma does not mediate TRIM. Similarly, integration of the five RCTs that compared recipients of allogeneic versus autologous blood demonstrated no increased risk of infection in association with ABT.

Association between non-leucocyte-reduced ABT and short-term mortality

The association of non-leucocyte-reduced ABT with short-term mortality from all causes started out as a data-derived hypothesis to account for an unexpected transfusion effect. The RCT of van de Watering *et al.* [6] (Figure 10.2) had been designed to investigate differences in postoperative infection between recipients of non-leucocyte-reduced versus leucocyte-reduced allogeneic RBCs. However, it detected, instead, differences in 60-day mortality between the arms (Figure 10.3). The authors suggested that non-leucocyte-reduced ABT may predispose to MOF, which, in turn, may predispose to mortality.

If 11 medically heterogeneous RCTs reported before 2005 and comparing recipients on non-leucocyte-reduced versus leucocyte-reduced ABT and reporting on short-term mortality were to be combined, there would be no increase in mortality in association with non-leucocyte-reduced ABT. These studies transfused to the non-leucocyte-reduced arm either buffy-coat-rich or buffy-coat-reduced allogeneic RBCs; as already discussed, the former should have

more of an effect than the latter. However, this theoretical prediction is the opposite of what the analysis actually showed. Across six RCTs transfusing buffy-coat-reduced RBCs to the non-leucocyte-reduced arm and pre-storage filtered RBCs to the leucocyte-reduced arm, there was a 60% increase in mortality in association with non-leucocyte-reduced ABT (summary OR = 1.60; 95% CI, 1.14–2.24; $p < 0.05$) (Figure 10.3a). In this analysis, pre-storage filtration appeared to abrogate an increased mortality risk, but the benefit from pre-storage filtration was not seen where more of an ABT effect would have been expected. Across the RCTs that transfused buffy-coat-rich RBCs to the non-leucocyte-reduced arm, no ABT effect was detected, although some 4500 subjects had been enrolled in these studies.

Perhaps the benefit observed in the analysis of studies transfusing buffy-coat-reduced versus pre-storage filtered RBCs (Figure 10.3a) was due to overrepresentation in that analysis of the cardiac surgery studies: three of the six RCTs included in that analysis (i.e. the studies by van de Watering *et al.* [6], Bilgin *et al.* [7] and Wallis *et al.* [5]) had been conducted in open-heart surgery. Across all five RCTs conducted in cardiac surgery (Figure 10.3b), there was a 72% increase in mortality in association with non-leucocyte-reduced ABT (summary OR = 1.72; 95% CI, 1.05–2.81; $p < 0.05$). In contrast, across the six RCTs conducted in other surgical settings, there was no ABT effect (summary OR = 0.99; 95% CI, 0.73–1.33; $p > 0.05$).

Thus, the ABT-related mortality risk, which is not seen in any other setting, may relate to another effect present in patients undergoing cardiac surgery. During open-heart surgery, blood is exposed to the extracorporeal circuit, as well as to hypothermia and to ischemic and reperfusion injury. These insults are potent inducers of a stress response, triggering a systemic inflammatory response syndrome (SIRS), which is immediately counteracted by a compensatory anti-inflammatory response syndrome (CARS) [8]. SIRS manifests with leukocytosis, capillary leakage and organ dysfunction; overwhelming SIRS causes a dormant state of metabolism referred to as multiple-organ dysfunction syndrome (MODS). CARS has an immune-paralysing effect characterized by anti-inflammatory cytokines, such as TGF-β1, IL-4 and IL-10. Through the intervention of CARS, the postperfusion SIRS of cardiac surgery generally resolves. However, any intervention by biologic

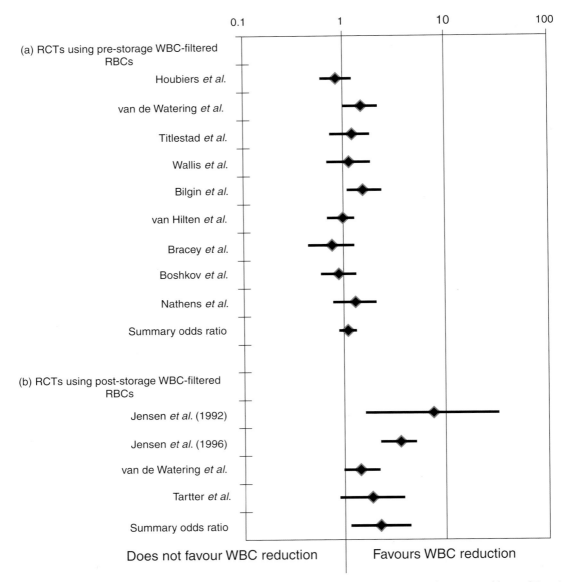

Fig 10.2 RCTs of ABT and postoperative infection administering (a) pre-storage leucocyte-filtered or (b) post-storage leucocyte-filtered allogeneic RBCs to the leucocyte-reduced arm. The figure shows the OR of postoperative infection, as calculated from an intention-to-treat analysis of each study, and the summary OR across the depicted RCTs, as calculated from a meta-analysis. A deleterious ABT effect (and thus a benefit from leucocyte reduction) is demonstrated by an OR > 1, provided that the effect is statistically significant ($p < 0.05$; i.e. provided that the associated 95% CI does not include the null value of 1). The RCT of van de Watering et al. included recipients of both pre-storage filtered and post-storage filtered RBCs and found no difference between these two arms. For the references to the listed studies, see Further reading, Vamvakas & Blajchman (2007).

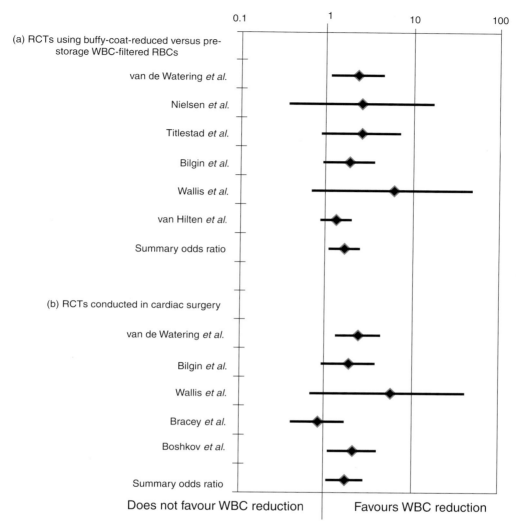

Fig 10.3 RCTs investigating the association of non-leucocyte-reduced ABT with (a) short-term (up to 3-month posttransfusion), all-cause mortality and transfusing buffy-coat-reduced versus pre-storage filtered allogeneic RBCs or (b) conducted in cardiac surgery. For each RCT, the figure shows the OR of short-term mortality, as calculated from an intention-to-treat analysis and the summary OR across the depicted RCTs, as calculated from a meta-analysis. A deleterious ABT effect (and thus a benefit from leucocyte reduction) is demonstrated by an OR > 1, provided that the effect is statistically significant ($p < 0.05$; i.e. provided that the associated 95% CI does not include the null value of 1). For the references to the listed studies, see Further reading, Vamvakas & Blajchman (2007).

response modifiers during an already existing inflammatory cascade can push the SIRS/CARS equilibrium towards SIRS, thereby leading to MODS, MOF and death. Leucocyte-containing ABT administered during cardiac surgery may provide this 'second hit', exacerbating the SIRS and potentially causing the patient's death [8]. However, this explanation is speculative as, hitherto, no cardiac surgery RCT has reported an association between non-leucocyte-reduced (versus leucocyte-reduced) ABT and MOF.

111

Adverse effects of the transfusion of 'old' RBCs

Since 2005, the controversy about the deleterious effects of 'old' (versus 'fresh') RBCs has supplanted the debate on the purported adverse TRIM effects. When non-leucocyte-reduced 'old' RBCs are considered, some of the same postulated biologic mechanisms (e.g. the effects mediated by leucocyte-derived, soluble mediators) are invoked for both the adverse TRIM effects and the adverse effects of old RBCs. For both the non-leucocyte-reduced and leucocyte-reduced 'old' RBCs, additional mechanisms have been proposed for the association between transfusion of old RBCs and increased risk of short-term mortality, in-hospital infection or MOF, which include the following:
- proinflammatory, procoagulant and/or immune effects of old (rather than fresh) RBCs secondary to the development of microparticles in old blood;
- an increase in iron load from haemolysed stored RBCs;
- activation of complement and neutrophils and/or depletion of nitric oxide or S-nitrosylated hemoglobin in stored RBCs, which reduces the ability of the transfused RBCs to induce vasodilation (thereby resulting in inadequate blood flow and impaired oxygen delivery).

In the words of Ness [9], the question whether 'old' RBCs are less safe than fresh RBCs is the most critical issue facing transfusion medicine today. If the associations of old (rather than fresh) RBCs with increased mortality, infection and/or MOF reported from observational studies are shown to be causal, the allowed storage period of RBCs (35 or 42 days) will have to be promptly reduced – depending on the findings of future studies – to 2, 3 or 4 weeks. In addition, greater reliance will have to be placed on approaches to patient blood management [10], including the appropriate conservation and management of a patient's own blood as a vital resource, because the patient's own freshly shed blood is the freshest blood possible. Several large RCTs comparing the frequency of common adverse outcomes between recipients of 'old' and 'fresh' RBCs are currently enrolling patients in North America.

Some experts have argued that it is injudicious to wait for the results of these RCTs before we reduce the allowed RBC storage period. Instead of waiting for the definitive evidence that the ongoing RCTs will provide, inference of cause should be made from passive observation (i.e. from the results of the available observational studies), so that policy decisions can be made in the manner that they are made in risk-factor epidemiology – an area in which policymakers deal with deleterious exposures such as asbestos or tobacco smoke [11]. A widely publicized, large retrospective study published in a prominent journal reported an association between transfusion of RBCs older than 14 days and significantly increased mortality [12]. However, the conclusions reached by the numerous available observational studies are not unanimous and the hitherto-completed pilot RCTs have produced no evidence that transfusion of 'old' (rather than 'fresh') RBCs is associated with increased mortality.

Most observational studies reported on the effect of a single RBC unit: the oldest RBC unit transfused during a patient's hospitalization. Yet, observational studies suffer from an inability to separate any effect of the oldest transfused RBC unit from the effect of the number of transfused RBCs. Because need for RBC transfusion reflects the presence of comorbidities, more severe illness and a poorer baseline prognosis, the number of transfused RBCs is the best predictor of adverse outcomes in observational studies. In addition, the number of transfused RBCs is associated – nonspecifically – with *any* adverse outcome (be it mortality or major morbidity such as in-hospital infection or MOF), because it reflects – nonspecifically – more severe illness. As illustrated by van de Watering *et al.* [13], as patients receive a total transfusion dose of 1, 2, 3, . . . , 10, or >10 RBC units, the oldest transfused RBC unit gets, progressively and without fail, older and older. This is because each time a request for transfusion is received by the blood bank, the blood bank issues for transfusion the oldest compatible unit in the inventory. Therefore, the more often a patient is transfused, the more likely he/she is to be issued blood at a time that the oldest compatible unit is 'old'.

To establish a valid association between the length of storage of the oldest transfused unit and adverse outcomes in observational studies, it is therefore necessary to adjust any reported relationship for the number of transfused RBCs. A meta-analysis showed that integration of *adjusted* results from the observational studies published before 31 December 2008 (which had reported on the same outcome – mortality or infection or MOF – in the same clinical setting and had defined transfusion of 'old' versus 'fresh' RBCs in the same manner) produced summary results across the studies that were negative (showing no effect of old blood) in six of eight analyses [14]. The two situations in which old blood was associated with a worse outcome did not integrate results of studies that had adjusted for the effect of the most important confounder (i.e. the number of transfused RBCs). Three additional systematic reviews concluded that the existence of the purported common adverse effects of 'old' RBCs *cannot* be adequately inferred from the available data [15–17].

Edgren *et al.* included all patients receiving RBCs in Denmark and Sweden between 1995 and 2002, thereby including 404 959 transfusion episodes in their study [18]. These investigators found no effect of 'old' RBCs on short-term (7-day) mortality – an outcome comparable to the in-hospital mortality recorded by the other observational studies. With >400 000 transfusions in their database, Edgren *et al.* were able to use elaborate statistical modelling to adjust for the effects of confounding factors (including the number of transfused RBCs, as they reported separately on recipients of 1–2, 3–4 or ≥5 units, as well as on all patients and on recipients of leucocyte-reduced units); and they offered unprecedented statistical precision, as well as maximum generalizability of their findings.

Three pilot RCTs, intended to investigate the feasibility of conducting large RCTs of the relationship between transfusion of 'old' (rather than 'fresh') RBCs and common adverse outcomes, have reported data on the mortality of recipients of 'old' versus 'fresh' RBCs. All three studies showed no difference in mortality between the two arms and no trial showed a trend towards increased mortality in association with the receipt of 'old' (rather than 'fresh') RBCs.

Conclusions

TRIM appears to be a real biologic phenomenon resulting in at least one established beneficial clinical effect in humans, the enhanced survival of renal allografts in patients receiving pretransplant ABT, but the existence of deleterious clinical TRIM effects manifest across other clinical settings has not yet been confirmed by adequately powered RCTs. Except for cardiac surgery, there is no setting where the results of the RCTs of deleterious TRIM effects have been consistent. In cardiac surgery patients, the use of non-leucocyte-reduced ABT has been consistently associated with increased mortality, but, even in this setting, the reasons for the excess deaths remain elusive [8].

The other TRIM effects shown in Figures 10.2b and 10.3a, the one on postoperative infection prevented by post-storage filtration and the one on short-term mortality mediated by non-leucocyte-reduced ABT of buffy-coat-reduced RBCs, appear to contradict current theories about TRIM pathogenesis, because they are not accompanied by similar (or larger) ABT effects prevented by pre-storage filtration or mediated by buffy-coat-rich RBCs [4]. The effect prevented by post-storage filtration may be due to the inclusion in that analysis of two early studies by Jensen *et al.* (Figure 10.2b) of transfused blood components no longer used today (non-leucocyte-reduced versus leucocyte-reduced allogeneic whole blood or post-storage filtered, leucocyte-reduced allogeneic RBCs). These studies reported extraordinarily large adverse TRIM effects (Figure 10.2b). No TRIM effect is detected if these studies are excluded from the meta-analysis.

The effect on mortality mediated by buffy-coat-reduced RBCs may be due to overrepresentation in that analysis of the cardiac surgery RCTs. Thus, the only adverse TRIM effect of non-leucocyte-reduced ABT that has been clinically documented in humans is increased mortality in cardiac surgery. Until further studies are conducted to pinpoint the mechanisms for these excess deaths (or to refute this association), all cellular blood components transfused in cardiac surgery should be leucocyte-reduced components. At this time, the totality of the evidence from RCTs does not support a policy of universal leucocyte reduction introduced specifically to prevent TRIM, although universal leucocyte reduction can be justified based on other clinical benefits of leucocyte reduction.

Dzik *et al.* [19] tested the benefit accrued from providing leucocyte-reduced (versus non-leucocyte-reduced) RBCs to all 2780 patients who were transfused over 6 months at a tertiary-care medical centre. No difference in mortality, use of antibiotics or hospital stay was found when leucocyte-reduced (versus non-leucocyte-reduced) RBCs were given indiscriminately to all patients, regardless of disease classification or indication for transfusion. The study was criticized because of a high (20%) proportion of protocol violations, whereby the wrong (as opposed to the assigned) RBC component was given to the enrolled patients; such protocol violations would have biased the estimate of the effect towards the null.

The evidence for implementing universal leucocyte reduction for the prevention of the TRIM effects may not be available, because the requisite adequately powered studies have not been conducted. The design of the available RCTs has not been based on specific hypotheses about the mechanisms of TRIM formulated in the preclinical studies. For example, animal models of ABT and tumour growth have convincingly documented that allogeneic blood containing functional dendritic cells can facilitate the growth of selected tumours. However, none of the available RCTs has transfused fresh, non-leucocite-reduced RBCs to test this theory or has enrolled patients with tumours whose growth could be augmented by ABT. Furthermore, to separate the TRIM mechanism in surgical patients from the TRIM mechanism in renal transplantation, Dzik *et al.* [20] proposed the existence of two different categories of TRIM effects: one operating on the innate immune response and one operating on the adaptive antigen-driven immune system. Although the innate and adaptive immune systems are linked by subsets of natural killer and dendritic cells, the difference in the clinical condition of a surgical patient versus a patient in a steady-state disease may be important and account for the various TRIM effects reported from different settings.

The latest shift in research focus has been from the investigation of the adverse TRIM effects to the investigation of the adverse effects of 'old' RBCs. Despite impressions that have been generated in North America from highly publicized results of observational studies, there is a paucity of evidence on any association between transfusion of 'old' (versus 'fresh') RBCs and the common adverse outcomes of mortality, in-hospital infection or MOF. Given this paucity of evidence, it would be injudicious for policy-makers to endorse any radical change in policy (mandating transfusion of 'fresh' rather than 'old' RBCs) without waiting for the definitive evidence to be produced by the RCTs currently underway in North America.

Key points

1 TRIM is a real biologic phenomenon, resulting in at least one established beneficial clinical effect in humans (enhancement of renal allograft survival).
2 The existence of deleterious clinical TRIM effects has not yet been confirmed by adequately powered RCTs.
3 In cardiac surgery, transfusion of leucocyte-reduced (compared with non-leucocyte-reduced) allogeneic RBCs appears to reduce short-term (up to 3 months posttransfusion) all-cause mortality, but the reasons for the observed excess deaths remain elusive.
4 Based on the available data, leucocyte reduction of all cellular blood components – introduced specifically for the prevention of adverse TRIM effects – is indicated in cardiac surgery.
5 There is a paucity of evidence on any association between transfusion of 'old' RBCs and the common adverse outcomes of mortality, in-hospital infection or MOF.

References

1 Opelz G, Sengar DP, Mickey MR *et al.* Effect of blood transfusions on subsequent kidney transplants. *Transplant Proc* 1973; 5: 253–259.
2 Collier A, Kalish L, Busch M *et al.* Leukocyte-reduced red-blood-cell transfusion in patients with anemia and human immunodeficiency virus infection. *J Am Med Assoc* 2001; 285: 1592–1601.
3 Escobar GA, Cheng AM, Moore EE *et al.* Stored packed red blood cell transfusion up-regulates inflammatory gene expression in circulating leukocytes. *Ann Surg* 2007; 246: 129–134.
4 Vamvakas EC. Why have meta-analyses of the randomized controlled trials of the association between non-white-blood-cell reduced allogeneic blood transfusion and postoperative infection produced discordant results? *Vox Sanguinis* 2007; 93: 196–207.
5 Wallis JP, Chapman CE, Orr KE *et al.* Effect of leucoreduction of transfused RBCs on postoperative infection rates in cardiac surgery. *Transfusion* 2002; 42: 1127–1134.
6 van de Watering LMG, Hermans J, Houbiers JGA *et al.* Beneficial effect of leukocyte depletion of transfused blood on post-operative complications in patients undergoing cardiac surgery: a randomized clinical trial. *Circulation* 1998; 97: 562–568.

7 Bilgin YM, van de Watering LMG, Eijsman L et al. Double-blind randomized controlled trial on the effect of leukocyte-depleted erythrocyte transfusions in cardiac-valve surgery. *Circulation* 2004; 109: 2755–2760.

8 Bilgin YM & Brand A. Transfusion-related immunomodulation: a second hit in an inflammatory cascade? *Vox Sanguinis* 2008; 95: 261–271.

9 Ness PM. Does transfusion of stored red blood cells cause clinically important adverse effects? A critical question in search of an answer and a plan. *Transfusion* 2011; 51: 666–667.

10 Hofmann A, Farmer S & Shander A. Five drivers shifting the paradigm from product-focused transfusion practice to patient blood management. *Oncologist* 2011; 16(Suppl. 3): 3–11.

11 Isbister JP, Shander RA & Spahn DR. Adverse blood transfusion outcomes: establishing causation. *Transfus Med Rev* 2011; 25: 89–101.

12 Koch CG, Li L, Sessler DI et al. Duration of red cell storage and complications after cardiac surgery. *N Engl J Med* 2008; 358: 1229–1239.

13 van de Watering L, Lorinser J, Versteegh M et al. Effects of storage time of red-blood-cell transfusions on the prognosis of coronary-artery bypass-graft patients. *Transfusion* 2006; 46: 1712–1718.

14 Vamvakas EC. Meta-analysis of clinical studies of the purported deleterious effects of 'old' (versus 'fresh') red blood cells: Are we at equipoise? *Transfusion* 2010; 50: 600–610.

15 Zimrin AB & Hess JR. Current issues relating to the transfusion of stored red blood cells. *Vox Sanguinis* 2009; 96: 93–103.

16 Lelubre C, Piagnerelli M & Vincent JL. Association between storage of transfused red blood cells and morbidity and mortality in adult patients: Myth or reality? *Transfusion* 2009; 49: 1348–1394.

17 van de Watering L. Red cell storage and prognosis. *Vox Sanguinis* 2011; 100: 36–45.

18 Edgren G, Kamper-Jorgensen M, Eloranta S et al. Duration of red-blood-cell storage and survival of transfused patients. *Transfusion* 2010; 50: 1185–1195.

19 Dzik WH, Anderson JK, O'Neill EM et al. A prospective randomized clinical trial of universal leukoreduction. *Transfusion* 2002; 42: 1114–1122.

20 Dzik WH, Mincheff M & Puppo F. An alternative mechanism for the immunosuppressive effect of transfusion. *Vox Sanguinis* 2002; 83(Suppl.): S417–S419.

Further reading

Blajchman MA & Bordin JO. Mechanisms of transfusion-associated immunosuppression. *Curr Opin Hematol* 1994; 1: 457–461.

Vamvakas EC. Equipoise and the continued transfusion of 'old' blood. *Decision-Making in Transfusion Medicine*. Bethesda, MD: AABB Press; 2011, pp. 235–263.

Vamvakas EC & Blajchman MA. Transfusion-related immunomodulation (TRIM): an update. *Blood Rev* 2007; 21: 327–348.

Vamvakas EC, Bordin JO & Blajchman MA. Immunomodulatory and proinflammatory effects of allogeneic blood transfusion. In: TL Simon, EL Snyder, BG Solheim et al. (eds), *Rossi's Principles of Transfusion Medicine*, 4th edn. Bethesda, MD: AABB Press; 2009, pp. 699–717.

van de Watering L. Pitfalls in the current published observational literature on the effects of red blood cell storage. *Transfusion* 2011; 51: 1847–1854.

11 Transfusion-associated graft-versus-host disease and microchimerism

Beth H. Shaz[1,2], *Richard O. Francis*[1,3] & *Christopher D. Hillyer*[1,4]

[1]New York Blood Center, New York, NY, USA
[2]Emory University School of Medicine, Atlanta, GA, USA
[3]Columbia University Medical Center, New York, NY, USA
[4]Weill Cornell Medical College, New York, NY, USA

Transfusion-associated graft-versus-host disease

Transfusion-associated graft-versus-host disease (TA-GVHD) is an uncommon yet highly fatal complication of cellular blood component transfusion; cellular components are defined as red blood cell (RBC), platelet and granulocyte components (not fresh frozen plasma). TA-GVHD is defined by the UK haemovigilance system Serious Hazards of Transfusion (SHOT) as fever, rash, liver dysfunction, diarrhoea and pancytopenia occurring 1–6 weeks after transfusion, without other apparent cause (similarly the US National Healthcare Safety Network Biovigilance system definition for definitive diagnosis is fever, rash, hepatomegaly, diarrhoea between 2 days and 6 weeks after transfusion with laboratory evidence of liver dysfunction, pancytopenia, leucocyte chimerism and findings of TA-GVHD on skin or liver biopsy). Development of TA-GVHD requires the product to contain immunologically competent lymphocytes and the recipient must express tissue antigens absent in the donor and must be incapable of mounting an effective immune response to destroy the foreign lymphocytes. Cellular blood products contain viable lymphocytes that can proliferate and result in TA-GVHD. Inactivation of these lymphocytes, usually through irradiation, prevents TA-GVHD. The identification of individuals at high risk for TA-GVHD, such as immune-impaired patients or those receiving products from relatives, and the subsequent requirement that these individuals receive irradiated products, reduces the incidence of TA-GVHD, but its elimination requires universal irradiation or lymphocyte inactivation of all cellular blood components.

Pathogenesis

TA-GVHD results from the engraftment of transfused donor T-lymphocytes in a recipient whose immune system is unable to reject them. The mechanism of TA-GVHD is similar to that of acute GVHD after haemopoietic stem cell (HSC) transplantation. Donor T-lymphocytes recognize recipient HLA antigens as foreign, resulting in activation and proliferation of the lymphocytes, which leads to host cell death and tissue destruction.

Clinical features

TA-GVHD is an acute illness characterized by fever, rash, pancytopenia, diarrhoea and liver dysfunction which begins 4–30 days (median 8–10 days) after transfusion and results in death within 3 weeks from symptom onset in over 90% of the cases [1]. In neonates the clinical manifestations are similar, yet the interval between transfusion and onset is longer; the

Practical Transfusion Medicine, Fourth Edition. Edited by Michael F. Murphy, Derwood H. Pamphilon and Nancy M. Heddle.
© 2013 John Wiley & Sons, Ltd. Published 2013 by John Wiley & Sons, Ltd.

median time of onset of fever is 28 days, rash 30 days and death 51 days [2]. In the typical scenario, fever is the presenting symptom followed by an erythematous maculopapular rash, which begins on the face and trunk and spreads to the extremities. Liver dysfunction manifests as an obstructive jaundice or an acute hepatitis. Gastrointestinal complications include nausea, anorexia or diarrhoea. Leucopenia and pancytopenia, the primary reason for death resulting from sepsis, candidiasis and multiorgan failure, develop later and progressively become more severe.

Diagnosis

The diagnosis of TA-GVHD is based on the characteristic clinical manifestations, pathologic findings on tissue biopsy, and, if possible, evidence of donor-derived lymphocytes in the recipient's blood or affected tissues. Laboratory data demonstrate pancytopenia and abnormal liver function tests. Skin biopsy changes include epidermal basal cell vacuolization and mononuclear cell infiltration. Liver biopsy findings include degeneration of the small bile ducts, periportal mononuclear infiltrates and cholestasis. The bone marrow is usually hypocellular or aplastic, which is the primary differentiating feature between TA-GVHD and GVHD occurring after HSC transplantation. The discovery of donor lymphocytes or DNA in the patient's peripheral blood or tissue biopsy with the appropriate clinical scenario confirms the diagnosis. Donor-derived DNA is usually detected using polymerase chain reaction (PCR)-based HLA typing; other methods include the use of amplified fragment length polymorphisms, variable-number tandem repeat analysis, short tandem repeat analysis, microsatellite markers and cytogenetics.

Treatment

Most treatments of TA-GVHD are largely ineffective including aggressive use of corticosteroids, antithymocyte globulin, ciclosporin and growth factors. However, spontaneous resolution and successful treatment with a combination of ciclosporin, steroids and OKT3 (anti-CD3 monoclonal antibody) or antithymocyte globulin have been reported. Transient improvement has been seen with nafamostat mesilate, a serine protease inhibitor that inhibits cytotoxic T-lymphocytes. There are case reports of successful treatment with autologous or allogeneic HSC transplantation.

Prevention

Since treatment options for TA-GVHD are mostly unsuccessful, patients at increased risk must be identified and transfused with lymphocyte inactivated products, usually by gamma-irradiation or pathogen inactivation technologies. Gamma-radiation is derived from decay of radioactive isotopes, such as caesium-137 or cobalt-60. Properly installed and maintained radioisotope instruments are safe, but their use requires appropriate security, radiation safety protocols and training (in the USA, blood irradiators are regulated by the Nuclear Regulatory Commission). Some pathogen reduction technologies have been shown in human clinical trials, mouse models and other lymphocyte proliferation assays to inactivate T-lymphocytes (Table 11.1). Gamma-irradiation is the most common method used for irradiation to prevent TA-GVHD; in Europe the use of pathogen inactivation for platelets is growing, and irradiation by X-ray generated by linear

Table 11.1 Potential methods for leucocyte inactivation.

Method	Leucocyte inactivation
Ultraviolet B	Inhibits TA-GVHD in dog transfusion model
8-Methoxypsoralen with UV	Inhibits activation and proliferation
Aminomethyl trimethylpsoralen with UVA	Inhibits activation and proliferation
Amotosalen (S-59) with UVA	Inhibits activation and proliferation
	Inhibits TA-GVHD in murine transfusion model
Methylene blue with light	Does not inactivate leucocytes
Dimethylmethylene blue with light	No data on leucocyte inactivation
Riboflavin with UV	Inhibits proliferation
Inactine (PEN 110)	Inhibits TA-GVHD in murine transfusion model
	Inhibits activation and proliferation
Thionine with UVB	Inhibits proliferation

Adapted by permission from Macmillan Publishers Ltd, *Bone Marrow Transplant* 2004, 33(1): 1–7, copyright 2004.

acceleration is increasing in the USA as a non radionuclide source.

Source and dose of ionizing radiation

Both gamma-rays and X-rays inactivate T-lymphocytes and can be used to irradiate blood components. Usually gamma-rays originate from caesium-137 or cobalt-60 while X-rays are generated from linear accelerators. Quality assurance measures should be performed, including dose mapping, adjustment of irradiation time to correct for isotopic decay, assurance of no radiation leakage, timer accuracy, turntable operation, preventive maintenance and a qualitative indicator label to confirm that blood products have been properly irradiated.

The dose of irradiation must be sufficient to inhibit lymphocyte proliferation but not significantly damage RBCs, platelets and granulocytes or their functions. Assays to assess the effect of irradiation on T-lymphocyte proliferation include mixed lymphocyte culture (MLC) assay and limiting dilution analysis (LDA). The recommended dose varies between 15 and 50 Gy (Table 11.2). Of note, there have been three patients transfused with irradiated blood products, two at doses of 20 Gy [3, 4] and one at 15 Gy [5], who developed TA-GVHD, but it is unknown if there was a process or dose failure.

Adverse effects of irradiation

At recommended doses, radiation causes some oxidation and damage to lipid components of membranes, which continues during storage. Products irradiated immediately prior to transfusion appear to be unaffected and have virtually normal function. In stored products, radiation modestly harms RBCs, but does not appear to affect platelet and granulocyte function significantly in the clinically utilized doses. The effects on RBCs include an increase in extracellular potassium and a decrease in posttransfusion RBC survival. The increase in extracellular potassium is usually not of clinical significance because of posttransfusion dilution of the potassium. However, there may be certain patients who are sensitive to the increased potassium resulting in transfusion-associated hyperkalemia, such as premature infants, infants receiving large RBC volumes and fetuses receiving intrauterine transfusions (IUT), neonatal exchange transfusions or intracardiac transfusions via central line catheters. The potassium increase can be prevented by either irradiating the RBC product within 24 hours of infusion or washing the RBC product prior to transfusion. Also RBC products stored in additive solutions have lower extracellular potassium than CPDA-1 units of a similar age. The *in vivo* viability of irradiated RBCs evaluated at 24-hour recovery is reduced by 3–10% compared to nonirradiated RBCs [6]. As a consequence, RBC product outdate is variably shortened to 14–28 days after irradiation (Table 11.2).

Blood component factors

Age of blood

Use of fresh blood increases the risk of TA-GVHD. A Japanese series of cases of TA-GVHD in immunocompetent patients found that 62% of patients had received blood less than 72 hours old [1] and a US series found about 90% of cases received blood less than 4 days old [10]. The increased risk with fresh blood is possibly due to the function and viability of lymphocytes as during storage these cells undergo apoptosis and fail to stimulate an MLC response. Therefore, older blood may be less likely to cause TA-GVHD.

Leucocyte dose

Leucocyte reduction of blood components may decrease the risk of TA-GVHD, but it does not eliminate it. SHOT data reported a decrease in the number of TA-GVHD cases following universal leucocyte reduction of blood components in the UK in 1999 [11].

Blood components

All cellular blood components, including RBCs, platelets, granulocytes, whole blood and fresh plasma (not frozen plasma) contain viable T-lymphocytes that are capable of causing TA-GVHD (Table 11.2). Granulocyte transfusions are the highest risk product because they have a high lymphocyte count and are administered fresh to neutropenic and immunosuppressed patients. Therefore, it is recommended that all granulocyte products undergo irradiation prior to transfusion and the remaining cellular blood components be irradiated for patients at increased risk.

Table 11.2 Comparison of irradiation guidelines, including dose and indications.

	UK [7]	USA [8]	Japan [9]
Techniques	Gamma-irradiation or X-rays	Gamma-irradiation or X-rays	Gamma-irradiation
Dose	Minimum 2500 cGy No part >5000 cGy	2500 cGy at centre of product Minimum 1500 cGy at any point Maximum 5000 cGy	Between 1500 and 5000 cGy

Type of product	All cellular products:
	  Whole blood
	  RBCs
	  Platelets
	  Granulocytes
		All cellular products:
		  Whole blood
		  RBCs
		  Platelets
		  Granulocytes
			All cellular products:
			  Whole blood
			  RBCs
			  Platelets
			  Granulocytes
			  Fresh plasma

Age of product	RBCs <14 days after collection For hyperkalaemia risk, e.g. exchange or intrauterine transfusion: <24 h before transfusion Platelets – any time during 5 day storage	RBCs – any time Platelets – any time	RBCs – ≤ 3 days – regardless of recipient ≤ 14 days – if clinically indicated At any time – if patient immunocompromised
Expiration	RBCs stored for 14 days after irradiation	RBCs stored for up to 28 days after irradiation or original outdate, whichever is sooner	Irradiated RBCs – up to 3 weeks after collection
General	All blood from relatives All HLA-selected products All granulocytes	All blood from relatives All HLA-selected products	All blood from relatives All HLA-selected products
Neonates	Intrauterine transfusions Exchange transfusions in IUT babies	IUT	All
Congenital immunodeficiency	All	All	All
Allogeneic HSC transplantation	All – at least 6 months post-BMT; longer in selected patients	All	All
Autologous HSC transplantation	All – at least 3 months post-BMT; 6 months if TBI used		
Leukaemia	No	*	To be considered
Hodgkin disease	All stages	*	To be considered
Purine analogues	All	*	Not discussed
Non-Hodgkin lymphoma	Not discussed	*	To be considered
Solid tumours	No	*	To be considered
Solid organ transplants	No	*	To be considered
Cardiovascular surgery	No	No	Yes
AIDS	No	No	No

*According to policies and procedures developed by the blood bank or transfusion service.

Table 11.3 Indications for irradiated cellular blood components to prevent TA-GVHD.

Clear indications

Congenital immunodeficiency syndromes (suspected or known)

Allogeneic and autologous haemopoietic progenitor cell transplantation

Transfusions from blood relatives

HLA-matched or partially HLA-matched products (platelet transfusions)

Granulocyte transfusions

Hodgkin disease

Treatment with purine analogue drugs (fludarabine, cladribine and deoxycoformycin)

Treatment with Campath (anti-CD52) and other drugs/antibodies that affect T-lymphocyte number or function

Intrauterine transfusions

Indications deemed appropriate by most authorities

Neonatal exchange transfusions

Pre-term infants/low birthweight infants

Infant/child with congenital heart disease (secondary to possible DiGeorge syndrome)

Acute leukaemia

Non-Hodgkin lymphoma and other haematologic malignancies

Aplastic anaemia

Solid tumours receiving intensive chemotherapy and/or radiotherapy

Recipient and donor pair from a genetically homogeneous population

Indications unwarranted by most authorities

Solid organ transplantation

Healthy newborns/term infants

HIV/AIDS

Patients at increased risk

Patient populations have varying risk factors for developing TA-GVHD (Table 11.3). It is difficult to quantify any of these risks because the number of these patients, the number who are transfused or the number of transfusions or type of products received are unknown. The risk is therefore derived from case reports or haemovigilance data, which is biased by underrecognition, misdiagnosis and under- and passive reporting.

Congenital immunodeficiency patients

The first reported cases of TA-GVHD occurred in the 1960s in children with T-lymphocyte congenital immunodeficiency syndromes. Children with severe congenital immunodeficiency syndromes (SCID) and with variable immunodeficiency syndromes, such as Wiskott–Aldrich and DiGeorge syndromes, have developed TA-GVHD. These children may be transfused prior to the recognition of these immunodeficiency syndromes, which has been reported in two infants in Canada. Because of the possibility of the patient not being known to be immunodeficient, it may be prudent to irradiate all blood components for children under a certain age. This is particularly true with infants undergoing cardiac surgery who may have unrecognized DiGeorge syndrome. In three reported cases of TA-GVHD in SCID patients, allogeneic HSC transplantation was successful in treating the disease. It is recommended that all patients with suspected or confirmed congenital immunodeficiency receive irradiated products.

Allogeneic and autologous HSC recipients

Both allogeneic and autologous HSC transplant recipients are at increased risk of TA-GVHD. Patients who undergo allogeneic HSC transplantation have received irradiated blood products routinely for over 40 years. Multiple organizations, including The European School of Haematology (ESH), European Group for Blood and Marrow Transplantation (EMBT) and Foundation for the Accreditation of Cellular Therapy (FACT), recommend irradiated blood products for allogeneic and autologous HSC recipients, but it is unclear for how long before and after transplantation these patients require irradiated blood products.

Leukaemia and lymphoma patients

Patients with haematologic malignancies are at increased risk for TA-GVHD, especially patients with Hodgkin disease (HD). Twenty cases were reported in patients with malignant lymphoma, 13 in association with HD and 7 with non-Hodgkin lymphoma (NHL), and all undergoing therapy for active disease at the time. Five of thirteen cases reported to SHOT were associated with haematologic malignancies (Table 11.4). In the 1970s and 1980s, cases of TA-GVHD occurred in patients with acute leukaemia undergoing chemotherapy; the majority of these patients had received granulocyte transfusions. It is recommended

Table 11.4 Cases of TA-GVHD reported to SHOT 1996 through 2001.*

Year	Number of cases	Case	Diagnosis and/or possible risk factor	RBCs and/or platelets leukodepletion	Donor-recipient HLA haplotype share
1996–1997	4	1	Immunodeficient neonate, not diagnosed at time of transfusion	No	Reported as haplotype share; no other details provided
		2	Epistaxis, age 88	No	NK
		3	B-cell NHL	No	NK
		4	B-cell NHL	No	NK
1997–1998	4	5	Waldenstom's macroglobulinaemia	No	Donor reported as homozygous; no other details provided; patient's HLA type not determined
		6	B-cell NHL	No	Yes; donor homozygous: A1; B8; DR17 Patient: A1, A31; B7, B8, Bw6; Cw7; DR17; DQ2
		7	CABG, RBCs less than 3 days old	No	Yes; donor homozygous: A*01; B*0801; DRB1*0301
		8	ITP, treated with prednisolone	No	NK
1998–1999	4	9	Myeloma, 6 units of RBCs, all less than 7 days old	Yes	NK
		10	Male, age 53; uncharacterized immunodeficiency; HIV negative	No	NK; 100% XX cells in marrow
		11	CABG, also received platelets	No	NK (32 donors)
		12	CABG	No	Donor homozygous: A*01; B*0801; Cw*0701/06/07; DRB1*0301; DQB1*0201/02 Patient: A*01, A*3301/03; B*0801, B*14202/03; Cw*0701/06/07; Cw*0802; DRB1*0301, DRB1*0701/03; DQB1*03032/06, DQB1*0201/02
1999–2000	0				
2000–2001	1	13	Relapsed ALL on UKALL R2. Died despite 'rescue' HSC allograft	Yes	NK; chimerism shown by variable-number tandem repeat analysis but no donor HLA typing performed
Total	13				

*No cases were reported from 2002 through 2010.
CABG, coronary artery bypass grafting; ITP, immune thrombocytopenia; NHL, non-Hodgkin lymphoma; HSC, haemopoietic stem cell; NKs, not known.
Reprinted with permission from Williamson *et al.* (2007) [11].

that patients with haematological malignancies receive irradiated products; however, it is less clear if this requirement should be only during active treatment.

Recipients of fludarabine and other purine analogues as well as other drugs/antibodies that affect T-lymphocyte number or function

TA-GVHD was initially reported in patients with CLL receiving fludarabine, a purine analogue that results in profound lymphopenia. There are nine cases of TA-GVHD in CLL, AML and NHL patients who received fludarabine up to 11 months prior to transfusion. In addition, TA-GVHD occurred in one patient who received fludarabine for autoimmune disease. Other purine analogues, including deoxycoformycin (pentostatin) and chlorodeoxyadenosine (cladribine), have been associated with the development of TA-GVHD. Thus, it is recommended that all patients who have received fludarabine or other purine analogues as well as Campath (anti-CD52) or other drugs/antibodies that affect T-lymphocyte function or number be transfused with irradiated products; however, it is unclear if this requirement should only be for at least one year and until recovery from the resulting lymphopenia following the administration of these drugs.

Fetus and neonate

Fetuses and neonates have immature immune systems and may be at increased risk of TA-GVHD. In neonates, most cases of TA-GVHD reported are in those with congenital immunodeficiency or that received products from related donors. At least ten cases have been reported after neonatal exchange transfusions; four occurred in infants who had previously received IUT. Seven cases were in preterm infants (excluding those who received a product from a relative). A single case report involved a full-term infant receiving extracorporeal membrane oxygenation (ECMO). The use of irradiated products for fetal and neonatal transfusions is recommended for exchange transfusions and IUT, preterm infants, infants with congenital immunodeficiency and those receiving products from relatives; its need is less clear for other neonatal transfusions.

Patients with aplastic anaemia

Since patients with aplastic anaemia are usually treated with intensive chemotherapy regimens and possible HSC transplantation, some authorities recommend they receive irradiated products, especially during myelosuppressive therapy or treatment with antithymocyte globulin.

Patients receiving chemotherapy and immunotherapy

TA-GVHD has occurred in patients with solid tumours, including neuroblastoma, rhabdomyosarcoma and bladder and small cell lung cancer, during intensive myeloablative therapy. Therefore, it is recommended that patients with solid tumours receive irradiated products, especially during myelosuppressive therapy.

Solid organ transplantation recipients

GVHD is a rare complication of solid organ transplantation, which usually results from the passenger lymphocytes contained within the solid organ and not from transfusion, even though these individuals are highly immunosuppressed and transfused. There have been four cases of TA-GVHD in solid organ transplant recipients; one was a liver transplant recipient with pre-existing pancytopenia, one a heart transplant recipient and two were inconclusive cases in kidney transplant recipients. The risk of TA-GVHD in solid organ transplant recipients appears low and the use of irradiated products is generally considered to be unwarranted.

Human immunodeficiency virus (HIV) and acquired immunodeficiency syndrome (AIDS) patients

HIV/AIDS is not considered a risk factor for TA-GVHD as there is only a single case report of a child with AIDS developing transient TA-GVHD. It is postulated that HIV infects the transfused T-lymphocytes and thus prohibits the donor lymphocytes from engrafting. The use of irradiated blood products in HIV/AIDS patients is not warranted, but approximately a quarter of institutions in the USA choose to take this precaution, probably because of the immunosuppresive nature of HIV/AIDS and the high degree of fatality of TA-GVHD.

Cardiovascular surgery patients

Prior to the Japanese changing their irradiation policies, their reported incidence of TA-GVHD following cardiovascular surgery was 0.15–0.47%. Fifty-six of the 122 cases of TA-GVHD reported in Japan from 1985 to 1993 were patients after cardiovascular surgery; 28% used blood from a relative and 72% used blood less than 72 hours old [1]. They also reported a lower risk for women than men, possibly secondary to women having previous exposure to leucocytes during pregnancy and childbirth. There are five cases reported in the UK (Table 11.4) and one in the USA [12]. Possible reasons for the increased risk are that the RBC products are usually less than 72 hours old and cardiac surgery may result in reduced cell-mediated immunity. The recommendation for irradiated products is warranted in Japan but not in the USA or UK at this time.

Immunocompetent patients

TA-GVHD has been reported in immunocompetent patients, especially those who received transfusions of blood products donated by close relatives. The majority of cases reported in immunocompetent patients occurred with the use of fresh whole blood from a close relative [13]. In a review of 122 cases of TA-GVHD in immunocompetent Japanese patients, 67% had not received products from a related donor and of the 66 noncardiovascular surgery patients, 39 had solid tumours and 27 had other conditions [1]. The risk of receiving a blood product from a homozygous donor is greatest in populations with limited HLA haplotype polymorphisms, such as Japan [14] (Table 11.5). The frequency of reported cases is sub-

Table 11.5 Frequency of homozygous HLA donors in various populations.

Frequency of transfusion from homozygous donors to potential heterozygous recipients

Population	Parent/child	Sibling	Unrelated
US Whites	1:475	1:920	1:7174
Japan	1:102	1:193	1:874
Canada Whites	1:154	1:294	1:1664
Germany	1:220	1:424	1:3144
Korea	1:183	1:356	1:3220
Spain	1:226	1:438	1:3552
South African Blacks	1:286	1:558	1:5519
Italy	1:434	1:854	1:12870
France	1:762	1:2685	1:16835

stantially lower than these estimates, which may be a result of unrecognized and/or unreported cases, lymphocytes in blood products that are either nonviable or insufficient to cause disease and/or recipients who may be able to destroy the donor lymphocytes based on minor HLA differences between the donor and recipient. Irradiation of products from close relatives and HLA matched products is recommended, but the risk is minimal for other immunocompetent patients.

Guidelines and requirements for irradiated products

In 1989, AABB institutional members were surveyed about their blood product irradiation practices [15]. Approximately 10.1% of the products transfused were irradiated, which has remained fairly constant. The indications included patients with allogeneic HSC transplantation (88%), autologous HSC transplantation (81.4%), congenital immunodeficiency syndrome (68.4%), premature newborn (53.9%), leukaemia (51.4%), organ transplantation (40.4%), HD (34.0%), NHL (32.0%), HLA matched product (31.0%), AIDS (24.5%), term newborn (24.0%) and solid tumour (20.0%). This survey highlighted the need for guidelines. In 1996, the American Society for Clinical Pathology and the UK published guidelines for the use of irradiation to prevent TA-GVHD; the UK guidelines were updated in 2010 [7] (Table 11.2). Japan has elected to irradiate all blood products.

Only two of the 13 TA-GVHD cases reported to SHOT fulfilled the current UK guideline criteria for irradiated blood products, which highlights the need to continually monitor and revise the definition of high-risk individuals. The remaining 11 patients may have had some degree of unrecognized immunosuppression or shared HLA haplotypes with the donors, potentially demonstrating the need for universal irradiation.

Universal irradiation

As case reports cited above indicate, TA-GVHD can occur in immunocompetent patients and individuals where the degree of immunocompromise was not known or properly identified prior to transfusion. Given that TA-GVHD is fatal in almost all cases and the risk of radiation of a product includes only minimal cost and effect on product potency, many authorities consider that the cost : benefit ratio is weighted in favour of universal irradiation. Consideration of universal irradiation should be undertaken on a local, regional or national basis, as appropriate.

Haemovigilance

Some countries have begun comprehensive tracking systems for adverse events of blood transfusion (Chapter 18). SHOT data from 1996 to 2005 revealed that 11 cases of TA-GVHD occurred with the use of non-leucocyte-reduced and two cases with leucocyte-reduced products (Table 11.4). No additional cases have been reported through 2010. In addition there were 405 reports where irradiated products were indicated and were not used due to error. From 1992 to 2000, two cases of TA-GVHD have been reported to Health Canada with the addition of 1–2 cases that were presented but not reported. Irradiated blood products were used in Canada for highly immunocompromised patients and patients receiving directed donation from close relatives. With this information, the risk of TA-GVHD in Canada is estimated to be less than 1 per million products transfused. The continued occurrence of TA-GVHD is likely to be from lack of agreement on the level of immunodeficiency that results in increased risk and patients with immunocompromised conditions who receive nonirradiated products either secondary to not being identified prior to transfusion or the product not being irradiated by error. On the other hand, the low incidence reported may be secondary to underreporting and/or underrecognition, the fact that lymphocytes are no longer capable of proliferating because the blood is older by the time of transfusion, the risk decreasing by leucocyte reduction of blood products and the genetic heterogeneity of Canadians.

Transfusion-associated microchimerism

Chimerism is defined as the presence of two genetically distinct cell lines in a single organism. Haemopoietic chimerism refers to the persistence of allogeneic donor lymphocytes in a recipient. Microchimerism (MC) occurs when these donor cells represent a small population (less than 5%) and can be a consequence of pregnancy, organ transplantation or transfusion. With increased sensitivity of methods, MC can be detected

not infrequently after transfusion, but the conditions that facilitate and consequences of this phenomenon are unknown.

Normal clearance of transfused lymphocytes

In a study investigating the clearance of lymphocytes in immunocompetent recipients, three phases were found: first, 99.9% of the lymphocytes were cleared over the first 2 days, second, there was a 1-log increase in the number of circulating donor lymphocytes on days 3–5 and, lastly, there was a secondary clearance [16]. It was postulated that this transient increase in donor lymphocytes represents one arm of an *in vivo* mixed lymphocyte reaction with activated donor T-lymphocytes proliferating in reaction to HLA-incompatible recipient cells.

Clinical data

TA-MC has been reported mostly in trauma patients [17], but has also been reported in sickle cell disease and thalassemia patients. HIV-positive individuals do not have sustained TA-MC. Irradiation of products prevents TA-MC. Leucocyte reduction of blood products is reported not to decrease the incidence of TA-MC among trauma patients [18]. In addition, TA-MC can be sustained for decades after transfusion [19]. Age, gender, injury severity score, splenectomy and number of units transfused did not correlate with the establishment of TA-MC in trauma patients. When patients were evaluated for symptoms suggestive of chronic GVHD several months after transfusion, TA-MC did not correlate with these symptoms. One study reported a decrease in donor-specific lymphocyte response in TA-MC trauma patients versus non-TA-MC patients [20]. TA-MC may occur, especially in trauma patients, but its conditions and consequences are unknown.

Testing for TA-MC

Detection of TA-MC requires the ability to detect small amounts of minor population DNA among large amounts of host DNA and selection of optimal genetic differences. One technique is to use real-time PCR. Initially this technique was used to detect the Y chromosome in women who received blood transfusions from at least one male donor. This has been expanded to a panel of 12 HLA-DR polymorphisms. A third improvement was the addition of a panel of 12 insertion/deletion (InDel) polymorphisms.

Testing limitations

The ability to detect TA-MC is limited by sample volume and sampling error. Large sample volume creates too much DNA and results in difficulties in testing. Sampling error is likely when an extremely low level of TA-MC exists. Techniques that look for the Y chromosome in women transfused with male blood components are of limited value, because this can result from the previous carrying of a male fetus. Because the clinical significance, if any, of TA-MC remains unknown, molecular testing is for research purposes.

Clinical consequences

To date, no clear relationship of TA-MC to clinical outcomes has been elucidated. To determine the association between TA-MC and autoimmune or other diseases, important confounding factors need to be considered, and long follow-up times are needed as these diseases can take years to develop and may result in vague symptoms. Currently, the conditions that facilitate TA-MC and its consequences remain to be established.

Key points

1 TA-GVHD is a rare yet highly fatal complication of cellular blood component transfusion.
2 TA-GVHD can be prevented by using irradiated or leucocyte-inactivated blood components.
3 Patients at increased risk for TA-GVHD include those who are immune impaired and those receiving blood components donated from relatives.
4 Leucocyte dose and age of the blood component, HLA matching between the donor and the recipient and immune state of the recipient contribute to the likelihood of developing TA-GVHD.
5 While there is strong data for providing irradiated blood components to prevent TA-GVHD in some patient populations, the need for irradiation in other disease states is less clear (refer to Table 11.3).

6 With increased sensitivity of methods to detect chimerism, microchimerism can be detected not infrequently after transfusion, but the conditions that facilitate it and its clinical consequences are unknown.

References

1 Ohto H & Anderson KC. Survey of transfusion-associated graft-versus-host disease in immunocompetent recipients. *Transfus Med Rev* 1996; 10: 31–43.
2 Ohto H & Anderson KC. Posttransfusion graft-versus-host disease in Japanese newborns. *Transfusion* 1996; 36: 117–123.
3 Drobyski S, Thibodeau S, Truitt RL *et al*. Third-party-mediated graft rejection and graft-versus-host disease after T-cell-depleted bone marrow transplantation, as demonstrated by hypervariable DNA probes and HLA-DR polymorphism. *Blood* 1989; 74: 2285–2294.
4 Sproul AM, Chalmers EA, Mills KI *et al*. Third party mediated graft rejection despite irradiation of blood products. *Br J Haematol* 1992; 80: 251–252.
5 Lowenthal RM, Challis DR, Griffiths AE *et al*. Transfusion-associated graft-versus-host disease: report of an occurrence following the administration of irradiated blood. *Transfusion* 1993; 33: 524–529.
6 Davey RJ, McCoy NC, Yu M *et al*. The effect of prestorage irradiation on posttransfusion red cell survival. *Transfusion* 1992; 32: 525–528.
7 Treleaven J, Gennery A, Marsh J *et al*. Guidelines on the use of irradiated blood components prepared by the British committee for standards in haematology blood transfusion task force. *Br J Haematol* 2011; 152: 35–51.
8 Roback JD (ed.). *Technical Manual: AABB*, 17th edn. Bethesda, MD: AABB; 2011, pp. 753–755.
9 Asai T, Inaba S, Ohto H *et al*. Guidelines for irradiation of blood and blood components to prevent post-transfusion graft-vs.-host disease in Japan. *Transfus Med* 2000; 10: 315–320.
10 Petz LD, Calhoun L, Yam P *et al*. Transfusion-associated graft-versus-host disease in immunocompetent patients: report of a fatal case associated with transfusion of blood from a second-degree relative, and a survey of predisposing factors. *Transfusion* 1993; 33: 742–750.
11 Williamson LM, Stainsby D, Jones H *et al*. The impact of universal leukodepletion of the blood supply on hemovigilance reports of posttransfusion purpura and transfusion-associated graft-versus-host disease. *Transfusion* 2007; 47: 1455–1467.
12 Triulzi D, Duquesnoy R, Nichols L *et al*. Fatal transfusion-associated graft-versus-host disease in an

immunocompetent recipient of a volunteer unit of red cells. *Transfusion* 2006; 46: 885–888.

13 Agbaht K, Altintas ND, Topeli A *et al.* Transfusion-associated graft-versus-host disease in immunocompetent patients: case series and review of the literature. *Transfusion* 2007; 47: 1405–1411.

14 Ohto H, Yasuda H, Noguchi M *et al.* Risk of transfusion-associated graft-versus-host disease as a result of directed donations from relatives. *Transfusion* 1992; 32: 691–693.

15 Anderson KC, Goodnough LT, Sayers M *et al.* Variation in blood component irradiation practice: implications for prevention of transfusion-associated graft-versus-host disease. *Blood* 1991; 77: 2096–2102.

16 Lee TH, Donegan E, Slichter S *et al.* Transient increase in circulating donor leukocytes after allogeneic transfusions in immunocompetent recipients compatible with donor cell proliferation. *Blood* 1995; 85: 1207–1214.

17 Utter GH, Owings JT, Lee TH *et al.* Blood transfusion is associated with donor leukocyte microchimerism in trauma patients. *J Trauma* 2004; 57: 702–708.

18 Utter GH, Nathens AB, Lee TH *et al.* Leukoreduction of blood transfusions does not diminish transfusion-associated microchimerism in trauma patients. *Transfusion* 2006; 46: 1863–1869.

19 Utter GH, Lee TZ, Rivers RM *et al.* Microchimerism decades after transfusion among combat-injured US veterans from the Vietnam, Korean, World War II conflicts. *Transfusion* 2008; 48: 1609–1615.

20 Utter GH, Owings JT, Lee TZ *et al.* Microchimerism in transfused trauma patients is associated with diminished donor-specific lymphocyte response. *J Trauma* 2005; 58: 925–932.

Further reading

Corash L & Lin L. Novel processes for inactivation of leukocytes to prevent transfusion-associated graft-versus-host disease. *Bone Marrow Transplant* 2004; 33: 1–7.

Hume HA & Preiksaitis JB. Transfusion associated graft-versus-host disease, cytomegalovirus infection and HLA alloimmunization in neonatal and pediatric patients. *Transfus Sci* 1999; 21: 73–95.

Marschner S, Fast LD, Baldwin WM *et al.* White blood cell inactivation after treatment with riboflavin and ultraviolet light. *Transfusion* 2010; 50: 2489–2498.

Mintz PD & Wehrli G. Irradiation eradication and pathogen reduction. Ceasing cesium irradiation of blood products. *Bone Marrow Transplant* 2009; 44: 205–211.

Moroff G & Luban NLC. The irradiation of blood and blood components to prevent graft-versus-host disease: technical issues and guidelines. *Transfus Med Rev* 1997; 11: 15–26.

Ruhl H, Bein G & Sachs UJH. Transfusion-associated graft-versus-host disease. *Transfus Med Rev* 2009; 23: 62–71.

Triulzi DJ & Nalesnik MA. Microchimerism, GVHD, and tolerance in solid organ transplantation. *Transfusion* 2001; 41: 419–426.

Utter GH, Reed WF, Lee TH & Busch MP. Transfusion-associated microchimerism. *Vox Sanguinis* 2007; 93: 188–195.

12 Posttransfusion purpura

Michael F. Murphy

University of Oxford and NHS Blood and Transplant and Department of Haematology,
John Radcliffe Hospital, Oxford, UK

In 1959, van Loghem and colleagues described a 51-year-old woman who developed severe thrombocytopenia 7 days after elective surgery [1]. The thrombocytopenia did not respond to transfusion of fresh blood, but there was a spontaneous recovery after 3 weeks. The patient's serum contained a strong platelet alloantibody, which enabled the description of the first human platelet antigen (HPA) (Zw, see Chapter 5). However, the relationship of platelet alloimmunization to posttransfusion thrombocytopenia was not recognized until 2 years later when Shulman and colleagues studied a similar case, naming the antibody anti-Pl^{A1} (later shown to be the same as anti-Zw), and coined the term posttransfusion purpura (PTP) [2].

Definition

PTP is an acute episode of severe thrombocytopenia occurring about a week after a blood transfusion. It usually affects HPA-1a-negative women who have previously been alloimmunized by pregnancy. The transfusion precipitating PTP causes a secondary immune response, boosting the HPA-1a antibodies, although the mechanism of destruction of the patient's own HPA-1a-negative platelets remains uncertain.

Incidence

PTP is considered to be a rare complication of transfusion. Over 200 cases had been reported in the literature till 1991 [3]. However, this may not reflect the true incidence of PTP, which is not known except through reporting to haemovigilance schemes. In the first 4 years of the Serious Hazards of Transfusion (SHOT) scheme, during which approximately 13 million blood components were transfused, 37 cases were reported, giving an approximate incidence of 1 case in 350 000 transfusions. In the following 10 years, after the introduction of universal leucocyte reduction of blood components in the UK, only 13 cases were reported to SHOT, giving an approximate incidence of 1 in 2 million blood components transfused [4].

The low incidence of PTP relative to the 2.5% of the population who are HPA-1a negative and at risk of the condition raises the question of individual susceptibility. As in neonatal alloimmune thrombocytopenia (NAIT), the antibody response to HPA-1a is strongly associated with a certain HLA class II type (HLA-DRB3*0101) (Chapter 5).

Clinical features

PTP typically occurs in middle-aged or elderly women (mean 57 years, range 21–80), although it has also been reported in a small number of males [5]. All patients, apart from rare exceptions, have had previous exposure to platelet antigens through pregnancy and/or transfusion. The interval between pregnancy and/or transfusion and PTP is variable, the shortest

Practical Transfusion Medicine, Fourth Edition. Edited by Michael F. Murphy, Derwood H. Pamphilon and Nancy M. Heddle.
© 2013 John Wiley & Sons, Ltd. Published 2013 by John Wiley & Sons, Ltd.

being 3 years and the longest 52 years. The initial maternal sensitization to platelet antigens during pregnancy in females subsequently developing PTP is rarely of sufficient degree to cause NAIT.

Blood components implicated in causing PTP are:
- whole blood;
- packed red cells; and
- red cell concentrates.

There are occasional case reports of PTP following the transfusion of plasma, presumably due to the presence of platelet particles expressing platelet antigens [5].

Severe thrombocytopenia and bleeding usually occur about 5–12 days after transfusion; shorter or longer intervals are rare. The onset is usually rapid, with the platelet count falling from normal to $<10 \times 10^9$/L within 12–24 hours. Haemorrhage is very common and sometimes severe. There is typically widespread purpura and bleeding from mucous membranes and the gastrointestinal and urinary tracts. In many cases the precipitating transfusion has been associated with a febrile nonhaemolytic transfusion reaction, probably due to the presence of HLA antibodies stimulated by previous pregnancy and/or transfusion. Megakaryocytes are present in normal or increased numbers in the bone marrow and coagulation screening tests are normal in uncomplicated PTP. In untreated cases the thrombocytopenia usually lasts between 7 and 28 days although it occasionally persists for longer.

Differential diagnosis

The rapid onset of severe thrombocytopenia in a middle-aged or elderly woman should arouse suspicion of PTP and a history of recent blood transfusion should be sought. The differential diagnosis includes other causes of acute immune thrombocytopenia such as:
- autoimmune thrombocytopenia;
- drug-induced thrombocytopenia, e.g. heparin-induced thrombocytopenia (HIT) (see Chapter 30);
- nonimmune platelet consumption, e.g. disseminated intravascular coagulation (DIC) and thrombotic thrombocytopenic purpura (TTP);
- a less likely possibility is passively transfused platelet-specific alloantibodies from an immunized blood donor when thrombocytopenia occurs within the first 48 hours after the transfusion [6, 7]; and

- pseudothrombocytopenia due to ethylenediamine tetra-acetic acid (EDTA)-dependent antibodies should be excluded in any patient with unexplained thrombocytopenia by examination of the blood film.

Laboratory investigations

A preliminary diagnosis of PTP on clinical grounds needs to be confirmed by the detection of platelet-specific alloantibodies. The majority (80–90%) of cases of PTP are associated with the development of HPA-1a antibodies in HPA-1a-negative patients [5, 8]. Antibodies against HPA-1b, HPA-3a, HPA-3b, HPA-4a, HPA-5a, HPA-5b, HPA-15b and Nak[a] have been associated with PTP, and occasionally multiple antibodies are present, e.g. anti-HPA-1a, anti-HPA-2b and anti-HPA-3a were found in one case.

HLA antibodies are often present in patients with PTP. There is no evidence that they are involved in causing PTP but their presence complicates the detection of platelet-specific antibodies. Modern platelet serological techniques such as the monoclonal antibody immobilization of platelet antigens (MAIPA) assay are useful for resolving mixtures of antibodies in patients with PTP (Chapter 5).

Pathophysiology

The time course of events in PTP is shown in Figure 12.1. A blood transfusion triggers a rapid secondary antibody response against HPA-1a and there is acute thrombocytopenia about a week after the transfusion. It is difficult to understand why the patient's own HPA-1a-negative platelets are destroyed. There remains no generally accepted mechanism to explain this although a number of suggestions have been made as follows.
- Transfused HPA-1a-positive platelets release HPA-1a antigen, which is adsorbed on to the patient's HPA-1a-negative platelets, making them a target for anti-HPA-1a. Support for this hypothesis comes from observations such as the elution of anti-HPA-1a from HPA-1a-negative platelets in some cases of PTP and the demonstration of the adsorption of HPA-1a antigen on to HPA-1a-negative platelets after

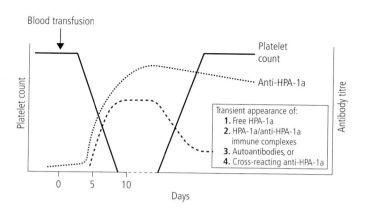

Fig 12.1 A typical time course of posttransfusion purpura. Purpura and severe thrombocytopenia occurred 5–10 days after a blood transfusion. The figure indicates the secondary antibody response of anti-HPA-1a and the postulated transient appearance of free HPA-1a antigen in the plasma, which binds to HPA-1a-negative platelets, HPA-1a/anti-HPA-1a immune complexes, platelet autoantibodies or crossreacting HPA-1a antibodies.

incubation with plasma from HPA-1a-positive stored blood [9].

• The released HPA-1a antigen forms immune complexes with anti-HPA-1a in the plasma and the immune complexes become bound to the patient's platelets, causing their destruction.

• The transfusion stimulates the production of platelet autoantibodies as well as anti-HPA-1a. Evidence in favour of this mechanism is the detection of positive reactions of some PTP patients' sera from the acute thrombocytopenic phase with autologous platelets.

• In the early phase of the secondary antibody response, anti-HPA-1a may be produced which has the ability to cross-react with autologous as well as allogeneic platelets.

Management

Immediate treatment is essential as the risk of fatal haemorrhage is greatest early in the course of PTP. In a review of 71 cases of PTP, five died within the first 10 days because of intracranial haemorrhage [5]. The main aim of treatment is to prevent severe haemorrhage by shortening the duration of severe thrombocytopenia.

No randomized controlled trials of treatment for PTP have been carried out. Comparison of various therapeutic measures is complicated because it may be difficult to differentiate a response to treatment from a spontaneous remission in individual cases.

High dose intravenous immunoglobulin (IVIgG) (2 g/kg given over 2 or 5 days) is the current treatment

of choice, with responses in about 80% of cases [10]; there is often a rapid increase in the platelet count within 48–72 hours [11] (Figure 12.2). Steroids and plasma exchange were the preferred treatments before the availability of IVIgG and plasma exchange, in particular, appeared to be effective in some but not all cases [5].

Platelet transfusions are usually ineffective in raising the platelet count but may be needed in large doses to control severe bleeding in the acute phase, particularly in patients who have recently undergone surgery before there has been a response to high dose IVIgG. There is no evidence that platelet concentrates from HPA-1a-negative platelets are more effective than those from random donors in the acute thrombocytopenic phase. There is no evidence to suggest that further transfusions in the acute phase prolong the duration or severity of thrombocytopenia.

Platelet transfusions have been reported to cause severe febrile and occasionally pulmonary reactions in patients with PTP; these were probably due to HLA antibodies reacting against leucocytes in non-leucocyte-reduced platelet concentrates.

Prevention of recurrence of PTP

Recurrence of PTP has been reported. However, it is unpredictable and has usually occurred following a delay of 3 years or more after the first episode. The patient should be issued with a card to indicate that he/she has previously had PTP and 'special' blood is required for future transfusions.

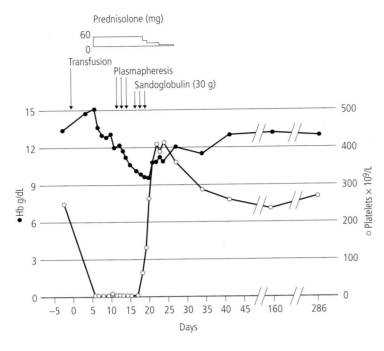

Fig 12.2 Haematological course of a patient with posttransfusion purpura showing the onset of profound thrombocytopenia 6 days after a blood transfusion. Initial treatment with random platelet concentrates caused rigors and bronchospasm, and there was no platelet increment. There was no response to prednisolone (60 mg/day) or plasma exchange (2.5 L/day for 3 days), but there was a prompt remission following high-dose IVIgG (30 g/day for 3 days). Redrawn with permission from Berney et al. [11].

Future transfusion policy should be to use red cell and platelet concentrates from HPA-compatible donors or autologous transfusion. If these are not available, leucocyte-reduced blood components are considered to be safe. There have been occasional reports of recurrence of PTP with leucocyte-reduced red cell concentrates, but the implicated components would not have complied with current standards for leucocyte reduction.

Key points

1 Posttransfusion purpura (PTP) is characterized by an acute episode of severe thrombocytopenia occurring about a week after a transfusion.
2 The pathophysiology remains uncertain.
3 PTP typically occurs in HPA-1a-negative women who have been alloimmunized by pregnancy.
4 Haemorrhage is common and sometimes severe, although the thrombocytopenia resolves spontaneously within a few weeks.
5 High dose intravenous immunoglobulin (IVIgG) (2 g/kg given over 2 or 5 days) is the current treatment of choice to shorten the duration of thrombocytopenia, with responses in about 80% of cases.

6 Universal leucocyte reduction of blood components in the UK has resulted in a marked reduction in the number of reported cases.

References

1 Loghem JJ van, Dorfmeijer H, Hart M van der & Schreuder F. Serological and genetical studies on a platelet antigen (Zw). Vox Sanguinis 1959; 4: 161–169.
2 Shulman NR, Aster RH, Leitner A & Hiller MC. Immunoreactions involving platelets. V. Post-transfusion purpura due to a complement-fixing antibody against a genetically controlled platelet antigen. A proposed mechanism for thrombocytopenia and its relevance in 'autoimmunity'. J Clin Invest 1961; 40: 1597–1620.
3 Shulman NR. Post-transfusion purpura: clinical features and the mechanism of platelet destruction. In: SJ Nance (ed.), Clinical and Basic Science Aspects of Immuno-haematology. Arlington, VA: American Association of Blood Banks; 1991, pp. 137–154.
4 Serious Hazards of Transfusion (SHOT) Steering Group. The 2010 Annual SHOT Report. www.shotuk.org.
5 Mueller-Eckhardt C. Post-transfusion purpura. Br J Haematol 1986; 64: 419–424.

6 Ballem PJ, Buskard NA, Decary F & Doubroff P. Post-transfusion purpura due to secondary transfer of anti-Pl^{A1} by blood transfusion. *Br J Haematol* 1987; 66: 113–114.

7 Solenthaler M, Krauss JK, Boehlen F, Koller R, Hug M & Lamlle B. *Br J Haematol* 1999; 6106: 258–259.

8 Kr von dem Borne AEG & van derPlas-van Dalen CM. Further observations on post-transfusion purpura. *Br J Haematol* 1985; 61: 374–375.

9 Kickler TS, Ness PM, Herman JH & Bell WR. Studies on the pathophysiology of post-transfusion purpura. *Blood* 1986; 68: 347–350.

10 Becker T, Panzer S, Maas D *et al.* High-dose intravenous immunoglobulin for post-transfusion purpura. *Br J Haematol* 1985; 61: 149–155.

11 Berney SI, Metcalfe P, Wathen NC & Waters AH. Post-transfusion purpura responding to high-dose intravenous IgG: further observations on pathogenesis. *Br J Haematol* 1985; 61: 627–632.

Further reading

Waters AH. Post-transfusion purpura. *Blood Rev* 1989; 3: 83–87.

13 Transfusion-transmitted infections

Roger Y. Dodd[1] & Susan L. Stramer[2]

[1] American Red Cross, Jerome H. Holland Laboratory for the Biomedical Sciences, Rockville, Maryland, USA

[2] American Red Cross, Scientific Support Office, Gaithersburg, Maryland, USA

Introduction

Transmission of infectious agents by blood transfusion has been a recognized risk since the identification of transmission and an introduced intervention for syphilis in the 1940s [1]. In particular, in the late 1960s, viral hepatitis was recognized among more than 10% of blood recipients [2]. Since that time, however, there have been continuous advances to the point at which the risk from posttransfusion hepatitis ranges from one infection per 350 000 units transfused for hepatitis B virus (HBV) to one infection per 1.15 million units transfused for hepatitis C virus (HCV) [3–5]. However, many other infections have been found to be transmitted via this route, with HIV being the most notable; the risk of infection with this virus has been reduced to less than one in 1.5 million units transfused [5]. This chapter describes posttransfusion infection and its recognition, details the means that are used to prevent or minimize the risk of such transmission and outlines those infectious agents known to be transmitted by this route. Emerging infections are discussed in Chapter 16 and the problem of bacterial contamination of blood components is reviewed in Chapter 14.

Transmission of infections by blood transfusion

A number of conditions must be met in order for a disease to be transmitted by blood transfusion [6]:

- an asymptomatic phase during which the agent is present in the bloodstream;
- ability of the agent to survive during the collection, processing and storage of the donation;
- infectivity via the intravenous route;
- a susceptible patient population;
- development of the disease in at least some infected recipients.

The infections discussed in this chapter are all well recognized as offering risk to transfusion recipients and all are subject to some measures to reduce such risk, but it must be recognized that, to date, no intervention is completely effective. In cases where testing has been implemented, risks are currently extremely low and it is clear that any residual risk is attributable to collection of blood during the so-called early window period after exposure, when the infectious agent may circulate but be undetectable by current methods. Testing has reduced this window period to a few days, reducing residual risk by many orders or magnitude [7, 8]. Another threat is the development of new strains or mutations that lead to agents that escape detection, but in most cases key agents are subject to multiple redundant tests, generally avoiding this problem. This also reduces the risk attributable to laboratory failures (which are themselves very rare). In cases where the principal intervention is a donor question, it is self-evident that a donor's failure to answer the questions correctly may lead to the collection of an infectious unit. It is also not generally possible to craft a question that is completely effective in segregating

Practical Transfusion Medicine, Fourth Edition. Edited by Michael F. Murphy, Derwood H. Pamphilon and Nancy M. Heddle.
© 2013 John Wiley & Sons, Ltd. Published 2013 by John Wiley & Sons, Ltd.

all those who are infected with a given organism while assuring that there is not an undue loss of donors.

Transfusion-transmitted infections: detection and management

Clinicians responsible for the care of transfused patients should be alert to the possibility of transfusion-transmitted disease or infection, even though this is now a rare event. Unfortunately, recognition of most transfusion-transmitted infections is not easy, for one or more of the following reasons [6]:

• Many transfusion-transmitted infections (TTIs) are asymptomatic.

• If disease symptoms occur, they tend to be nonspecific (fever, flu-like illness).

• The incubation period may be prolonged, in some cases extending out to months or even years.

• The patient's underlying disease may mask or modulate evidence of other infections.

• There may be pre-existing risk factors for, or infection with, the disease agent that is thought to have been transfusion transmitted.

• Exotic infections may be transmitted by transfusion; they may be unexpected, unfamiliar or hard to recognize or diagnose.

Effective investigation of a potential TTI is relatively complex, time consuming and does not always lead to a definitive conclusion. Nevertheless, care should be taken to avoid inappropriate designation of the source of an infection temporally linked to transfusion. The following activities may contribute to the proper investigation of a suspected TTI:

• clinical diagnosis of the transfusion-associated disease;

• use of serological and/or nucleic acid testing to diagnose the disease definitively and to identify the infecting agent.

• Investigation of the patient's pretransfusion blood samples to establish the absence of infection prior to transfusion.

• Investigation of the patient's risk history to eliminate the possibility of alternate routes of infection.

• Investigation of all implicated blood donors for evidence of current or recent infection with the relevant agent; this will require the cooperation of the blood provider.

• Comparison of the agent isolated from the patient with that isolated from the donor by nucleic acid sequencing.

• Alert, or consult with, infectious disease specialists and/or public health agencies as appropriate.

• Early reporting of cases to the blood provider is critical and is usually required, so that other blood components from the implicated donor can be identified and recovered.

This chapter is concerned with those infections known to be transmitted by transfusion, the individual agents responsible and the diseases that they cause. However, it is worth noting that the presentation of a disease in a transfused patient may offer some clues. A patient may react very rapidly (e.g. even during administration) to the transfusion of a blood component that is contaminated with significant levels of bacteria; this topic is discussed in Chapter 14.

Viruses

Early manifestations (a few days to three weeks) are not common and if they occur they most likely reflect transmission of a virus that causes acute infection, such as West Nile virus or even dengue virus [9, 10]. Such an event is most likely to be associated with a known outbreak of the disease in question [11]. The most common symptoms are likely to be fever and headache, muscle pain, malaise, possibly with more severe manifestations typical of the virus itself [9]. In the case of the B19 parvovirus, infection may result in red cell aplasia or even an aplastic crisis in addition to viral syndromes [12]. Interestingly, infection with HIV can also result in an early acute viral syndrome, although the manifestations of AIDS are not likely to occur until many years after infection.

Hepatitis was, for many years, the most common infectious complication of transfusion, but is now very infrequent. HBV and HCV infections are usually asymptomatic initially and if there is any clinically apparent disease, it will not occur until several months after transfusion [2]. Transfusion-transmitted hepatitis A virus (HAV) is rare, but occasional cases have been reported, as is also the case for hepatitis E virus (HEV). These agents tend to have a shorter incubation period and generally cause an acute, rather than chronic, form of hepatitis [13].

As with hepatitis viruses, transfusion transmission of retroviruses is also extremely rare. As pointed out above, there may be an acute viral syndrome shortly after infection with HIV-1, but there is no such early response to infection with HTLV-1 or -2. In the absence of treatment, HIV infection almost invariably will lead to the eventual development of AIDS many years after the original infection, but only a minority of those infected with HTLV will develop symptomatic disease (tropical spastic paraparesis or adult T-cell leukaemia).

Thus, detection of transfusion-transmitted retroviral infection, or indeed hepatitis virus infection, is almost entirely dependent on laboratory testing. However, because most blood collection organizations actively trace recipients of prior donations from repeat donors who are newly found to be infected with these viruses, transfusion services may be notified that an earlier blood component may be infectious and are asked to identify and test the affected recipients. This approach has been responsible for the detection of essentially all confirmed transfusion transmissions of HIV and HCV in the USA since 1999, when nucleic acid testing of all blood donors was implemented.

Parasites

A number of protozoan parasites are transmissible by transfusion, most notably *Plasmodium* spp. (the agents of malaria), *Babesia* spp. and *Trypanosoma cruzi* (the agent of Chagas disease) [13]. Malaria and babesia infection may present with typical flu-like symptoms a few weeks to a few months after transfusion and may progress to the typical manifestations of the disease. Asplenic patients are at particular risk of disease from babesia infection. In many cases, posttransfusion infection with these agents may be detected by examination of blood smears. Posttransfusion babesia infection is not uncommon in the USA, particularly in areas where the parasite is endemic, but is rare elsewhere in the world [14, 15]. In the USA, transfusion-transmitted babesia may be mistaken for malaria. Posttransfusion *T. cruzi* infection may occur in Latin America, where the parasite is endemic (although control programmes are reducing the threat), but is also recognized in areas where there is significant immigration from endemic areas [16]. Transfusion-transmitted *T. cruzi* may be asymptomatic but can result in severe or fulminant disease in immune compromised patients. The incubation period for acute infection ranges from 20 to 40 days; fever that is unresponsive to antibiotics is the most common symptom, followed by lymphadenopathy and splenomegaly. The parasite may be detectable in blood films in some cases.

Prions

It is now clear from experience in the UK that the prion that causes variant Creutzfeldt–Jakob disease (vCJD) may be transmitted by transfusion and four such transmissions have been clearly documented (Chapter 15). There is, as yet, no evidence for transmission of other prions. Detection of transfusion transmission of the vCJD prion was dependent upon a carefully designed surveillance programme and such an event is not likely to be observed in routine clinical practice, as the incubation period is in excess of several years [13, 17].

Interventions to minimize the impact of transfusion-transmitted infection

A variety of methods and processes are used to control TTIs. In general, they involve: the identification of appropriate donor populations and the selection of safe donors; testing blood donations for markers of infection or infectivity; treatment of the donation and, in some circumstances, treatment of the blood recipient. Many of these interventions are required by laws and regulations and/or by voluntary standards [18, 19].

Donor populations are selected implicitly by location of collection sites and by voluntary nonremuneration policies and explicitly by avoidance of collection from a variety of institutions (particularly prisons). Asking presenting donors questions relating to medical, travel and behavioural histories is used to assess donor suitability. These questions are intended to identify those at higher risk of certain infections. Typically, donors are asked about [18]:
• a history of selected diseases or infections, such as viral hepatitis, HIV/AIDS, selected parasitic diseases;
• intimate or family exposure to specific infectious diseases;

- exposure to blood or body fluids through illicit injection or routine transfusion;
- receipt of potentially infectious vaccines or therapeutic agents;
- behavioural risk factors, particularly involving male–male sex or payment or exchange of drugs for sex;
- travel to locations or areas offering risk of exposure to (for example) malaria or the vCJD prion.

Depending upon the responses to these questions, the presenting donor will be temporarily or permanently deferred from donation and the deferral will be recorded so that the risk may be identified should the donor try to present again during the time of deferral. The efficacy of these measures to select safer donors can be evaluated by comparing the prevalence and incidence of positive TTI test results among donors, with those seen in the general population. In the USA, studies suggest that donor prevalence rates for key TTIs are some 6- to 20-fold lower than those for the general population, while incidence rates may be 4- to 20-fold lower than community rates [20]. Testing each donation for markers of infection or infectivity using serologic and/or nucleic acid tests is a critical step in assuring safety from infections where such tests are available and suitable; this aspect is covered in Chapter 20.

To some extent, routine postcollection processing of blood components may impact their infectivity. There is some evidence that infectivity for some agents may vary by component, with infectivity for malaria and babesia being found primarily (but not exclusively) in red cell concentrates [13]. Conversely, infectivity for *T. cruzi* seems to be confined to platelet concentrates [16]. The infectivity titre for some agents (most notably HTLV-1) clearly declines with product storage, although this is not considered to be a safety measure in its own right. However, leucocyte reduction of blood components clearly reduces the risk of transmission of CMV and probably that of other cell-associated viruses including HTLV [13]. Most promising, of course, is the application of formal pathogen reduction methods, which are currently available in many countries for the treatment of platelet concentrates and plasma for transfusion [6]. Methods for whole blood and for red cell concentrates remain under development.

Transfusion-transmitted infectious agents

Viruses

Hepatitis A virus (HAV)

HAV is a small (27–32-nm diameter) nonenveloped virus with a single strand of positive sense RNA, 7.5 kb in length, in the family Picornaviridae, genus *Hepatovirus*. The primary transmission route is faecal-oral, sometimes through food or water or close personal contact. Single-source outbreaks are not uncommon. The incidence of infection in the general population tends to be relatively low at less than 7 per 100 000 annually, although seroprevalence rates are 29 to 34% in the USA [13]. The incubation period is 10 to 50 days, with a mode of one month. The course of disease is almost always acute, typically with anorexia, relatively mild fever, fatigue, vomiting, leading to typical hepatitis with varying degrees of transaminase elevation and icterus. Overall, the disease tends not to be severe with fulminant or fatal cases infrequent – usually much less than 1%. There is a 7- to 14-day period of viremia prior to the appearance of symptoms and, during this time, blood is likely to be infectious via transfusion. Tests for IgG and IgM antibodies and for viral RNA are available. A handful of transfusion-transmitted HAV cases have been reported, some with secondary transmission [13]. Testing of whole blood donations is not warranted because transmission is so rare, but plasma for further manufacture is tested for HAV RNA by pooled NAT. Blood donors are usually asked to notify the collection site if they become sick shortly after donation and such postdonation information has led to the identification and recovery of at least some potentially infectious units.

Hepatitis B virus (HBV)

HBV is a small enveloped spherical virus 42 to 47 nm in diameter, with a partially double-stranded, circular DNA genome 3.2 kb in length with overlapping reading frames, in the family Hepadnaviridae, genus *Hepadnavirus*. Transmission routes are primarily sexual, parenteral and perinatal. An unusual feature of HBV infection is the overproduction of viral coat material that can circulate at high concentrations. This is termed hepatitis B surface antigen (HBsAg); its presence is indicative of active infection (acute or chronic) and it is the primary analyte for blood donor screening. Antibodies to HBsAg (anti-HBs) are generally indicative of past infection, but antibodies to the inner core of the virus (anti-HBc) appear earlier and may also indicate some risk of infectivity. IgM anti-HBc in combination with HBsAg are markers of infection within the last 6 months [21]. Detectable HBV DNA in the plasma is associated with varying levels of infectivity, depending upon the phase of the infection; the early window phase when DNA is the only detectable marker appears to be the most infectious. The estimated incidence of infection in the USA is approximately 12 per 100 000 whereas the prevalence is 4 to 5% [22]. Since the introduction of an effective vaccine in the USA, the incidence has decreased by 80%. The global burden of chronic HBV infection is as high as 400 million individuals. The incubation period from exposure to infection is from one week to six months. While many infections are asymptomatic, the range of disease manifestations is extensive, from mild acute symptoms to life-threatening or fatal fulminant cases. Symptoms are generally similar to those described for HAV infection. Chronic infection results more frequently from infection early in life and chronic disease may lead to cirrhosis and/or liver cancer. Diagnostic tests include serum transaminase measurement and detection of HBV antibodies, particularly IgM anti-HBc. Nucleic acid testing may also be of value.

The risk of transfusion transmission varies widely, but in the USA has been estimated as approximately one case per 350 000 units transfused [3, 4]. However, the number of confirmed reported cases is considerably less than would be anticipated from this figure. The major interventions to reduce the risk of transmission include donor questioning for a history of viral hepatitis, close contact with a case and risk behaviours for sexual and parenteral exposure. Donations are tested for markers of HBV infection; most important is the use of sensitive immunoassays for HBsAg. In addition, in some countries donors are tested for anti-HBc, which identifies a small number of additional infectious donations. Such testing is not practical in areas with a high prevalence of HBV infection. Increasingly, donors are also being tested for HBV DNA, using triplex tests that are also designed to detect HIV and HCV RNA. However, the incremental impact of such testing on HBV safety appears to be limited if performed in mini-pools [4].

Hepatitis D virus (HDV) is a very small RNA virus that only infects those with on-going HBV infection. HDV coinfection increases the severity of disease in those with chronic hepatitis B [13]. Because HDV is dependent on HBV for replication, measures to prevent HBV transmission are also effective against HDV.

Hepatitis C virus (HCV)

HCV is a small, enveloped spherical (55–65 nm in diameter) virus with a single positive strand of RNA, 9.6 kb in length, in the family Flaviviridae, genus *Hepacivirus*. The transmission route is primarily parenteral. The incidence of new infections in the USA is estimated at approximately 6 per 100 000 annually and the prevalence is 1.3 to 1.9% [22]. Most infections are chronic and lifelong; around 20% of infections may resolve. The incubation period is typically 4 to 12 weeks, with an extended range of 2 to 24 weeks. Most infections are asymptomatic, but when symptoms occur they include fever, fatigue, loss of appetite and abdominal pain among others. Chronic disease may lead to cirrhosis and, in some cases, liver cancer after many years. The incidence has declined significantly over recent years. Although the virus was not specifically identified until 1989, it was recognized as the predominant causative agent of posttransfusion hepatitis [2]. The development, progressive improvement and universal implementation of tests for anti-HCV in donors have profoundly reduced the impact of this virus on blood safety, with a further significant improvement attributable to the implementation of testing for HCV RNA [23]. Nucleic acid testing has reduced the infectious window period from around 70 days to about 7 days [8]. In the USA, the current risk of transmission of HCV by transfusion is 1 per 1 150 000 units [5]. Fewer cases of posttransfusion HCV infection are observed than would be predicted from this figure. Diagnostic tools include serum transaminase testing, antibody and RNA detection.

Interventions to reduce the transmission of HCV by transfusion include questioning donors about a history of viral hepatitis, exposure to a case or risk behaviours involving parenteral exposure to blood. All donations are tested for antibodies to HCV and, in some cases, also to the core antigen of the virus. Nucleic acid testing for HCV has been in place in a number of countries since the late 1990s and has been instrumental in decreasing the residual risk.

Hepatitis E virus (HEV)

HEV is a small, nonenveloped icosahedral (30–34 nm in diameter) virus with a single, positive strand of RNA, 7.2 kb in length, in the family Hepeviridae, genus *Hepevirus*. The transmission routes are primarily faecal-oral, often waterborne, but apparently also foodborne, with cases attributable to consumption of raw or undercooked pork [13]. There are four genotypes representing a single serotype; the genotypes have varying geographic distribution and pathogenicity for humans. HEV1 and HEV2 are restricted to humans and transmitted via contaminated water in developing countries and HEV3 and HEV4 infect humans as well as pigs and other mammals; HEV3 and HEV4 are of lower human pathogenicity and are responsible for the localized sporadic, mostly foodborne, HEV cases worldwide. Incidence data are not readily available, but prevalence rates of 20 to 40% are found in endemic regions. However, similar rates have been observed in the USA and other nonendemic regions: it is likely that these high rates are attributable to serotypes of low human pathogenicity. The incubation period is usually 3 to 8 weeks and infection may result in a wide spectrum of disease from unapparent to fulminant, with apparently increased severity in pregnant women [13]. Transfusion transmission has been noted rarely in nonendemic areas and with some frequency in endemic areas, such as Hokkaido in Japan [13]. Nucleic acid testing of presenting donors has been implemented as a preventative measure in some areas of concern, but there seems to be little justification for widespread application of this intervention.

Human immunodeficiency virus (HIV)

HIV is an enveloped, more or less spherical (106–183 nm in diameter) virus, with two linear, positive sense strands of RNA, 9.2 kb in length, in the family Retroviridae, genus *Lentivirus*. There are two major species, HIV-1 and HIV-2, although HIV-2 is much less common and less virulent than HIV-1. HIV-1 has multiple distinct clades [13]. The predominant transmission routes are sexual, perinatal and parenteral. Prevalence and incidence rates vary widely, with prevalence and incidence rates as high as 20% and 1–2% in parts of sub-Saharan Africa. Prevalence in the USA is estimated at about 0.4% and incidence rates are about 16 per 100 000 annually [24]. Rates in Western Europe and other highly developed countries are generally somewhat lower. The incubation period to the acute retroviral syndrome averages about 21 days, but may range from 5 to 70 days. It is now known that HIV RNA becomes detectable around 9 days after infection using current NAT assays. Sensitive tests for antibodies to HIV will become positive about 3 weeks after infection [8]. These periods represent the window periods for nucleic acid and antibody testing. Most infections are asymptomatic and the acute retroviral syndrome, when it occurs, tends to be relatively mild, with a short (a week or two) period of fever, fatigue and possibly lymphadenopathy and rash. Typically, patients recover and are asymptomatic for many years thereafter, until the symptoms of full-blown AIDS emerge. Diagnosis of infection may be based upon tests for antibodies to HIV and/or the presence of HIV RNA in the plasma. Currently the risk of transmission of HIV by transfusion has been estimated as approximately 1 case per 1 500 000 units [5]. Again, however, transfusion-transmitted HIV infections are not recognized as frequently as this risk estimate would suggest. It is of interest to note that two of the five transmission events noted in the USA since 1999 have involved infection from a transfusable plasma unit, but not from the accompanying red cell concentrate, suggesting that the sensitivity of nucleic acid testing is approaching the infectious dose of HIV offered by a red cell concentrate [4].

While the AIDS epidemic has been a medical and human disaster, it stimulated the current stringent approach to blood safety and continuous quality improvement. All donors are directly asked about a history of AIDS-related symptoms and about possible exposure to infection. Questions about behavioural risk are asked and individuals acknowledging such risk are permanently or temporarily deferred. Some of the questions, particularly those relating to male-to-male sexual activity, have been challenged as discriminatory, particularly when accompanied by permanent deferral. Nevertheless, the rights of the patient to receive safe blood also have to be recognized and policies differ from one country to another, but almost always involve some period of deferral for those considered to be at increased risk of HIV infection. All donations are, at a minimum, tested for antibodies to HIV and, in many areas, also for HIV RNA. Testing for the HIV p24 antigen may be performed as an alternative to testing for RNA, but this approach offers lesser sensitivity [23].

*Human T-lymphotropic viruses 1 and 2
(HTLV-1 and -2)*

HTLV is an enveloped, spherical (150–200 nm in diameter) virus, with two linear, positive-sense, single strands of RNA, 8.5 kb in length, in the family Retroviridae, genus *Deltaretrovirus*. There are two different viruses, HTLV-1 and HTLV-2, and at least two additional variants have been described [13]. The primary routes of transmission are sexual and perinatal (via breast milk) and parenteral transmission (particularly via injecting drug use) has been widely documented, especially for HTLV-2. Prevalence rates vary widely, but tend to be very low in developed Western countries. There are pockets of high prevalence in Japan, the Caribbean and Africa (HTLV-1) and among some native populations in the Americas (HTLV-2). Infection is most often asymptomatic; for HTLV-1, there is a lifetime risk of a few percent for the eventual development of adult T-cell leukaemia/lymphoma or tropical spastic paraperesis, but only the latter has ever been associated with transfusion. Less is known about disease associations for HTLV-2. Transfusion transmission of these viruses has been recognized for many years. In the USA and a number of other countries, donations are tested for antibodies to HTLV-1 and -2, using a single combination test. There is no evidence of residual transmission although it may be estimated that there is a risk of one transmission per several million units [7]. Leucocyte reduction seems to eliminate the risk of transmission, which also declines during refrigerated storage of red cell components.

Cytomegalovirus (human CMV, HHV-5)

CMV is an enveloped, spherical beta herpesvirus 200 to 300 nm in diameter, with a double-stranded DNA genome of 235 kb pairs, in the family Herpesviridae, genus *Cytomegalovirus*. Seroprevalence rates vary by age and location but are on the order of 30 to 40% among blood donors in the USA and Western Europe [13]. There are no good measures of incidence rates, but the presence of antibodies to CMV implies that the virus is present, albeit often in a latent form. The normal transmission route is by contact, droplets or body fluid exposure, but it is also transmissible from mother to fetus and by blood transfusion and organ transplant. In general, healthy individuals are asymptomatic or show only mild symptoms (fever, lymphadenopathy, mononucleosis-like disease), but vulnerable individuals, including the fetus, low birth-weight infants, transplant patients and those with severe immune deficiencies may suffer serious or fatal disease, including pneumonia, multiorgan disease, etc. Infection during pregnancy may have profound effects on the fetus including developmental problems. TTI is typically recognized one to two months posttransfusion. There are two primary interventions to reduce or eliminate posttransfusion CMV infection: leucocyte reduction and/or the use of seronegative blood components for those at risk. Studies have suggested that both methods have similar efficacy in reducing risk but that breakthrough infections may still be seen [25]. There are a number of explanations for such breakthrough cases, including failure of testing or leucocyte reduction, the presence of extracellular virus in early infection and the possibility that at least some hospital-acquired infections may be mistaken for transfusion transmissions. Lastly, reactivation of latent CMV infection triggered by transfusion probably accounts for most reported cases of transfusion-transmitted CMV [26].

Other human herpesviruses

Two other human herpesviruses, Epstein–Barr virus (EBV) and human herpes virus-8 (HHV-8) are known to be transmissible by transfusion [13]. EBV is an almost ubiquitous virus, associated with mononucleosis, and in some locations, especially in Africa, Burkitt's lymphoma and nasopharyngeal carcinoma in Asia. Evidence is increasing for its role in the causation of lymphoproliferative disease among transfused immunocompromised patients, but other than leucocyte reduction, there is little in the way of an intervention, at least in the absence of pathogen reduction. HHV-8 is the causative agent of Kaposi's sarcoma and there is evidence for its transmissibility by transfusion, at least in parts of Africa, where it is endemic. To date, however, there does not appear to be any evidence for transfusion-transmitted HHV-8 disease; reductions in viral loads are most likely the result of leucocyte reduction [13].

West Nile virus (WNV)

WNV is an enveloped, spherical (40–60 nm in diameter) virus with a linear, single strand of positive-sense RNA, 11 kb in length, in the family Flaviviridae, genus *Flavivirus* (Japanese encephalitis complex). The primary transmission route is via (mainly culicine) mosquitoes and the amplifying hosts are primarily birds. Humans are accidental, dead-end hosts, although the virus is readily transmitted via blood transfusion [11]. At the peak of the new epidemic, which emerged in the USA in 1999, several hundred thousand individuals were naturally infected each year; the largest WNV outbreaks ever recorded worldwide occurred in the USA in 2002 and again in 2003 but the number of cases have declined and appear to have reached a stable number until a resurgence in 2012. The virus is endemic in parts of Africa, the Middle East and parts of Southern Europe where smaller outbreaks frequently occur. Infection results in a range of outcomes from asymptomatic, through flu-like symptoms occurring in approximately 25% of infected individuals. Symptoms include headache, weakness, new rash, fever muscle joint and eye pain, and is referred to as West Nile fever [9]. A more severe neurologic disease involving meningoencephalitis, with outcomes sometimes leading to death, occurs in between 1 in 150 and 1 in 200 infected individuals [9]. The incubation period is 2 to 14 days with a period of early viremia of about 7 to 10 days during which the blood of the patient may be infectious; low levels of viremia may be detectable for a longer time. In the USA, cases occur mainly between April and October. In 2002, there was a report of 23 well-characterized transfusion-transmitted cases of WNV infections and within less than a year, universal donor screening for WNV RNA by pooled nucleic acid testing was implemented [27]. Experience showed that such testing was insufficiently sensitive to detect all infectious donations so measures were established to perform single donation testing in areas and times with a high incidence of WNV activity [28]. Outside the USA, there has not been widespread testing, but donor deferral based upon travel to endemic areas has been implemented in some countries. Testing has been implemented in parts of Europe in response to a number of discrete outbreaks.

Other arboviruses

WNV illustrated two somewhat unexpected facts: the ability of arthropod-borne viruses (arboviruses) to establish huge, unprecedented outbreaks in previously unaffected areas and efficient transmission of an acute infection via blood transfusion. Accordingly, unexpected intense outbreaks of infection with chikungunya virus (an alphavirus transmitted by *Aedes* spp. mosquitoes) resulted in specific measures designed to prevent transfusion transmission in some affected areas; however, although explosive outbreaks occurred, transfusion transmission was never documented [6, 13]. In contrast, three clusters of transfusion transmission of dengue virus have been reported from Hong Kong, Singapore and Puerto Rico [13]. Donor testing has been implemented in Puerto Rico and may be considered elsewhere in the future, particularly in countries in which this virus is not endemic but outbreaks may occur [10].

Human B19 parvovirus (B19V)

B19V is a small, nonenveloped, icosahedral (23–26 nm in diameter) virus with a linear, negative-sense, single strand of DNA, 5.6 kb in length, in the family Parvoviridae, genus *Erythrovirus*. The primary transmission routes are respiratory and transplacental [13]. The virus is transmitted by blood transfusion and, at least in the past, via some plasma-derived products. Levels of viraemia during acute infection can be extremely high, sometimes exceeding 10^{12} DNA copies per mL. The virus is ubiquitous, often causing seasonal outbreaks of mild disease, particularly among children. Seroprevalence rates are around 50% in adults and incidence rates can be 1.5%. Most infections are asymptomatic, but the virus causes erythema infectiosum (fifth disease) in children and occasional arthropathy in adults. Of particular concern is transient aplastic crisis in patients with shortened red cell survival or haemolytic anaemias; in some cases there may be pure red cell aplasia or pancytopenia. Infection in pregnant women may result in hydrops fetalis. Symptomatic infection from transfusion transmission is extremely rare. Nevertheless, in some countries (such as Germany and Japan), donor blood is routinely screened for viral DNA or by haemagglutination to eliminate the transfusion of components with high titres of virus. Currently, plasma for further manufacture is tested in pools for B19 DNA in order to minimize the levels of virus in manufacturing pools. Such testing is becoming available through rapid, high throughput procedures and this may lead to expansion of routine blood donation testing.

Bacteria

Currently, the major blood safety risk from bacteria results from contamination of components and subsequent outgrowth, resulting in septic reactions in the patient. This is discussed in Chapter 14. However, a small number of bacterial species may be transmitted from donor to recipient by blood, leading to infection and the development of disease. The best-known (but least-frequent) example of this is syphilis, although there has been no reported case in the literature since 1960. The rarity of such transmission is likely to be due to a combination of factors, including donor selection and testing and to the fragility of *Treponema pallidum* (the infectious spirochete) in stored components, along with the frequent use of antibiotics among patients. Recently, there has been concern about the potential for transmission of Q fever (caused by the small bacterium *Coxiella burnetii*) as a result of large, focused outbreaks of human infection in the Netherlands [13]. The infection resulted from human exposure to airborne bacteria associated with intensive goat farming. Investigations demonstrated bacteraemia in some patients and a small amount of suggestive evidence for rare transfusion transmission. In times and in areas of concern, donations were tested for *C. burnetii* by PCR. Veterinary public health measures have, however, essentially eliminated the outbreaks. Other tickborne rickettsia-like bacteria have engendered some concern, but to date there have been several reports of transfusion transmission of *Anaplasma phagocytophilum* [13]. There has been no evidence of transmission of *Borrelia burgdorferi* (the agent of Lyme disease) by this route [13].

Parasitic diseases

Malaria

Human malaria is caused by intraerythrocytic protozoan parasites of the genus *Plasmodium*, namely *P. falciparum*, *P. vivax*, *P. ovale* and *P. malariae*; recently, some cases have also been attributed to the primate parasite, *P. knowlesi* [13]. The parasites are transmitted by anophelene mosquitoes. The parasites may be present in the circulation during a prolonged asymptomatic period and are readily transmitted by blood transfusion. Such transmission is thought to be quite common in the endemic areas in the tropics, but is also a significant risk in nonendemic countries, as a result of collection of blood from donors infected as a result of travel from endemic areas. Disease symptoms include periodic fever, rigors and chills, headache, myalgias, arthralgias, splenomegaly and haemolytic anaemia. Although the typical incubation period is usually a few weeks, this period may be extended in blood recipients and recognition and diagnosis may not be easy. In general, the most severe forms of the disease are attributable to *P. falciparum*. Diagnosis may be achieved through microscopic inspection of blood smears and serological testing; research-level nucleic acid tests are also available. In nonendemic countries, transfusion-transmitted malaria is controlled by questioning donors about a history of malaria and of travel from, or residence in, malarious areas. Policies differ somewhat, but in general casual travel by residents of nonendemic countries is not a major risk, provided that such travellers are deferred for a few months. On the other hand, those who have resided for long periods in malarious areas may be partially immune and can be infectious for a number of years. Many donors are deferred for travel histories, with a negative impact on blood availability, and in some European countries and in Australia deferred donors may be tested for antibodies to *Plasmodium* spp.; if nonreactive they are permitted to donate after a shortened deferral period [29].

Babesiosis

Babesia is also an intraerythrocytic protozoan parasite and the causative agent of babesiosis; a variety of species may be found throughout the world [13, 15]. *Babesia* spp. are transmitted by ticks and primarily affect mammals, with humans as an accidental host. Babesiosis has symptoms similar to those of malaria, but the disease is more severe in the elderly and those patients without a functioning spleen. Transfusion-transmitted babesiosis may be confused with malaria, as the characteristic 'Maltese cross' appearance of the parasite in red cells is quite infrequent. *B. microti* is most often associated with human disease and with transmission by transfusion, which is most often seen in the USA, with a recent report detailing 162 cases since 1979 [14]. Few cases have been reported from any other countries. The disease is generally treatable, but, nevertheless, transfusion-transmitted cases have a significant fatality rate. At the time of writing, there has been no effective intervention available, as donor questioning regarding tick bite or clinical disease is insensitive and licensed donation tests are not available. Infection may be diagnosed by serologic and nucleic acid tests, or by examination of blood films.

Chagas disease

Chagas disease is caused by the protozoan parasite *Trypanosoma cruzi*, which infects numerous mammalian hosts [13]. It is transmitted to humans by reduviid bugs, generally as a result of exposure to the parasites in the bug's faecal material, which may be rubbed into mucous membranes, or the site of a bite from the bug itself. The parasite is endemic in the Americas, generally between latitudes 40 N and 40 S. Most human infections occur in rural or underdeveloped areas of Latin America where there are more opportunities for interactions between humans and the vector insects, which tend to colonize substandard housing. The parasite often infects infants and children and infection may be lifelong. Infected individuals may be asymptomatic over periods of many years and their blood can transmit the infection via transfusion. Transplacental infection may also occur, sometimes across more than one generation. Population movements have introduced the infection into nonendemic countries, especially the USA, Canada and Spain. Initial symptoms after infection may involve localized swelling and mild fever. Over the longer term, hepatomegaly and cardiac or gastrointestinal symptoms may emerge. Fulminant disease may occur in immunocompromised patients, particularly in the case of transfusion transmission. Diagnosis may be achieved through the use of serological tests, although infections are occasionally recognized on examination of blood films. Prevention of transfusion transmission relies primarily upon blood donor testing for antibodies to *T. cruzi*. Such testing is widespread in Latin America and was implemented in the USA in 2007. Subsequent evaluation of the testing programme in the USA suggested that selective testing was effective and, currently, blood donors are tested only once and if nonreactive subsequent donations are accepted without any testing. In other countries, notably Canada and Spain, presenting donors are asked about prolonged travel, residence or birth in Chagas-endemic countries and whether their mothers or grandmothers were born in such an area. If so, the donors are tested for *T. cruzi* antibodies and may donate if such tests are nonreactive. The number of transfusion-transmitted cases is limited and has been described primarily from platelets [16].

Prions

Variant Creutzfeldt–Jakob disease (vCJD) (see Chapter 15)

Variant CJD is the human form of bovine spongiform encephalopathy (BSE, mad cow disease), transmitted to humans through ingestion of tissues from infected cattle [13]. The disease was first recognized as a distinct entity in 1996. Although similar to classic CJD, vCJD occurs primarily among younger individuals, presents with psychiatric symptoms and generally has a longer course from diagnosis to death. The pathology typically involves unusual, florid plaques in the brain. About 220 cases have occurred, mostly in Great Britain. The frequency of reported cases has been declining over the past 5 or more years. Careful review of surveillance data has shown that there have been four instances of transmission of the vCJD agent by transfusion. Three such cases resulted in the development of vCJD in the recipient and the fourth occurred in an individual who died of underlying disease but was found to harbour the agent in the spleen and at least one lymph node [17]. One other possible case of transmission has been reported, attributed to receipt of Factor VIII concentrates. Although these events are infrequent, they do reflect a high transmission rate among exposed recipients. Because of concern about such transmissions, a number of preventative measures had been implemented well before the recognition of any transmissions. In the USA, such measures included permanent deferral from donation of individuals judged at risk of exposure to BSE by virtue of residence or prolonged cumulative travel to the UK and Western Europe and similar measures were taken elsewhere. In the UK, universal leucocyte reduction of blood components was implemented, domestic plasma was eliminated for transfusion or fractionation and there have been considerable efforts to reduce the overall use of donor blood. There has been a prolonged effort to develop pre mortem tests for infection with vCJD, but at the time or writing, no such test was available. To date, there has been no evidence that the classic form of CJD is transmissible by transfusion [13].

Key points

1 A number of pathogens, including viruses, bacteria, protozoan parasites and one prion are known to be transmitted by transfusion.
2 Measures are in place to control such transmission, including blood donor selection, deferral, laboratory testing and component treatment.
3 These measures have reduced the incidence of key TTIs to very low levels, usually less than one case per million components transfused.
4 TTIs are difficult to detect and diagnose.
5 Careful studies involving the patient and all implicated donors are necessary in order to confirm that an infection is attributable to transfusion.
6 TTI should be appropriately reported to blood providers and other agencies, as required by regulation or practice.

References

1 Dodd RY. Germs, gels and genomes: a personal recollection of 30 years in blood safety testing. In: SL Stramer (ed), *Blood Safety in the New Millennium*. Bethesda, MD: AABB; 2001, pp. 97–122.
2 Alter HJ & Houghton M. Hepatitis C virus and eliminating post-transfusion hepatitis. *Nature Med* 2000; 6: 1082–1086.
3 Zou S, Stramer SL, Notari EP, Kuhns MC, Krysztof D, Musavi F, Fang CT & Dodd RY. Current incidence and residual risk of hepatitis B infection among blood donors in the United States. *Transfusion* 2009; 48: 1609–1620.
4 Stramer SL, Wend U, Candotti D, Foster GA, Hollinger FB, Dodd RY, Allain J-P & Gerlich W. Nucleic acid testing to detect HBV infection in blood donors. *New Engl J Med* 2011; 364: 236–247.
5 Zou S, Dorsey KA, Notari EP, Foster GA, Krysztof DE, Musavi F, Dodd RY & Stramer SL. Prevalence, incidence and residual risk of human immunodeficiency virus and hepatitis C virus infections among United States blood donors since the introduction of nucleic acid testing. *Transfusion* 2010; 50: 1495–1504.
6 Stramer SL, Hollinger FB, Katz LM, Kleinman S, Metzel PS, Gregory KR & Dodd RY. Emerging infectious disease agents and their potential threat to transfusion safety. *Transfusion* 2009; 49 (Suppl.): 1S–235S.
7 Dodd RY, Notari EP & Stramer SL. Current prevalence and incidence of infectious disease markers and estimated window-period risk in the American Red Cross blood donor population. *Transfusion* 2002; 42: 975–979.
8 Busch MP, Glynn SA, Stramer SL, Strong DM, Caglioti S, Wright DJ, Pappalardo B, Kleinman SH, NHLBI-REDS NAT Study Group. A new strategy for estimating risks of transfusion-transmitted infections based on rates of detection of recently infected donors. *Transfusion* 2005; 45: 254–264.
9 Zou S, Foster GA, Dodd RY, Petersen LR Stramer, SL. West Nile fever characteristics among viremic persons identified through blood donor screening. *J Infect Dis* 2010; 202: 1354–1561.
10 Stramer SL, Linnen JL, Carrick JM *et al.* Dengue viremia in blood donors identified by RNA and detection of dengue transfusion transmission during the 2007 dengue outbreak in Puerto Rico. *Transfusion* 2012; first published online: 17 February 2012. DOI: 10.1111/j.1537-2995.2012.03566.x.
11 Pealer LN, Marfin AA, Petersen LR *et al.* Transmission of West Nile virus through blood transfusion in the United States. *New Engl J Med* 2003; 349: 1236–1245.
12 Dodd RY. B19: benign or not? *Transfusion* 2011; 51: 1878–1879.
13 AABB: Emerging Infectious Diseases Fact Sheets. http://www.aabb.org/resources/bct/eid/Pages/eidpostpub.aspx.
14 Herwaldt BL, Linden JV, Bosserman E, Young C, Olkowska D & Wilson M. Transfusion-associated babesiosis in the United States: a description of cases. *Ann Int Med* 2011; 155: 509–519.
15 Leiby DA. Transfusion-transmitted *Babesia* spp.: bullseye on *Babesia microti. Clin Microbiol Rev* 2011; 24: 14–28.
16 Benjamin RJ, Stramer SL, Leiby DA, Dodd RY, Fearon M & Castro E. *Trypanosoma cruzi* infection in North America and Spain: evidence in support of transfusion transmission. *Transfusion* 2012; first published online: 10 February 2012. DOI: 10.1111/j.1537-2995.2011.03554.x.
17 Hewitt PE, Llewelyn CA, Mackenzie J & Will RG. Creutzfeldt–Jakob disease and blood transfusion: results of the UK transfusion medicine epidemiological review study. *Vox Sanguinis* 2006; 91: 221–230.
18 Eder A & Bianco C (eds). *Screening Blood Donors*. Bethesda, MD: AABB Press; 2007, pp. 1–287.
19 AABB. *Standards for Blood Banks and Transfusion Services*, 27th edn. Bethesda, MD: AABB Press; 2011, pp. 1–118.
20 Dodd RY. Current estimates of transfusion safety worldwide. *Dev Biol (Basel)* 2005; 120: 3–10.
21 Hollinger FB. Hepatitis B virus infection and transfusion medicine: science and the occult. *Transfusion* 2008; 48: 1001–1026.

22 Centers for Disease Control. Viral Hepatitis Surveillance – United States, 2009; http://www.cdc.gov/hepatitis/Statistics/2009Surveillance/index.htm.

23 Stramer SL, Glynn SA, Kleinman SH *et al*. Detection of HIV-1 and HCV infections among antibody-negative blood donors by nucleic acid-amplification testing. *New Engl J Med* 2004; 351: 760–768.

24 Centers for Disease Control Fact Sheets; http://www.cdc.gov/hiv/resources/factsheets/us.htm.

25 Vamvakas EC. Is white blood cell reduction equivalent to antibody screening in preventing transmission of cytomegalovirus by transfusion? A review of the literature and meta-analysis. *Transfus Med Rev* 2005; 19: 181–199.

26 Drew WL & Roback JD. Prevention of transfusion-transmitted cytomegalovirus: reactivation of the debate? *Transfusion* 2007; 47: 1955–1958.

27 Stramer SL, Fang CT, Foster GA, Wagner AG, Brodsky JP & Dodd RY. West Nile virus among blood donors in the United States, 2003 and 2004. *N Engl J Med* 2005; 353: 451–459.

28 Biggerstaff BJ & Petersen LR. A modeling framework for evaluation and comparison of trigger strategies for switching from minipool to individual-donation testing for West Nile virus. *Transfusion* 2009; 49: 1151–1159.

29 Seed CR, Kee G, Wong T, Law M & Ismay S. Assessing the safety and efficacy of a test-based, targeted donor screening strategy to minimize transfusion transmitted malaria. *Vox Sanguinis* 2010; 98: e182–e192.

Further reading

Alter HJ & Klein HG. The hazards of blood transfusion in historical perspective. *Blood* 2008; 112: 2617–2626.

Barbara JAJ, Regan FAM & Contreras MC (eds). *Transfusion Microbiology*. Cambridge: Cambridge University Press; 2008, pp. 1–390.

Bern C, Kjos S, Yabsley MJ & Montgomery SP. *Trypanosoma cruzi* and Chagas' disease in the United States. *Clin Microbiol Rev* 2011; 24: 655–681.

Busch MP. Transfusion-transmitted viral infections: building bridges to transfusion medicine to reduce risks and understand epidemiology and pathogenesis. *Transfusion* 2006; 46: 1624–1640.

Perkins HA & Busch MP. Transfusion-associated infections: 50 years of relentless challenges and remarkable progress. *Transfusion* 2010; 50: 2080–2099.

Petersen LR & Hayes EB. Westward Ho? The spread of West Nile virus. *New Engl J Med* 2004; 351: 2257–2259.

14 Bacterial contamination

Sandra Ramírez-Arcos & Mindy Goldman
Canadian Blood Services, Ottawa, Ontario, Canada

Incidence of bacterial contamination

Transfusion-associated septic events have been reduced in recent years by the introduction of several interventions including improved donor screening and skin disinfection methods, as well as implementation of first aliquot diversion and bacterial testing. However, recent reports of severe, even fatal reactions, indicate that bacterial contamination of blood components continues to be the most prevalent transfusion-associated infectious risk in Europe and North America. The UK Serious Hazard of Transfusion (SHOT) scheme documented 11 confirmed adverse transfusion reactions (ATRs) due to bacterial contamination of platelet concentrates (PCs) and red blood cells (RBCs) between 2005 and 2009, while only three possible bacterial ATRs were reported in 2010 [1, 2]. From 2005 to 2010, the US Food and Drug Administration (FDA) reported 24 fatalities caused by blood components contaminated with bacteria [3]. In Canada, the Transfusion Transmitted Injuries Surveillance System Program Report for 2004–2005 described 12 serious ATRs with eight of the cases relating to contaminated RBCs [4]. Since 2004, Canadian Blood Services has received six reports of ATRs due to bacterial contamination of blood components including PCs and RBCs (personal communication).

The current incidence of bacterial contamination in PCs varies from 1/1000 to 1/5000, with an estimated risk of transfusion-transmitted septic reactions of ~1/100 000 and a fatality rate of ~1/million [5, 6], while the prevalence of bacterially contaminated RBCs is ~1/30 000 with a septic reaction rate of ~1/500 000 and a fatality rate of ~1/10 million [7].

Blood components implicated in adverse transfusion reactions

Platelet concentrates

Platelet concentrates are the blood components most susceptible to bacterial contamination due to their storage conditions. PCs are stored with constant agitation at $22 \pm 2°C$ in oxygen-permeable plastic containers. The anticoagulant solutions added during PC production provide a physiological pH and a glucose content of ~500 mg/dL. All of these conditions offer an ideal environment for bacterial growth. The initial levels of bacteria in PCs are usually exceedingly low (<10 colony forming units, CFU) but clinically significant levels (10^5 CFU/ml) can be reached after 3–5 days of storage depending on the organism [5, 8, 9].

Clinical sequelae of transfusing bacterially contaminated PCs are variable and may be acute or delayed, depending on the severity of the recipient's medical condition, the type and concentration of the contaminant organism and the timing of transfusion. It is accepted that sepsis due to bacterial contamination of PCs is underrecognized and patients developing severe

Practical Transfusion Medicine, Fourth Edition. Edited by Michael F. Murphy, Derwood H. Pamphilon and Nancy M. Heddle.
© 2013 John Wiley & Sons, Ltd. Published 2013 by John Wiley & Sons, Ltd.

or fatal infections are more likely to be diagnosed and reported [5, 8].

Red blood cells

Storage of RBC units at low temperatures (1–6°C) is believed to limit bacterial growth and decrease the risk of adverse posttransfusion events. However, psychrophilic (grow optimally at refrigeration temperatures) pathogenic bacteria can proliferate from very low levels of contamination to clinically significant concentrations under RBC storage conditions.

Reactions associated with transfusion of bacterially contaminated RBC units are usually severe, due to infused endotoxin (lipopolysaccharide) associated with the cell wall of Gram-negative bacteria. Clinical symptoms may include fever over 38.5°C, hypotension, nausea and vomiting starting during the transfusion. Septic shock with complications such as oliguria and disseminated intravascular coagulation may occur [7, 8].

Plasma and cryoprecipitate

The incidence of ATRs due to contaminated plasma or cryoprecipitate is very low. Only a few reports are found in the literature documenting cases of products being contaminated during thawing in waterbaths. Recipients developed severe infections including endocarditis and septicaemia several days posttransfusion [80].

Contaminant bacterial species

Platelet concentrates

Gram-positive bacteria are the predominant PC contaminants. Although these bacteria have the ability to survive and proliferate during PC storage, most of them are considered to be nonpathogenic. Coagulase negative staphylococci and propionibacteria are the predominant bacterial contaminants of PCs with *Staphylococcus epidermidis* being the species most commonly isolated [5, 10]. Transfusions with fatal outcomes due to platelets contaminated with *Staphylococcus epidermidis* have been reported in Canada, the USA and Europe [8]. Missed detection of *Staphylococcus epidermidis* is attributed to low initial concen-

tration, its characteristic slow growth under platelet storage conditions and the ability of some strains to form slimy bacterial aggregates attached to the platelet containers known as biofilms [8, 11]. Other Gram-positive bacteria often identified as PC contaminants include corynebacteria, *Staphylococcus aureus*, *Bacillus* spp. and *Streptococcus* spp. [5, 8, 10]. Most of the PC contaminants are either aerobic or facultative anaerobic bacteria; however, there have been reports of septic reactions associated with strict anaerobic organisms such as *Clostridium perfringens* [10]. The anaerobe *Propionibacterium acnes* is a common platelet contaminant and, although mild transfusion reactions with this organism have been reported, its clinical relevance in transfusion settings is still under debate [10].

Although less commonly recognized as PC contaminants, Gram-negative bacteria can be present and will cause severe and often fatal infections due to the potent septic shock reaction induced by the endotoxin, which elicits an uncontrolled inflammatory response in the recipient. The most frequently identified Gram-negative PC contaminants include *Escherichia coli*, *Klebsiella pneumoniae*, *Enterobacter* spp. and *Serratia* spp. [6, 8–10].

Red blood cells

RBCs are the most frequently transfused blood component. The predominant RBC contaminants are Gram-negative bacteria of the family Enterobacteriacea, with *Yersinia enterocolitica* being the predominant species. Recovering donors who had *Yersinia enterocolitica* infections can be asymptomatic due to the low bacterial content in their bloodstream (<10 CFU/ml). *Yersinia* growth in RBCs is supported by the storage conditions; being a psychrophilic organism, this bacterium proliferates well at 1–6°C, reaching concentrations >10^8 CFU/ml after 3 weeks of incubation. *Yersinia enterocolitica* lacks siderophores for iron acquisition, which results in a long lag phase (from 1 to 3 weeks) until free haemin is available from spontaneous RBC haemolysis. Glucose and adenine, used as energy sources by this organism, are provided by the RBC anticoagulant solutions. Transfusion of RBC units heavily contaminated with *Y. enterocolitica* results in severe septic shock due to high levels of endotoxin [12].

Table 14.1 Sources of bacterial contamination and prevention strategies. Reproduced from Ramirez-Arcos S, Goldman M & Blajchman MA. Bacterial contamination. In: MA Popovsky (ed.), *Transfusion Reactions*. Bethesda, MD: American Association of Blood Banks; 2007, pp. 163–206 [8].

Source of contamination	Possible control measures
Blood donor • Silent bacteraemia • Respiratory flora	• Donor screening • Pretransfusion detection • Pathogen reduction technologies
Blood collection procedures • Normal and transient skin flora • Collection practices and equipment	• Skin disinfection • First aliquot diversion • Pretransfusion detection • Pathogen reduction technologies
Blood processing procedures	• Improved quality control • Pretransfusion detection • Pathogen reduction technologies

Other RBC Gram-negative bacterial contaminants include *Serratia* spp., *Pseudomonas* spp., *Enterobacter* spp., *Campylobacter* spp. and *Escherichia coli*, all of which have the potential to cause endotoxic shock in recipients [6, 8–10].

Plasma and cryoprecipitate

Burkolderia cepacia (previously known as *Pseudomonas cepacia*) and *Pseudomonas aeruginosa* have been implicated in ATRs due to contaminated plasma and cryoprecipitate [8].

Sources of contamination

Contaminant bacteria of blood components can originate from the donor or the blood collection and processing procedures (Table 14.1).

Blood donor

The predominant blood component bacterial contaminants are aerobic and anaerobic Gram-positive bacteria that are part of the normal skin flora and, more rarely, Gram-negative bacteria that can originate from silent donor bacteremia or be part of the transient skin flora. It is impossible to completely decontaminate human skin and it has been reported that normal skin flora organisms such as *Staphylococcus epidermidis* can adhere firmly to human hair despite skin disinfection [5, 6, 8–10].

Different bacteria can be part of the transient skin flora. *Clostridium perfringens*, which is part of faecal flora, was implicated in a fatal ATR. The microorganism was isolated from the arm of a donor who frequently changed his children's diapers. A *Salmonella enterica* isolate, which caused two transfusion-associated sepsis events, was found in a stool sample of the pet boa owned by the donor implicated in this case. Although not confirmed, it was speculated that the bacterium was present on the donor's skin at the time of donation [8].

On the odd occasion, asymptomatic donor bacteraemia may lead to contamination of blood components. Low level bacteraemia may occur in the incubation or recovery phase of acute infections after procedures such as tooth extraction. Chronic, low grade infections, such as osteomyelitis, have been associated with contaminated platelet products, as have gastrointestinal disorders such as diverticulosis and colon cancer [13].

Blood collection and production processes

Blood collection and production processes can also be sources of bacterial contamination. Three cases of *Serratia marcescens* sepsis following platelet transfusions were linked to contaminated vacuum tubes used for blood collection [8]. *Burkolderia cepacia* and *Pseudomonas aeruginosa* implicated in ATRs due to contaminated plasma and cryoprecipitate were isolated from the waterbaths used to thaw the products [8].

Although rare, unusual practices during blood collection could also result in blood component contamination. A cool cloth contaminated with *Pseudomonas fluorescens*, which was used by a donor with low pain tolerance, led to heavy contamination of an RBC unit that was transfused, causing a severe transfusion reaction [8].

Investigation of transfusion reactions (also see Chapter 6)

Symptoms of transfusion-associated septic reactions usually appear during the first four hours after the transfusion was initiated. If a septic reaction is suspected, the transfusion should be stopped immediately and the open port of the blood component must be covered immediately to avoid environmental contamination. Remaining component, intravenous solutions and blood samples from the recipient should be sent to a microbiology laboratory for investigation. Septic transfusion reactions are confirmed if the same bacterium is isolated from the recipient and the implicated blood component. Associated components to the concerned blood component should be recalled, and if available, also cultured. If the contaminant organism is not part of the normal skin flora, the donor should be contacted and followed up. Donor deferral might be necessary but it should be based on medical judgement depending on the laboratory results and the microorganism identified [13].

Donors with silent bacteraemia identified during routine platelet screening should also be investigated. The donor's health should be considered as well as the possibility of recurrent contaminated donations. Depending on the results of the investigation, donor deferral from future donations might be required [14].

Prevention strategies

Strategies used to decrease the levels of bacterial contamination in blood components include donor screening, skin disinfection, first aliquot diversion, pretransfusion detection and pathogen reduction technologies (Table 14.1).

Donor screening

Most transfusion centres have established methods for donor screening to avoid collection of potentially contaminated blood components. Donor screening includes body temperature determination and answering a questionnaire that includes questions related to the donor's general health and potential signs of infection or silent bacteraemia, such as the occurrence of recent dental work, gastrointestinal diseases or malaise.

Skin disinfection

Since the majority of bacteria found in contaminated blood components are part of the skin flora, optimal skin disinfection of the phlebotomy site is essential to maximize the inactivation of contaminant bacteria during blood donation.

Several factors affect the efficacy of skin disinfection including: the type and concentration of antiseptic used, the mode of application (scrub, swab, applicator or ampoule), whether there is a single or two-step method, the time that the antiseptic is in contact with the skin and the training of the personnel applying the disinfectant. A two-step method involving a scrub with a 0.75% povidone–iodine compound followed by an application of a 10% povidone–iodine preparation solution is recommended by the AABB. For donors sensitive to iodine, the use of 2% chlorhexidine and 70% isopropyl alcohol is optional and, for donors that react to both iodine and chlorhexidine, using only isopropyl alcohol should be considered. Currently, a one-step 2% chlorhexidine and 70% isopropyl alcohol skin cleansing kit is being used in the UK, the USA, Australia and Canada. The Australian Red Cross reported a 99% reduction in bacterial load after implementing the use of a one-step swab containing a chlorhexidine–alcohol antiseptic. Similarly, rate reductions have been observed in the UK and the USA upon implementation of the enhanced method [5, 8].

First aliquot diversion

Diversion of the first 30–40 ml of blood at the point of collection has been associated with significant reduction in contamination by skin flora. The diverted blood sample is either discarded or used for viral and immunohaematology testing. Significant reductions of the whole blood bacterial contamination rate as a result of the implementation of a diversion bag have been reported by the Sanquin Blood Blank, the Québec Hemovigilance System, the American Red Cross and the Japanase Red Cross [6, 8, 15].

Single donor apheresis versus pooled platelet concentrates

An increased risk of bacterial contamination has been traditionally associated with pooled PCs in comparison to single donor apheresis PCs due to a potential pooling of microorganisms [6]. However, nowadays apheresis donors may donate by a double or triple platepheresis procedure and therefore multiple contaminated therapeutic units can be produced, counterbalancing the 'pooling' effect of whole-blood-derived PCs. Studies from other countries such as Canada and Germany have shown that the rate of contamination of apheresis PCs and buffy coat platelet pools is similar [16, 17].

Bacterial detection methods

Routine testing for bacterial contamination has been implemented in several countries to screen apheresis and whole-blood-derived PCs. RBCs or plasma are not tested for bacterial contamination; however, RBC and/or plasma units associated with contaminated whole-blood-derived PCs are removed from the inventory, if available. There is evidence that only 40% of RBC and plasma units associated with bacterially contaminated PCs would test positive [8].

Detection of bacteria in transfusable blood components is more complex than viral detection since bacterial concentrations increase over time under routine blood component storage conditions. Factors that should be considered prior to the implementation of a bacterial screening method include: the time of testing, the method used for sample collection, the sample volume to be tested, the time required to perform the test and whether the blood component should be quarantined prior to testing. Since initial bacterial loads are usually very low (<1 CFU/mL), a very sensitive technique should be used in the blood collection centre shortly after collection. However, less sensitive methods may be used at the hospital end for blood component screening prior to transfusion.

Pretransfusion detection methods used by blood component suppliers

The BacT/ALERT® 3D system (bioMérieux, Marcy l'Etoile, France) and the Pall enhanced Bacterial Detection System (eBDS, Pall Corporation, New York, USA) are culture systems that have been licensed in Europe and North America to detect bacterial contamination in PCs [5, 6, 8].

The BacT/ALERT System uses liquid aerobic and anaerobic culture bottles with a colorimetric sensor at the bottom that changes colour from green to yellow when pH decreases as a result of the metabolic activity of growing bacteria. The culture bottles are inoculated with 8–10 mL of PC samples and are incubated at 36°C for one to six or seven days depending on the centre. It is reported that this system can detect 1–10 CFU/mL of most common platelet contaminants. The BacT/ALERT system has been widely used for bacterial testing of apheresis and whole-blood-derived PCs. When an initial positive culture is confirmed by repeat testing of the implicated blood component, a retention sample and/or samples from the recipient, it is considered to be a true (confirmed) positive. Table 14.2 summarizes the rate of contamination in selected blood centres that use the BacT/ALERT system for platelet screening. True positive rates vary from 1/134 to 1/7 536 (Table 14.2).

Despite its high sensitivity, several reports of missed bacteria detection in apheresis and whole-blood-derived PCs tested by the BacT/ALERT system have been reported worldwide. Examples of microorganisms that were implicated in false negative cases include: *Salmonella, Serratia marcescens,* Group A

Table 14.2 Prevalence of bacterial contamination in platelet concentrates in selected blood centres.

Centre	Number of units/ pools tested	Initial positives	Confirmed positives		Reference
			Number	Rate per 1000	
American Red Cross Regional Blood Centers	1 786 142	1285	351	0.2 (1/5088)	19
Belgian Red Cross	107 827	1030	803	7.4 (1/134)	8
Canadian Blood Services	489 847	476	65	0.1 (1/7536)	16
Copenhagen Transfusion Service	22 165	50	34	1.5 (1/651)	8
Department of Immunology and Transfusion Medicine, Norway	36 896	88	12	0.3 (1/3074)	8
Funen Transfusion Service, Denmark	22 057	84	21	1.0 (1/1050)	8
Welsh Blood Services	54 828	257	38	0.7 (1/1442)	20

Streptococcus, Staphylococcus aureus and coagulase negative *Staphylococcus* in Canada [16] and *Staphylococcus aureus*, coagulase negative staphylococci, *Streptococcus* spp., *Serratia marcescens, Escherichia coli, Klebsiella oxytoca, Morganella morgannii* (previously known as *Proteuns morganii*) and the anaerobe *Eubacterium limosum* in the USA [3]. All of these false negatives resulted in severe or fatal reactions. It is likely that many false negative results were not recognized because no reactions occurred or signs and symptoms of a reaction were mild. Attempts to decrease the likelihood of false negative cultures include the use of a two-bottle (aerobic and anaerobic) culture system and/or retesting components after 3–4 days of storage.

Most centres are routinely testing for aerobic bacteria, as the majority of clinically significant organisms belong to this group. Centres using the two-bottle system have reported an increase in the detection rate of bacterial contamination in PCs since anaerobic culture bottles allow the capture of strict anaerobic bacteria such as *Propionibacterium acnes* and *Staphylococcus saccharolyticus*. Although cases of transfusion-transmitted *Propionibacterium acnes* have been reported, none of them have resulted in severe transfusion reactions. However, there are reports of severe and fatal ATRs due to the presence of the anaerobes *Eubacterium limosum* and *Clostridium perfringens*. It has also been documented that some platelet contaminants including *Staphylococcus* spp. and *Serratia marcescens* can be preferentially recovered from anaerobic culture media and not from aerobic cultures. Implementation of anaerobic bacterial cultures is still controversial due to the doubtful clinical relevance of *Propionibacterium acnes*, the most common anaerobic platelet contaminant, and the high incidence of false positive results obtained with anaerobic culture bottles [3, 5, 8, 10].

The Pall Bacterial Detection System uses the decrease in oxygen concentration as an indicator of bacterial growth in PCs. Between 4 and 6 mL of PC samples are transferred into an incubation bag. After 24–30 hours of incubation, the oxygen concentration of this bag is measured with an oxygen analyser. A decrease in the percentage of oxygen to $\leq 19.5\%$ is indicative of bacterial growth. This system only detects aerobic Gram-positive and Gram-negative bacteria at the levels of 100–500 CFU/mL with a sensitivity of 96.5%. The Pall eBDS system has been validated for bacteria detection in both leucocyte-reduced PCs and RBCs [5, 6, 8].

Other methods developed to detect bacterial contamination in PCs include detection of bacterial 16S rRNA genes by reverse transcriptase polymerase chain reaction and pH monitoring [6, 8]. However, these methods are neither sensitive nor specific enough to be an alternative for the automated culture-base methods currently used by the blood production centres.

Bacterial detection methods to be used prior to transfusion
Methods to be used at the hospital end can be less sensitive detecting bacteria in the range of 10^3–10^4 CFU/mL, but such tests need to be rapid and specific. The new AABB Interim Standard 5.1.5.1.1 requests the use of methods that have been either validated or approved by the Food and Drug Administration (FDA). Therefore, subjective, nonsensitive and/or complex and time-consuming methods such as visual examination, staining of platelet smears and multi-reagent strip testing are no longer recommended in the US.

The easy-to-use rapid immunoassay Verax PGD test has been licensed by the FDA as a point-of-use assay for bacterial detection in apheresis and whole-blood-derived PCs that have been previously tested with an approved culture-based test. The PGD assay can detect aerobic and anaerobic bacteria based on the existence of conserved bacterial cell wall antigens. The test has a sensitivity of 8.2×10^3 to 8.6×10^5 CFU/mL depending on the contaminant microorganism and a specificity of 98.4–99.7% depending on the platelet type. Recent studies showed that the PGD test detected contaminated PCs that had been released as negative by initial screening with automated culture systems, demonstrating the utility of this assay as a point of release test [18].

Pathogen reduction technologies

In contrast to testing, pathogen reduction technologies (PRT) involve the treatment of PCs as soon as possible after collection with a process to inactivate or reduce the level of contaminating bacteria, viruses, parasites and residual leucocytes. Two technologies, Mirasol® (TerumoBCT, CO, USA) and INTERCEPT Blood System (Cerus Europe BV, Amersfoort, The Netherlands) have received CE (Conformité Européenne) Mark

149

registration and have been introduced into routine use by several European countries. Neither of these technologies has been licensed in North America. Both of these processes utilize photochemical techniques with different mechanisms of action. A third technology, THERAFLEX UV Platelets technology, which utilizes UVC light without a photochemical compound, is in clinical development and has not been introduced into routine use [5].

The INTERCEPT process is used within the first 24 hours after collection and utilizes a synthetic psoralen, amotoslaen HCl, which targets nucleic acid and utilizes UVA light (3 J/cm^2: 320–400 nm) to form covalent adducts with nucleic acids. INTERCEPT inactivates a broad spectrum of Gram-positive and Gram-negative bacterial species associated with ATRs but cannot inactivate bacterial spores. In countries where the system has been used for several years, no ATRs related to bacterial contamination have been reported [5].

The Mirasol® system uses riboflavin (vitamin B2, 50 μg per 300 ml) with UVC, UVB and a portion of UVA light (265–375 nm). The efficacy of this process is based on the association of riboflavin with nucleic acids and the generation of reactive oxygen species, leading to nucleic acid disruption rather than adduct formation. In a spiking study, the efficacy of Mirasol to inactivate Gram-positive and Gram-negative bacteria ranged from 33 to 100% but not all bacterial strains were completely inactivated; no data have been reported regarding bacterial spore destruction [5].

Key points

1 Bacterial contamination of blood components poses the most prevalent transfusion-transmitted infectious risk.
2 Platelet concentrates are the blood components most susceptible to bacterial contamination due to their storage conditions.
3 Interventions such as improved donor screening and skin disinfection, first aliquot diversion and bacterial testing have decreased the occurrence of transfusion-associated septic events.
4 Gram-positive skin flora are the predominant blood component contaminants.
5 Gram-negative bacteria originated from silent donor bacteraemia or transient skin colonization,

are less frequently found as blood component contaminants, but they pose the major infectious risk due to their production of endotoxin.
6 Platelet concentrates are the only blood component that is routinely tested for bacterial contamination.
7 The BacT/ALERT and Pall eBDS automated culture systems are the only methods currently licensed for routine testing of platelet concentrates by blood component suppliers in Europe and North America.
8 Recommended bacterial detection methods to be used prior to transfusion at the hospital end include repeat culture and the new immunoassay PGD test.
9 Despite high sensitivity of the current testing methods, contaminated PC units still escape detection, resulting in false negative transfusion cases.
10 Pathogen reduction technologies are the ultimate approach to prevent bacterial contamination of blood components.

References

1 Serious Hazards of Transfusion SHOT. Summary of Annual Report 2009 [homepage on the Internet]. Available from: http://www.shotuk.org/shot-reports/report-and-summary-2009/ (last accessed 6 October 2011).
2 Serious Hazards of Transfusion (SHOT). Summary of Annual Report 2010 [homepage on the Internet]. Available from: http://www.shotuk.org/shot-reports/report-and-summary-2010-2/ (last accessed 6 October 2011).
3 Fatalities Reported to FDA Following Blood Collection and Transfusion. Annual Summary for Fiscal Year 2010 [homepage on the Internet]. Available from: http://www.fda.gov/downloads/BiologicsBloodVaccines/SafetyAvailability/ReportaProblem/TransfusionDonationFatalities/UCM254860.pdf (last accessed 6 October 2011).
4 Transfusion Transmitted Injuries Surveillance System Program Report 2004–2005 [homepage on the Internet]. Available from: http://www.phac-aspc.gc.ca/hcai-iamss/tti-it/pr-re0405/pdf/ttiss-ssit0405-eng.pdf. (last accessed 6 October 2011).
5 Corash L. Bacterial contamination of platelet components: potential solutions to prevent transfusion-related sepsis. *Expert Rev Hematol* 2011; 4(5): 509–525.
6 Palavecino EL, Yomtovian RA & Jacobs MR. Bacterial contamination of platelets. *Transfus Apher Sci* 2010; 42(1): 71–82.

7 Chen CL, Yu JC, Holme S, Jacobs MR, Yomtovian R & McDonald CP. Detection of bacteria in stored red cell products using a culture-based bacterial detection system. *Transfusion* 2008; 48(8): 1550–1557.

8 Ramirez-Arcos S, Goldman M & Blajchman MA. Bacterial contamination. In MA Popovsky (ed.), *Transfusion Reactions*. Bethesda, MD: American Association of Blood Banks (AABB), 2007, pp. 163–206.

9 Jacobs MR, Good CE, Lazarus HM & Yomtovian RA. Relationship between bacterial load, species virulence, and transfusion reaction with transfusion of bacterially contaminated platelets. *Clin Infect Dis* 2008; 46(8): 1214–1220.

10 Walther-Wenke G, Schrezenmeier H, Deitenbeck R, Geis G, Burkhart J, Höchsmann B et al. Screening of platelet concentrates for bacterial contamination: spectrum of bacteria detected, proportion of transfused units, and clinical follow-up. *Ann Hematol* 2009; 89: 83–91.

11 Greco C, Martincic I, Gusinjac A, Kalab M, Yang AF & Ramírez-Arcos S. *Staphylococcus epidermidis* forms biofilms under simulated platelet storage conditions. *Transfusion* 2007; 47(7): 1143–1153.

12 Guinet F, Carniel E & Leclercq A. Transfusion-transmitted *Yersinia enterocolitica* sepsis. *Clin Infect Dis* 2011; 53(6): 583–591.

13 Public Health Agency of Canada. Guideline for Investigation of Suspected Transmitted Bacterial Contamination [homepage on the Internet]. Available from: http://www.phac-aspc.gc.ca/publicat/ccdr-rmtc/08vol34/34s1/34s1-eng.php (last accessed 6 October 2011).

14 Eder AF & Goldman M. How do I investigate septic transfusion reactions and blood donors with culture-positive platelet donations? *Transfusion* 2011; 51(8): 1662–1668.

15 Robillard P, Delage G, Itaj NK & Goldman M. Use of hemovigilance data to evaluate the effectiveness of diversion and bacterial detection. *Transfusion* 2011; 51(7): 1405–1411.

16 Jenkins C, Ramírez-Arcos S, Goldman M & Devine DV. Bacterial contamination in platelets: incremental improvements drive down but do not eliminate risk. *Transfusion* 2011; 51(12): 2555–2565.

17 Schrezenmeier H, Walther-Wenke G, Müller TH, Weinauer F, Younis A, Holland-Letz T et al. Bacterial contamination of platelet concentrates: results of a prospective multicenter study comparing pooled whole blood-derived platelets and apheresis platelets. *Transfusion* 2007; 47(4): 644–652.

18 Jacobs MR, Smith D, Heaton WA, Zantek ND & Good CE; PGD Study Group. Detection of bacterial contamination in prestorage culture-negative apheresis platelets on day of issue with the PAN Genera Detection test. *Transfusion* 2011; 51(12): 2573–2582.

19 Eder AF, Kennedy JM, Dy BA, Notari EP, Skeate R, Bachowski G et al. Limiting and detecting bacterial contamination of apheresis platelets: inlet-line diversion and increased culture volume improve component safety. *Transfusion* 2009; 49(8): 1554–1563.

20 Pearce S, Rowe GP & Field SP. Screening of platelets for bacterial contamination at the Welsh Blood Service. *Transfus Med* 2011; 21(1): 25–32.

Further reading

AABB Association Bulletin #04-07. Actions Following an Initial Positive Test for Possible Bacterial Contamination of a Platelet Unit [homepage on the Internet]. Available from: http://www.aabb.org/resources/publications/bulletins/Pages/ab04-07.aspx (last accessed 7 October 2011).

AABB Association Bulletin #05-02. Guidance on Management of Blood and Platelet Donors with Positive or Abnormal Results on Bacterial Contamination Tests [homepage on the Internet]. Available from: http://www.aabb.org/Content/Members_Area/Association_Bulletins/ab05-2.htm (last accessed 7 October 2011).

AABB Association Bulletin #10-05. Suggested Options for Transfusion Services and Blood Collectors to Facilitate Implementation of BB/TS Interim Standard 5.1.5.1.1 [homepage on the Internet]. Available from: http://www.aabb.org/resources/publications/bulletins/Pages/ab05-02.aspx (last accessed 7 October 2011).

AuBuchon& Prowse CV (eds). Pathogen Inactivation. *The Penultimate Paradigm Shift*. Bethesda, MD: AABB Press; 2010.

Blajchman MA, Beckers EAM, Dickmeiss E, Lin L, Moore G & Muylle L. Bacterial detection of platelets: current problems and possible resolutions. *Transfus Med Rev* 2005; 19: 259–272.

Brecher ME & Hay SN. Bacterial contamination of blood components. *Clin Microbiol Rev* 2005; 18: 195–204.

Dumont LJ, Kleinman S & Murphy JR. Screening of single-donor apheresis platelets for bacterial contamination: the PASSPORT study results. *Transfusion* 2010; 50: 589–599.

INTERCEPT Blood System by Cerus Corporation [homepage on the Internet]. Available from: http://www.interceptbloodsystem.com/ (last accessed 6 October 2011).

Mirasol® Pathogen Reduction Technology [homepage on the Internet]. Available from: http://www.caridianbct.com/location/emea/products-and-services/Pages/mirasol-pathogen-reduction-technology.aspx (last accessed 6 October 2011).

Platelet PGD test http://www.fda.gov/downloads/biologicsbloodvaccines/bloodbloodproducts/approvedproducts/substantiallyequivalent510kdeviceinformation/ucm190504.pdf (last accessed 7 October 2011).

15 Variant Creutzfeldt–Jakob disease

Marc L. Turner

Scottish National Blood Transfusion Service, Edinburgh, Scotland, UK

A variety of transmissible spongiform encephalopathies or prion diseases are described in animals and humans (Table 15.1). Scrapie, an endemic disease of sheep and goats, was first described over 250 years ago. Chronic wasting disease is spreading in deer and elk in the USA. Bovine spongiform encephalopathy (BSE) was first described in cattle in the UK in 1986, though in retrospect the first cases probably appeared as early as 1982 [1, 2]. It remains unclear whether BSE arose from scrapie in sheep or from a sporadic case of prion disease in cattle, but it is thought that it was transmitted through the food chain via rendered meat and bonemeal. In the UK over 180 000 clinical cases of BSE have been described, with around 300 cases in other European countries, and occasional cases elsewhere in the world, probably related to exported UK cattle or meat and bonemeal. The UK epidemic peaked in 1992 and has now subsided as a result of a ban on the use of ruminant protein in cattle feed. However, mathematical projections suggest that 1–2 million infected cattle could have entered the human food chain before showing evidence of disease. Unlike scrapie, BSE has proved itself capable of crossing species barriers by infecting a number of other animals including exotic and domestic cats (feline spongiform encephalopathy) and exotic ruminants in zoos (exotic ungulate encephalopathy).

In humans several forms of prion disease have been described. Sporadic or classical Creutzfeldt–Jakob disease (CJD) was first described in the early 1920s. It presents at a median age of 68 years as a rapidly progressive dementia with a duration of illness of around 6 months. The incidence of CJD is around 1 per million per annum throughout the world, with no clear link to the incidence of prion disease in other animals.

In the 1950s, a form of prion disease called kuru was described in the Foré people of the highlands of Papua New Guinea. This disease presented at a much younger age, with cerebellar ataxia as a prominent feature and a more prolonged clinical course. Kuru was transmitted from person to person, probably through the cannibalistic funeral rites practised by the tribe at that time. It is informative to note that children died from kuru and that although cannibalistic feasts discontinued around 1959–1960, there are still occasional patients presenting with the clinical disease. This points to a very wide range of incubation periods, with an upper limit of 40–50 years or perhaps even beyond the normal human lifespan.

In the 1980s a number of iatrogenic transmissions of CJD were described. These fell broadly into two groups. Direct central nervous systems (CNS) transmission due to contaminated neurosurgical instruments, EEG electrodes and dura mater grafts led to a rapidly progressive dementia reminiscent of sporadic CJD after a short incubation period of around 2 years and death within about 6 months of presentation. Peripheral transmission from cadaveric pituitary-derived growth- and follicle-stimulating hormone gave rise to a clinical picture reminiscent of

Practical Transfusion Medicine, Fourth Edition. Edited by Michael F. Murphy, Derwood H. Pamphlon and Nancy M. Heddle.
© 2013 John Wiley & Sons, Ltd. Published 2013 by John Wiley & Sons, Ltd.

Table 15.1 Prion diseases.

Animals	Human
Scrapie	Sporadic Creutzfeldt–Jakob disease
Chronic wasting disease	Kuru
Transmissible mink encephalopathy	Iatrogenic Creutzfeldt–Jakob disease
Bovine spongiform encephalopathy	Variant Creutzfeldt–Jakob disease
Feline spongiform encephalopathy	Familial Creutzfeldt–Jakob disease
Exotic ungulate encephalopathy	Gerstmann–Sträussler–Scheinker disease
	Fatal familial insomnia

kuru, with a prolonged incubation period of some 13–15 years.

Finally, a number of familial forms of CJD have been described including familial CJD, Gerstmann–Sträussler–Scheinker (GSS) disease and fatal familial insomnia (FFI), which arise due to polymorphisms in the gene for prion protein (PrP).

Prion diseases are therefore interesting from an aetiological perspective in that they can arise spontaneously, are transmissible and can also arise due to genetic polymorphism.

Variant CJD

The UK government instituted routine surveillance for CJD in 1989 in response to the BSE epidemic, with the aim of monitoring any change in the incidence or pattern of disease in the UK population. In 1995 the first cases of variant CJD were described. The clinical features differ from those of sporadic CJD. Patients are younger, with a median age at presentation of 28 years (range 12–74 years). They often present with behavioural change, such as depression and anxiety, or with dysaesthesia. Untreated, the disease progresses to cerebellar ataxia, involuntary movements, dementia and death over a period of 7–38 months. In the UK 176 cases of variant CJD have been described thus far, though the incidence of new cases appears to be falling. Elsewhere there have been 27 cases described in France, 5 in Spain, 4 in the Republic of Ireland,

3 in the USA and the Netherlands, 2 in Portugal, Canada and Italy, and 1 in Japan, Saudi Arabia and Taiwan. Two of the American and Irish patients, and one each of the French, Canadian and Taiwan patients had spent a considerable time in the UK, whereas the others did not, and probably contracted the disease in their own countries. Though original estimates of the number of people who may eventually develop the disease gave very high upper limits, the recent downturn in the number of new cases in the UK has led to a revised prediction of just over 70 cases. However, retrospective studies of appendix samples in the UK recorded suggest a prevalence of subclinical disease of around 1/2000 (95% confidence interval (CI), 1/1250–1/3500). These individuals should be assumed to be at risk of passing infection to others via contaminated surgical instruments or blood transfusion.

A considerable amount of epidemiological, clinical, neuropathological and experimental data now supports the view that variant CJD is the same strain of disease as BSE [4] and that these are different from the prion strains that give rise to other forms of CJD in humans or scrapie and chronic wasting disease in animals.

Aetiology and pathophysiology

Prion diseases are associated with a change in the secondary structure of PrP. PrP is a widely expressed 30–35 kDa glycoprotein with two N-linked oligosaccharides. It is normally linked to the cell membrane by a glycosylphosphatidylinositol (GPI) anchor, though transmembrane anchorage has also been described. The normal secondary structure of PrP contains around 40% α-helices and 3% β-pleated sheets, with the membrane-distal part of the molecule largely unstructured. The development of prion disease is associated with a change in the secondary structure of the PrP glycoprotein, with an increase in the proportion of β-pleated sheets to some 40–50% of the molecule largely at the expense of the unstructured region (PrP^{TSE}) (Figure 15.1). This changes the physicochemical characteristics of the molecule, giving it increased resistance to both physical and biological degradation. *In vitro* treatment with proteinase-K removes the membrane-distal part of the molecule, but is unable to digest the 30–32 kDa core (PrP^{Res}).

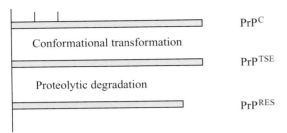

Fig 15.1 The prion hypothesis. PrP^C (top) is a 30–35 kDa glycoprotein with two N-linked glycosylation sites, anchored by glycosylphosphatidylinositol to the cell membrane, with 40% α-helix and 3% β-pleated sheet. Prion diseases are associated with conformational change in the secondary structure, with an increase in the amount of β-pleated sheet to some 40–50% of the molecule (PrP^{TSE}) (middle). This changes the physicochemical and biological properties of the molecule, rendering it resistant to degradation by enzymes such as proteinase-K (PrP^{RES}) (bottom).

PrP^{TSE} accumulates *in vivo*, leading to the deposition of amyloid plaques. The pathophysiology of the disease remains debated. Some authorities propose the presence of a small DNA molecule associated with PrP^{TSE} (termed a virion), but this has not yet been identified and the infectious agent does appear to be resistant to physical conditions that would normally degrade DNA. The prion hypothesis proposes that the abnormal isoform of the protein is itself the infectious agent, changing the structure of the normal form either through heterodimer formation or though a physicochemical process of nuclear polymerization.

Accumulation of amyloid plaques consisting of PrP^{TSE} leads to the classical neuropathological features of neuronal death, astrogliosis and spongiform degeneration of the CNS (Plates 15.1 and 15.2 in the plate section). In sporadic, iatrogenic and familial forms of CJD, abnormal PrP accumulation appears to be confined to the CNS. In variant CJD, abnormal PrP^{TSE} accumulation has been demonstrated in follicular dendritic cells (FDCs) in the tonsil, spleen, cervical, mediastinal, paraaortic and mesenteric lymph nodes and gut-associated lymphoid tissue of the appendix up to 2 years prior to the onset of clinical disease (Plate 15.3 in the plate section). This observation is consistent with what we know about the pathophysiology of transmission of prion diseases by peripheral routes in experimental animals.

Experimental peripheral transmission of scrapie strains in murine models leads to the presence of infectivity and/or PrP^{TSE} in the spleen and lymph node from a very early stage of infection, well before detection of infectivity of PrP^{TSE} in the CNS. Interestingly, immunosuppression and splenectomy have long been known to decrease the efficiency of peripheral transmission, whereas irradiation and thymectomy do not. A series of experiments has demonstrated that mice with severe combined immunodeficiency are resistant to peripheral but not central prion challenge and that sensitivity is regained after allogeneic bone marrow transplantation. Similarly, PrP-negative mice with a PrP-positive CNS implant can be infected only by peripheral transmission following PrP-positive allogeneic bone marrow transplant, whereas PrP-positive mice develop resistance to peripherally transmitted disease following PrP-negative bone marrow transplant. Detailed knockout experiments have demonstrated that Rag 1, Rag 2 and μMT knockout mice are resistant to peripheral challenge whereas CD4, CD8, β-microglobulin and perforin knockout models display normal sensitivity. These data led to the suggestion that B-lymphocytes were essential to peripheral transmission whereas T-lymphocytes were not. However, B-lymphocytes are also essential for FDC survival and more recent studies have demonstrated that PrP-positive FDCs are essential to peripheral transmission whereas PrP-positive B-lymphocytes are not. Indeed, peripheral transmission can be inhibited even by temporary FDC inactivation by lymphotoxin β-receptor blockade and also by depletion of complement receptors. These data convincingly support the seminal role of FDCs in the early stages of peripheral transmission.

Assessing peripheral blood infectivity in animal models

It has been demonstrated that PrP is present in the peripheral blood of normal individuals at a concentration of 100–300 ng/mL [5], with the majority found in platelets and plasma. PrP^{TSE} accumulation has recently been demonstrated in the peripheral blood of humans with clinical variant CJD [6], though it has not proved possible to detect infectivity in this context, probably because of limitations in the volumes of blood that can be inoculated into experimental animals and the species barrier between man and rodents. Most of the information on peripheral blood infectivity comes from animal experiments where it has proved possible to demonstrate infectivity in the peripheral blood of sheep and rodents with experimental scrapie and BSE, and in rodents with experimental GSS, during both the clinical and incubation phases of disease [7–10]. However, no infectivity has been demonstrated in natural scrapie in sheep and goats, natural transmissible mink encephalopathy or natural or experimental BSE in cattle. The reason for these differences is not clear. Levels of peripheral blood infectivity have been investigated in the Fukuoka-1 strain of GSS in experimental mice and have been found to be on the order of 100 infectious units/mL during the clinical phase of disease and 5–10 infectious units/mL during the incubation period. A fourfold to fivefold higher level of infectivity was demonstrated in the buffy coat (containing the leucocytes and platelets) compared with plasma. Plasma itself showed a 10-fold higher concentration of infectivity compared with any of the Cohn fractions in an experimental fractionation system. The distribution of infectivity in blood was similar during the incubation phase of disease. Similar findings have been described in the 263K scrapie hamster model, where a little infectivity is associated with (purified) red cells or platelets, around 40% is associated with leucocytes and the remainder is in the plasma. Indeed, more recent data from the same group suggests that washing the leucocytes removes most of the associated infectivity.

In a different model, sheep experimentally infected with BSE or scrapie by oral ingestion have been bled during the incubation and clinical phases of the disease and whole-blood donations administered intravenously to secondary recipients [11]. Up to 50% of the secondary recipients in both cohorts have subsequently developed the relevant prion disease, amounting to proof of the principle that certain forms of prion disease can be transmitted by blood transfusion.

Clinical transmission of CJD from the peripheral blood of patients

In humans, of 37 reported attempts to transmit sporadic CJD from peripheral blood of patients with clinical disease by intracerebral inoculation into rodents, there have been five positive reports. Interestingly,

transmission of CJD from human peripheral blood to primates by intracerebral inoculation has not proved possible and this has thrown some doubt on the validity of the rodent data. Thus far, there have been no successful transmissions of variant CJD from human peripheral blood to rodents or primates.

There have been three anecdotal case reports of patients who have developed sporadic CJD some time after receiving blood components or plasma products. In none of these, however, has it been shown that the donors themselves developed CJD. In comparison a large number of epidemiological case-control, look-back and surveillance studies over the past 25 years have shown little evidence of increased risk of sporadic CJD in blood or plasma product recipients, even where a donor is known to have subsequently developed sporadic CJD. One recent study has suggested an increased risk of transfusion more than 10 years before the clinical onset in sporadic CJD patients, though the significance of this remains uncertain.

In contrast, there are now 18 patients identified with variant CJD who, in the past, were blood donors; 67 recipients of blood components and plasma products from these donors have been traced of whom 17 are alive and 50 deceased [12]. Thus far three of the recipients have developed clinical variant CJD and one has shown evidence of abnormal prion accumulation in the spleen and a cervical lymph node [13, 14].

Strategies for risk containment

Blood services have felt it prudent to implement precautionary policies to contain the risk of transmission of variant CJD. However, such policies require careful evaluation, both in terms of likely efficacy in reducing the risk of secondary transmission by blood transfusion and in terms of the potential increase in other risks including that of blood shortages. Consideration also needs to be given to the cross-impact of different policies and the opportunity costs incurred.

Donor selection

The UK blood services use a number of criteria to exclude blood and tissue donors who may be at increased risk of sporadic, iatrogenic or familial CJD

Table 15.2 UK criteria for excluding blood and tissue donors who have, or may have had contact with, sporadic, iatrogenic, or familial CJD.

Obligatory
Permanently exclude donors with CJD or other
  prion-associated disorder
Permanently exclude anyone identified at high risk of
  developing a prion-associated disorder
Recipients of dura mater, corneal or scleral grafts
Recipients of human pituitary-derived extracts such as
  growth hormone and gonadotrophins
Individuals at familial risk of prion-associated diseases
This includes individuals who have had two or more blood
  relatives develop a prion-associated disease and
  individuals who have been informed that they are at risk
  following genetic counselling

Exceptions
Individuals who have had two or more blood relatives
  develop a prion-associated disease but who, following
  genetic counselling, have been informed that they are not
  at risk. This requires confirmation by the consultant with
  responsibility for donors

(Table 15.2). There are no epidemiological risk factors described thus far that would discriminate a high-risk group for development of variant CJD within the UK. For example, there is no evidence that veterinary surgeons, cattle farmers, abattoir workers or others with a high risk of exposure to infected bovine materials are at higher risk of developing variant CJD than the general population. In comparison, some individuals who have been vegetarians for prolonged periods have developed variant CJD. A number of countries have taken the precautionary step of excluding blood donors who have spent more than a defined period in the UK between the beginning of 1980 and the end of 1996. The defined period varies depending on the frequency and pattern with which indigenous donors visit the UK and the likely prevalence of subclinical variant CJD in the general population. These are factors that impact upon the efficacy of UK donor exclusion in terms of risk reduction and on the likely negative impact on the blood donor base.

Subsequent to the evidence of transmission of variant CJD by blood transfusion, the UK blood services moved in April 2004 to defer blood donors who have themselves received blood transfusions in order to reduce the risk that tertiary and higher order transmissions would lead to a self-sustaining outbreak. This led to the loss of approximately 5–10% of the donor base.

Importation of blood components

An alternative approach would be to source blood components from countries with a low incidence of BSE and variant CJD. It is impractical to source all red blood cell concentrates for the UK (some 2.5 million components per annum) from overseas volunteer nonremunerated donors. The short shelf life of platelet concentrates also mitigates against this approach. Consideration needs to be given to the risk of other infectious agents in the proposed alternative donor population and long-term security of supply. It is possible to source plasma from overseas since surplus clinical plasma is generated by red cell collection programmes and the product can be virus inactivated and cryopreserved for transportation with a 2-year shelf life.

In the UK it has been decided to import methylene blue-inactivated plasma for neonates and children born since 1st January 1996. Neonates in particular receive a proportionately high number of blood components due to prematurity and surgery for congenital disorders. They are likely to have a low primary exposure to BSE through the food chain and they have the longest prospective lifespan during which to develop clinical variant CJD should they become infected. More recently solvent-detergent fresh frozen plasma has been imported for patients exposed to large volumes of plasma (such as patients undergoing plasma exchange for thrombotic thrombocytopenic purpura).

Development of peripheral blood assays for donor screening

There is no conventional immune response to prion infection and no DNA has been detected in association with transmission of these diseases. Hence, conventional serological and molecular approaches to the development of peripheral blood assays, utilized to such good effect in screening for microbiological disease, are not applicable to prion diseases.

A number of nonspecific markers of CNS damage are known to be elevated in the peripheral blood of patients with CJD, including 14-3-3 and S100, but given that patients with CNS damage are excluded by donor selection criteria, it seems unlikely that these would have much to offer in the context of screening normal healthy blood donors.

Surrogate markers could allow exclusion of individuals at risk of development of variant CJD. Reduced transcription of erythroid differentiation-associated factors (EDAF) has been described in the bone marrow and peripheral blood of scrapie-infected sheep and rodents and of BSE-infected cattle. However, these findings do not appear to have been borne out in humans.

The gold standard would be, of course, infectivity bioassays. However, not only is it impractical to use such an approach for primary screening but also, as noted above, infectivity is not detectable in the peripheral blood of patients with variant CJD despite the fact that it is clearly transmissible. This implies that total reliance will need to be placed on any *in vitro* assay since there may be no other way of establishing whether the test-positive individual is 'truly' infected or will develop clinical disease in the future.

Detection of PrP^{TSE} in the peripheral blood is the only practical way forward, although there are a number of fundamental problems. First is the analytical sensitivity likely to be required. If one assumes infectivity in human blood to be on the order of 1–10 infectious units/mL during the incubation period of disease (an extrapolation from the rodent models) and that the ratio of infectivity to PrP^{TSE} is similar to that seen in animal models, then the concentration of PrP^{TSE} in infected peripheral blood will be on the order of 0.01–0.1 pg/mL (in the context of 100–300 ng/mL of PrP^C). Moreover, there are uncertainties around the physicochemical form of PrP^{TSE} in blood and indeed the exact relationship between PrP^{TSE} and infectivity.

Nevertheless, a number of assays are under development based on a combination of proteinase-K digestion, the use of chaotropic agents, high affinity ligands or monoclonal antibodies as capture or detection agents and/or *in vitro* amplification, which are beginning to approach the levels of sensitivity required. Some of these approaches use PrP^{TSE} concentration steps to further increase the analytical sensitivity of the assay. A recent publication describes a prototype assay with an analytical sensitivity of 10^{-7} to 10^{-10} of variant CJD infected brain homogenate capable of detecting PrP^{TSE} in 15 out of 21 blood samples from patients with clinical variant CJD [6].

A second problem is the validation of such assays given that normally this would involve samples from patients with the disease in question. Variant CJD assays will have to be validated using animal model systems and human blood spiked with homogenized prion-infected tissues, given the limited volumes of blood available from patients with variant CJD.

Moreover, the diagnostic sensitivity and specificity of an assay is dependent not only on its analytical features but also on the population under study. An assay that has a high level of specificity in the clinical context of a patient with suspected disease may have a very low level of specificity (i.e. have a high false-positive rate) in the context of healthy blood donors. This point is made in Figure 15.2, which illustrates the consequences of screening 1 million blood donors with an assay with 99% sensitivity and specificity. Assuming a prevalence of subclinical variant CJD of 1 in 10 000 (as an example), around 99 infected individuals would be detected (true positives), whilst 1 would be missed (false negative). The majority of donors would of course be true negatives, but a sizeable minority (just under 10 000) would be falsely positive.

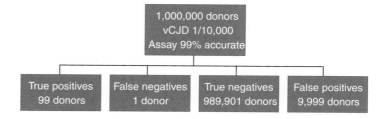

Fig 15.2 Likely impact of a putative variant CJD assay with 99% sensitivity and specificity.

- Negative predictive value: 99.99989%
- Positive predictive value: 0.98%

157

This brings into perspective the requirement for confirmatory assays, based on different analytical principles. Even with confirmatory assays it may still be very difficult to predict whether a test-positive individual will ever go on to develop clinical variant CJD (and/or whether they are infective to others).

Test-positive individuals would have to be informed and deferred. The psychological and social impact on the donor and the overall impact on donor recruitment and retention should not be underestimated.

Component processing

Universal leucocyte reduction was introduced in the UK in July 1998, predicated on the thesis that if variant CJD infectivity was present in the peripheral blood, it was likely to be mainly associated with the mononuclear leucocyte population. Modern leucocyte-reduced filters remove 3–4 $\log_{10}$ of leucocytes with no evidence of selective subset removal or cellular fragmentation. However, experimental studies in rodents suggest that only 40–70% of the infectivity in peripheral blood is removed by leucocyte reduction, with little impact on plasma-associated infectivity as expected. Under most scenarios, sufficient infectivity would therefore remain to allow transmission to a recipient. Several companies are now developing prion removal devices that may be able to remove additional 3 log infectivity from red cells concentrates and thereby impact on transmission risk (Table 15.3) [15, 16].

Plasma products

Plasma product recall is not indicated if a blood donor develops sporadic CJD, based on the accumulated clinical evidence of a low risk of transmission in look-back and surveillance studies. In December 1997 the UK Committee for the Safety of Medicines recommended product recall if a donor became infected with variant CJD in view of the uncertainties surrounding transmissibility of the disease. In Autumn 1999 the use of UK plasma for fractionation was discontinued altogether because of the recognition that a significant number of cases of variant CJD among donors would lead to multiple recalls and critical product shortages irrespective of the transmissibility of the disease. Other European plasma fractionation centres continue to use their own plasma.

Most studies suggest a significant reduction in infectivity by the Cohn fractionation process. Studies with 263K and 301V spikes using Western blot, DELFIA and infectivity bioassays as readouts suggest that cold ethanol precipitation, depth filtration, ion-exchange chromatography and nanofiltration all give several $\log_{10}$ reductions in infectivity titre, though whether these steps are additive is unclear. Criticisms of these studies surround the use of homogenized brain as the spike because infectivity may not be in the same physicochemical form as that seen in naturally infected blood. The studies of Brown et al. referred to earlier, using plasma from mice infected with the Fukuoka 1 strain of GSS, have shown an overall reduction of up to 3–4 $\log_{10}$, though the starting levels of infectivity are low and so estimates of the reduction in infectivity by serial plasma processing steps are likely to be conservative.

A number of patients with variant CJD have donated plasma for product manufacture. The implicated batches have been identified and, where possible, the recipients traced, notified and managed as 'at risk for public health purposes'. One patient with haemophilia has shown evidence of abnormal prion

Log reduction in infectivity	Residual leucocytes	Residual plasma	Total residual infectivity	Risk of transmission
Leucocyte reduction alone	0.2	130	130.2	Certain
1 log	0.2	13	13.2	Certain
2 log	0.2	1.3	13.2	Certain
3 log	0.2	0.13	0.33	1/3
4 log	0.2	0.013	0.213	1/5

Table 15.3 ikely impact of leucocyte reduction and prion reduction devices on variant CJD infectivity and transmissibility.

accumulation in the spleen following exposure to UK blood components and plasma products over an extended period of time [17]. However, no plasma product recipients have thus far developed clinical variant CJD [18].

Optimal use of blood components

There remains a need to reduce blood use and outdating both to manage the risk of unnecessary exposure to variant CJD and to reduce pressure on the blood supply at a time when a significant reduction in the number of blood donors due to the introduction of new donor selection or screening criteria is a real possibility. Key issues to be addressed include better evidence of the efficacy of current clinical transfusion practice, reduction in blood outdate and discard rates, and adoption of approaches for blood conservation.

Cell, tissue and organ transplantation

Though the level of infectivity associated with other cell and tissue products is unknown, in almost all cases the mass of tissue transplanted is sufficiently large that the concentration of infection required to effect transmission would be well below the sensitivity of current assays. A precautionary assumption should therefore be made that these tissues will also transmit infection should the donor be infected.

Key points

1 To date, there have been four cases of variant CJD prion transmission by red cell components.
2 The prevalence of subclinical disease may be significantly higher than that suggested by the incidence of clinical cases.
3 A number of precautionary measures have already been taken, including donor deferrals, universal leucocyte reduction and sourcing of plasma for fractionation from outside the UK.
4 Further precautionary measures are under consideration, including prion reduction filters and prion assays.
5 Such measures require careful evaluation in terms of likely efficacy, associated risks and opportunity costs.

References

1 Collee JG & Bradley R. BSE: a decade on. Part 1. *Lancet* 1997; 349: 636–641.
2 Collee JG & Bradley R. BSE: a decade on. Part 2. *Lancet* 1997; 349: 715–721.
3 Hilton DA, Ghani AC, Conyers L *et al*. Prevalence of lymphoreticular prion protein accumulation in UK tissue samples. *J Pathol* 2004; 203: 733–739.
4 Brown P, Will RG, Bradley R *et al*. Bovine spongiform encephalopathy and variant Creutzfeldt–Jakob disease: background, evolution and current concerns. *Emerg Infect Dis* 2001; 7: 6–16.
5 Macgregor I. Prion protein and developments in its detection. *Transfusion* 2001; 11: 3–14.
6 Edgeworth JA, Farmer M, Sicilia A *et al*. Detection of prion infection in variant Creutzfeldt–Jakob disease: a blood-based assay. *Lancet* 2011; 377: 487–493.
7 Brown P, Rohwer RG, Dunstan BC *et al*. The distribution of infectivity in blood components and plasma derivatives in experimental models of transmissible spongiform encephalopathy. *Transfusion* 1998; 38: 810–816.
8 Brown P, Cervenakova L, McShane LM *et al*. Further studies of blood infectivity in an experimental model of transmissible spongiform encephalopathy with an explanation of why blood components do not transmit Creutzfeldt–Jakob disease in humans. *Transfusion* 1999; 39: 1169–1178.
9 Brown P. The pathogenesis of transmissible spongiform encephalopathy: routes to the brain and the erection of therapeutic barriers. *Cell Molec Life Sci* 2001; 58: 259–265.
10 Brown P, Cervenakova L & Diringer M. Blood infectivity and the prospects for a diagnostic screening test in Creutzfeldt–Jakob disease. *J Lab Clin Med* 2001; 137: 5–13.
11 McCutcheon S, Richard A, Blanco A, Houston EF, de Wolf C, Tan BC, Smith A, Groschup MH, Hunter N, Hornsey VS, MacGregor IR, Prowse CV, Turner M & Manson JC. All clinically relevant blood components transmit prion disease following a single blood transfusion: a sheep model of vCJD. *PLOS ONE* 6(8): e23169. DOI: 10.1371/journal.pone.0023169.
12 Hewitt PE, Llewelyn CA, McKenzie J *et al*. Creutfeldt–Jakob disease and blood transfusion: results of the UK Transfusion Medicine Epidemiology Review study. *Vox Sanguinis* 2006; 91: 221–230.
13 Llewelyn CA, Hewitt PE, Knight RS *et al*. Possible transmission of variant Creutzfeldt–Jakob disease by blood transfusion. *Lancet* 2004; 363: 417–421.
14 Peden AH, Head MW, Ritchie DL *et al*. Preclinical vCJD after blood transfusion in a PRNP codon 129 heterozygous patient. *Lancet* 2004; 364: 527–529.

15 Gregori L, McCombie N, Palmer D *et al.* Effectiveness of leucoreduction for removal of infectivity of transmissible spongiform encephalopathies from blood. *Lancet* 2004; 364: 529–531.

16 Sowemimo-Coker SO, Demczyk CA, Andrade F & Baker CA. Evaluation of removal of prion infectivity from red blood cells with prion reduction filters using a new rapid and highly sensitive cell culture-based infectivity assay. *Transfusion* 2010; 50: 980–988.

17 Peden A, McCardle L, Head MW *et al.* Variant CJD infection in the spleen of a neurologically asymptomatic UK adult patient with haemophilia. *Haemophilia* 2010; 16: 286–304.

18 Zaman SMA, Hill FGH, Palmer B *et al.* The risk of variant Creutzfeldt–Jakob disease amongst UK patients with bleeding disorders, known to have received potentially contaminated plasma products. *Haemophilia* 2011; 1–7. DOI: 10.1111/j.1365-2516.2011.02508.x.

Further reading

Blajchman MA, Goldman M, Webert KE *et al.* Proceedings of a Consensus Conference: the screening of blood donors for variant CJD. *Transf Med Rev* 2004; 18: 73–92.

Collinge J. Variant Creutzfeldt–Jakob disease. *Lancet* 1999; 354: 317–323.

Dodd RY. Prions and precautions: be careful for what you ask. *Transfusion* 2010; 50: 956–958.

Foster PR. Prions and blood products. *Ann Med* 2000; 32: 501–513.

Ludlam CA & Turner ML. Managing the risk of transmission of variant Creutzfeldt–Jakob disease by blood products. *Br J Haematol* 2005; 132: 13–24.

Peden A, Head MW, Jones M *et al.* Advances in the development of a screening test for vCJD. *Expert Opinion on Medical Diagnostics* 2008: 2: 207–219.

Turner ML (ed.). *Creutzfeldt–Jakob Disease: Managing the Risk of Transmission by Blood, Plasma and Tissues.* Bethesda, MD: AABB Press; 2006.

Turner ML & Ludlam CA. An update on the assessment and management of the risk of transmission of variant Creutzfeldt–Jakob disease by blood and plasma products. *Br J Haematol* 2008: 144: 14–23.

Zhou S, Fang CT & Schonberger LB. Transfusion transmission of human prion diseases. *Transf Med Rev* 2008; 22: 58–69.

16 Emerging infections and transfusion safety

Roger Y. Dodd

American Red Cross, Jerome H. Holland Laboratory for the Biomedical Sciences, Rockville, Maryland, USA

The Institute of Medicine in the USA has defined emerging infections as those whose incidence in humans has increased within the past two decades or threatens to increase in the near future. Emergence may be due to the spread of a new agent, the recognition of an infection that has been present in the population but has gone undetected or the realization that an established disease has an infectious origin. Emergence may also be used to describe the reappearance (or re-emergence) of a known infection after a decline in incidence. A proportion of such emerging infections have properties that permit their transmissibility by blood transfusion; perhaps the most notable example has been HIV/AIDS, although there are others, such as West Nile virus (WNV), dengue virus, babesia and malaria. This chapter will explain the basis for emergence of infectious agents and discuss their recognition and management in the context of the safety of the blood supply.

Emerging infections

There is no single reason to account for the emergence of infections, although it is possible to establish relatively broad groupings [1].
• Failure of existing control mechanisms, including the appearance of drug-resistant strains, vaccine escape mutants or cessation of vector control accounts for a large group of agents.

• Environmental change can have profound effects, whether through global warming, changes in land utilization or irrigation practice, urbanization or even agricultural practices.
• Population movements and rapid transportation can introduce infectious agents into new environments where they may spread rapidly and without constraint, as has been the case for WNV in the USA.
• Human behaviours can contribute in a number of ways: new agents have been introduced into human populations by contact with, or even preparation and consumption of, wildlife; many infections have been spread widely though extensive sexual networks and armed conflicts have led to extensive disease spread.

Of course, many of these factors may also work in combination. Key points are that new or unexpected diseases can appear in any location at any time and that an appropriate understanding of the epidemiology of such diseases can assist in the development of appropriate interventions.

In order to be transmissible by transfusion, an agent must have certain key properties [2].
• Most importantly, there must be a phase when the agent is present in the blood in the absence of any significant symptoms. Until recently, it was generally thought that such infectivity would reflect a long-term carrier state for the agent in question, as exemplified by HIV, HBV or HCV, although there had been a few cases of transmission of hepatitis A virus, which

Practical Transfusion Medicine, Fourth Edition. Edited by Michael F. Murphy, Derwood H. Pamphilon and Nancy M. Heddle.
© 2013 John Wiley & Sons, Ltd. Published 2013 by John Wiley & Sons, Ltd.

provokes an acute infection with a relatively short period of asymptomatic viraemia. However, the finding of transfusion transmission of WNV showed that, in epidemic outbreaks, acute infections could be readily transmitted by transfusion.

• A secondary requirement is that the agent must be able to survive component preparation and storage.

• Finally, the agent should have a clinically apparent outcome in at least a proportion of cases of infection or it will lack clear relevance to blood safety and its transmission will not generally be recognized. There are some examples of transfusion-transmissible agents that do not seem to cause any significant outcomes, such as GB virus type C/hepatitis G virus (GBV-C/HGV) and torque tenovirus (TTV).

Table 16.1 lists a number of emerging infections that are known, or suspected, to be transfusion transmissible and also notes the factors thought to be responsible for their emergence.

Approaches to the management of transfusion-transmissible emerging infections

As far as it is possible, emerging infections that do, or may, impact on blood safety should be managed in a systematic fashion. In general, this will be the responsibility of agencies that are charged with the maintenance of public health, or the management of the blood supply or its regulation. However, there are a number of areas in which individual professionals can contribute. One of these is the first step, which is the recognition of a transfusion-transmitted infection and its subsequent investigation. It is, in fact, unlikely that the first occurrence of an emerging infection will be seen in a transfused recipient, so it is therefore important that there be a system of assessing the threat and risk of emerging infections for their potential impact on blood safety. This implies a process for evaluating each emerging infection for its transmissibility by this route and for estimating the severity and potential extent of the threat. The risk assessment should help to define the need for and urgency of development and implementation of interventions to reduce the risk of transmission of the agent. Such interventions, if implemented, should be evaluated for efficacy and modified as appropriate.

Assessing the risk and threat of transfusion transmissibility

It is important to have a general awareness of the status of new and emerging infections, with particular reference to your own country or area. Such awareness may involve familiarity with a number of sources of information, ranging from news media, through alerts from local, national and global public health agencies, to specialized resources such as ProMED Mail (an Internet listserver and website that tracks and comments on disease outbreaks) [3]. Other tools continue to become available; e.g. the American Association of Blood Banks (AABB) has developed and is maintaining a listing of potentially transfusion-transmissible infectious agents that has been published in print and on their website: the listing also contains much of the information discussed below, along with a ranking of threat level. Other agencies (e.g. the Centers for Disease Control and Prevention and the World Health Organization) provide general, current information about emerging infectious agents on their websites.

Table 16.2 outlines questions that serve to define the risk of transfusion transmission of each agent and the potential extent and severity of that risk. The primary question is whether or not the disease agent can, in fact, be transmitted by blood. As pointed out above, this is dependent on the presence of an asymptomatic phase during which the disease agent is present in the bloodstream. In some cases, of course, there may already be documentation of transfusion transmission of the agent in question or there may be suggestive evidence, such as transmission by organ transplantation. However, in the latter case, such evidence may not be definitive, as rabies has been transmitted by organ transplantation but is almost certainly not transmissible by blood. The answer to this question is not always readily obtainable, but may often be inferred by considering what is known about the natural transmission route of the infection or from the properties of closely related organisms. The duration of the blood phase of the infection will have a direct impact on the risk of transmission, reflecting the chance that an individual will give blood during the infectious phase.

The actual risk of transmission is a function of the frequency of the infection in the donor population and the length of the period of bloodborne infectivity [4]. The period of infectivity may not, however, be identical to the period during which the infectious

Table 16.1 Selected emerging infections potentially or actually transmissible by blood transfusion.

Agent	Basis for emergence	Notes
Prions		
vCJD	Agricultural practice: feeding meat and bonemeal to cattle	Of most concern in UK; apparently coming under control
Viruses		
Chikungunya	Global climate change, dispersion of mosquito vector, travel	Rapid emergence in a number of areas, including Italy; surveillance indicated
Dengue	Global climate change, dispersion of mosquito vector, travel	Similar properties to WNV; surveillance indicated
HBV variants	Selection pressure resulting from vaccination	Mutants may escape detection by standard test methods
HHV-8	Transmission between men who have sex with men and perhaps by intravenous drug use	Transmission by transfusion and transplantation known
HIV	Interactions with wildlife, sexual networks, travel	Classic example of an emerging infection
HIV variants	Viral mutation, travel	May escape detection by standard tests
Influenza	Pandemic anticipated as a result of antigenic change	Possible threat to blood safety, major impact on availability
SARS	Explosive global epidemic, wildlife origin, spread by travel	No demonstrated transfusion transmission, epidemic over
Simian foamy virus	Exposure to monkeys, concern about species jumping and mutation	Regulatory concern over blood safety, intervention in Canada
WNV	Introduction into the USA (probably via jet transport), rapid spread across continent	Recognition of transfusion transmission in 2002 led to rapid implementation of NAT for donors
Bacteria		
Anaplasma phagocytophilum	Tickborne agent expanding its geographic range	One potential transfusion transmission reported
Borrelia burgdorferi	Tickborne agent expanding its geographic range and human exposure	No transfusion transmission reported
Parasites		
Babesia spp.	Tickborne agent expanding its geographic range and human exposure	More than 160 transfusion-transmission cases reported
Leishmania spp.	Increased exposure to military and others in Iraq, Afghanistan	Unexpected visceral forms potentially transmissible
Plasmodium spp.	Classic re-emergence, in part due to climate change, travel	Re-emergence threatens value of travel deferral
Trypanosoma cruzi	Imported into nonendemic areas by population movement	Transfusion transmissible, preventable by donor testing

agent can be detected in the blood. For example, in the case of WNV, periods of viraemia in excess of 100 days have been measured occasionally, but the actual infectious period may be limited to the week or two prior to the appearance of IgG antibodies.

Another difficulty is that the frequency of disease and the frequency of infection may differ greatly, as is again the case with WNV. Nevertheless, it is abundantly clear that individuals who do not develop symptoms may be infectious via their blood donations.

163

Table 16.2 Key questions to assess risk of transfusion transmissibility of an infectious agent.

1 Have transfusion-transmitted cases been observed?

2 Does the agent have an asymptomatic, bloodborne phase?

3 Does the agent survive component preparation and storage?

4 Are blood recipients susceptible to infection with the agent?

5 Does the agent cause disease, particularly in blood recipients?

6 What is the severity, mortality and treatability of the disease?

7 Are there recipient conditions, such as immunosuppression, that favour more severe disease?

8 Is there a meaningful frequency of infectivity in the potential donor population?

9 Is this frequency declining, stable or increasing?

10 Are there reasons to anticipate any changes in the frequency of donor infectivity?

11 What is the level of concern about the agent and its disease among professionals, public health experts, regulators, politicians, media and the general population?

12 Are there rational and accessible interventions to eliminate or reduce transmission by transfusion?

Consequently, it may be important to estimate the size of the infected (and infectious) population by laboratory testing rather than through disease reporting. Indeed, organized studies of prevalence rates of infection among donor populations have been used in many circumstances in order to assess the level of risk and to predict the impact of a testing intervention. Examples of this approach include studies on HTLV, trypanosomes (*Trypanosoma cruzi*), babesia and, more recently, dengue virus, where assessments of the frequency of viraemia are proving valuable. Another important factor is the dynamics of the outbreak. Is the frequency of infection stable or increasing and, if increasing, is change linear or logarithmic and what is the rate of increase? Obviously, rapid increase, as seen in the case of WNV, would imply a need for a more rapid response than would a slow, linear increase, as in the case of *T. cruzi*.

The severity of disease that may result from a transfusion-transmitted infection is also an important guide to the extent and speed of implementation of any intervention. There are both objective and subjective aspects to such an assessment. Clearly, the severity of the disease and its associated mortality can be defined, but it may also be important to judge the public concern around the disease, which may be disproportionate to its actual public health impact [2]. Another factor that is often presented as important is the extent to which a transfusion-transmitted infection might result in further or secondary infections. In actual fact, transmission of an infection by transfusion will almost certainly not lead to any magnification of an epidemic but, nevertheless, it is something that should be considered.

A word of caution is in order with respect to efforts to use modern laboratory methods to identify previously unrecognized infectious agents. There is increasing enthusiasm for this approach, but it is important to recognize that without any established relationship to a disease state, the results of such searches can be misleading. At this time, for example, it does not appear that either TTV or GBV-C/HGV have any relationship to any disease state and do not seem to offer risk to blood recipients, despite clear evidence of their transmissibility. It is unclear how many other such orphan viruses are awaiting discovery.

The recent recognition and management of a new retrovirus, XMRV, originally thought to be associated with prostate cancer and chronic fatigue syndrome (CFS), is instructive. It was suggested that this virus was a threat to transfusion safety and an organized programme was put in place to evaluate this possibility [5, 6]. A complication was that CFS advocates actively promoted the concept of transfusion risk as a means to establish legitimacy (and perhaps funding) for the disease. A key activity was a careful, blinded evaluation of a number of different tests for XMRV, including those used by the laboratories responsible for the original discoveries. This evaluation, along with other studies, revealed that the available tests could not reliably identify the virus or related ones, either in patient samples or negative controls [7]. The original observations were eventually shown to be due to various forms of contamination and XMRV itself was revealed to be a laboratory artefact. While early intervention for an emerging infection may be necessary and appropriate, care should be taken to avoid reacting to situations involving incomplete or imperfect science.

Recognition of transfusion transmission of emerging infections

There is no simple formula for recognizing that a transfusion-transmitted infection has occurred, particularly in the case of a rare or unusual disease agent. Nevertheless, many such events have been recognized by astute clinicians. Knowledge of the potential for transmission of an emerging infection can be valuable and very likely contributed to the relatively early recognition of transfusion transmission of WNV [8]. Unusual posttransfusion events with a suspected infectious origin should be brought to the attention of experts in infectious diseases or public health agencies for assistance in identification and follow-up. Appropriate investigation of illness occurring a few days or more after transfusion can reveal infections through identification of serologic or molecular evidence of infectious agents in posttransfusion samples. However, such detection is by no means definitive. It is helpful if a pretransfusion patient sample is also available, as this will reveal whether the condition predated the transfusion. Also, recall and further testing of implicated donors will reveal whether one or more of them was the likely source of the infection. Ideally, if the responsible organism can be isolated from both donor and recipient, molecular analyses such as nucleic acid sequencing can demonstrate (or exclude) the identity of the agent from the two sources. There are significant problems in recognizing that infections with a very long incubation period may have been transmitted by transfusion; this was illustrated by HIV/AIDS, which did not result in well-defined illness until many years after exposure. This prevented early recognition of transfusion-transmitted AIDS and further concealed the actual magnitude of the infectious donor population and of the population of infected blood recipients. This implies that, for emerging infections that appear to have lengthy incubation periods, it would be wise to assess transfusion transmissibility by serologic or molecular evaluation of appropriate donor–recipient sample repositories or to engage in some form of active surveillance, such as that used to identify the transmission of variant Creutzfeldt–Jakob disease (vCJD) by transfusion in England [9]. Haemovigilance programmes may contribute to the identification of posttransfusion infections, although they are generally designed to identify well-described outcomes.

Interventions

In the event that an emerging infection is found to be transfusion transmissible and public and professional concern implies a need to protect the safety of the blood supply, there are a number of interventions that could be considered.

A possible, but rather unsatisfactory approach is to focus on the recipient by diagnosing and treating cases that occur. This, of course, works only for treatable infections. It is de facto part of the approach to manage transfusion babesiosis in the USA at this time.

Most interventions are focused on the donor or the donation. In the absence of a test, it may be possible to devise a question that would identify some proportion of donors at risk of transmitting the infection. Such measures are usually neither sensitive nor specific, but may have value, particularly where the disease is localized so that a travel history is sufficient to identify those at risk.

The development and implementation of a test for infectivity in donor blood is usually a more sensitive and specific approach than questioning and for some infections may be the only valid solution. In the past, serologic tests were relied upon, but now nucleic acid testing is also available and may be a better solution, as was the case for WNV. Indeed, a test for WNV RNA was developed and implemented in less than a year in the USA [10]. However, this is not always the optimal solution. For example, some parasitic diseases in particular result in long-term, antibody-positive infection with very low levels of infectious agent in the bloodstream, resulting in only intermittent NAT-positive findings. This is particularly true of Chagas disease, and as most individuals were infected early in life, antibody tests are preferable for identifying potentially infectious donors [11].

An emerging technology that offers some promise is that of pathogen reduction, which is a treatment that inactivates infectious agents in blood while retaining the biological activities of the blood itself. Methods are currently available for plasma and for platelet concentrates and are in use in some countries. It should be noted that available methods may have differing efficacies for different infectious agents and that they may not be fully successful in eliminating very high levels of infectivity for some agents, although this has not been established in practice. A real disadvantage is that no method is currently available for red cells.

A pathogen reduction method was implemented for platelets in the island of La Reunion during a large outbreak of chikungunya virus infection.

The precautionary principle is often cited when decisions about interventions to reduce the risk of transfusion-transmitted infections are discussed. In general, it is suggested that, in the absence of any specific information about the efficacy of an intervention, it is appropriate to implement it, as long as it does no harm. This position may be arguable, particularly as commentary on the precautionary principle suggests that it should not be invoked without some evaluation to give assurance that the measure is not extreme and does not exceed other measures taken in known circumstances. In fact, significant measures were taken to reduce the potential risk of transmission of vCJD even before it was known that it was transmissible by transfusion. It can be argued that subsequent events justified the precautions taken, but this may not always be the case [12].

Key points

1 Some emerging infections may threaten the safety of the blood supply.
2 Those responsible for maintaining the safety of the blood supply should be familiar with emerging infections.
3 Physicians responsible for the care of transfused patients should be alert for signs of unexpected infections.
4 The nature and extent of the safety threat offered by emerging infections may be assessed by examination of a fairly simple sequence of questions.
5 If interventions are needed, consideration should be given to the use of donor questions and/or laboratory tests.
6 Care must be taken to balance public concern against good science.

References

1 Morens DM, Folkers GK & Fauci AS. Emerging infections: a perpetual challenge. *Lancet Infect Dis* 2008; 8: 710–719.
2 Stramer SL, Hollinger FB, Katz LM, Kleinman S, Metzel PS, Gregory KM & Dodd RY. Emerging infectious disease agents and their potential threat to transfusion safety. *Transfusion* 2009; 49 (Suppl.): 1S–233S.
3 http://www.promedmail.org/.
4 Glynn SA, Kleinman SH, Wright DJ & Busch MP. NHLBI Retrovirus Epidemiology Study. International application of the incidence rate/window period model. *Transfusion* 2002; 42: 966–972.
5 Klein HG, Dodd RY, Hollinger FB, Katz LM, Kleinman S, McCleary KK, Silverman RH & Stramer SL, for the AABB Interorganizational Task Force on XMRV. Xenotropic murine leukemia virus-related virus (XMRV) and blood transfusion: Report of the AABB Interorganizational XMRV Task Force. *Transfusion* 2011; 51: 654–661.
6 Simmons G, Glynn SA, Holmberg JA, Coffin JM, Hewlett IK, Lo SC, Mikovits JA, Switzer WM, Linnen JM & Busch MP, for the Blood XMRV Scientific Research Working Group (SRWG). The blood xenotropic murine leukemia virus-related virus scientific research working group: mission, progress, and plans. *Transfusion* 2011; 51: 643–653.
7 Simmons G, Glynn SA, Komaroff AL, Mikovits JA, Tobler LH, Hackett Jr J, Tang N, Switzer WM, Heneine W, Hewlett IK, Zhao J, Lo SC, Alter HJ, Linnen JM, Gao K, Coffin JM, Kearney MF, Ruscetti FW, Pfost MA, Bethel J, Kleinman S, Holmberg JA & Busch MP, for the Blood XMRV Scientific Research Working Group (SRWG). Failure to confirm XMRV/MLV in the blood of patients with chronic fatigue syndrome: a multilaboratory study. *Science* 2011; 334: 814–817.
8 Biggerstaff BJ & Petersen LR. Estimated risk of West Nile virus transmission through blood transfusion during an epidemic in Queens, New York City. *Transfusion* 2002; 42: 1019–1026.
9 Hewitt PE, Llewelyn CA, Mackenzie J & Will RG. Creutzfeldt–Jakob disease and blood transfusion: results of the UK Transfusion Medicine Epidemiological Review study. *Vox Sanguinis* 2006; 91: 221–230.
10 Dodd RY. Perspective: emerging infections, transfusion safety and epidemiology. *New Engl J Med* 2003; 349: 1205–1206.
11 Benjamin RJ, Stramer SL, Leiby DA, Dodd RY, Fearon M & Castro E. *Trypanosoma cruzi* infection in North America and Spain: evidence in support of transfusion transmission. *Transfusion* 2012. Early online publication, DOI: 10.1111/j.1537-2995.2011.03554.x.
12 Wilson K & Ricketts MN. The success of precaution? Managing the risk of transfusion transmission of variant Creutzfeldt–Jakob disease. *Transfusion* 2004; 44: 1475–1478.

Further reading

Alter HJ, Stramer SL & Dodd RY. Emerging infectious diseases that threaten the blood supply. *Semin Hematol* 2007; 44: 32–41.

Biggerstaff BJ & Petersen LR. Estimated risk of transmission of the West Nile virus through blood transfusion in the US, 2002. *Transfusion* 2003; 43: 1007–1017.

Dodd RY & Leiby DA. Emerging infectious threats to the blood supply. *Annual Rev Med* 2004; 55: 191–207.

Mackenzie JS, Gubler DJ & Petersen LR. Emerging flaviviruses: the spread and resurgence of Japanese encephalitis, West Nile and dengue viruses. *Nat Med (Suppl.)* 2004; 10(12): S98–S108.

Stramer SL, Fang CT, Foster GA, Wagner AG, Brodsky JP & Dodd RY. West Nile virus among blood donors in the United States, 2003 and 2004. *N Engl J Med* 2005; 353: 451–459.

Tomashek KM & Margolis HS. Dengue: a potential transfusion-transmitted disease. *Transfusion* 2011; 51: 1654–1660.

Weiss RA & McMichael AJ. Social and environmental risk factors in the emergence of infectious disease. *Nat Med (Suppl.)* 2004; 10(12): S70–S76.

17 Regulatory aspects of blood transfusion

William G. Murphy[1], *Louis M. Katz*[2] *& Peter Flanagan*[3]

[1]Health Service Executive, Clinical Strategy and Programmes, and University College Dublin, Dublin, Republic of Ireland
[2]America's Blood Centers, Washington, DC, USA
[3]New Zealand Blood Service, Auckland, New Zealand

Introduction

Blood is an irreplaceable medicine used in life saving circumstances. Because it is necessary to source the material for this medicine from biologically and behaviourally heterogeneous humans, absolute uniformity of product and its absolute safety cannot be guaranteed, no matter how extensively we test or how energetically we process the material. Ultimately pragmatic compromises must be reached between adequate safety and adequate supply. It is by now generally accepted that each country's government must ensure that its citizens and visitors are provided with an adequate supply of safe and effective blood for transfusion as these compromises are made. The World Health Organization (WHO) has identified the importance of a well-legislated and regulated blood transfusion service as a crucial component in assuring safety [1].

However, there is at best a weak international consensus on what that responsibility implies and how it may be discharged. What is adequate in terms of supply of red cells in Canada, for example, would be disastrously inadequate in Germany. What is permissible in France may be unthinkable in the USA, and vice versa. The Food and Drug Administration (FDA) in the USA takes a substantially different position from the European Commission in deciding what donor screening assays should be done on its territory. In the USA the stringency of, and the resources

needed for, the Biologics License Application (BLA) process required for approval of a donor screening test thwarts the availability of a broad menu of tests, while generally resulting in assays with superb performance characteristics. In Europe a minimum only is specified and individual blood services can and do use additional tests or technologies as they consider fit, although within Europe the German authorities (the Paul Ehrlich Institute) are as rigorous and controlling as the FDA.

Nevertheless, within each state or jurisdiction, the Government, its regulatory agencies, the blood transfusion services and the hospital blood services form a publicly accountable process that is subject to regulation and regulatory oversight to a greater or lesser degree. The degree of public accountability that gives rise to and gives legitimacy to the regulatory process is demonstrated by the scale of public inquiry in several countries into systematic failures in blood safety in the late 20th century. In several cases the regulatory agencies were found wanting to a comparable degree as the blood services they were supposed to oversee.

While there are considerable differences between medicines in general and blood components in particular, regulation tends to apply the pharmaceutical paradigm to blood transfusion services. There are, however, some critical differences between the two processes. Medicine regulation normally involves a government regulator assessing pharmaceutical products manufactured by commercial organizations. A

Practical Transfusion Medicine, Fourth Edition. Edited by Michael F. Murphy, Derwood H. Pamphilon and Nancy M. Heddle.
© 2013 John Wiley & Sons, Ltd. Published 2013 by John Wiley & Sons, Ltd.

decision to approve a new medicine in no way implies an expectation that all patients will receive it. Health organizations and individual doctors will determine what is right and affordable. Blood, on the other hand, often, though not always, involves regulation of government owned or funded entities (the Blood Transfusion Services) and decisions around safety standards are incremental; i.e. once a decision is made the standard of the component changes for all recipients. The impact of regulation and the need for good decision making is therefore particularly important for blood.

Importantly, however, research and development, which are the real drivers of quality, efficacy and safety, are generally outside the regulatory process, and except within a humanitarian and professional ethos no one is held accountable if these things are not done, or not done well.

In the field of blood transfusion, separate national regulations cover the licensing of devices, kits and other materials used in the collection of blood donations, in testing or the preparation, storage and transport of blood components. These will generally be similar to the regulations covering other medical devices and tests or manufactured items put on the market within a State. This is an important mechanism whereby governments and regulators can control standards in the blood sector.

The extent of the role of regulatory authorities can be explored through the following questions:
• Who is responsible if there is insufficient blood on hospital shelves?
• Who is responsible if the blood on hospital shelves is not of appropriate quality?
• Who is responsible if the blood supply or the blood supplied does not improve in response to emerging clinical science – if, for example, it fails to be adequately modified to meet a newly emerging threat or a better understanding of clinical efficacy?

Who is responsible if there is insufficient blood on hospital shelves?
It is the people's *problem* ultimately and therefore, hopefully, the Government's, but the *fault* could lie with:
• the regulatory agency – excess stringency in applying limits for donor haemoglobin for example;
• the blood service – inadequate skill in reaching potential donors effectively, or in managing its supply

chain or customer base, or in identifying and implementing new strategies or techniques;
• the clinical services – excess use of blood over real need as defined by a growing evidence base;
• the hospital blood banks – excess wastage through overstocking;
• the Departments of Health or Finance for failing to provide enough resources;
• Government, through poor structuring and oversight of the healthcare system.

Who is responsible if the blood on hospital shelves is not of adequate quality?
• The Government, through the regulatory agencies, has explicit and primary responsibility. The agencies will discharge their duties and purge their fault through inspections, accreditation and sanctions, but ultimately they have the authority to ensure the public safety and they will, or should, be held accountable for failure to do so. Nevertheless, blood suppliers should also be considered to have an ethical and professional responsibility to go beyond the minimum regulatory or legal requirements in the interest of safety if the regulator does not require sufficient quality, and in any event they have a responsibility to ensure that standards are met in a consistent manner.

Who is responsible if the blood supply or the blood supplied does not improve in response to emerging clinical science – if, for example, it fails to be adequately modified to meet a newly emerging threat or a better understanding of clinical efficacy?
• The Blood Services (and their professional societies to the degree they influence blood operations);
• the Regulatory Agency where it takes on a role of scientific leadership, such as the FDA in the United States, the Paul Erhlich Institute (PEI) in Germany and the French Agency for Safety of Health Products (AFSSAPS – Agence Française de Sécurité Sanitaire des Produits de Santé);
• the Government if it fails to invest in the intellectual and scientific capacity of its blood services (though it will take a major inquiry to apportion fault in this way if it exists).

An explicit and documented 'National Blood Policy' along the lines of the WHO's recommended approach [1], where the responsibilities of each of the stakeholders is clearly documented, and ideally captured in legislation, may be the most secure route to success in ensuring that regulation is integrated into a national approach to blood safety.

The functional components of regulation

Regulation is made up of several components:
• *Guiding principles and law.* National or international law, which has the force of justice and humanity, and which is defined and enacted by legitimate representatives of the society concerned, governs the regulations of blood components in a jurisdiction. A competent system of regulation must be backed by such law, which specifies and limits the scope and power of the regulator. The law should be explicit and production of blood for transfusion in a state should be expressly governed by statute. Within the EU member states, the national statutes are subject to the Blood Directives – a set of laws developed over several years between 1996 and the present that are binding on all the member states of the Union. There is a core or parent Directive [2] and a set of subsidiary ones covering donors and donations and component specifications [3], traceability and haemovigilance [4] and quality systems [5]. Additional updates and modifications may appear in response to emerging threats or technical advances. Elsewhere national, federal, provincial and state laws almost invariably provide a basis for regulation, though in several parts of the world such laws and regulations may be merely aspirations [6].

Guiding principles may be explicit or implicit. For example, the EU specifies the otherwise-unexplained 'Principles of Good Practice' as the principles covering the quality systems in blood establishments (Article 11 of 2002/98/EC – the core EU Directive on Blood Transfusion), although it does specify 'Good Manufacturing Practice' as an overall guiding principle in the Preamble [2]. The Preamble also contains other statements of principle, scope and intent, and these may have a legal function in the event of dispute. It states, for example, that the intent of the regulations is to ensure public health, thereby forever giving blood safety in the EU primacy over legitimate commercial interests in the drafting and execution of regulations. The Therapeutics Goods Administration (TGA) in Australia produces a specific Code of GMP for blood and tissues. This includes both quality and technical

standards that must be met. The FDA states that Good Manufacturing Practices (GMPs) are the guiding principles in the functioning of blood services. GMPs (generally called just GMP outside of North America) are a dynamic and very comprehensive set of overall directions, principles, rules and regulations that reduce the entropy in a complex system, and thereby the likelihood of mishap. (Regulators, however, by definition draft regulation as well as enforce it, and may and do increase complexity beyond any possibly meaningful improvement in safety. This requires a constant dynamic in the regulatory process: see below.)

The Precautionary Principle emerged in the 1980s as a statement of best practice when faced with serious but unquantifiable risks. This principle was enshrined at the 1992 Rio Conference on the Environment and Development, as 'Where there are threats of serious or irreversible damage, lack of full scientific certainty shall not be used as a reason for postponing cost-effective measures to prevent environmental degradation.' Since then it has come to be explicitly adopted for health protection, for example in the European Union [7] and in Canada [6, 8]. It continues to develop and evolve and to gather increased force of law through case law in Europe and elsewhere.

In European law, according to the European Commission, 'the precautionary principle may be invoked when a phenomenon, product or process may have a dangerous effect, identified by a scientific and objective evaluation, if this evaluation does not allow the risk to be determined with sufficient certainty'. An explicit statement of precaution appears in the core Blood Directive [2]: 'The availability of blood and blood components used for therapeutic purposes is dependent largely on Community citizens who are prepared to donate. In order to safeguard public health and to prevent the transmission of infectious diseases, all precautionary measures during their collection, processing, distribution and use need to be taken making appropriate use of scientific progress in the detection and inactivation and elimination of transfusion transmissible pathogenic agents.' This rather stringent application of the principle results in interventions to mitigate risk that will not be considered cost-effective in other clinical venues (vide infra).

Most formulations of the precautionary principle include rather explicit acknowledgement that decisions taken under its aegis are subject to reconsideration and modification as more complete data are accrued. This results in tensions over what constitutes sufficient evidence to undertake amendment of long-standing regulatory decisions.

• *Standards*. Professional advisory bodies as well as technical standards bodies such as the International Standards Organization may set standards to be attained for accreditation, whereas regulators define rules and regulations that blood component and service providers must comply with to operate within the law. Regulators may, however, mandate accreditation by other bodies as a regulation to be complied with. In this way standards of the International Standards Organization (ISO standards) and national technical standards bodies or of professional bodies such as AABB and the College of American Pathologists (CAP) in the USA may be explicitly applied to blood component or transfusion service providers and may be given force of law. Standards used for accreditation and regulatory purposes need to be current; they also need a firm, functioning and explicit mechanism of review and change as scientific knowledge accrues, circumstances change and experience informs.

• *Application and Enforcement of Regulations*. A regulation is of limited value if it cannot be enforced, either because the rule of law is lax, the enforcing agency is weak or the standard is unrealistic or unrealistically expensive. There are three levels of application of regulations and of standards in the regulatory setting.

  ○ *Inspection/accreditation/licensing*. In most countries with a robust health system all bodies participating in the business of providing blood for transfusion are required to be visible and accountable through an official process, usually by registration, accreditation or licensing. Self-inspection, or accreditation by peer review, is generally no longer considered acceptable in isolation. Different scales of licensing requirements often apply to facilities that collect and test blood from donors than to hospital blood banks, who either store blood for transfusion and issue it or who conduct minimal processing. Licences are time-limited and require renewal with re-inspection typically every one to three years.

  ○ *Vigilance: haemovigilance/feedback/market surveillance*. It has become obvious that clinical trials cannot be powered to measure the safety of transfusion. Very large-scale systematic well-organized surveys of clinical outcomes over tens or hundreds of thousands of recipients are required to track the occurrence and even to establish the existence of problems with the function, safety and quality of medicines, devices or processes. Within blood transfusion practice this is known as haemovigilance; originally mandated in France and voluntary in the United Kingdom, it has evolved to become mandatory throughout the European Union, and in several other countries, though it is at a relatively early stage of implementation in the decentralized blood systems of the USA. In the EU haemovigilance also extends to adverse effects in blood donors. This will force changes in approaches to donor care as more valid statistics of the incidence of very rare events emerge, as well as leading to mandatory approaches to such common events as iron deficiency.

  ○ *Enforcement*. The rule of law demands compliance. Regulatory authorities can and do apply fines, sometimes of millions of dollars, to blood establishments for failure to comply with legal requirements. Hospital blood banks may be closed for serious quality failures. Blood transfusion staff may be arrested and jailed, though usually as a result of egregious events rather than for systematic failures detected through routine application of regulatory methods.

  ○ *Threat surveillance*. Some regulatory agencies have adopted a formal threat surveillance role, by which they generally mean infectious disease threat surveillance. For example, the FDA works closely with the Center for Disease Control and other agencies in the Department of Health and Human Services in the USA, and in Europe the European Commission works with the European Centre for Disease Control. Haemovigilance systems augment this approach.

• *Cost effectiveness*. Blood for transfusion is perceived as a reasonably cheap medicine, compared to similar therapeutic agents. However, the constant evolution of techniques and tests, along with the implications of the results of haemovigilance and clinical studies of safety and efficacy, inexorably drive up the costs and the price of blood components. While most countries and unions adopt some benchmark of cost-effective healthcare, regulatory agencies have a responsibility to assure quality, safety and efficacy and do not generally have a duty to ensure that their approaches and requirements do not result in unrealistic costs to the healthcare system. In the USA, for example, the FDA is specifically enjoined from considering cost as they promulgate rules, regulations and guidances, while in Australia the Jurisdictional Blood Committee takes responsibility for deciding whether new initiatives should be funded, independent from the regulatory agency, the TGA. Overall responsibility for deciding what is affordable must lie with the Government. Within the USA, Centers for Medicare and Medicaid Services (CMS) which pays for well over half of care in the USA and sets the benchmarks for third-party payers, does not pay for the cost of blood but for episodes of care by diagnosis and adjusts payment only with a substantial time lag to reflect increased costs. This results in some safety interventions being unfunded mandates for substantial intervals.

In assessing cost effectiveness, a measure such as an incremental quality-adjusted life year (QALY) with a defined monetary value can be used to decide whether to pay for a new drug in the community - how many years of what degree of benefit will this therapy provide per taxpayer's dollar? The cut-off value for buying the treatment for the community will vary on the country's economic state and culture, but by any measure in use worldwide NAT testing of blood donations provides a very poor return by several orders of magnitude. A general consensus on how to resolve this conflict, due in some measure to the public's perception of blood safety and the blood industry after the HIV and HCV disasters of the last century, has yet to emerge. Ultimately the decision is a political one on whether to mandate a costly change in practice. Professionals in the field of blood transfusion should do their best to ensure that the political decision-making process is publicly visible and recorded, perhaps especially in the event of an explicit political decision not to fund a new safety step.

The regulatory bodies (Table 17.1)

There are several types of bodies involved in the regulatory framework or structure in blood transfusion. They contribute either to the formulation or application of the law, the formation, application or review of standards, or they can enforce the regulations.
• *National Statutory bodies with powers of enforcement.* Most high and medium development index countries have a more-or-less functioning National Medicines Agency that sets and applies standards for

drugs being prescribed, imported and sold in that country. Similar bodies, in many cases the same body, set and apply standards for blood components. They have the force of law and can seek to imprison or fine those who break the law. A person setting up their own blood collection service within the EU, for example, without a licence from the relevant Government agency would face serious charges. Examples are the Food and Drug Administration (FDA) in the USA, the Medicines and Healthcare Products Regulatory Agency (MHRA) in the UK, Agence Française de Sécurité Sanitaire des Produits de Santé (AFSSAPS) in France, the Paul Erhlich Institute (PEI) in Germany, Therapeutic Goods Administration (TGA) in Australia, Health Canada and the various national agencies in the EU and other European countries. They are not all the same – some, notably the FDA, the PEI and AFSSAPS, have developed roles as scientific leaders in blood transfusion science and participate actively in developments in the field. In several countries, including some of the older Eastern bloc members of the EU, the agency within the State responsible for regulation (in the EU these agencies are called 'Competent Authorities') is also the National Transfusion Service, reflecting older Communist structures. In these cases it is very difficult to maintain the perception of separation of conflicting interests.
• *Supranational agencies with statutory powers.* The European Commission in the European Union – essentially the civil service of the European Union – has very broad powers in the field of consumer safety and citizens' health, including explicit powers under the founding treaty in ensuring blood safety. A series of laws (Directives) were enacted since 2002 that cover licensing of blood establishments, accreditation of hospital blood banks and technical specifications, from donor qualification to component transportation. In addition the Directives address traceability and haemovigilance. The Commission has very little in-house expertise in blood transfusion and uses industry expertise, sourced mainly through the Departments of Health in the member states, to provide support.

The FDA in the USA is of a similar scale and scope – insofar as it has a remit across the 50 States, a number of territories and commonwealths, and the district of Columbia. The USA carries substantial weight in the industry far beyond other national statutory agencies. It has a very mature and heavily resourced

Table 17.1 Agencies involved in regulatory processes in blood transfusion.

Type of agency	Name	Role	Further information
Multinational agency with statutory powers	The European Commission	Drafts laws for implementation in European Union member states. These laws include technical specifications for blood components, for example. Oversees the application of those laws through national authorities – the 'competent authorities'	Lacks a well-defined structure for scientific analysis of the impact of the laws on healthcare and health economic implications of practices; has a limited but developing ability to adapt to advances in the field
National agency with statutory powers, with significant scientific/ developmental/leadership roles	The Food and Drug Administration (USA); Paul Ehrlich Institute (Germany); AFSSAPS (French Agency for the Safety of Health Products, France)	Defines national rules and regulations and licenses the blood establishments in national or federal setting. Conducts scientific programmes aimed at developing the field of blood banking and the scientific basis of regulation, and publishes their work in a peer reviewed environment	Within the EU the member states have to comply with the basic requirements of the EU laws; beyond that they are free to impose other requirements and standards. Germany, through the PEI, licenses blood components as medicines, as does Austria. In the USA, the FDA establishes minimum requirements for safety, purity and potency and licenses and inspects facilities against them, and maintains an active research program in support of good regulation and guidance
National agency with regulatory powers, but without significant in-house scientific activity, though in some cases they provide scientific leadership through structured partnerships between the regulator, BTS and government agencies	Health Canada, the Therapeutic Good Agency (Australia), Medicines and Healthcare Products Regulatory Agency (MHRA) [9] (UK), South Africa, New Zealand, other EU member states, Brazil, etc.	Inspects and licenses blood banks and blood transfusion services on their territory in accordance with national laws (in the EU these national laws are subservient to EU law and must include all the EU requirements as a minimum)	
National agency that also manages the blood supply	In several of the old Communist bloc countries, for example, a combined central power base was established at the national blood service provider, who then assumed the role of regulator in the EU setting	Both provider and regulator. Very difficult to avoid the impression of failure of separation of responsibilities	

Table 17.1 (*Continued*)

Type of agency	Name	Role	Further information
International treaty-defined agencies with considerable leverage in national and international blood banking policies and regulations	The World Health Organization/Pan-American Health Organization	The WHO requires member states to develop policies and standards in national blood transfusion systems	The WHO carries considerable force is many parts of the world, but much less so in high development index areas. In several countries dependent on aid for blood transfusion development, the WHO approach has quasi-regulatory status
	The Council of Europe* (The European Directorate for the Quality of Medicines and Health Care, EDQM)	The Council of Europe has for many years produced an annual technical guideline, which attempted to raise the bar of quality in member states in an iterative fashion. This function has now devolved to the EDQM under the influence of the European Commission. The Guide is now published every two years. Recent editions have begun to separate Standards from Principles. Increasingly EDQM is attempting to position itself as the technical organization managing the technical aspects of the Directives. This in many ways mirrors its work in managing the European Pharmacopeia	This situation is in evolution – the EDQM is developing a more formal link with the European Commission in this function – i.e. providing the technical expertise the Commission needs to maintain regulation in blood transfusion (the only country to date to give the Council of Europe Guide regulatory force is Australia)
Supranational incorporated bodies that have no statutory powers, but seek to provide scientific leadership and define standards of professional practice	AABB, ISBT		
Supranational incorporated bodies that have no statutory powers but have a lobbying and advocacy function	ABC, ABO, EBA, IPPC, IPFA, PPTA, International Federation of Red Cross and Red Crescent Societies		

(*continued*)

Table 17.1 (*Continued*)

Type of agency	Name	Role	Further information
Patient organizations	Groups representing patients who depend on a safe and adequate supply of blood components for health – including people with haemophilia, thalassaemia, immune deficiencies or antitrypsin deficiency	Organization to put pressure on blood services, commercial suppliers and politicians to address patients' needs for an adequate supply of good quality safe medicines	Can be very powerful campaigners for change in the legislation or regulation of blood components, especially where supply and safety may be compromised
Donor organizations	FIODS (International Federation of Blood Donor Organizations)	Promotes voluntary unpaid donation; strong supporters of blood collection programmes	Influence and activity varies considerably from country to country
Other groups who involve themselves in public debates and political activity in relation to blood transfusion	Notably LBGT (lesbian, bisexual, gay and transgender) groups and supporting allied groups such as student unions	Address perceived inequalities and discrimination in donor deferral policies or in access to services and products	In several jurisdictions such groups have been successful in changing restrictions banning men who have sex with men from donating blood

*The Council of Europe is not the European Council – the former is a union to promote humanitarian values and principles in law, rights and health, among other areas, and produces advice and works by recommendation and peer pressure between states; the latter is an administrative arm of the European Union. (The other two administrative arms are the Commission – essentially a very powerful civil service – and the Parliament. While all EU member states belong to the Council of Europe not all Council of Europe member states belong to the EU.)

function in defining standards, direction of research and, uniquely, decides which tests or other technologies must and may be applied within its jurisdiction.

• *Supranational agencies with treaty-defined powers and remits.* There are two – the World Health Organization (including the Pan American Health Organization, PAHO) and the Council of Europe. They may exclude countries from membership, but in reality their power is soft and their function is essentially advisory, though they can provide support with funding or with channelling of funding from others. While the WHO involvement in blood transfusion carries considerable weight in medium and low development index countries, this is not the case in high index ones. The WHO's approach is essentially to promote national policies around a central nationally coordinated blood transfusion service with accountability to government.

• *Professional organizations within the blood transfusion community itself that set or define professional standards.* These bodies have no statutory powers.

Examples include the AABB and ISBT (the International Society of Blood Transfusion), and national professional organizations. They have an important regulatory function in providing professional support including defined standards for the state agencies.

• *Other agencies.* There are other agencies with more limited input into the regulatory process, especially those with a lobbying role at Government or international level: the International League of Red Cross and Red Crescent Societies, America's Blood Centers (ABC), the European Blood Alliance (EBA), the Alliance of Blood Operators (ABO) and professional trade associations such as the International Plasma Producers Congress (IPPC), the Plasma Protein Therapeutics Association (PPTA) and the International Plasma Fractionation Association (IPFA).

• *Patient involvement.* The voice of the patient in regulation of blood transfusion, where expressed, is generally through the political process and the governance arrangements for regulators, hospitals and blood suppliers. In addition, several well-organized

groups representing users of blood components – people with thalassaemia and sickle cell anaemia – and plasma products – people with haemophilia or primary immune deficiencies – have valid concerns and often formal input into regulatory processes [10].
• *Donor involvement.* Donor associations exist as separate entities to blood transfusion services in several countries and have an international body – the International Federation of Blood Donor Associations. From time to time these groups may lobby regulators, governments and blood suppliers.
• *Other groups.* Public bodies, for example lesbian, bisexual, gay and transgender groups rights and allied groups, may become involved in public debates and issues surrounding blood transfusion from time to time.

The role of blood transfusion agencies and health professionals vis-à-vis regulatory agencies

Laws, regulations, ethics and social values evolve. What is accepted as ethical and proper in one time and place may not be legal in another. Laws governing gender and sexuality are but one example. So while the law as it is must be observed and respected, it need not be revered as complete, correct or immutable. Neither should it be seen to be outside the sphere of influence of the public to whom it applies. In contrast, it is the civic duty of citizens of a state and the ethical duty of scientists and physicians everywhere to attempt to correct deficits or address shortcomings in the law, whether through contributing to the drafting of new statutes, correcting technical errors, including omissions, in the law itself or advocating repeal when the prevailing conditions render laws obsolete. This must be effected through legal and transparent processes, perhaps ideally through competent and legal organization for this purpose, including, in blood transfusion, the AABB, ABC, EBA and similar bodies.

In almost no country are the regulatory authorities concerned with improvements in the efficacy of red cells or platelets, or with treatment protocols and guidelines. These remain the preserve of the professionals in the field. Blood remains a problematic medicine; regulation tends by its nature to be very conservative and tends to preserve the status quo at the expense of development. This may give rise to a natural and often constructive tension between regulators and practitioners, to whom it is obvious that there is much to be improved.

Regulatory compliance is always part of professional and scientific integrity and endeavour, but it is never all of it, and much less a substitute for it.

Key points

1 A well-legislated and regulated blood transfusion service is a crucial component in assuring safety of the blood supply within a country or state, although there are large differences among different jurisdictions in how this is addressed.
2 Regulations should, but do not always, address issues of adequacy of supply and availability of blood within a State, as well as quality, safety and scientific developments.
3 Regulations are based in law, which should be explicit in statute, and are governed by guiding principles, often in practice a version of the Precautionary Principle and the principles and rules of Good Manufacturing Practice.
4 State regulatory agencies apply Standards; these are often set by national accreditation or standards bodies, or by professional bodies within the field.
5 The nature and scope of regulations may be influenced by forces inside or outside blood transfusion – lobbying by professional groups, trade organizations, patients and groups and other interested bodies can apply pressure for change at the political and public level.

References

1 World Health Organization. Resolutions relating to blood safety adopted by WHO governing bodies. WHO 2006. Available at: www.who.int/bloodsafety/en, accessed March 2012.
2 Directive 2002/98/EC of 27 January 2003 of the European Parliament and of the Council setting standards of quality and safety for the collection, testing, processing, storage and distribution of human blood and blood components and amending Directive 2001/83/EC. *Official Journal of the European Union* 2003; L 33/30.
3 Commission Directive 2004/33/EC of 22 March 2004 implementing Directive 2002/98/EC of the European

Parliament and of the Council as regards certain technical requirements for blood and blood components. *Official Journal of the European Union* 2004; L 91/25.

4 Commission Directive 2005/61/EC of 30 September 2005 implementing Directive 2002/98/EC of the European Parliament and of the Council as regards traceability requirements and notification of serious adverse reactions and events. *Official Journal of the European Union* 2005; L 265/32.

5 Commission Directive 2005/62/EC of 30 September 2005 implementing Directive 2002/98/EC of the European Parliament and of the Council as regards Community standards and specifications relating to a quality system for blood establishments. *Official Journal of the European Union* 2005; L 256/41.

6 Epstein J, Seitz R, Dhingra N, Ganz PR, Gharehbaghian A, Spindel R, Teo D & Reddy R. Role of regulatory agencies. *Biologicals* 2009; 37: 94–102.10.

7 Europa.eu. Summaries of EU legislation. The Precautionary Principle. Available at: http://europa.eu/legislation_summaries/consumers/consumer_safety/l32042_en.htm. 2011 (accessed March 2012).

8 Vamvakas EC, Kleinman S, Hume H & Sher GD. The development of West Nile virus safety policies by Canadian blood services: guiding principles and a comparison between Canada and the United States. *Transfus Med Rev* 2006; 20: 97–109.

9 Medicines and Healthcare Products Regulatory Agency (MHRA). *Rules and Guidance for Pharmaceutical Manufacturers and Distributors (The Orange Guide)*. London: Pharmaceutical Press; 2007.

10 O'Mahony B & Turner A. The Dublin Consensus Statement 2011 on vital issues relating to the collection and provision of blood components and plasma-derived medicinal products. *Vox Sanguinis* 2012, February; 102: 140–143.

18 The role of haemovigilance in transfusion safety

James P. AuBuchon[1] & *Katharine A. Downes*[2]

[1] Puget Sound Blood Center and University of Washington Seattle, Seattle, Washington, USA
[2] University Hospitals Case Medical Center and Case Western Reserve University, Cleveland, Ohio, USA

Introduction

In the last decade the quality improvement movement in healthcare has engendered many adages while increasing our ability to improve the delivery of services and patient outcomes. One of these is especially pertinent to haemovigilance: 'If you can't measure it, you can't improve it.' This concept sums up the rationale behind the creation of a haemovigilance system in most developed nations over the last decade and the excitement associated with the data they are generating. By defining the frequency of problems encountered in the transfusion system from vein to vein, i.e. from the time of collection through the consequences of transfusion, and documenting any failures to achieve the desired goal of safe and efficacious transfusion *every time*, we can begin to identify where our attention and resources should be directed in order to allow transfusion medicine to participate fully in modern medicine's attempt to provide care through robust systems that yield dependable outcomes.

Although different entities have applied slightly different definitions to haemovigilance, that of the International Haemovigilance Network (IHN) is one of the most encompassing:

Haemovigilance is a set of surveillance procedures covering the entire transfusion chain (from the donation of blood and its components to the follow-up of recipients of transfusions), intended to collect and assess information on unexpected or undesirable effects resulting from the therapeutic use of labile blood products, and to prevent the occurrence or recurrence of such incidents.

Recognition that transfusion hazards may accrue from any of the multiple steps along the complex pathway from donor selection to recipient transfusion requires that a haemovigilance system maintain a broad, all-encompassing scope in order to define these risks. Inclusion of the expectation that steps will be taken to reduce these risks is critical, since merely collecting data will not prompt improvements in the transfusion system. In essence, then, haemovigilance systems provide the engine through which transfusion systems can improve their services and patient outcomes.

Origin and impetus

Haemovigilance systems arose out of a confluence of events that questioned the safety of the healthcare system to deliver treatment without causing unnecessary harm and the ability of the blood supply system to deliver components with minimal risk. Increasing recognition that the reliability of medical care systems is suboptimal led to broad efforts to reduce the substantial risks associated with delivery of all aspects of healthcare. These efforts alone might have

Practical Transfusion Medicine, Fourth Edition. Edited by Michael F. Murphy, Derwood H. Pamphilon and Nancy M. Heddle.
© 2013 John Wiley & Sons, Ltd. Published 2013 by John Wiley & Sons, Ltd.

stirred blood bankers into action, but the earlier public debates, commissions of inquiry and prosecutions (and convictions) stemming from how the nascent HIV risk of the 1980s had been handled provided additional impetus for the field to assess the safety of its services through ongoing risk assessment measures. As the infectious disease risks of HIV and HCV that captivated our attention through the 1980s and 1990s were documented to have been greatly diminished through concerted multifaceted interventions, the field of transfusion medicine felt increasingly able to redirect its attention to problems that had been known to exist for many years but that had never been definitively or effectively addressed.

The legal framework and the organizational structure of these systems vary from country to country. An early system was reported to have been established in Japan in 1992 [1]. In Europe the first system was established about the same time in France as a mandatory system in which the reporting of all untoward outcomes from transfusions was required [2]. The second European system implemented arose through the efforts of transfusion medicine professionals in the UK and was organized through the Royal College of Pathologists as a voluntary reporting system focused on Serious Hazards of Transfusion (SHOT) [3]. Subsequently, systems have been created and implemented in most developed nations as a hybrid of these approaches. Some of these reside within and derive reporting mandates from a national ministry of health while others are primarily organized through professional societies or the country's blood collection system with sharing of data among all concerned parties. The European Community currently requires implementation of a haemovigilance system in each member state with reporting to a central office [4]. Development of a voluntary hemovigilance system in the USA evolved through efforts of numerous stakeholder organizations from the private and public sectors.

Although each country's system has characteristics unique for its own healthcare and transfusion systems, these systems bear multiple similarities and have yielded similar results [5], as will be discussed in the next section.

Coincident with these occurrences, more and more healthcare organizations, including blood collection organizations and transfusion services, have recognized the value of applying lean process improvement methodology. By focusing attention on where processes add value that is important to the end customer (the patient, in the case of transfusion) or where they fail to do so, improvements in the system that could add useful benefits can be targeted. Haemovigilance systems identify circumstances where value – in terms of safety and, in some cases, also efficiency – is lost from the transfusion process. Therefore, the experience garnered from a haemovigilance system adds useful information to the attempts by transfusion professionals to provide increased safety to the entire process.

Key elements and residual questions

The structure and content of haemovigilance systems vary by country, but the successful show several similarities in important facets of their philosophy and function (Table 18.1).

Definitions and terminology

Whether dealing with clinical events, such as transfusion reactions or near-miss incidents, a standardized lexicon must be adopted. Clear and precise definitions must be utilized and terms resistant to misinterpretation must be employed to decrease the chance of a misapplication of a classification scheme that would degrade the value of the system's data.

The importance of data conventions and data standardization cannot be overstated [6]. Standardization of data elements and terminology, as well as uniformity in data capture and reporting methods, are required to ensure data integrity for comparative analyses and also enable (1) consistent tracking of

Table 18.1 Important features of a haemovigilance system.

Confidentiality of submitted data
Broad participation, supported by education
Use of standardized definitions and terminology
Nonpunitive evaluation of data
Reporting of *rates* of occurrences
Sufficient detail to make effective recommendations for improved practices
Focus on improved safety and outcomes
Simple and efficient operations
Sustainable organization

internal performance over time, (2) benchmarking across institutions and (3) assessment of outcomes of process improvements. The importance of this standardization for comparison between systems was recognized early on by the IHN, and a working party of the International Society of Blood Transfusion (ISBT) has been developing definitions of transfusion reactions that could be used to achieve commonality and facilitate meaningful comparisons of data between countries. Some systems have taken the additional step of interposing a review of the details of a reported event to ensure that it meets the definitions used in that reporting system. While this rigour adds robustness to the reports of the system, larger systems or those with relatively fewer resources need to depend on participants' accurate application of the definitions embedded in the classification scheme.

Unexpected value from clearly defining the elements of a transfusion reaction have been reported from early implementation of the US Biovigilance Network. In addition to providing a standardized means through which reaction rates could truly be compared between institutions, the standardized definitions that were applied provided a framework through which reactions previously regarded as 'uncategorizable' could be tallied appropriately as well as uniformly. The standardized definitions thus provided benefit to the system and to the local transfusion specialist as well as to the practitioner who previously had to deal with the patient without clear guidance. The field of anatomic pathology has long recognized the importance of a clearly enunciated set of diagnostic criteria for diagnosis and grading of pathologic lesions; the transfusion segment of clinical pathology now is applying the same methodology to achieve better uniformity in describing untoward outcomes, thus informing the individual clinician as well as the system as a whole.

Detection and reporting of adverse events

Common to all haemovigilance systems is development and/or application of a system to capture events of interest directly from the site of the transfusion recipient or the hospital transfusion service. Many of the countries that first implemented haemovigilance systems had most of their transfusion expertise headquartered in blood centres and few transfusion medicine specialists located in hospitals. They generally did not have a history of capturing transfusion

reaction events in real time for investigation, accumulation and (local) analysis. To provide information for the new haemovigilance network, France identified a 'rapporteur' or 'haemovigilance officer' in each hospital (usually a physician, such as a haematologist or anaesthesiologist), the UK trained a cadre of nurses as 'specialized practitioners of transfusion' and Québec established a network of 'transfusion safety officers' (TSOs, usually nurses) in the larger hospitals who also oversaw reporting of events from nearby smaller facilities. In countries with a more established transfusion medicine professional presence at the hospital level, these new assignments or positions would not be required. For example, the haemovigilance reporting system in the USA is based on the pre-existing transfusion reaction reporting system extant in hospitals of all sizes that reports to the hospital's transfusion service and to the facility's transfusion committee. Regulatory and accreditation requirements strongly influence many of the components and requirements of such transfusion reaction reporting systems in US healthcare organizations.

For any reporting system to be reliable, those charged with capturing the event must be cognisant of the commonly recognized signs and symptoms of transfusion reactions as well as remaining alert to events that 'just don't seem right' during or after a transfusion. Simply dismissing an unusual sign or an unexpected symptom as causally unrelated to the transfusion will deprive not only the patient of steps that might prevent a recurrence in a future transfusion but also the transfusion system of the knowledge of an event that might disclose a significant new phenomenon. Ensuring that those likely to be the first to identify problems with a transfusion will report the occurrence is a critical first step in creating and maintaining a useful and credible haemovigilance system. Tying haemovigilance reporting to a bedside system that captures standardized and complete data from every transfusion undoubtedly improves the penetration of the haemovigilance system and the believability of the data it generates as well.

Despite the diligence of such efforts, however, haemovigilance systems will always be challenged to tally untoward outcomes that occur long after a transfusion because of the loss of an obvious temporal relationship (Table 18.2). For example, identifying transfusion transmission of an infectious disease would require recognition of the lack of other means of

Table 18.2 Limitations of haemovigilance systems.

Incomplete reporting
Detection of transfusion relationship of late events,
    including infections
Limited details
Variation in terminology and definitions
Influence of healthcare system's or institution's 'culture'
    regarding compliance, process improvement and
    reporting
Acceptance of nonstandard definitions and terminology
Inability to track cases back to their source to ensure that
    correct and complete reporting has occurred

Table 18.3 Variations among haemovigilance systems.

Scope	Serious events or all events?
	Events causing harm or also 'near-miss' events?
Breadth	Labile transfusible components
	Plasma derivative products
	Tissues and/or organs for transplantation (biovigilance)
Analysis	System level
	Institutional level
	Healthcare system level, comparison with all hospitals – locally, regionally, nationally and/or internationally?
	Comparison with (anonymous) peer institution subset
	Appropriateness of analysis of incidents and events
	Access to full details of incidents and events

transmission to the recipient and relative rarity of the disease entity in order for the transfusion connection to be recognized, and then the physician caring for the patient would need to contact the transfusion service in order for an investigation and possibly a report to the haemovigilance system to be generated. Haemovigilance-like investigations led to the detection of transmission of West Nile virus (WNV) through transfusion relatively early in the US outbreak of this disease, but making the connection between poor patient outcome and transfusion exposure of an organ donor would have been much more difficult had the incubation period been longer. Additional utility of a haemovigilance system is seen, however, through real-time assessment of regional risk through donor testing and revision of donor testing protocols in response to this information, as is being done in the USA with West Nile virus testing.

Scope of reporting

The scope of haemovigilance systems, however, is varied (Table 18.3). The SHOT system clearly specifies its interest only in the *serious* hazards and precludes reporting febrile and urticarial reactions, for example. This restriction provides natural focus on the hazards that have the largest potential impact on a particular recipient but at some risk of missing events of lesser morbidity that may affect a larger number of patients or that may be harbingers of more serious sequelae after transfusion. The more common approach of seeking to capture all transfusion reactions, on the other hand, risks 'system fatigue' from overwhelmed personnel or reporting and analysis tools through which events of major clinical significance

are obscured from view by the more numerous but less-informative reports of 'minor' events.

The extension of haemovigilance systems to incidents that are not directly associated with a reaction or an untoward outcome for a recipient is an important means of detecting problems in the *transfusion system* and preventing these from harming patients. Whether called an incident, a deviation or an error, these failures to adhere to standard procedures may represent human frailty or limitations, inadequate training, unique features of a patient's situation or a combination of factors that aligned with weak points in the transfusion system. The most notable among these has been patient and sample identification errors in pretransfusion testing. Inclusion of 'near-miss' events where the error is detected and remedied and/or where it does not cause harm to the recipient quickly causes such occurrences to become the most commonly reported events in a haemovigilance system. Although these occurrences may individually appear to be of minor importance, they represent a critical view into the workings of a transfusion system and allow preventive actions to be taken to bolster system safeguards.

Analysis of incident reports

The ability of an individual hospital or some other relevant unit of the healthcare system to assess the outcomes of its transfusions is important in addition to the national review of problems in the transfusion system. At the smallest division in which policies are common and practice is (presumed to be) universal, an analysis of reports of transfusion reactions and transfusion practice should be undertaken in order to understand how this microsystem compares to the larger whole, such as national comparators. In most situations, this analysis would be at the hospital level since enforcement of uniformity of practice outside of one's immediate reach is often difficult. Identification of where one's system is not being applied faithfully is critical knowledge that can be used to strengthen the system and remove ambiguity or opportunities for imprecise or incorrect actions to occur (or at least to go unnoticed). The individual hospital that participates in a national haemovigilance system that captures these kinds of data can benefit by comparing their experience to that of others working in the same type of system. Understanding where in the transfusion chain differences in practice are occurring may identify those steps in the process that are truly critical to be performed with a high degree of fidelity and also identify transfusion practices associated with superior outcomes.

There are several features of haemovigilance systems and hospital 'cultures' that are presumed to be associated with higher rates of reporting compliance. The degree to which an institution focuses on outcome improvement and adherence to policies is probably an important determinant of the acceptance of a reporting system such as represented by a haemovigilance system. Related to this may be the extent to which an 'open learning culture' is supported in the institution. Similarly, the more that 'incidents' are recognized as failures of the (imperfect) system rather than of those working within it, the more likely that staff will feel comfortable reporting the occurrences. When these reports lead to improvements in the process (and particularly when those affected by the incident have been able to participate in the improvement of the transfusion system), the satisfaction that is generated also empowers further reporting towards the end of improving operations and outcomes.

Encouragement of active participation in haemovigilance

This leads naturally to a discussion of whether reporting to a haemovigilance system should be 'voluntary' or 'mandatory'. In all likelihood, a mixture of incentives is most salutary. Error reporting will suffer in a system where reporting may be 'required' but more frequently leads to punishment of those caught in a cumbersome, error-prone system rather than to change in that system. The lack of nonpunitive reporting would clearly limit the ability of the haemovigilance system to effect improvements. A nonpunitive approach to reporting – for the individual reporting the case as well as for those involved in it and the institution itself – is essential to compliance. On the other hand, voluntary reporting, even when coupled with confidentiality safeguards, is unlikely to attract respondents unless the importance of their actions is well understood and they see the fruits of their efforts through system reports and process changes. All systems have noted a continual rise in the number of reports submitted over their first few years, as more staff 'on the front lines' become aware of the system, its importance and the logistics of reporting; those systems with more extensive educational infrastructure appear to have the most rapid attainment of extensive penetration. Endorsement of participation by a professional association or the ministry of health may boost participation, particularly if the system is easy for participants to use and has already established its credibility. In a legal system where the involved person or institution is subject to liability damages from an 'error', assurance of confidentiality for the details of the report and freedom from compelled disclosure are absolutely essential for enabling reporting. Even if no harm befell a patient from an incident, an institution would understandably require assurance that its 'dirty laundry' could not be used against it by a plaintiff's attorney alleging a pattern of inappropriate practices.

Whether participation in haemovigilance is voluntary or mandatory, thorough preparation within the participating organization is a key success factor. Effective preparation includes detailed review of current processes and procedures for adverse reaction reporting and interpretation and gap analysis compared to what will be expected for the haemovigilance programme. Such a review optimally includes representation from all stakeholder groups including physicians, nurses, laboratory staff and information system support staff. Sufficient time must be set aside for creating the necessary, locally appropriate definitions, e.g. transfusion location codes, in the computer system(s) and adequate testing. Training requirements, particularly for busy clinician groups, can be easily underestimated or overlooked. Pilot implementation at a hospital may be a useful way to uncover issues for correction prior to data entry into a haemovigilance system.

Data management

Simplicity of reporting is also the key to high participation rates. Most haemovigilance systems began with paper reports but are converting or have converted to electronic submission systems. This approach not only facilitates data management by the coordinating office but also simplifies the reporting mechanism for the participant; an intelligent, web-based data capture system could display only those items that were pertinent to the case's report as it unfolded rather than frightening a respondent with multiple pages of data elements, many of which would not be pertinent in any one particular case. Such a context-sensitive system could also check for completeness and prevent logging of an incomplete case or check for internal congruity in a case and prevent clearly erroneous entry errors. The extent to which a system wishes to go to ensure that its definitions are being followed may be dependent on assumptions made about the support available for data entry. For example, does the system require entry of pre- and posttransfusion temperatures and a check to see if the definition of a febrile transfusion reaction has been met, or does the system expect that the respondent is applying the definition correctly? The former approach would provide better assurance of data integrity but would require more time for data entry. The quality of analysis possible from computerized databases depends upon the appropriateness of the definitions of the data elements that are established in the database and the consistency with which data entry is accomplished.

Optimally, the national haemovigilance system would be interfaced to a facility's internal error management software (such as MERS-TM [7]) and be able to accept the report of the necessary elements of a case automatically. Most haemovigilance systems have not reached that level of sophistication, but centrally coordinated healthcare systems may be able to integrate laboratory information, error management and haemovigilance systems to accomplish this. Since the capabilities of many transfusion services to analyse and report their experience with incidents and events are limited in their laboratory information system, the ability of the national haemovigilance system to construct the tables and graphs illustrating the experience of the reporter's institution and overlay the system's experience (in aggregate form or from institutions with similar characteristics) may reward (and thus encourage) participation.

The extent of data collection ultimately affects the richness of the system's data. The more detail of an incident or a reaction that is captured by a system, the greater the impact on policy development the reports may offer. Capturing detail about where an incident occurred may help identify 'high-risk clinical areas', and identifying the steps in the transfusion process that were vulnerable to error will similarly help direct attention to the part of the transfusion process where improvements will have the greatest impact. The performance of a root-cause analysis is beyond the purview of a national haemovigilance system, but capturing the results of such an analysis and estimating the probability of a recurrence and its impact can also help focus attention on 'big payoff' targets.

A critical category of data elements in a haemovigilance system is the 'denominator data'. Although tallying the number of units of each component type transfused or the number of pretransfusion specimens tested does not inform us about transfusion safety, this information is essential in turning reported occurrences into rates. Only through a comparison of the rates of events can we compare meaningfully across institutions and countries of different sizes and different transfusion activity levels. As different countries – or, indeed, different regions within one country – account for outdated and discarded units differently, depending solely on reports from blood centres for component volumes may lead to inaccuracy in calculation of transfusion rates.

Breadth of the system

An analogous consideration is the breadth of the system. What products should be included in the system's tracking? The IHN's definition of haemovigilance focuses on labile components, but there remains much to be learned about the use of and reactions to plasma derivative products, and in some jurisidictions these are handled through the same transfusion service system. In such a case, as in Canada, valuable information can be gleaned through extending the system to these additional components. Should haemovigilance systems be further expanded to incorporate tissues and organs to become *bio*vigilance systems? The principles of haemovigilance – including product traceability, learning from one's practice and a commitment to continual improvement – are applicable to transplantation as well as to transfusion, and transfusion services handle these products in some countries as well. Efforts to create systems applicable to tissues have already begun in earnest in the USA, again spurred by safety concerns, and marrow transplant organizations have for many years been tracking the outcomes of their efforts in order to find keys to improving patient outcomes. The extent to which these efforts will be interdigitated with haemovigilance systems rather than standing alone as complimentary systems will be determined by the extent to which the participating institutions and physicians contribute directly to both fields and whether their systems are mutually supportive. At the least, transfusion medicine specialists should be aware of these parallel efforts in related fields so that, whenever possible, their systems can be made compatible and congruent, even if not communicating directly.

However, inclusion of donor operations should be regarded as integral to a haemovigilance system. Not only are there important donor and patient safety elements to be gleaned from taking a holistic view of the transfusion process, but a system that spans the same vein-to-vein reach of the transfusion process will be better positioned to 'connect the dots' to unravel dilemmas and inform policy changes. Already enlightening have been data on the frequency of postdonation reaction rates with different blood volumes collected and delineation of the rate of postdonation death among donors assumed to be healthy. As with the recipient-focused end of the system, standardized terminology and definitions are needed to ensure comparability of recorded observations.

Learning from experience

Haemovigilance systems are sufficiently mature in multiple countries that the medical literature is providing an increasing number of reports of their observations. By their nature, these are observational, but they still provide interesting insights into the problems faced by different transfusion systems and the risks borne by their donors and recipients. It is beyond the scope of this chapter to attempt to replicate all the available data, but the reader is referred to several recent, thorough reports to understand the scope of information available (see Further reading).

Several important, common themes are evident from reviewing these data and some of these observations have led to recommendations that have improved transfusion safety, the intention of haemovigilance systems in the first place.

1 Transfusion of the incorrect unit or component is the most frequent system problem encountered. The problem may manifest as the patient not receiving precisely the component (sub)type that was ordered or may manifest as a fatal haemolytic transfusion reaction. Clearly, inadequate and/or inaccurate identification of the patient or sample/unit at the time of pretransfusion sampling and at transfusion are frequent problems that defy simple solutions but that merit more attention and more capable technology. As shown in the Canadian experience, almost half of all high severity incidents were related to pretransfusion sample collection, and a third of all high severity events where harm occurred were associated with transfusion of the incorrect unit.

2 The greatest mortality risk in most systems currently appears to be transfusion-related acute lung injury (TRALI), although assessment of the frequency of this complication is complicated due to subtle differences in the definitions applied and understanding that significant 'underrecognition' is undoubtedly occurring. This highlights again a potentially important role for TSOs in clinician education for the benefit of the transfusion recipient as well as for improved reporting and understanding of the reaction.

3 Data from haemovigilance systems have been helpful not only in defining the frequency of bacterial contamination of platelets but also in investigating the frequency of certain types of contamination after identification of a cluster of incidents and in documenting the effects of implementing interventions to address the problem.

Several applications of haemovigilance data from the SHOT system have been particularly noteworthy in improving the safety of that transfusion system and show the power of haemovigilance systems when their data are applied thoughtfully through evidence-based recommendations (see Further reading). Reports of mistransfusion due to identification problems continued unabated until the recognition that delineation of the problem alone would not effect an improvement. Subsequent implementation of augmented approaches to patient, sample and unit identification was associated with, for the first time, a decline in the number of reported deaths due to mistransfusions. Similar results of interventions have been reported from other systems, such as in France, where ABO-incompatible transfusions were reduced by three-quarters.

Similarly, recognition of the magnitude of the problem posed by TRALI and the high frequency of association of TRALI cases with the plasma of female donors prompted the UK's National Blood Service to reduce the proportion of plasma for transfusion coming from female donors with a subsequent marked reduction in the number of deaths attributable to TRALI. Recognition in one reporting period that transfusion-associated circulatory overload (TACO) was the most common cause of posttransfusion mortality in Québec [8] prompted an increase in education of clinicians on this problem and additional clinical attention to the complication such that a subsequent decline in its frequency was seen.

Haemovigilance data have also led to some unexpected, intriguing observations. Thirteen fatal cases of graft-versus-host disease (GVHD) were reported in a 10-year time span through SHOT, all of them prior to the implementation of universal leucocyte reduction and all but two of them in patients who did not meet usual indications for use of irradiated components [9]. Also, universal leucocyte reduction was associated with a marked reduction in the number of posttransfusion purpura (PTP) cases reported and an apparent shift of these from predominantly red cell recipients (57% from 3%) to include more platelet recipients. This information may be useful in exploring the pathophysiology of these reactions and provide information that may be relevant to blood supply systems not currently employing this approach to component production. Without a haemovigilance system operating 'in the background' to amass this experience, these findings might have been missed due to the relative infrequency of GVHD and PTP.

Haemovigilance systems could also be applied to address important yet unanswered questions through the large number of events that they track. For example, the utility of routine premedication with antipyretics and antihistamines has been challenged, but many clinicians continue to believe in their importance. A haemovigilance system could seek to generate a database of sufficient size to address this issue within one jurisdiction or healthcare system so that clinicians could not simply dismiss the data as not being applicable to them. Conversely, the large experience of multiple nations might be able to determine whether the incidence of TRALI is affected by all the plasma in a platelet unit originating from a single donor versus multiple but smaller exposures. There is also considerable interest in applying the power of a haemovigilance system's large purview for 'Phase IV' or 'postmarketing surveillance' studies to help assess the safety of new interventions, such as pathogen inactivation. This could be accomplished by ensuring that appropriate questions were included on the posttransfusion report form completed by transfusionists or through targeted studies utilizing special reporting tools.

In addition to the evidence-based benefits outlined above, haemovigilance programmes have resulted in number of 'intangible' benefits. Participation in a coordinated, standardized programme aimed at improving patient care around transfusions engenders confidence in laboratory and clinical staff, and, particularly for laboratory staff, greater recognition of the role they play in patient care. The benchmarking inherent in haemovigilance is of interest to clinical departments and hospital administrators looking for such data. Computerizing formerly paper-based processes reduces inefficiencies of manual processes. Overall, participating in such national (and international) efforts offers satisfaction from being involved in an even greater good.

Although the stated intention of haemovigilance systems is to improve the safety of transfusion recipients, such systems are also excellently positioned to improve the practice of haemotherapy through the assessment of patient outcomes. There remains wide variation in the application of indications for transfusions and the lack of adoption of published guidelines is sometimes blamed on lack of evidence of their clinical applicability. The data necessary to address these questions are not readily available to most transfusion services at present, but further expansion and integration of laboratory information systems with electronic medical records and linkage with recipient registries may allow future versions of haemovigilance systems wider access to data that could address these and other important transfusion-related questions.

Key points

1 'If you can't measure it, you can't improve it', but measurement alone will not improve systems. Concerted action to improve transfusion systems and reduce transfusion risks is necessary.

2 Haemovigilance systems are most effective when they are based on data reported by clinical practitioners trained to be observant for transfusion-related problems and reported consistently using standardized nomenclature and definitions.

3 Including 'near-miss' incidents in haemovigilance reporting provides insights into weak points of the transfusion process and the opportunity to improve the system by reducing the potential for human error to cause harm.

4 The most common problem reported across multiple haemovigilance systems is the transfusion of an 'incorrect blood component' and the most dangerous problems encountered frequently relate to sample and patient identification errors.

5 Recognition of serious problems followed by action directed at their cause can improve transfusion safety, as has been seen in steps taken to reduce the frequency of TRALI and ABO-related acute haemolytic events.

6 Haemovigilance systems may be extended to provide important information about haemotherapy decisions and follow-up of new transfusion approaches.

References

1 Juji T, Nishimura M, Watanabe Y, Uchida S, Okazaki H & Tadokoro K. Transfusion-associated graft-versus-host disease. *ISBT Sci Ser* 2009; 4: 236–240.

2 Rebibo D, Hauser L, Slimani A, Hervé P & Andreu G. The French haemovigilance system: organization and results for 2003. *Transfus Apher Sci* 2004; 31: 145–153.

3 Stainsby D, Jones H, Asher D *et al.* (on behalf of the SHOT Steering Group). Serious hazards of transfusion: a decade of hemovigilance in the UK. *Transfus Med Rev* 2006; 20: 273–282.

4 Faber JC. The European blood directive: a new era of blood regulation has begun. *Transfus Med* 2004; 14: 257–273.

5 Faber J-C. Work of the European haemovigilance network (EHN). *Transfus Clin Biol* 2004; 11: 2–10.

6 Robillard P, Chan P & Kleinman S. Hemovigilance for improvement of blood safety. *Transfus Apher Sci* 2004; 31: 95–98.

7 Callum JL, Merkley LL, Coovadia AS, Lima AP & Kaplan HS. Experience with the medical event reporting system for transfusion medicine (MERS-TM) at three hospitals. *Transfus Apher Sci* 2004; 31: 133–143.

8 Engelfriet CP & Reesink HW. Haemovigilance. *Vox Sanguinis* 2006; 90: 207–241.

9 Williamson LM, Stainsby D, Jones H *et al.* (on behalf of the Serious Hazards of Transfusion Steering Group). The impact of universal leukodepletion of the blood supply in hemovigilance reports of posttransfusion purpura and transfusion-associated graft-versus-host disease. *Transfusion* 2007; 47: 1455–1467.

Further reading

AuBuchon JP & Whitaker BI. America finds hemovigilance! *Transfusion* 2007; 47: 1937–1942.

Callum JL, Kaplan HS, Merkley LL *et al.* Reporting of near-miss events for transfusion medicine: improving transfusion safety. *Transfusion* 2001; 41: 1204–1211.

de Vries RR, Faber JC, Strengers PF, Board of the International Haemovigilance Network. Haemovigilance: an effective tool for improving transfusion practice. *Vox Sanguinis* 2011; 100(91): 60–67.

Williamson LM. Transfusion hazard reporting: powerful data, but do we know how best to use it? *Transfusion* 2002; 42: 1249–1252.

Donors and blood collection

Ellen McSweeney[1] *& William G. Murphy*[1,2]

[1]Irish Blood Transfusion Service, National Blood Centre, Dublin, Republic of Ireland
[2]Health Service Executive, Clinical Strategy and Programmes, and University College Dublin, Republic of Ireland

Collecting blood from people for transfusion to others is not optional – it is an essential part of healthcare. A developed healthcare system needs to provide approximately 30–40 therapeutic units of red cells and up to six therapeutic doses of platelets annually per thousand of the population it serves. There is no satisfactory alternative therapy in most cases and no prospect of any such alternative emerging soon.

Blood donors: paid, directed, payback and altruistic

People can be motivated to donate blood in three different ways: (1) as a direct response to the needs of an individual they care about, (2) for an economically valued reward or (3) as an altruistic act. All three methods are in wide use today. All have their drawbacks. However, it has by now become clear that societies that succeed in establishing a mature programme of altruistic donations generally gain a more secure and stable supply of safer blood for transfusion than those that do not. There is compelling evidence that the incidence and prevalence of infectious diseases are higher among donors who donate for personal economic gain. There is also some evidence that individuals who are directly approached by a relative or friend to donate for a particular patient are more likely to withhold critical information about their personal infectious risk history that may compromise the safety of the recipient of the donation.

Motivation, recruitment and retention of altruistic donors are not easy or cheap. In most developed nations 5% or less of the population donates per year. While donors will queue for hours in times of clear perception of need, such as in a major disaster, most of the time blood services need to work hard to maintain supply. Establishing a mature altruism-based blood donation and collection programme requires a high degree of social cohesion and an immense effort in education and communication. Maintaining a programme once it is established may also need considerable effort and expense. Many successful national or regional programmes based on altruism were set up around the middle of the 20th century, at a time of national need in conflict or post-conflict. The appeal of sharing health and well-being was relatively easily conflated with national military or civil requirements at that time. Countries that did not establish altruism-based blood services to begin with have tended to find it much more difficult to establish one afterwards, and often remain dependent on nonaltruistic donations. Huge efforts are currently being made to redress this throughout the developing world, often directed towards younger adults (Chapter 24).

Paying blood donors will provide a supply of blood, but it requires enough people in the population for whom the payment on offer provides sufficient motivation. Students or other economically marginalized

Practical Transfusion Medicine, Fourth Edition. Edited by Michael F. Murphy, Derwood H. Pamphilon and Nancy M. Heddle.
© 2013 John Wiley & Sons, Ltd. Published 2013 by John Wiley & Sons, Ltd.

individuals will often provide blood or plasma for payment, but the strategy will limit overall supply where there are not enough economic marginals in the community to respond. In more developed economies the balance of high demand for blood for transfusion with limited numbers of people who will be motivated by the rewards on offer often makes paying for donations an inadequate strategy. In addition, paying for blood also undermines the alternative, more successful motivation of altruism in these economies.

Apart from the problems of supply, paid donors are, in general, a less safe source than volunteer donors. Data comparing disease markers between paid and nonpaid donors reflect this difference in safety. In an analysis of 28 published data sets, it was found that while the incidence of disease markers had diminished over the years between 1977 and 1996 for paid and unpaid donors alike, unpaid donors were on average 5–10 times safer than paid donors and that this difference had not changed over time (see van der Poel *et al.*, in Further Reading). The logic is compelling: people who genuinely feel well, and have no great incentive to donate other than genuine regard for their fellow humans, will tend not to withhold risk information, or at least not return regularly even if they do. People who need money or items of small economic value at the level they may be offered by blood services will have more pressing needs and are more likely to withhold relevant risk information. In addition, increased at-risk exposure from drug addiction or sex working occurs more frequently at the lower economic margins of a Westernized society.

A system of directed and payback donations, where donors are recruited among the relatives and friends of the patient requiring blood transfusions, also provides some supply. Such an approach will generally be insufficient to support a well-developed healthcare system and is prone in places to covert payments to donors, including professional donors.

European Union (EU) Directive 2002/98/EC (see Further reading) instructs member states to promote community self-sufficiency in human blood and blood components and to encourage voluntary unpaid donations of blood and blood components.

Whereas starting a career as a blood donor is mainly driven by external stimuli, becoming a committed regular donor requires a high level of intrinsic motivation. It is essential that the donor sees him/herself as a dedicated donor and that donating becomes a habit. Key strategies that blood services must consider in blood donor retention programmes include active communication with the donor from the beginning, making donation convenient, reducing donor anxiety and adverse reactions, having well-trained and motivated staff, and encouraging temporarily deferred donors to return as soon as possible following the expiry of their deferral period. These measures enable blood services to convert first-time donors to regular committed donors, a primary goal of donor management [1].

Challenges still remain in recruiting donors from ethnic minorities. Migrant populations have different disease patterns with different transfusion demands. Added to this, data suggest that migrants tend not to become blood donors in their new country. A number of factors may contribute to the proportionally low representation of minorities in the donating population, including culture, lack of social/ethnic identification, fear and lack of information.

Donor management in Europe

Almost 50 blood establishments from 34 European countries contributed to the development of the DOMAINE Donor Management in Europe Project (see Further reading) to analyse practices in donor management in Europe. The project compiled a *Donor Management Manual* and developed a Training Programme to provide tools for blood establishments to optimize practice in their local context. The manual covers development and usage of donor recruitment and retention strategies, organization of blood donor sessions, blood donor data management and donor counselling, in addition to donor management in relation to patients needing multiple transfusions, human resources issues, training, information technology and ethical issues.

Risks to the blood donor

Blood donation is generally very safe. Most people can readily tolerate venesections of approximately 10% of their blood volumes without apparent harm or significant physiological compromise. However, it is not a trivial undertaking and requires considerable care to minimize the risk to the donor. This is particularly the case since there is no proven health benefit to the donor except in the treatment, inadvertent or otherwise, of haemochromatosis. The risks associated with blood donation are listed in Table 19.1.

An internationally accepted description and classification of adverse events and reactions was proposed by the European Haemovigilance Network (EHN) and the International Society of Blood Transfusion (ISBT) in 2004 and refined in 2008. They classified complications into two main categories: those with predominately local symptoms, such as haematomas, nerve injuries and tendon injuries, and those with predominately generalized symptoms, such as vasovagal reactions. Complications specific to apheresis procedures were categorized separately. Complications were further graded into mild, moderate and severe, and were assigned an imputability score for the likelihood of blood donation being the cause of the reaction.

Some complications are specific to apheresis donations, e.g. citrate reactions, haemolysis, air emboli and allergic reactions to ethylene oxide used in the sterilization of the harness. The majority of apheresis donors experience mild citrate reactions, such as a metallic taste or tingling in the lips. This is an accepted occurrence, considered to be an inevitable effect of the anticoagulant. Most blood establishments will only report citrate effects if they are severe or if they result in the donation being discontinued.

Longer term consequences of donation, such as iron depletion with or without associated anaemia, psychological consequences of false positive reactions in screening assays or increased bone resorption, as has been reported in apheresis donors, are not currently reported as complications of donation, but this may change given time.

The overall incidence of complications directly related to blood donation is often quoted as being approximately 1%, though the reported rate of reactions may be much less than the true reaction rate. One study where information on adverse events was actively sought on follow-up rather than relying on passive collection of spontaneous reports by donors reported that from 1000 randomly selected donors three weeks after donation 36% of donors had had one or more adverse events: fatigue (7.8%), vasovagal symptoms (5.3%), nausea and vomiting (1.1%), along with bruising (22.7%), soreness (10%) and haematomas (1.7%) at the venepuncture site [2]. Of complications collated by the EHN/ISBT Working

Group 99% belonged to four categories: vasovagal reactions (86% of all complications), haematomas (13%), nerve injuries (1%) and arterial punctures (0.4%) [3].

Rarely severe complications arise, such as accidents related to vasovagal reactions and nerve injuries with long-lasting symptoms. These can have serious consequences for the donor and can impact on his/her daily life. Vasovagal reactions that occur after the donor has left the session are of particular concern. Such delayed reactions are thought to account for 10% of all vasovagal reactions and occasionally death has been attributed to accidents following them. A retrospective analysis of Danish data relating to 2.5 million donations found that severe complications occurred with an incidence of 19 per 100 000 procedures; two-thirds of which were due to vasovagal reactions with loss of consciousness and one-third due to needle insertion [4].

Young age, first time donor status and low total blood volume are independent predictors of higher reaction rates. A complication rate of 10.7% in 16 and 17 year olds, 8.3% in 18 and 19 year olds and 2.8% in donors aged 20 years and older has been observed, as has a higher incidence of donation-related injury (particularly physical injury from syncope-related falls) in 16 and 17 year olds compared with older donors. Syncope occurred in 4 in 1000 donations and injury in 6 in 10 000 donations in this age group and almost half of the injuries that occurred in American Red Cross regions involved 16 to 17-year-old whole blood donors [5].

It is unlikely that the risks to blood donors can ever be reduced to zero. Coupled with the societal necessity for blood donations, this places a significant ethical burden on blood services to use their best endeavours to reduce the risks. This includes particular attention to detail, careful collation and analysis of data on the incidence and nature of adverse events or reactions, and proper management of the information derived, e.g. by sharing and comparing data among blood services to identify and promote best practices. The uneven risk-to-benefit ratio for blood donors also places an ethical responsibility on healthcare givers, the users of blood donations, to avoid wastage and unnecessary use of blood transfusions.

Several strategies can be taken to reduce the risk of complications occurring during and after donation. Efforts to improve the donation experience are

Table 19.1 Adverse events or reactions in blood donors.

Type of event or reaction	Incidence
Vasovagal events or reactions	
Dizziness, nausea, simple fainting, severe faint with prolonged loss of consciousness and convulsions; associated trauma from falls or vehicle accidents	1.4–7% moderate reactions rate* 0.1–0.5% severe reaction rate*
Hospitalization rate	1 per 198 000 donations* Two-thirds of these are due to vasovagal reactions
Needle injury	
Sore arm	12.5% females, 6.9% males*
To the vein, causing pain and bruising, which may be extensive, thrombophlebitis, thrombosis	9–23%*
To the artery, causing extensive bruising, fistula, aneurysm, distal ischaemia, compartment syndrome	0.003–0.011%*
To the nerve, causing pain, and motor and sensory loss, which can be prolonged	0.016–0.9%* 0.0022% (disablement)*
To a tendon, causing acute and intense pain	Rare
Serious cardiovascular events or reactions	
Angina, myocardial infarction, cerebrovascular accident	Very rare; may or may not be causally related to the donation; always associated with underlying pre-existing disease
Iron deficiency with or without anaemia	
Even in the absence of anaemia, tissue iron deficiency may be associated with mild disturbance of cerebral function, such as impaired concentration, and with sleep disturbance/restless legs	Regular blood donors: iron depletion >20%* Absent iron stores 15%* Frequent donors: Absent iron stores: males 16.4%, females 27.1%*
Allergic reactions/anaphylaxis	
Reactions may be to the skin preparation materials or adhesives, or to latex in the attendants' gloves	Rare
In apheresis donors in addition to the above	
Citrate toxicity from the anticoagulant	Mild reactions are common 80%* Severe reactions are rare 0.4%*
Thrombocytopenia and protein deficiency from excessive platelet or plasma donations respectively	Rare and easily prevented
Allergic reactions to ethylene oxide used in the sterilization of the harness	Rare
Haemolysis/air embolus due to errors in the procedure or problems with the manufacturing of the harness	Very rare
For granulocyte donors: allergic reactions to hetastarch if used as a sedimentation agent or adverse drug reactions to steroids or growth factors used to raise the donor's leucocyte count	Mild reactions including bone pain are common with the use of growth factors and steroids in donors. Many blood services do not provide granulocytes by apheresis. Pooled buffy coats provide an alternative that is logistically simpler, safer for the donor, and may be equally efficacious

*When marked with an asterisk, the figure is from Reference [10].

crucial not only to ensure the health and well-being of blood donors but to sustain an adequate blood supply. Even minor reactions discourage donors from donating again and syncope, particularly if associated with injury, profoundly decreases the return rate of donors. Good needle insertion techniques are critical to reduce the incidence and severity of venepuncture-related complications. Other successful strategies include pre-donation education, optimizing the session environment, appropriate selection criteria (particularly as regards estimated blood volume), vigilant supervision of donors by staff, water ingestion before donation, distraction techniques and muscle tension during phlebotomy, and post-reaction instructions to donors [6].

Donor selection and exclusion

Prospective blood donors are subjected to a process, often specified in national legislation, intended to minimize the risks to the donor and to the eventual recipient of the donated blood. This involves a donor history to identify clinical conditions in the donor that may suggest increased risk to the donor of a serious adverse event/reaction if the donation goes ahead or any recognizable risk in the donor for transmitting infectious agents to the recipient. Infectious risks from donors are listed in Table 19.2, along with available donor exclusion strategies to address these risks.

In some services the donor undergoes some form of physical examination, but this is often cursory and abbreviated and, among altruistic donors at least, is of doubtful value in someone who has provided satisfactory answers to a detailed history.

Donors generally undergo a measurement of their haemoglobin level at some point, either prior to the donation or, in some countries, on a sample taken at the same time as the donation. This is either from a skin puncture ('capillary sample') or a venous sample. This measurement of haemoglobin serves two purposes – it provides some protection to the donor against having a pre-existing anaemia made worse by donating and it helps ensure that the final therapeutic product will have a minimum red cell content. It might also help prevent acute adverse reactions or events in the donor, but there is no evidence that this is the case. The cut-off levels for the allowable haemoglobin level in the donor vary between blood services and regulatory authorities and are empirically derived. Often, as in the European Union (EU) rules

(Directive 2004/33/EC, see Further reading) a different level is used for males and females, with the allowable minimum haemoglobin level set 1 g/dL higher for males than for females. Haemoglobin levels vary in the same individual between capillary and venous blood [7], with the seasons and the time of day, and with posture and activity. In addition, measuring haemoglobin levels does not provide protection against nonanaemic iron deficiency.

Where a blood service is subject to legally binding regulations, donor exclusions may be specified by law. In the EU the specifications are generally interpreted as a minimum requirement by the member states or the national blood services; in the USA and other jurisdictions, in contrast, the specifications are generally regarded as a maximum requirement by the blood service operators, who rarely add to them on their own initiative. The EU requirements for permanent and temporary exclusion of donors are listed in Table 19.3; the blood services in many countries routinely exceed these requirements, sometimes on the basis of local epidemiological risks and sometimes on the basis of national or regional perceptions of best practice. For example, exclusions on the basis of sexual risk, travel, haemochromatosis or previous transfusions vary from country to country in the EU, while remaining within the legal specification defined in the EU Directives.

Deferral rates vary in different blood services. Reported deferral rates in EU blood services range from 0.5 to 25.2% of donors, with a mean of 10.9%. The lowest deferral rates are in countries where the public knowledge of blood donation selection criteria is high – where donors may register online and complete an eligibility questionnaire in advance. A low haemoglobin level is typically the commonest reason for deferral, accounting for nearly 40% of deferrals. Other factors include relative proportions of new and regular donors, urban versus rural venues and sessions with a majority of younger donors in whom deferrals for skin piercing, tattooing and travel are higher.

Iron deficiency in blood donors

Blood donation results in a significant iron loss of approximately 200–250 mg per donation. Both iron deficiency causing anaemia and iron deficiency in the absence of anaemia are common among donors, particularly though by no means exclusively, in females of

Table 19.2 Infections risks from blood donors.

Categories of risks	Examples of infections	Donor exclusions that may reduce risk
Failure of a test to detect an infectious agent where it should have done so: while this risk is very low, it is not zero and provides a reason to continue strict exclusion practices in the presence of increasingly sensitive testing methods	HIV 1 and 2, hepatitis C, hepatitis B	Excluding at-risk donors identified by questions about risk activities in the past: e.g. drug use or high risk sexual activity at any time in the past
Window-period infections: a donor is infectious with an agent for which the donation is routinely tested, but the infection was acquired so recently that the donor does not yet have detectable infectivity in the blood	HIV 1 and 2, hepatitis C, hepatitis B	Excluding at-risk donors identified by questions about risk activities in the recent past: e.g. recent at-risk sexual activity, recent tattoos or piercings or recent invasive procedures
Infections for which donors are not routinely tested	Malaria, West Nile virus, Chagas' disease, visceral leishmaniasis, vCJD, dengue	Excluding donors, where possible, on the basis of travel or previous residence. This is very difficult in areas of high prevalence and endemicity, and requires additional testing where possible
	Any recently acquired infection that the donor has not yet cleared and that may have a viraemic or bacteraemic phase	Excluding donors on the basis of a recent history of any febrile illness; excluding donors who have recently had a live virus vaccination
Known diseases in the donor's past that may have an unknown transmissible element	Cancer, autoimmune diseases	Excluding donors with a previous history of cancer, with the exception of some localized and cured forms
		Excluding donors with a history of a multisystem autoimmune disease
Risks from unrecognized yet-to-emerge infectious agents	In the recent past HIV and HCV were extensively spread by blood transfusions before the true nature of the diseases became apparent. A similar fate could have arisen with vCJD	Excluding donors with a history of conditions strongly associated in the past with the early and extensive spread of emerging diseases with long incubation periods. Such donors include sex workers and intravenous drug users
		More contentiously, excluding men who have previously had sex with men at any time in their past
		Excluding donors who have previously received blood transfusions
		Excluding xenotransplant recipients
Risk from transmissible spongiform encephalopathies	All prion diseases are considered to have the possibility of an infectious blood phase	Excluding donors who have a strong family history of spongiform encephalopathy
		Excluding donors who have been treated with human-derived pituitary hormones or dura mater
		Outside the UK and Europe, exclusion on the basis of residence in higher risk countries during the BSE epidemic
		In some European countries previous recipients of blood transfusions are excluded to try to limit the risk of transfusion-acquired vCJD

Table 19.3 Deferral criteria for donors of whole blood and blood components. Reproduced from Commission Directive 2004/33/EC of 22 March 2004 implementing Directive 2002/98/EC of the European Parliament and of the Council as regards certain technical requirements for blood and blood components, OJ L 91, 30.3.2004, http://eur-lex.europa.eu, © European Union, 1998–2012.

1 Permanent deferral criteria for donors of allogeneic donations

Cardiovascular disease

Prospective donors with active or past serious cardiovascular disease, except congenital abnormalities with complete cure

Central nervous system disease

A history of serious CNS disease

Abnormal bleeding tendency

Prospective donors who give a history of a coagulopathy

Repeated episodes of syncope or a history of convulsions

Other than childhood convulsions or where at least 3 years have elapsed since the date the donor last took anticonvulsant medication without any recurrence of convulsions

Gastrointestinal, genitourinary, haematological, immunological, metabolic, renal or respiratory system diseases

Prospective donors with serious active, chronic or relapsing disease

Diabetes

If being treated with insulin

Infectious diseases

Hepatitis B, except for HBsAg-negative persons who are demonstrated to be immune

Hepatitis C

HIV-1/2

HTLV I/II

Babesiosis (*)

Kala-azar (visceral leishmaniasis) (*)

Trypanosomiasis cruzi (Chagas' disease) (*)

Malignant diseases except *in situ* cancer with complete recovery

Transmissible spongiform encephalopathies (TSEs) (e.g. Creutzfeldt–Jakob disease, variant Creutzfeldt–Jakob disease)

Persons who have a family history that places them at risk of developing a TSE, or persons who have received a corneal or dura mater graft, or who have been treated in the past with medicines made from human pituitary glands. For variant Creutzfeldt–Jacob disease, further precautionary measures may be recommended.

Intravenous (IV) or intramuscular (IM) drug use

Any history of nonprescribed IV or IM drug use, including bodybuilding steroids or hormones

Xenotransplant recipients

Sexual behaviour

Persons whose sexual behaviour puts them at high risk of acquiring severe infectious diseases that can be transmitted by blood

2 Temporary deferral criteria for donors of allogeneic donations

2.1 *Infections.* Duration of deferral period

After an infectious illness: prospective donors shall be deferred for at least 2 weeks following the date of full clinical recovery. However, the following deferral periods shall apply for the infections listed in the table:

Brucellosis (*): 2 years following the date of full recovery

Osteomyelitis: 2 years after confirmed cured

Q fever (*): 2 years following the date of confirmed cured

Syphilis (*): 1 year following the date of confirmed cured

Toxoplasmosis (*): 6 months following the date of clinical recovery

Tuberculosis: 2 years following the date of confirmed cured

Rheumatic fever: 2 years following the date of cessation of symptoms, unless evidence of chronic heart disease

Fever > °C: 2 weeks following the date of cessation of symptoms

Table 19.3 (*Continued*)

Flu-like illness: 2 weeks after cessation of symptoms

Malaria (*):

  – individuals who have lived in a malarial area within the first 5 years of life:
  3 years following return from last visit to any endemic area, provided person remains symptom free; may be reduced to 4 months if an immunologic or molecular genomic test is negative at each donation;

  – individuals with a history of malaria: 3 years following cessation of treatment *and* absence of symptoms; accept thereafter only if an immunologic or molecular genomic test is negative;

  – asymptomatic visitors to endemic areas: 6 months after leaving the endemic area unless an immunologic or molecular genomic test is negative;

  – individuals with a history of undiagnosed febrile illness during or within 6 months of a visit to an endemic area: 3 years following resolution of symptoms; may be reduced to 4 months if an immunologic or molecular test is negative.

West Nile virus (WNV) (*): 28 days after leaving an area with ongoing transmission of WNV to humans.

2.2 *Exposure to risk of acquiring a transfusion-transmissible infection:*

  – endoscopic examination using flexible instruments;
  – mucosal splash with blood or needlestick injury;
  – transfusion of blood components;
  – tissue or cell transplant of human origin;
  – major surgery;
  – tattoo or body piercing;
  – acupuncture unless performed by a qualified practitioner and with sterile single-use needles;
  – persons at risk due to close household contact with persons with hepatitis B;
  defer for 6 months or for 4 months provided a NAT test for hepatitis C is negative;
  – persons whose behaviour or activity places them at risk of acquiring infectious diseases that may be transmitted by blood; defer after cessation of risk behaviour for a period determined by the disease in question and by the availability of appropriate tests.

2.3 *Vaccination*

Attenuated viruses or bacteria: 4 weeks

Inactivated/killed viruses, bacteria or rickettsiae: no deferral if well

Toxoids: no deferral if well

Hepatitis A or hepatitis B vaccines: no deferral if well and if no exposure

Rabies: no deferral if well and if no exposure. If vaccination is given following exposure defer for 1 year

Tickborne encephalitis vaccines: no deferral if well and if no exposure

2.4 *Other temporary deferrals*

Pregnancy: 6 months after delivery or termination, except in exceptional circumstances and at the discretion of a physician

Minor surgery: 1 week

Dental treatment:

Minor treatment by dentist or dental hygienist (note that tooth extraction, root-filling and similar treatment is considered as minor surgery): defer until next day

Medication: based on the nature of the prescribed medicine, its mode of action and the disease being treated

3 Deferral for particular epidemiological situations

Particular epidemiological situations (e.g. disease outbreaks):

Deferral consistent with the epidemiological situation (these deferrals should be notified by the competent authority to the European Commission with a view to Community action)

(continued)

Table 19.3 (*Continued*)

4 Deferral criteria for donors of autologous donations
  Serious cardiac disease: depending on the clinical setting of the blood collection
  Persons with or with a history of:
  – hepatitis B, except for HBsAg-negative persons who are demonstrated to be immune
  – hepatitis C
  – HIV-1/2
  – HTLV I/II
  Member states may, however, establish specific provisions for autologous donations by such persons. Active bacterial
    infection.

The tests and deferral periods indicated by an asterisk (*) are not required when the donation is used exclusively for plasma for fractionation.

child-bearing age. Iron depletion below a ferritin level of 12 μg/L can be present even when there is no evidence of iron-deficient erythropoiesis. It may cause poor concentration and sleep disturbances, and has been associated with restless legs syndrome. Iron deficiency also arises in donors of plasma or platelets by apheresis due to the red cell losses from blood samples and from the residual amounts of blood in the collection harness. A study of 1535 male and 1487 female Australian blood donors showed that 5.3% of males and 18.9% of females who met the EU criteria for haemoglobin levels were iron deficient as defined by a serum ferritin level of less than 12 μg/L. The prevalence of iron deficiency among the general female population in Australia is 5–7% and is negligible among the general male population [8]. Similar findings were noted in a US study [9].

Iron deficiency among donors may be prevented or treated by adequate intake of oral iron. However, optimum regimens for iron prophylaxis or therapy among blood donors have not been generally defined and practice varies considerably. Options include regular measurement of blood or plasma indices of iron deficiency, routine provision of iron supplements, particularly to female donors, and dietary advice. Fears about the risk of serious iron toxicity in children who accidentally take a donor's iron tablets are probably well founded: iron should be dispensed with adequate warnings, packaging and advice when it is supplied.

Large-scale studies and technical developments will be required to optimize the approach to screening donors to prevent morbidity from anaemia and iron deficiency.

The blood collection/donation process

Assessing the donor, collecting and storing the information obtained, collecting the unit of blood and the accompanying blood samples, and storing and transporting the collected blood are all critical manufacturing steps in the preparation of the final therapeutic product. The entire process needs to be controlled within a functioning quality system, while maintaining the humanity of the process, and especially the dignity of the donor. The venue must be clean, warm, but not excessively so, uncluttered, bright and without excessive noise. Staff should not be distracted or distressed by extraneous events. There must be appropriate space available for confidential discussions between donors and staff. The flow of the donor from reception through registration, interview, haemoglobin check if done, and venesection should be orderly and unidirectional. Allocation of numbers and labels for the units collected must be rigorously controlled; a mix up in labels between units or between samples is a potentially fatal error. Materials used in the collection clinic – bags, antiseptic wipes, mixer-weighers, haemoglobinometers, etc. – must all be controlled.

Several blood services do not take a blood collection from a donor on their first attendance. Instead, they take a sample for blood group, blood count and virus screen. This practice almost guarantees that a unit of blood will not be mislabelled with the wrong ABO group provided an automated check against historical donor records is in place; it also provides some protection against window period donations from people who are donating for the purposes of getting an

HIV or hepatitis test. It is, however, very costly – a significant proportion of blood in most services come from first time and once-only donors.

Preparation of the venepuncture site must also be rigorously controlled to reduce the risk of bacterial contamination; this is discussed in Chapter 14. This process and indeed all collection activities should be subject to regular audit.

Donors may be recruited or retained to donate for apheresis as well as, or instead of, whole blood. Apheresis may be for red cells, usually as a double dose from larger donors, platelets or plasma, or combinations of these. Donor acceptance or rejection criteria are similar to those for whole blood donors, though plasma donors may be exempted for some infectious risks (Table 19.3). Platelet and plasma donation intervals are shorter. Since patients receiving apheresis platelets, and to a lesser extent apheresis red cells, receive fewer donor exposures, there is a benefit to using these components as much as possible. For selected products, such as HPA-1a negative platelets, apheresis is the only viable approach. Apheresis is generally a more expensive method of providing components than whole blood collection and processing, but the economics vary from place to place. In addition, apheresis donation can be a very effective way of maximizing the return to a blood service from many of its committed donors.

Much of the plasma used in the manufacture of blood components comes from apheresis donors, many of whom are paid and who can donate up to twice weekly. Populations of paid plasma donors have a higher prevalence and incidence of infectious disease markers than nonremunerated donors, but since the early 1990s blood component manufacture has had a very good safety record from the point of view of transmission of infectious diseases. This has been achieved by increased donor screening and exclusion procedures, advances in testing, including the introduction of nucleic acid testing for viruses, and effective methods of pathogen removal or inactivation, such as pasteurization, solvent detergent treatment and nanofiltration. As things stand at present, the supply of manufactured blood components worldwide could probably not be maintained without paid plasma donation, though several countries have in the past supplied their national needs for blood components from nonremunerated donors, and several of these still do.

Obligations to donors

Although donors are well and are not seeking care, they are subjected to a healthcare intervention from the moment they begin to complete the history questionnaire. The blood service enters a contract with them and develops an ethical obligation to them from the very start of the first attendance. The service's main duty of care is to the recipient of the donation, and it cannot compromise that, but it has obligations to the donor that must also be discharged. Donation is not a right, but rights accrue to the donor once the process is embarked upon.

The donor has a right:
• to confidentiality and autonomy;
• to informed consent;
• to protection from harm – this includes not being made to feel unhealthy when they are merely outside donation specifications;
• to receive the results of tests when these are of significance to their health;
• they are entitled to receive direction and counselling around the results of such tests;
• they must be protected as much as possible from adverse events or reactions by the use of adequate facilities, adequately trained staff, provision of clear and accurate information, and 24-hour access to advice after donation.

In turn, donors are required:
• to identify themselves correctly;
• to be truthful in their answers to the screening questions – in some countries this obligation is explicitly stated to have the force of the law behind it; and
• to inform the blood service if any change arises in their health after they have donated.

In some services, donors are also provided with a form or a phone number they can use if they have knowingly withheld important information during the screening process that they have been too embarrassed to give at interview. This process, termed confidential unit exclusion, is still in use in some countries. It may provide some protection against donations in the window period, but it may also encourage donors to withhold information at the point where it should be given; this in turn would compromise blood safety.

Donors also have some rights in relation to the use of their donation – the consent that they give must include the possibility that the donation may not be used for the therapeutic use that they assume, but that it might expire unused or be used for control purposes. Where a unit of blood is collected specifically for control, test or calibration purposes, the donor is entitled to be asked to give explicit consent for that. Lastly, donors have a right to expect that healthcare providers will take account of the unique nature of the medicine that they are using, and ensure ethical and appropriate use.

Key points

1 The incidence and prevalence of infectious diseases are higher among donors who donate for personal economic gain.
2 Iron deficiency is common among donors; it can occur in the absence of anaemia and even of iron-deficient erythropoiesis and may cause symptoms such as poor concentration and sleep disturbances.
3 Assessing the donor, collecting and storing the information obtained, collecting the unit of blood and the accompanying blood samples, and storing and transporting the collected blood are all critical manufacturing steps in the preparation of the final therapeutic product.
4 The donor has a right to confidentiality and autonomy, informed consent and protection from harm.
5 Clinicians should take account of the unique nature of blood components as a medicine, so as to avoid wastage and ensure appropriate use.

References

1 Ringwald J, Zimmermann R & Eckstein R. Keys to open the door for blood donors to return. *Transfus Med Rev* 2010; 24: 295–304.
2 Newman PH & Roth AJ. Estimating the probability of a blood donation adverse event based on 1000 post donation interviewed whole-blood donors. *Transfusion* 2005; 45: 1715–1721.
3 Sorensen B & Jorgensen J. International bench marking of severe complications related to blood donation. *Vox Sanguinis* 2010; 99: 294.
4 Sorensen BS, Johnsen SP & Jorgensen J. Complications related to blood donation: a population-based study. *Vox Sanguinis* 2008; 94: 132–137.
5 Eder AF, Hillyer CD, Dy BA, Notari 4th EP & Benjamin RJ. Adverse reactions to allogeneic whole blood donation by 16- and 17-year-olds. *J Am Med Assoc* 2008, May 21; 299(19): 2279–2286.
6 Eder AF. Improving safety for young blood donors. *Transfus Med Rev* 2012; 26: 14–26.
7 Tong E, Murphy WG, Kinsella A, Darragh E, Woods J, Murphy C & McSweeney E. Capillary and venous haemoglobin levels in blood donors: a 42-month study of 36,258 paired samples. *Vox Sanguinis* 2010, May; 98(4): 547–553.
8 Farrugia A. Iron and blood donation – an under recognised safety issue. *Dev Biol (Basel)* 2006; 127: 137–146.
9 Bryant BJ, Yau YY, Arceo SM, Daniel-Johnson J, Hopkins JA & Leitman SF. Iron replacement therapy in the routine management of blood donors. *Transfusion* 2012; 52: 1566–1575.
10 Amrein K, Valentin A, Lanzer G & Drexler C Adverse events and safety issues in blood donation – a comprehensive review. *Blood Rev* 2012; 26: 33–42.

Further reading

Council of Europe. Final Report – Collection, testing and use of blood and blood products in Europe in 2003. Strasbourg: Council of Europe Publishing. Available at: http://www.edqm.eu/medias/fichiers/2003_Report_on_the_collection_testing_and_use_of_blood_and_blood_products_in_Europe.pdf.

Crusz TAM. Adverse events of blood donation. *Blood Matters* 2007; 22. NHS Blood and Transplant. Available at: www.blood.co.uk/pdfdocs/blood_matters_22.pdf.

European Commission. Commission Directive 2004/33/EC of 22 March 2004 implementing Directive 2002/98/EC of the European Parliament and of the Council as regards certain technical requirements for blood and blood components. *Official Journal of the European Union* 2004; L9: 25–39.

ISBT Working Party on Haemovigilance. Standard for Collecting and Presentation of Data on Complications Related to Blood Donation. 2007. Available at: www.isbt-web.org/documentation.

Van der Poel CL. Remuneration of blood donors: new proof of the pudding? *Vox Sanguinis* 2008; 94(3): 169–170.

Van der Poel CL, Seifried E & Schaasberg WP. Paying for blood donations: still a risk? *Vox Sanguinis* 2002; 83(4): 285–293.

20

Blood donation testing and the safety of the blood supply

Richard Tedder[1], Simon J. Stanworth[2] & Mindy Goldman[3]

[1]NHSBT/HPA Epidemiology Unit, NHS Blood and Transplant, Colindale, London, UK
[2]University of Oxford and NHS Blood and Transplant and Department of Haematology, John Radcliffe Hospital, Oxford, UK
[3]Canadian Blood Services, Ottawa, Ontario, Canada

Introduction

This chapter describes the aims and methods of laboratory testing of blood donations. It focuses not only on the range of tests currently employed but also on operational aspects crucial for the safe and efficient application of this process to the thousands of samples received in a blood centre laboratory each day [1, 2]. Testing is dealt with under three headings:
- red cell serological testing;
- microbiological testing and donor follow-up;
- operational and quality control issues.

Red cell serological testing

It is mandatory to test every blood donation for:
- ABO blood group;
- RhD blood group; and
- presence of irregular red cell antibodies.

The results from these tests are necessary for safe transfusion practice in order to reduce the risk of premature destruction of the transfused donor red cells in a recipient's circulation due to immunological incompatibility towards the major red cell antigens. Correct ABO blood group typing is critical, since naturally occurring antibodies can cause intravascular hemolysis and severe transfusion reactions if incompatible components, particularly red cells, are transfused. The RhD antigen is highly immunogenic and RhD negative recipients should only be transfused with RhD antigen negative red cells to avoid alloimmunization.

A more extensive red cell phenotype, including full Rh and Kell typing, may be performed on the entire inventory or a subset of donations, with variable practice between blood services. More extensively phenotyped red cells are needed for transfusion support of particular patient groups (e.g. thalassaemia, sickle disorders) where risks of alloimmunization are high because of the patient requirement for multiple red cell transfusions. Some blood services, such as the National Health Service Blood and Transplant (NHSBT) supplying hospitals in England and North Wales, have current policies to perform full Rh and Kell phenotyping on all donations, largely for operational reasons; others operate phenotyping on selected units for specific patient groups to prevent alloimmunization by selecting Rh and Kell compatible blood.

Samples

Tests are carried out on anticoagulated venous blood samples collected at the time of donation. The samples are identified by a unique bar-coded identification system, which in most countries is an International Society for Blood Transfusion (ISBT) 128 number consistent with the aims of international conformity in blood

---

Practical Transfusion Medicine, Fourth Edition. Edited by Michael F. Murphy, Derwood H. Pamphilon and Nancy M. Heddle.
© 2013 John Wiley & Sons, Ltd. Published 2013 by John Wiley & Sons, Ltd.

group labelling and which ensures that each donation has a unique number. Detailed specifications and guidance on the testing reagents required for blood grouping can be found in appropriate documents, such as the UK Blood Transfusion Service Guidelines ('Red Book') or the AABB Standards for Blood Banks and Transfusion Services. The following paragraphs highlight some key operational principles.

ABO grouping

Donor red cells are tested with monoclonal anti-A and anti-B antibodies, which are capable of detecting all subgroups of these red cell glycoproteins. A reverse grouping is also performed by testing the donor plasma with A and B reagent cells. The exact cells specified varies by blood transfusion service (e.g. NHSBT uses Group A1 and B reagent red cells for new donations).

Most blood services make use of automated systems for serology testing where batched samples are divided into separate microtitre plate wells. The test results are read photometrically and the pattern of results obtained from testing donor red cells and donor plasma analysed by microprocessors to establish the ABO blood group result for a particular donation. The forward and reverse ABO group must be concordant in order to assign a donor blood group. In the case of repeat donors, such a system also allows the results for ABO groupings to be compared with those generated previously.

RhD grouping

RhD grouping is performed by testing donor red cells with two different highly sensitive monoclonal anti-D reagents. In many countries, RhD-negative first-time donors undergo further testing using an alternative method to confirm that they are D-negative. Use of sensitive reagents and repeat testing are done to optimize the detection of weak or partial D-bearing red cells. This would include all the weaker Rh variants, including category D^{VI}. It is felt to be essential that blood services identify and consider all such donors as RhD positive in view of the highly immunogenic capability of the D antigen, even if some of these donors may be considered as D-negative if they were transfusion recipients or prenatal patients.

Detection of irregular blood group antibodies

Donor samples are tested to exclude the presence of red cell antibodies that could cause reduced red cell survival or haemolysis when transfused into recipients whose red cells are positive for the relevant antigen(s). This test is termed an antibody screen and involves the mixing and testing of donor plasma with group O R_1R_2 K-positive red cells, which are also positive for the majority of other red cell antigens thought to be clinically significant.

Blood services are largely concerned with the detection of high levels of clinically significant antibodies in donations. Methods and reagent cells used to detect antibodies are less sensitive than those used for pretransfusion testing in hospitals. Red cell units for transfusion are suspended in anticoagulant nutritive solutions and, depending on the manufacturing and processing process in use, will contain only a small volume of plasma. Weak antibodies in donor plasma will therefore be considerably diluted during processing or transfusion. In contrast, hospital blood bank practice initially requires stringent detection of any antibodies in a potential recipient, irrespective of the level, in part due to the possibility of developing a secondary immune response on re-exposure to the same antigen.

In some blood services, such as in the UK, blood for neonatal transfusion is tested for irregular antibodies to a higher level of sensitivity than standard testing for all other blood in order to further minimize the very small risk of transfusion reactions due to passive transfer of antibodies in this specific group of patients.

High titre anti-A and anti-B

Some group O donors may have (unexpectedly) high titres of anti-A and anti-B in their plasma that could cause lysis of A and/or B cells, particularly where large volumes of plasma are transfused. Recipients should receive group-specific or AB plasma to avoid haemolytic reactions.

Standard practice in hospitals is to transfuse group-specific red cells to all recipients. However, group O red cells may be transfused to certain groups of patients, such as neonates and patients requiring urgent transfusion before their blood group is known. In practice, because most red cell units are stored in additive solutions for preservation, the amount of plasma ultimately transfused is very small, so any risks of haemolysis for a transfusion of group O red cells with high-titre anti-A and anti-B are very low. It might be considered important to screen for hemolysins for large-volume red cell transfusions when planned for neonates.

Since platelets for transfusion have a short shelf life, it is not always possible to provide group-specific platelet transfusions. Several cases of haemolysis have been reported in group A recipients receiving group O platelets and, more rarely, in group B recipients receiving group O platelets; paediatric/neonatal patients appear to be at highest risk.

Plasma containing high-titre haemolysins can be screened in the blood service laboratory by observing the reactions between donor plasma and a diluted sample of reagent A_1B red cells; products that are negative for testing for high titre haemolysins are then labelled for issue. This can be done using automated systems.

Very occasionally, high titre anti-A may be found in group B donations (and vice versa). Recent refinements to testing for high titre haemolysins include methods to assess only the more clinically relevant IgG (rather than a combination of IgG and IgM) fraction. There is no standard method of testing for high titre haemolysins and the acceptable cut-off titre varies greatly with the technique used, thereby requiring local assessment of the procedures used.

Supplementary testing

Not infrequently, anomalies appear in some of the above test results and will preclude accurate conclusions based on the test results. For example, it has been estimated that 1 in 10 000 blood donors have a positive direct antiglobulin test (DAT) at the time of donation, which could interfere with some of the above assays. Weakly positive DAT may also not be detected in the routine grouping tests, which include a control for donor red cells mixed with inert serum. These donations may cause problems in hospital blood banks, since they would appear incompatible after crossmatching by indirect antiglobulin test (IAT). Subsequent donations from these donors will be 'flagged' and monitored as the positive DAT may be transient. Donors with positive DAT results on several donations may be deferred and advised to see their physician in order to have an evaluation done for possible clinical significance and underlying disorders.

In some cases where samples from donations give anomalous automated blood grouping results, the blood service laboratory may have to resort to manual techniques to identify the blood group or antibodies correctly. In general, only antibodies reacting in the IAT are considered to be clinically significant. In the case of some donations with, for example, identified anti-D or anti-c at low levels, the red cells may still be released for transfusion, since during component preparation the amount of antibody-containing plasma will be very small and diluted with an additive storage solution.

Phenotyped red blood cells

Many blood services undertake a more comprehensive red cell antigen phenotyping service in order to identify donors whose red cells could be used for transfusion to alloimmunized recipients or to patients at high risk of forming multiple alloantibodies, e.g. sickle cell disease. This involves phenotyping for Rh C/E and Kell, if not routinely done on all units, as well as for S, s, $Fy^{a/b}$, $Jk^{a/b}$, Kp^a and Lu^a. Where donations are tested and found negative for the antigens listed above, this information may be printed on the blood group label to aid hospitals with selection of blood for patients with antibodies.

In other selected groups of donations, different specific red cell phenotyping may be arranged. Testing may be done on individuals of Afro-Caribbean origin, to meet the needs of sickle cell anaemia patients for antigen-matched units. For example, the U antigen is far more likely to be absent in Afro-Caribbean individuals than in Caucasians. This facilitates the provision of U-negative blood required for transfusion to those individuals who have developed anti-U, which is a clinically relevant antibody.

Increasingly, molecular biology microarray technology is being used to perform mass genotyping of donors for multiple blood group systems. Results for donors missing a high frequency antigen, or with a combination of antigen negative alleles, are then reconfirmed using serological methods, since genotyping methods are not currently licensed.

Testing for HbS may be performed on a subset of units with particular phenotypes likely to be used for transfusion support for patients with sickle cell disease or to neonates during exchange transfusions. The need for a sickle cell screening test depends on the prevalence of HbS within the donor population. An additional consideration is the need to provide counselling support to inform donors found to be carriers of HbS. Of recent interest, it has been found that sickle trait (HbAS) blood significantly interferes with the function of some filters currently used for leucocyte reduction (Chapter 21). Such 'failed' donations would be discarded, but the pattern of red cell antigens in these individuals could be unique and very useful as a transfusion resource. In addition, HbAS units do not freeze well using current methods.

Microbiological testing of blood donations and donor follow-up

A wide range of infectious agents have been documented as transmissible by blood transfusion and these are described in Chapter 13. Donor selection criteria and the use of established guidelines to defer individuals at risk of infection are the important first steps aimed at reducing the risk of collecting blood donations with the potential to transmit infection. For some agents, no laboratory testing is currently available and donor criteria are the only means of deferring at-risk donors. Where testing is available, donor criteria are still important, particularly with respect to the collection of blood from donors who may be in the 'window period' of an infection where they are asymptomatic and have negative testing results, but are still infectious. Laboratory screening tests form the core of the process to identify infected blood components prior to transfusion [3].

Samples

Tests are usually carried out on serum or plasma venous samples collected at the time of donation and sent to highly automated centralized donor testing laboratories. In certain European countries, such as the Netherlands, donors undergo an initial screening process where eligibility is assessed using a questionnaire and blood samples are taken for testing without the collection of a unit of blood. In other countries this happens at the time of the first and all subsequent donations. As with samples for serological blood grouping, correct labelling of microbiological samples to ensure traceability of results is extremely important. Most tests are performed on individual donor samples, but nucleic acid testing (NAT) is often performed on small pools of samples from 6 to 24 donors, termed minipool testing; serological testing for HTLV infection may also be conducted on minipools.

Testing process and donor management

Sensitivity and specificity are important test attributes. Sensitivity refers to the ability of the test to identify truly infected individuals correctly. From the perspective of the transfusion recipient, sensitivity is the most important criterion for a laboratory screening test, i.e. the test will accurately identify infected donors. Specificity refers to the ability of the test to identify correctly donors who are not infected. Specificity is important both to avoid discarding donations from donors who are actually not infected and to reduce the resulting confirmatory workload necessary to provide appropriate donor counselling of those whose samples are reactive in a screening assay. Although most currently used screening assays show remarkably high levels of both specificity and sensitivity it is essential that additional assays are available to confirm infection in the donor.

Principles of investigating a repeat-reactive sample

If an initial screening test is reactive, it will be repeated on the same sample. If the repeat test, in duplicate, is negative, the overall result is considered negative, the blood donation will be used and the donor may continue to donate. If the repeat test is again reactive, a confirmatory or supplementary test is performed to establish whether the screening test result represents a true positive donor sample. Since donors usually constitute a low prevalence population, despite the high specificity of screening tests, there will be significant numbers of samples from donors being identified as repeatedly reactive on screening but who are not confirmed to be positive on supplementary testing (termed false-positive or nonspecific reactions). These donors are deferred from further donation, although some blood services permit donors with false-positive results to be re-tested after a defined deferral period and to be re-integrated as donors if all test results are negative or where supplemental testing indicates that a reaction is falsely positive and an alternative assay of similar sensitivity is negative. These algorithms are termed donor re-entry protocols.

Blood services must have policies for notifying donors with repeat reactive test results and particularly for those where the reactions indicate a donor to be infected. A post-test discussion may be carried out by blood service personnel or information may be forwarded to the donor's general practitioner or physician for further discussion of the results and advice regarding any personal, family and public health measures. In addition, in some countries, the law requires forwarding of details on a first identification of an infected person for some infections, such as HBV, to public health authorities. For donors with false-positive test results, it can be difficult to explain that although the test almost certainly represents a false-positive reaction, the individual may be deferred as a blood donor. This may be explained by an understandable wish to avoid all the very necessary activity undertaken by a transfusion service every time a 'reactive' donor is encountered.

When a sample from an established donor is found to be repeat reactive for one of the mandatory microbiology tests, e.g. HIV or HBV, components from previous donations that may still be in the inventory will be retrieved and discarded on the basis of wishing to exclude a potential window infection at the time of the earlier donation. If the donor is confirmed to be infected, any components remaining in the inventory will be recalled. On a case-by-case basis recipients of earlier components from the donor will be identified, notified and offered relevant testing and management, a process termed 'lookback'. Archived samples of plasma from the last negative donation may also be retrieved and tested with assays more proficient in identifying window infections. Where it is found that an infective plasma donation may have entered a plasma pool prior to fractionation, the fractionators should be informed. Again, on a case-by-case basis, all involved products should be identified and consideration given to their removal from inventory and notification of recipients. With improvements in testing and shortening of the window period, the likelihood of identifying an infected recipient and an infectious component/product on lookback investigation has decreased substantially.

Principles of infectious disease testing methodology

Screening tests may detect the host immune response to the microbial agent (such as antibody to HCV), a microbial antigen (such as the hepatitis B surface antigen, HBsAg) or the nucleic acid of the microbe (NAT). For bacteria, although NAT could be applied, screening tests may detect a component of the organism or a by-product of bacterial growth. Testing for bacterial growth is covered in Chapter 14.

Immunoassays

Immunoassay principles, using enzyme or chemiluminescent techniques of detection, have formed the basis for infectious disease testing [4, 5]. Traditionally, donor plasma at a fixed dilution is incubated over a solid phase where an antigen–antibody interaction occurs. After incubation and then washing, the products of the antigen–antibody interaction are detected by a revealing agent. Detection may involve a conjugate linked to an enzyme, usually peroxidase, which can be detected photometrically after addition of substrate, which produces colour, or by chemiluminescence, in which the optical measuring device detects photons emitted by the chemiluminescent reaction. Until relatively recently, serological assays were constructed to detect either antibody, the most commonly used modality, or antigen, a modality almost exclusively used for detection of HBsAg. The recognition of viral antigenaemia as a feature of early window infections spawned the development initially of antigen-only assays for HIV (p24Ag) and then for HCV (p22Ag). Though not analytically as sensitive as NAT they have proved useful diagnostically.

The more recent development of combined antigen and antibody assays, often referred to as 'Combo assays', provides operationally convenient single well tests for the detection of infection in the acute window phase as well as the antibody response to infection. Many blood services adopted the HIV Combo assay but few, if any, have taken up the HCV Combo assay in view of already having established HCV NAT. The sensitivity reduction of NAT through pooling renders sensitive antigen-only assays on individual donation testing an analytic advantage, such that HBsAg assays are similar in proficiency to HBV DNA NAT for detecting acute phase infections. However, the assay conditions for combined antigen/antibody detection disfavour the antigen modality and the resulting analytic sensitivity for antigens in the Combo assays appear somewhat reduced. Nevertheless, in situations where the frequency of incident (i.e. acute) infections is common Combo assays may still have merit if NAT assays are not available.

Antibody assays for donor screening must be of the highest sensitivity for detecting early serologic responses in the acutely infected donor. Since the *in vivo* development of detectable antibody is a host response to microbial antigens this marker is invariably delayed in the infection time course, which has led to the use of a term 'antibody window' – hence the phrase 'window infection' used previously. Proficiency at this stage requires characterization of the early antibody response and enhancement of the detection of the specific early antibodies, e.g. anti-p24 in HIV and in some cases enhancing detecting IgM class antibody. Once the antibody response has matured the remaining concerns centre around whether the antibody response to extreme microbial variants can still be detected on the 'routine' assay. One example was the realization that HIV 2 infection could not be reliably detected by early HIV tests based on HIV 1 components; similarly, the detection of malarial antibodies is influenced by the infecting species.

All immunoassays depend on the interaction between microbial antigens and antibodies. Where an antibody is a component reagent of the detection system there has been a shift to the use of monoclonal antibodies. These are chosen to have high avidity and are often directed at 'conserved' antigenic epitopes. The resulting narrow specificity is an advantage in terms of driving down background rates of nonspecific reaction, but this comes at a cost of susceptibility to mutations in the target epitope, rendering the antigen undetectable. Assays for HBsAg detection used in donor screening must be secure in detecting HBsAg mutants, especially the classical vaccine escape variant G145R.

Nucleic acid testing (NAT)

In NAT, nucleic acid is extracted from the donor plasma. A nucleic acid amplification test such as polymerase chain reaction (PCR) or transcription-mediated amplification (TMA) is then used to amplify and detect microbial genetic sequences. Testing is usually done on small pools of from 6 to 24 donor samples, termed minipools, depending on the methodology used. Single-donor testing may be considered in particular circumstances to enhance sensitivity but such a policy will increase unit costs. Single-sample

testing may also be required for resolution of a reactive pool to determine which donor sample contains the microbial target. Testing may be done for each agent individually or to identify several agents (HIV, HBV and HCV) simultaneously in a single reaction, when they are termed multiplex assays. Newer, completely automated platforms have reduced the operational complexity of testing. NAT, like antigen testing, reduces the window period when donors may be infectious but have negative serologic testing results in the period before the immune response becomes detectable. Window periods using serological assays are estimated in the order of 59 days for anti-HCV, 15 days for anti-HIV and 67 days for HBV. Window periods using minipool NAT are estimated in the order of 8 days for HCV, 9.5 days for HIV and 38 days for HBV. The utility of NAT depends on the incidence of these acute infections in the donor population, which in turn determines the incidence of window period donations that would be missed on antibody-only serologic testing. In countries such as the UK, Canada and the USA, where incidence rates are extremely low, the NAT yield, i.e. the number of infectious donations detected by NAT alone, has been extremely low, in the order of 1 in 1 million donations or lower. In contrast, the NAT yield has been considerably higher in countries such as South Africa, with a higher incidence of HIV infection in donors. The changing epizoology of arthropod-borne infections, e.g. West Nile and Chikungunya viruses, and other zoonotic infections, e.g. hepatitis E virus, are targets for discretionary NAT, the introduction being mandated by disease activity in any location. In each of these examples the infectious donors are those in the preclinical preantibody phase of acute infection, accessible only to either antigen or NAT assays.

Screening tests and donor–recipient matching

Table 20.1 lists the screening tests used in transfusion microbiology in different countries [6–8]. Some tests are mandatory and used to screen all donations. Other tests may be discretionary and used on selected groups of donors who are identified as being at particularly high risk for infection. In some situations additional testing may be required to mitigate transfusion transmission risks. CMV antibody testing may be done on a subset of donations in order to provide CMV

Table 20.1 Screening tests on blood donations in five countries as of 2011 (adapted from O'Brien *et al.* [2]).

Infection	Test	USA	Canada	France	UK	Australia
HIV 1,2	HIV antibody	✓	✓	✓	✓	✓
	HIV NAT	✓	✓	✓	✓	✓
HCV	HCV antibody	✓	✓	✓	✓	✓
	HCV NAT	✓	✓	✓	✓	✓
HBV	HBV surface antigen (HBsAg)	✓	✓	✓	✓	✓
	HBV NAT	Most centres	✓	✓	✓	✓
	Antibody to HBV core antigen (anti-HBC)	✓	✓	✓	Selective	Selective
HTLV I/II	HTLV antibody	✓	✓	✓	✓(Pooled)	✓
Syphilis	*Treponemal* antibody	✓	✓	✓	✓	✓
Malaria	Malarial antibody	No	No	Selective	Selective	Selective
Chagas	*Trypanosoma cruzi* antibody	Selective	Selective	Selective	Selective	No
West Nile virus	West Nile virus NAT	✓	✓	No	No	No

✓Indicates testing on all donations.

seronegative components for immunosuppressed or other susceptible patients at risk of severe CMV infection on the assumption that this strategy removes the risk CMV viraemia. Such a policy does not, however, remove the risk posed by incident CMV and some services prefer to use blood from CMV seropositive donors who are known to have been seropositive from previous donations. Other herpes viruses including the gammaviruses EBV and HHV8 might justify screening on occasion. The conditions of storage of blood or blood components, in particular plasma, and the manufacture of components into blood products will materially affect the transmissibility of an infection; so too will leucocyte reduction, which removes the majority of leucocytes that may harbour cell bound viruses such as the HTLV agents. Pooling of plasma may also require additional NAT testing of the start pool for a range of agents including HAV, HEV and parvovirus B19. The decision to implement a particular screening test in a country depends on consideration of a number of factors, including the incidence and prevalence of the infectious disease in the donor population, the available testing technologies and the known or anticipated morbidity associated with transfusion-transmitted infection. Regulatory requirements for testing and the availability of test kits specifically licensed for donor screening also play an important role.

Quality framework and operational issues

Ultimately, the microbiological and blood group safety of the blood supply depends on the input and interaction of a number of quality and operational factors.

A formal quality management system is an important part of ensuring that blood donation testing is adequately performed. The quality system needs to meet the requirements of a 'Competent Authority' under EU blood safety directives. Inspections are carried out by the Medicines and Healthcare Products Regulatory Authority (MHRA) in the UK. In the USA, there are both Food and Drug Administration (FDA) regulations and extensive requirements from professional accrediting organizations such as the AABB regarding quality requirements. Testing must be performed only by staff trained in approved standard operating procedures (SOPs). Document control systems must be in place to ensure that only current procedures are used and any changes documented and approved. Any errors that occur in laboratory procedures must be logged using a quality incident report (QIR) system, which requires corrective and preventative action to be taken.

The levels of process control now employed by the blood centre donation testing laboratories give a very high level of confidence that the test result for a donation is both valid and correct and that any potentially hazardous material will be discarded.

Most transfusion services have surveillance programmes for monitoring the rate of transmissible infections in blood donors, while haemovigilance schemes in place in several countries monitor transmission of transfusion-transmissible agents. The reporting of serious adverse events and reactions resulting from transfusion is an essential component of blood safety and is regarded as such by international agencies including the WHO and in Europe by its Commissioners.

Key points

1 It is mandatory to test every blood donation for ABO blood group, RhD blood group and the presence of irregular red cell antibodies.
2 A wide range of infectious agents have been documented as transmissible by blood transfusion, and laboratory screening tests form the core of the process to identify infected blood components prior to transfusion.
3 A knowledge of the donor panel demography and protocols for donor deferral and investigation of potentially infectious donors remain important components for maintaining blood safety.
4 Processes must be in place to communicate infectious disease marker results to donors.
5 Many of the newer techniques and kits currently used in blood centres to identify infected blood components show high levels of both specificity and sensitivity.
6 Both immunoassays and nucleic acid testing are used to identify possibly infectious units.
7 A quality framework is important for the accuracy of all laboratory testing.

Acknowledgements

Pat Hewitt, Ian Reeves and Richard Moule (NHS Blood and Transplant).

References

1 *Guidelines for the UK Blood Transfusion Services*, 7th edn. London: HMSO; 2005.
2 Safe Supplies: Focusing on Epidemiology. Annual Review from the NHS Blood and Transplant/Health Protection Agency Colindale Epidemiology Unit, 2010, London, September 2011. Available at: http://www.hpa.org.uk/Topics/InfectiousDiseases/ReferenceLibrary/BIBDReferences/.
3 Galel SA. Infectious disease screening. In: D Roback (ed.), *AABB Technical Manual*, 17th edn. Bethesda, MD: AABB Press; 2011, pp. 239–270.
4 Barbara J, Ramskill S, Perry K, Parry J & Nightingale M. The National Blood Service (England) approach to evaluation of kits for detecting infectious agents. *Transfus Med Rev* 2007; 21(2): 147–158.
5 UK Infection Surveillance Annual Report. Available at: http://www.hpa.org.uk/infections/topics_az/BIBD/publications.htm.-.
6 Transfusion-transmissible infections in Australia, Surveillance Report; 2011. Available at: www.med.unsw.edu.au.
7 Zou S *et al*. Donor testing and risk current prevalence, incidence, and residual risk for transfusion-transmissible agents in US allogeneic donations. *Transfus Med Rev* 2012; 26: 119–128.
8 O'Brien SF, Zou S, Laperche S, Brant LJ, Seed CR & Kleinman SH. Surveillance of transfusion-transmissible infections – comparison of systems in five developed countries. *Transfus Med Rev* 2012; 26: 38–57.

Further reading

Advent ND. Large-scale blood group genotyping: clinical implications. *Br J Haematol* 2009; 144: 3–13.
Campell-Lee SA. The future of red cell alloimmunization. *Transfusion* 2007; 47: 1959–1960.
Hillyer CD, Shaz BH, Winkler AM & Reid M. Integrating molecular technologies for red blood cell typing and compatibility testing into blood centers and transfusion services. *Transfus Med Rev* 2008; 22: 117–132.
Josephson CD, Castillejo MI, Grima K & Hillyer CD. ABO-mismatched platelet transfusion: strategies to mitigate patient exposure to naturally occurring hemolytic antibodies. *Transfus Apher Sci* 2010; 42: 83–88.
Kiely P & Wood E. Can we improve the management of blood donors with nonspecific reactivity in viral screening and confirmatory assays? *Transfus Med Rev* 2005; 19(1): 58–65.

21 Production and storage of blood components

Rebecca Cardigan[1] & Stephen Thomas[2]
[1]NHS Blood and Transplant, Cambridge, UK
[2]NHS Blood and Transplant, Brentwood, UK

Whole blood and its processing to components

Guidelines from the UK, Council of Europe and AABB define a blood donation as 450 mL ± 10% of blood collected into citrate anticoagulant also containing phosphate and dextrose. There are no absolute indications for transfusion of whole blood and the vast majority of blood units collected are processed to components – red cell and platelet concentrates, and plasma. Such plasma is suitable for either fractionation to plasma derivatives or freezing as whole fresh frozen plasma (FFP).

Component production from whole blood consists of centrifugation to separate out plasma and cells of different density, followed by manual or automated transfer of components from the primary collection pack to transfer packs. Collection and transfer packs are manufactured as a single closed unit to maintain sterility.

Whole blood donations from which platelets are to be harvested must be held and processed at 20–24°C, but, for other donations, pre-processing storage and centrifugation can be at either 22 or 4°C. Some countries hold all blood overnight at 22°C prior to component production, which yields components of acceptable quality.

There remains a small but finite risk of transmission of viruses via single-unit or small pool blood components. Techniques for pathogen inactivation of FFP and platelets are now available in Europe and are under development for red cells. These are discussed in the appropriate sections below.

Collection of components by apheresis

Apheresis involves separation of the blood into components during collection on specially designed equipment, the harvesting of specific blood elements and return of the rest of the blood to the donor. Because there is less loss of iron, plasma and platelet apheresis donors can donate monthly, and plateletpheresis permits collection of 1–3 adult doses/procedure, depending on the donor. Apheresis has been regarded as a more risky procedure than whole blood donation and tended to be undertaken only in donor clinics with trained nursing and medical staff available. However, apheresis equipment has developed into small portable machines drawing only a low extracorporeal volume so that they can be used safely on mobile sessions. Such equipment can be programmed flexibly to collect red cells and platelets or plasma, with double red cell collection being another option. An advantage of red cell collection by apheresis is that the haematocrit and haemoglobin content is much more consistent and predictable than in those produced from whole blood donations. In addition, double red cell collections could reduce the number of donors to whom recipients are exposed, which may be particularly relevant for transfusion-dependent and paediatric patients. Thus, the distinction between whole blood donation and apheresis is becoming less,

Practical Transfusion Medicine, Fourth Edition. Edited by Michael F. Murphy, Derwood H. Pamphilon and Nancy M. Heddle.
© 2013 John Wiley & Sons, Ltd. Published 2013 by John Wiley & Sons, Ltd.

and it is likely that 'near donor processing' will expand in future years.

Regulations, specifications and quality monitoring

Specifications for the key parameters of each component type are generally set out in a national guideline, such as those published by the UK Transfusion Services or AABB. European Guidelines published by the Council of Europe are not legally binding, but intended to promote improvements in practice. However, in 2005, the EU directive 2002/98/EC, Setting standards of quality and safety for the collection, testing, processing, storage and distribution of human blood and blood components, became legally binding in the UK as the Blood Safety and Quality Regulations (BSQR) 2005. In the UK, compliance of Blood Establishments with UK Guidelines and the BSQR is regulated by the Medicines and Healthcare Regulatory Authority (MRHA) – for more details see Chapter 17.

Many countries sample a proportion of blood components for quality monitoring to assess compliance with set specifications. The proportion tested is usually determined by statistical process control, but would typically be about 1% of components produced. Statistical process control identifies systems that are capable or performing well and also highlights trends towards poor performance at an early stage so that corrective action can be put in place to address the problem.

Leucocyte reduction of blood components

Many developed countries (although notably not the USA) have implemented universal leucocyte reduction (LR) of blood components. In the UK and Ireland, the risk that variant Creutzfeldt–Jakob disease (vCJD) might be transmissible by blood, and in particular by leucocytes, was the major factor in this decision in 1998 (Chapter 15). In other countries, additional benefits, such as a reduction in immune-related complications and removal of cell-associated viruses, were considered equally important. Adverse immunological effects attributed to leucocytes include HLA alloimmunization, transfusion-associated graft-versus-host disease (TA-GvHD) and immunosuppression, which in turn may lead to increased postoperative sepsis and tumour recurrence. However, universal LR may remove some of the beneficial effects of transfusion-induced immunomodulation, such as improved survival of transplanted kidneys, and suppression of Crohn's disease. These are discussed in detail in Chapter 10.

Production of leucocyte-reduced blood components

LR is completed prior to component storage while the cells are still intact, usually within 48 hours of donation. For whole blood donations this is achieved by filtration, whereas an LR step by centrifugation/elutriation is integral to some apheresis technologies. Most whole blood LR filters remove >2 logs of platelets in addition to >4 logs of leucocytes; therefore, only FFP and red cells can be produced by centrifugation of leucocyte-reduced whole blood (Figure 21.1). To produce platelet concentrates, each component (red cells, plasma or platelets) must be filtered after their separation from whole blood (Figure 21.1). The same processing options apply for

(a) Whole-blood filtration

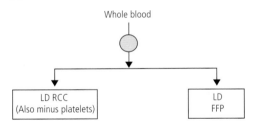

(b) Component filtration

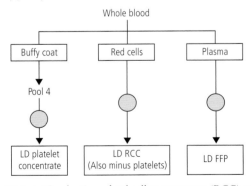

Fig 21.1 (a) Production of red cell concentrates (RCC) and plasma from blood donations. (b) Production of red cell concentrates, platelet concentrates and plasma from blood donations.

Table 21.1 Specifications for leucocyte-reduced blood components.

	UK	Council of Europe/ European Directive	AABB
Level of residual leucocytes	$<5 \times 10^6$/U	$<1 \times 10^6$/U	$<5 \times 10^6$/U for red cells and apheresis platelets $<8.3 \times 10^5$/U for PRP platelets
Percentage of components in which this must be attained	99	90	95
Statistical confidence that this is attained	95%	Not stated	Not stated

non-leucocyte-depleted components, except that the filters are omitted. LR results in a 10–15% loss of volume of whole blood or processed component, but has minimal adverse effects on the quality of blood components.

The specification for leucocyte-reduced components reflects the current capability of LR systems, the fact that only a fraction of components are tested for residual leucocytes and that the limit of sensitivity of current counting methods by flow cytometry is around 0.3×10^6/U. Specifications set by the UK, Council of Europe and AABB appear to be different, but are in fact broadly similar (Table 21.1). Despite advances in technology, LR systems occasionally fail. The risk that an LR system will result in blood components being issued that fail to meet the required specification for residual leucocytes is dependent on a number of factors: the capability of the LR system, potential manufacturing defects in the LR filter or pack system, the proportion of components that are tested for residual leucocytes and donor-related causes. Although most donor-related causes of filter failure are poorly understood, it is known that donors with a sickle cell trait are more likely to either block LR filters or fail to remove leucocytes effectively, and 100% of these donations are therefore usually assessed for residual leucocytes.

Removal of cell-associated viruses and prions by leucocyte reduction

Viruses associated with different leucocyte subtypes include cytomegalovirus (CMV), mainly in monocytes, and other DNA herpes viruses such as Epstein–Barr virus and human herpes virus 8 (in B cells) and T-cell viruses, such as human T-cell lymphotropic virus (HTLV) I and II. Most studies of pre-storage LR have demonstrated its efficacy in preventing transfusion-transmitted CMV, but a recent study has suggested that if enough patients are studied, a small increase in risk might emerge. Bedside filtration appears to be unreliable in this regard. The Council of Europe, the AABB and the British Committee for Standards in Haematology all consider that components leucocyte-reduced before storage are equivalent in safety to those tested as CMV seronegative. A recent review by the Advisory Committee on the Safety of Blood, Tissues and Organs (SaBTO) in the UK has concluded that LR should be considered to offer sufficient CMV protection for most CMV negative patients, with a number of notable exceptions where the risks of transmission remain the same but the consequences of a transmission could be more severe [1]. Information on removal of other viruses by LR is limited, although one study of HTLV-I removal showed incomplete clearance of virus from some asymptomatic carriers [2]. Studies in a rodent red cell transfusion model of vCJD suggest that LR only reduces infectivity by $<50\%$ [3] and LR does not prevent transmission of infectivity in a sheep model [4].

Red cell components (for specifications, see Table 21.2)

For the vast majority of red cell components, an additive solution is introduced following separation, to achieve a haematocrit of 50–70% and maintain red cell quality during storage. Red cells used for intrauterine transfusions (IUT) and exchange transfusion of neonates are normally stored or reconstituted in plasma. The most important changes that occur during storage are loss of intracellular potassium and a reduction in red cell recovery following transfusion. Red cell concentrates in additive solution

211

Table 21.2 Specification and typical values for volume and haemoglobin content for leucocyte-reduced (LR) red cell components.

	Specification						Typical values*		
	Volume (mL)			Hb content (g/unit)					
	UK	EU	AABB	UK	EU	AABB	Volume (mL)	Hb (g/unit)	Plasma volume (mL)
Red cells in additive solution, LR, apheresis	>75%; 220–340 mL	NS	>95%; >128 mL red cells	>75%; >40 g	>40 g	>95%; >42.5	273 ± 17	53 ± 4	22
Red cells in plasma, LR for exchange	NS			>75%; >40 g	NS		338 ± 25	61 ± 4	116
Red cells in additive solution, LR buffy coat removed	>75%; 220–340 mL	NS	NS	>75%; >40 g	>40 g	NS	250 ± 19	49 ± 6	6
Red cells in additive solution, LR	>75%; 220–340 mL	NS	NS	>75%; >40 g	>40 g	NS	304 ± 17	58 ± 5	28

*Based on quality monitoring data from England.

have a 35–42-day shelf life (depending on the how the red cells are produced and the storage solution), at a controlled temperature of 2–6°C. Red cells which are stored only in plasma have a 21–35-day shelf life. To minimize the possibility of bacterial proliferation and maintain viability, red cells should be removed from refrigeration as little as possible. For patients with severe febrile or anaphylactic reactions to red cells or those with immunoglobulin A (IgA) deficiency, red cells are washed and resuspended in saline or an approved additive solution. The objective of washing is to remove as much plasma as possible, as such reactions can be due to antibodies to plasma proteins. At least one closed system for cell washing is now available, which allows red cells to be stored after washing, albeit with a shortened shelf life. Red cells from donors with rare phenotypes or from occasional patients with multiple red cell alloantibodies, for whom provision of compatible donor blood is extremely difficult, can be stored frozen for 30 years. Prior to transfusion, frozen red cells are thawed and washed to remove the cryoprotectant used to store them.

Pathogen inactivation in red cells

Red cells present a challenge for photochemical pathogen inactivation methods due to the high degree of light absorption by haemoglobin. Two systems are currently in development and show some promise. The first, the Intercept system, uses a compound that does not depend on light activation, instead using a long incubation period (18 hours) to allow binding of a linker to the DNA, preventing pathogen replication. The in vitro quality and in vivo recovery of the red cells appears to be satisfactory at the end of their shelf life [5]. However, this was also true for a previous version of the same system, for which phase III chronic transfusion studies were suspended. This was due to antibodies being detected in a small number of recipients – these reacted with red cells after, but not before, pathogen inactivation, raising concern that the treatment step resulted in the formation of neoantigens on red cells. The manufacturer has since modified the system to reduce this risk and phase III trials are currently underway. An alternative system, Mirasol, is being developed to treat whole blood, using riboflavin and a high dose of UV light. It is initially being developed for military use and studies on components produced from inactivated whole blood are ongoing, with the

recovery of red cells in vivo shown to be acceptable [6]. It is likely that it will be 2–5 years before either system for red cells is licensed for routine use.

Prion reduction in red cells

Since leucocyte reduction alone is unlikely to render units free of PrP^{sc}, there is considerable interest in alternative methods to reduce the risk of transmission of vCJD by transfusion. Filters that remove prion protein from red cell concentrates are well advanced in their development, with the P-Capt filter developed by PRDT in collaboration with Macopharma now licensed in Europe. As yet, there are no prion removal filters for whole blood, platelets or single donor plasma. The P-Capt filter requires prior LR, so is associated with a further 10–15% loss of haemoglobin. Prion removal and LR may be combined into one filter in the future, with more than one company working on such an approach. On the basis of current working assumptions on levels of infectivity and prevalence of infection in the UK population, it is predicted that at least 3 log removal of infectivity (in addition to LR) would be needed to provide clinical benefit in terms of preventing transmission of vCJD. The P-Capt prion removal filter has been reported to remove 3–4 logs of infectivity from red cells spiked with scrapie-infected hamster brain and >1.2 log (to below the limit of detection) of infectivity from the blood of hamsters infected with scrapie [7]. The UK transfusion services have also commissioned an independent assessment of the efficacy of prion reduction, since evidence to date has been generated solely by the manufacturers. The P-Capt filter has been shown to have negligible effect on the in vitro quality of red cells, the expression of common red cell antigens or recovery of red cells following transfusion to healthy volunteers. In the UK, SaBTO has recommended that prion filtration be implemented for patients born after 1 January 1996, subject to satisfactory results from a clinical safety study in surgical patients. Post-marketing surveillance would be instigated to monitor unexpected reactions and alloimmunization, with baseline data being collected for 6 months prior to any implementation of prion filtration. The safety study (PRISM) is now complete, and no adverse effects on the safety of transfusion were attributed to the PCapt filter. However, SaBTO has deferred review of the recommendation to implement filtration until the independent evaluation of efficacy is complete. The outcome of the review is expected in 2013.

Platelet concentrates

Platelet production and storage

Platelets may be produced either from whole blood donations or by apheresis, in which platelets with or without plasma are collected and the red cells returned to the donor. Specifications for platelet yield and residual leucocyte count are similar for the two methods (see Table 21.3). Apart from exposing the patient to fewer donors and the possibility of HLA/HPA matching with the patient, apheresis platelets are not intrinsically of higher quality. Platelet production from whole blood may be carried out either from pooled buffy coats generated by bottom and top processing or from platelet-rich plasma (PRP) as an intermediate step (Figure 21.2). Buffy coat-derived platelets have long been favoured in Europe, are standard in the UK and have recently been adopted in Canada, while the PRP method is standard in the USA. LR by filtration may be routinely incorporated into either process. An adult therapeutic dose of platelets ($2.5-3.0 \times 10^{11}$) can be manufactured from buffy coats, or by the PRP method, from four to six whole blood donations. In contrast, with the appropriate selection of donors, 1–3 adult doses can be harvested from a single donor during one apheresis collection procedure.

Platelets are stored with agitation in incubators set at 20–24°C for 5 days, which may be extended to 7 days if a bacterial screening or pathogen inactivation method is used. Platelet concentrates should never be placed in the refrigerator as this impairs the recovery and survival of platelets following transfusion. With pre-storage LR and modern storage packs, platelets stored for 7 days in plasma maintain their *in vitro* function well. Apheresis platelets stored in plasma for 7 days have shown acceptable recovery and survival and several countries are performing additional clinical studies to assess the functionality of platelets stored beyond 5 days. During storage, platelets undergo a fall in pH due to accumulation of lactate, show increased surface expression of activation markers such as P-selectin (CD62P) and change from discoid to round. Many different laboratory assays have been advocated to monitor development of this so-called 'platelet storage lesion' but few have been demonstrated to correlate with *in vivo* survival. pH remains the only quantitative change that must be monitored routinely and must be above 6.2–6.4 at outdate. Visual inspection to look for the 'swirling' effect of discoid platelets has been recommended, but this is highly subjective and changes only when the platelets have been grossly damaged.

For patients with severe anaphylactic-type reactions, which are usually due to plasma proteins, it is possible to prepare platelets to be virtually plasma free by centrifuging the platelet concentrate, removing the supernatant plasma and replacing it with storage medium. The component is sometimes referred to as 'washed platelets', although there is no actual wash step, as this is unnecessary and may lead to platelet activation. Platelet storage media differ from red cell additive solutions in containing some or all of potassium, magnesium, acetate, citrate, phosphate, gluconate and chloride. In Europe, platelets in 100% storage medium have only a 24-hour shelf life, although it is possible that this could be extended using newer solutions containing glucose that are in development. A different component, containing approximately 70% storage medium and 30% plasma is now in production in a number of countries. This strategy makes more plasma available for fractionation, appears to reduce minor allergic reactions and allows a normal shelf life. Clinical data to day 7 and beyond are limited. These solutions have great potential, but require careful validation, which may need to include volunteer and patient studies.

Pathogen reduction in platelets

In order to mitigate the risk of bacterial growth in platelet concentrates stored at 20–24°C and other viral risks, a number of technologies have been developed using UV light, with or without specific additives, to inactivate pathogens. The mode of action of these technologies is to modify nucleic acid, thus preventing replication. This technology has no effect on prions, which lack nucleic acid.

Amotosalen, which belongs to a group of naturally occurring compounds called psoralens, is employed in one system for pathogen inactivation of platelet concentrates (Intercept, S-59). Amotosalen/UV-A treatment results in a high degree of killing of the major transfusion-transmitted viruses HIV, HCV and HBV, and intracellular pathogens such as CMV and HTLV.

Table 21.3 Specification and typical values for volume and platelet content for LR platelet components.

Platelet processing method	Number of donors per dose	Specification								Typical values*	
		Volume (mL)[†]			Platelet content (×10⁹ per unit)					Volume (mL)	Platelet content (×10⁹ per unit)
		UK	EU	AABB	UK	EU	AABB				
PRP	5–10	–	>40 mL per 60 × 10⁹ platelets	Not specified	–	>60	>55[§]				
Apheresis	1–2	Locally defined	>40 mL per 60 × 10⁹ platelets	Not specified	>240[§]	>200	>300[‡]			199 ± 18	278 ± 42
Buffy coat-derived pooled	4–8	Locally defined	>40 mL per 60 × 10⁹ platelets	Not specified	>240[§]	>200	–			296 ± 27	313 ± 48

*Based on quality monitoring data from England.
[†]The volume is also partly dictated by a requirement to keep the pH of platelet components above 6.4 during storage.
[‡]>90% of components must meet this criterion.
[§]>75% of components must meet this criterion.

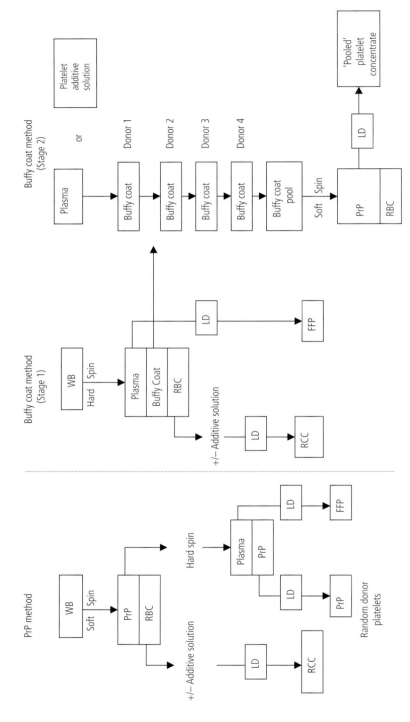

Fig 21.2 Production of platelet components from whole blood.

Following the treatment step, it is necessary to remove the amotosalen from the component prior to storage. A number of randomized clinical trials have been performed and have shown that amotosalen-treated platelets, whether prepared by apheresis or from pooled buffy coats, are effective in preventing haemorrhage in thrombocytopenic patients with haematological malignancies. However, platelet increments and intertransfusion intervals were less favourable than in control patients, raising the possibility that increased numbers of platelet units might be required to support such patients [8, 9]. This question can be answered only by further large-scale clinical studies. A recent study reported an increased risk of bleeding in the treatment group, although the study was open label and not powered with bleeding as the primary endpoint [10].

An alternative system for pathogen reduction in platelets, called Mirasol, has been developed using riboflavin (vitamin B_2) and UV light. A removal step following treatment is not needed. Platelets treated using this system show good *in vitro* quality, and acceptable recovery and survival in healthy subjects. However, as with Intercept-treated platelets, a clinical trial of the component showed lower count increments in the treatment group and more frequent transfusions being necessary, although noninferiority was not demonstrated [11]. A third system in development – the Theraflex system – uses no additive and exposure to UV-C light. *In vitro* studies and recovery and survival studies in healthy volunteers appear acceptable, and phase II/III clinical safety and efficacy studies are now in progress [12].

Both the Intercept and Mirasol systems are licensed in Europe, but not by the FDA in the USA. They are in routine use in some European countries, but not yet the UK. In addition to their inactivation of pathogens, inactivation of leucocytes offers an alternative to irradiation of components to prevent TA-GvHD. Pathogen inactivation of platelets would obviate the need for irradiation and CMV testing of components and for some systems permit a 7 day shelf life; this would simplify platelet stock management and reduce wastage. Their broad range of activity against viruses would also be expected to confer protection against new emerging infections that may be transmitted by transfusion. However, until a red cell pathogen inactivation system is also available, some of these benefits cannot be realized in full.

Fresh frozen plasma

Definition and specification

FFP is the plasma from a single donation, usually 250–300 mL, which has been frozen soon after collection without pooling. FFP can also be derived from apheresis collections, in 300 or 600 mL volumes. It is used primarily as a source of multiple coagulation factors in situations such as massive transfusion, disseminated intravascular coagulation and liver disease (Chapters 26 and 27). The permitted shelf life (12 months to 7 years) depends on the storage temperature. In Europe, FFP must be monitored for levels of factor VIII (Table 21.4). Although most FFP is prescribed for patients with normal or elevated factor VIII levels, it is selected for quality-monitoring purposes, as it is labile and hence sensitive to exposure to adverse conditions. FFP is thawed (in a protective overwrap to prevent bacterial contamination) in a waterbath, a purpose-designed microwave oven or dry heat source. Once thawed, FFP should be used as soon as possible since the levels of labile coagulation factors decline during further storage. Some countries permit thawed plasma to be used for up to 5 days if it is labelled as a different component.

Pathogen inactivation

Four systems for producing pathogen-inactivated FFP are now available and licensed in Europe. Three are suitable for single donor plasma: methylene blue (MB), amotosalen and riboflavin. The other, solvent–detergent (SD) treatment, is applied to pools of plasma. All methods offer good virus protection, but all are associated with loss of clotting factors [13]. The key features of pathogen inactivated FFP are shown in Table 21.5.

MB is a phenothiazine dye which, when exposed to white light, generates reactive oxygen species that damage nucleic acids, preventing viral replication. Treatment is applied to single units of plasma and requires prior removal of leucocytes by filtration or freeze–thawing. The MB is contained in or added to the integral pack system, mixed with the plasma and then placed on a light box for activation. The MB is removed using an adsorption filter prior to final storage of the component, leaving residual MB concentrations of $<0.3\ \mu M$. At these concentrations, no toxicity has been demonstrated or is predicted.

Table 21.4 Specifications and typical values for residual cellular and coagulation factor content of frozen plasma components.

Specification	Residual cellular content ($\times 10^9$/L)*			Coagulation factor content		
	UK†	EU	AABB	UK†	EU	AABB
FFP	Platelets <30 Red cells <6	Platelets <50 Red cells <6	None	FVIII > 0.70 IU/mL	FVIII > 0.70 IU/mL	None
Cryoprecipitate	None	None	None	Fibrinogen > 140 mg/unit FVIII > 70 IU/unit	Fibrinogen > 140 mg/unit FVIII > 70 IU/unit vWF > 100 IU/unit	Fibrinogen > 150 mg/unit FVIII > 80 IU/unit
Cryoprecipitate-depleted plasma	None	None	None	None	None	None

Typical values‡	Residual cellular content	Coagulation factor content	Total volume (mL)
FFP	Platelets < 3×10^9/L Red cells $0.63 \pm 0.50 \times 10^9$/L	FVIII 0.83 ± 0.22 IU/mL	274 ± 14
Cryoprecipitate	–	FVIII 105 ± 29 IU/unit Fibrinogen 396 ± 129 mg/unit	43 ± 4
Cryoprecipitate-depleted plasma	–	–	305 ± 31

*Specifications for residual leucocytes are as per Table 21.1.
†>75% of components must meet these criteria.
‡Based on quality-monitoring data from England.

Table 21.5 Comparison of pathogen inactivation methods for plasma.

	Solvent–detergent	Methylene blue	Intercept	Mirasol
Volume	Depends on supplier, produced from pool of donations	235–315 ml pre-treatment	385–680 ml pre-treatment (need to treat a double dose)	170–360 ml pre-treatment
Treatment step	1% TNBP 1% Tritonx100	1μM MB + visible light 30 min	150 μM amotosalen + UVA 4 min	50 μM riboflavin + UV 4–10 min
Removal step for residual chemicals?	Yes	Yes	Yes	No
Treat liquid or frozen–thawed FFP?	N/A	Yes	Yes	Yes
Shelf life – frozen/once thawed	4 years/ 8 hours	2 years/ 24 hours	2 years/ as validated	2 years/ 6 hours
Possible to make cryoprecipitate?	Yes	Yes, used in UK	Yes	Yes
Coagulation factor losses	Depends on supplier. In UK batches tested for V, VIII, XI all >0.50 IU/ml	20–30% loss of FVIII and fibrinogen, others less affected	20–30% loss of FVIII & fibrinogen, others less affected	20–30% loss of FVIII & fibrinogen, others less affected
Clinical studies performed	Observational studies: congenital coagulation deficiency	Observational studies: congenital coagulation deficiency and cardiac surgery	Observational studies: congenital coagulation deficiency	No published clinical data
	RCTs: liver disease and cardiac surgery	No large RCTs	RCTs: liver disease and TTP	
Indications	As for FFP	As for FFP Not TTP	As for FFP	As for FFP
TRALI risk	Very low – no cases reported	Low if selected from male or nulliparous females	Low if selected from male or nulliparous females	Low if selected from male or nulliparous females
Safety profile from haemovigilance data	Good	Good*	Good	No active HV
Total usage in Europe	>7 million	>4.5 million	>450 000	<32 000

*See text.

Glucose 6 phosphate dehydrogenase deficiency is not a contraindication to use of this product. The amotosalen and riboflavin treatment systems are similar to those described for platelets.

SD treatment can be applied only to pools of several hundred ABO-identical units; as the treatment destroys the lipid envelope of red cells, no RhD matching is required. Exposure to SD destroys the lipid envelope of HIV, HBV and HCV, and no such transmissions have been reported. Non-lipid-coated viruses such as parvovirus B19 and hepatitis A are not specifically inactivated, but their titre may be reduced in downstream processing. In addition, plasma pools with high genomic titres of these viruses are rejected and pools contain specified levels of viral antibodies, which may be at least partially protective. No increase in clinical cases of hepatitis A virus or B19 in SD FFP recipients is evident. Concerns have been expressed in the United States that SD FFP might be associated with increased thrombotic risk in certain clinical situations, attributed to loss of proteins C and S during SD treatment. However, these complications have not been prominent in recipients of SD FFP manufactured by the European method, which results in greater preservation of these proteins. A variant of SD FFP in which ABO groups are mixed is in development. By neutralization of A and B substances by anti-A and anti-B, it is intended to produce a 'universal FFP' that could be given to patients of any ABO group. A lyophylized SD FFP product is also in development.

The French regulatory authority have recently announced a phased withdrawal of MB FFP in response to haemovigilance data suggesting that severe allergic reactions are more common than to untreated or SD FFP. Their investigations suggest that in some cases these appear to be reactions to MB itself rather than plasma proteins. Other European countries that use MBFFP have not observed higher rates of allergic reactions to MB FFP compared with untreated FFP.

vCJD and FFP

In animal studies, plasma was found to contain infective prion. Therefore, a precautionary measure for the UK was announced in 2002 whereby FFP for children born on or after 1 January 1996 would be imported from a country with a low risk of vCJD. This was implemented in 2004, with plasma coming from volunteer donors extensively tested for transfusion-transmitted viruses. Plasma is treated with the MB pathogen inactivation process following arrival in the UK. In 2005, the use of imported MB FFP was extended to patients under the age of 16, and in 2012 the recommendation was made to continue its supply to those born on or after 1 January 2012.

Cryoprecipitate and cryosupernatant

Cryoprecipitate is manufactured by slowly thawing single units of FFP overnight at 4°C. This precipitates out the so-called cryoproteins, namely factor VIII, fibrinogen, fibronectin and factor XIII. By removing most of the supernatant plasma ('cryosupernatant'), a component providing a high concentration of these clotting factors is obtained (Table 21.4). Although originally developed for factor VIII deficiency (haemophilia A), most cryoprecipitate is now prescribed to treat congenital or acquired hypofibrinogenaemia, usually in the context of liver disease, disseminated intravascular coagulation or massive transfusion. An adult dose of 10–12 packs is generally indicated once the fibrinogen level falls below 0.5–1.0 g/L. Some countries pool 5 units of cryoprecipitate to facilitate its administration. An alternative product would be a virus-inactivated fibrinogen concentrate, but in many countries this is only licensed for congenital deficiency and clinical studies demonstrating efficacy of either cryoprecipitate or fibrinogen concentrate for acquired deficiency are lacking. Cryosupernatant has been used successfully as a replacement fluid in plasma exchange procedures for thrombotic thrombocytopenic purpura (TTP). It was thought to have theoretical advantages over FFP, possibly because it lacks the highest molecular weight multimers of the von Willebrand factor, although recent studies suggest that FFP is equally effective.

Virus inactivation of cryoprecipitate and cryosupernatant

Production of cryoprecipitate from SD FFP has been performed experimentally. Such cryoprecipitate contains insufficient von Willebrand factor to treat patients with von Willebrand's disease, but acceptable levels of fibrinogen. Cryoprecipitate produced from MB plasma is routinely used in the UK for patients under the age of 16. Intercept and Mirasol-treated plasma can also be used to produce cryoprecipitate.

Granulocytes for transfusion

The use of transfused granulocytes is uncommon. They are sometimes used for severely neutropenic patients (granulocyte count $<0.5 \times 10^9$/L) with focal bacterial or fungal infection refractory to antimicrobial therapy, but there are difficulties in obtaining sufficient functional cells from donors and administering them frequently enough to the patient. Granulocytes can either be collected by apheresis or produced from whole blood. Animal studies suggest that $>1 \times 10^{10}$ granulocytes once or twice daily are required to treat an adult, but apheresis usually produces no more than 0.5×10^{10}/dose unless donors are stimulated with granulocyte colony-stimulating factor (G-CSF). Therefore, unstimulated apheresis granulocytes are not suitable for adults. There has been renewed interest in the use of granulocytes by studies of granulocyte colony-stimulating factor (G-CSF) mobilized granulocytes collected by apheresis. Administration to the donor of a single subcutaneous injection of 10 μg/kg G-CSF plus oral dexamethasone 8 mg 12–24 hours prior to apheresis raises the peripheral leucocyte count to $>25 \times 10^9$/L. This, coupled with starch sedimentation, allows collection of a therapeutic dose of granulocytes of $5–20 \times 10^8$ granulocytes/kg body weight of the recipient. This can result in a measurable rise in the peripheral granulocyte count in the patient and recovery of migrated cells from saliva.

Clinical trials of such granulocytes are ongoing. At present, use of G-CSF for granulocyte collection is permitted in volunteer donors unrelated to the patient in the USA but not in other countries.

Some European countries transfuse buffy coats as a source of granulocytes. A dose of 1×10^{10} can be achieved from 10 buffy coats. A pooled granulocyte component made from 10 buffy coats has been developed in the UK and its safety assessed in clinical studies. The main advantage of the pooled component over standard buffy coats is a reduction in red cell contamination and volume, and that it is issued as a single unit.

All granulocyte preparations should be released for issue as soon as possible after collection, which may mean that certain time-consuming screening assays such as HCV genome testing cannot be done prior to release. They must be gamma irradiated to prevent TA-GvHD and should be administered to the patient without delay. If a short period of storage is unavoidable, this should be at 22°C without agitation. Because of red cell contamination, a red cell cross-match should be performed.

Components for intrauterine transfusion and for neonates and infants

General requirements (see Table 21.6)

Cellular components for these recipients should be selected or processed to reduce the risk of CMV transmission. Components other than those in additive solution must be free of clinically significant red

Table 21.6 UK specifications for red cells for intrauterine transfusion (IUT), exchange/large volume transfusions and 'top-up' transfusions for neonates.

	IUT	Exchange transfusion	Top-up transfusion
Previous virology-negative donation in previous 2 years	Yes	Yes	Yes
Free of high titre anti-A, anti-B	Yes	Yes	No
Use of additive solution permitted	No	No	Yes
Leucocyte reduced	Yes	Yes	Yes
Irradiation	Yes	Yes*	Yes
Haemoglobin S negative	Yes	Yes	No
CMV seronegative	Yes	Yes	Yes
Shelf life	24 h post-irradiation and <5 days total	24 h post-irradiation and <5 days total	35 days

*Provided it does not delay the procedure.

221

cell antibodies, including high titre anti-A and anti-B. Irradiation is required for intrauterine and exchange transfusions providing it does not unnecessarily delay the procedure. Red cells for 'top-up' transfusions need be irradiated only if there has been a previous intrauterine transfusion (IUT), in severe T lymphocyte deficiency syndromes or if the component is prepared from a family member. Family donations are not encouraged except in rare cases of fetomaternal alloimmunization where the infant's requirements cannot be met from donor blood. Although components are leucocyte depleted at source, they should still be administered through a 170–200-μm filter to remove any microaggregates formed during storage.

Intrauterine/exchange/large-volume transfusion of neonates

Red cells are given *in utero* to treat severe fetal anaemia due to haemolytic disease of the fetus and newborn (HDFN) or parvovirus B19 infection. Red cells for IUT are prepared from plasma-reduced blood to a haematocrit of 0.7–0.85. In cases of fetomaternal alloimmunization to platelets, transfusions of selected platelets (usually HPA-1a and HPA-5b negative) may be given *in utero* (Chapter 5). Apheresis of genotyped donors can be used to produce a hyperconcentrated platelet for this indication. Alternatively, platelets can be concentrated from a whole blood donation.

Exchange transfusion is undertaken to treat hyperbilirubinaemia due to either haemolytic disease or prematurity (Chapter 32). Either whole blood or partially packed red cells with a haematocrit of 0.5–0.6 may be used. Red cells in additive solution are not recommended by some paediatricians for exchange transfusion, because of concerns regarding the adverse effects of mannitol. Some countries use red cells in additive solution for large-volume transfusion of neonates and infants without adverse effect (see Chapter 32). To reduce the risk of hyperkalaemia, red cells for exchange or IUT should be administered within 24 hours of irradiation and by the end of day 5 from donation.

Top-up transfusions for neonates

Premature neonates are among the most heavily transfused patients in any hospital. Most red cell transfusions are given to replace repeated samples taken for laboratory testing. As each infant may require multiple small transfusions, adult packs are split into four to eight 'paedipacks' of 30–60 mL, which can be allocated to one infant for the duration of transfusion dependence. Such a strategy reduces donor exposure considerably. For these small-volume transfusions, red cells in additive solution may be used, up to their normal shelf life. Studies of RhEpo in premature infants have not convincingly shown a reduction in transfusion requirements.

Platelet concentrates and FFP

Platelets are most simply prepared from apheresis donations. Multiple aliquots can be allocated to the same infant if required. An alternative strategy for platelets is to prepare a platelet concentrate from a single buffy coat or from a unit of whole blood using the PRP method. These components are generally used for sick babies with multiple coagulation defects. Platelets from a panel of HPA-1a and 5b-negative donors can be used in suspected cases of neonatal alloimmune thrombocytopenia (Chapter 5).

Key points

1 There are no recognized indications for the transfusion of whole blood and therefore blood is separated into its components for transfusion (red cells, plasma and platelets).
2 Blood components can be produced from whole blood donations or collected directly from the donor by apheresis technology.
3 In the UK and some other countries, all blood components are leucocyte-reduced but others such as the USA have a variable proportion of leucocyte-reduced blood components.
4 Systems are now available in Europe to inactivate pathogens in plasma or platelet components prior to storage.
5 Filters have been developed that are designed to remove prion protein from red cells to reduce the risk of transmission of vCJD.

References

1 Advisory Committee on the Safety of Blood, Tissues and Organs. Position statement on CMV transmission by blood transfusion. http://www.dh.gov.uk/health/about-us/public-bodies-2/advisory-bodies/sabto/.

2 Pennington J, Taylor GP, Sutherland J, Davis RE, Seghatchian J, Allain JP & Williamson LM. Persistence of HTLV-I in blood components after leukocyte depletion. *Blood* 2002; 100: 677–681.

3 Gregori L, McCombie N, Palmer D *et al.* Effectiveness of leucoreduction for removal of infectivity of transmissible spongiform encephalopathies from blood. *Lancet* 2004; 364: 529–531.

4 McCutcheon S, Alejo Blanco AR, Houston EF, de Wolf C, Tan BC, Smith A, Groschup MH, Hunter N, Hornsey VS, MacGregor IR, Prowse CV, Turner M & Manson JC. All clinically-relevant blood components transmit prion disease following a single blood transfusion: a sheep model of vCJD. *PLoS One* 2011; 6(8): e23169. Epub 17 August 2011.

5 Cancelas JA, Dumont LJ, Rugg N, Szczepiorkowski ZM, Herschel L, Siegel A, Pratt PG, Worsham DN, Erickson A, Propst M, North A, Sherman CD, Mufti NA, Reed WF & Corash L. Stored red blood cell viability is maintained after treatment with a second-generation S-303 pathogen inactivation process. *Transfusion* 2011; 51: 2367–2376.

6 Cancelas JA, Rugg N, Fletcher D, Pratt PG, Worsham DN, Dunn SK, Marschner S, Reddy HL & Goodrich RP. *In vivo* viability of stored red blood cells derived from riboflavin plus ultraviolet light-treated whole blood. *Transfusion* 2011; 51: 1460–1468.

7 Gregori L, Gurgel PV, Lathrop JT, Edwardson P, Lambert BC, Carbonell RG, Burton SJ, Hammond DJ & Rohwer RG. Reduction in infectivity of endogenous transmissible spongiform encephalopathies present in blood by adsorption to selective affinity resins. *Lancet* 2006; 368: 2226–2230.

8 Snyder E, McCullough J, Slichter SJ, Strauss RG, Lopez-Plaza I, Lin JS, Corash L & Conlan MG; SPRINT Study Group. Clinical safety of platelets photochemically treated with amotosalen HCl and ultraviolet A light for pathogen inactivation: the SPRINT trial. *Transfusion* 2005; 45: 1864–1875.

9 van Rhenen D, Gulliksson H, Cazenave JP, Pamphilon D, Ljungman P, Klüter H, Vermeij H, Kappers-Klunne M, de Greef G, Laforet M, Lioure B, Davis K, Marblie S, Mayaudon V, Flament J, Conlan M, Lin L, Metzel P, Buchholz D & Corash L; euroSPRITE trial. Transfusion of pooled buffy coat platelet components prepared with photochemical pathogen inactivation treatment: the euroSPRITE trial. *Blood* 2003; 101: 2426–2433.

10 Kerkhoffs JL, van Putten WL, Novotny VM, Te Boekhorst PA, Schipperus MR, Zwaginga JJ, van Pampus LC, de Greef GE, Luten M, Huijgens PC, Brand A & van Rhenen DJ; Dutch–Belgian HOVON Cooperative Group. Clinical effectiveness of leucoreduced, pooled donor platelet concentrates, stored in plasma or additive solution with and without pathogen reduction. *Br J Haematol* 2010; 150: 209–217.

11 Mirasol Clinical Evaluation Study Group. A randomized controlled clinical trial evaluating the performance and safety of platelets treated with MIRASOL pathogen reduction technology. *Transfusion* 2010; 50: 2362–2375.

12 Mohr H, Steil L, Gravemann U, Thiele T, Hammer E, Greinacher A, Müller TH & Völker U. A novel approach to pathogen reduction in platelet concentrates using short-wave ultraviolet light. *Transfusion* 2009; 49: 2612–2624.

13 Rock G. A comparison of methods of pathogen inactivation of FFP. *Vox Sanguinis* 2011; 100: 169–178.

Further reading

American Association of Blood Banks. *Standards for Blood Banks and Transfusion Services*, 27th edn. Bethesda, MD: AABB Press; 2011.

British Committee for Standards in Haematology. Guidelines for the use of platelet transfusions. *Br J Haematol* 2003; 122: 10–23.

British Committee for Standards in Haematology. Transfusion guidelines for neonates and older children. *Br J Haematol* 2004; 124: 433–453.

British Committee for Standards in Haematology. Guidelines for the use of fresh-frozen plasma, cryoprecipitate and cryosupernatant. *Br J Haematol* 2005; 126: 11–28.

Council of Europe. *Guide to the Preparation, Use and Quality Assurance of Blood Components*, 16th edn. Strasbourg: Council of Europe Publishing; 2010.

McClelland DBL (ed.). *Handbook of Transfusion Medicine*, 4th edn. London: The Stationery Office; 2007.

United Kingdom Blood Transfusion Services/National Institute for Biological Standards and Control. *Guidelines for the Blood Transfusion Services in the United Kingdom*, 7th edn. London: The Stationery Office; 2005. Available at: www.transfusionguidelines.org, UK.

Webert KE, Cserti CM, Hannon J, Lin Y, Pavenski K, Pendergrast JM & Blajchman MA. Proceedings of a Consensus Conference: pathogen inactivation-making decisions about new technologies. *Transfus Med Rev* 2008; 22: 1–34.

22 Medicolegal aspects of transfusion practice

Patricia E. Hewitt

NHS Blood and Transplant, London, UK

Ethical principles

The International Society of Blood Transfusion (ISBT) some years ago instituted a code of ethics setting out the guiding principles for blood donation and transfusion. Following revision, this code of ethics was adopted by the World Health Organization (WHO). It was also used to support ethical standards in the drafting of the European Blood Directive. It is recommended that all blood transfusion provision is in accordance with the principles included in this code. The main provisions are listed below.
- There should be no coercion to donate blood.
- Both donors and recipients must be adequately informed.
- Confidentiality must be maintained.
- Adequate standards should be enforced.
- Clinical need must be the determinant of transfusion therapy.

Regulatory framework in the UK (also see Chapter 17)

The regulatory framework encompassing blood transfusion will necessarily differ according to the legal situation in the country concerned. The framework in the UK is briefly described. Similar arrangements are in place in all developed countries.

Medicines Act 1968

The Medicines Act provides the framework for the regulation and control of all dealings with medicinal products. Prior to the Blood Safety and Quality Regulations (2005), both cellular blood components and fractionated blood components were included within the terms of the Act. Fractionated components (e.g. albumin, coagulation factor concentrates and intravenous immunoglobulin preparations) are individually licensed. The provision of labile blood components (red cells, platelets, fresh frozen plasma and cryoprecipitate) was enabled by means of an organizational licence awarded to individual blood centres by the Medicines and Healthcare Products Regulatory Agency (MHRA) following appropriate inspection and demonstration of compliance with the standards of good manufacturing practice. Such inspections of 'blood establishments' are now covered under the Blood Safety and Quality Regulations.

Consumer Protection Act 1987

The Consumer Protection Act creates a strict liability action against manufacturers and suppliers when physical injury or property damage is caused by a defective product.

The Consumer Protection Act 1987 was enacted as a result of a European Community Directive in 1985 and clearly includes within its terms the provision of all blood components and blood products. Its

Practical Transfusion Medicine, Fourth Edition. Edited by Michael F. Murphy, Derwood H. Pamphilon and Nancy M. Heddle.
© 2013 John Wiley & Sons, Ltd. Published 2013 by John Wiley & Sons, Ltd.

Table 22.1 Relevant UK statutes.

Act	Terms
Medicines Act 1968	Regulates medicinal products
Consumer Protection Act 1987	Encompasses all aspects of provision of blood and blood components from donation to hospital blood bank
NHS Act 1999 and Health and Social Care Act 2006	Concentrates on clinical quality of care
Blood Safety and Quality Regulations 2005	Regulates collection, testing, processing and storage of blood, traceability, reporting of adverse events and quality systems.

premise is the principle of product liability, i.e. that there is no need to prove that a negligent action has taken place, but merely that the end product is defective and has caused harm. In Section 3 (1) of the Act, a 'defect' is defined as follows: 'There is a defect in the product ... if the safety of the product is not such as persons generally are entitled to expect. ... ' Blood providers can be held liable under the terms of the Act as producers, suppliers or keepers. The liability therefore extends from the blood centre producing the product to the hospital blood transfusion laboratory, which stores and issues products. There are possible defences within the terms of the Act, such as the 'state-of-the-art defence'. In essence this means that if a product is found to be defective based on current knowledge, that information cannot be used to prove that the same product was defective sometime previously when the current knowledge was not available (Table 22.1). This defence was not held to apply in the case of the hepatitis C litigation in England, since the defect (the transmission of hepatitis C) was apparent at the time of the claimants' transfusions (1988–1991), although the means of detecting the defect (the availability of a hepatitis C test) was not necessarily available during the whole period.

NHS Act 1999 and Health and Social Care Act 2006

The 1999 Act modernized the NHS in England, Wales and Scotland. Raising standards in the quality of NHS care was at its heart. A statutory duty of quality was placed on all NHS providers, monitored by means

of the Healthcare Commission. The spur to set up these statutory provisions had been inequality in care. All aspects of healthcare, including blood transfusion, came under the remit of the Healthcare Commission. Subsequent legislation, in the form of the Health and Social Care Act 2006, brought together existing health and social care regulators into one organization, the Care Quality Commission, with tough new powers to ensure safe and quality care. Additionally, the National Institute for Health and Clinical Excellence (NICE) was set up in 1999 to set standards for high quality healthcare in the UK, to produce clinical guidelines and to produce public health guidelines on how to improve people's health. NICE has produced little guidance in relation to blood transfusion therapy, but other organizations, such as the British Committee for Standards in Haematology (BCSH) regularly produce and review guidelines relating to transfusion practice.

European Blood Safety Directives (2002/98)

The European Blood Safety Directive (2002/98) [1] sets standards relating to blood collection, testing, processing and storage. A 'daughter' Directive (2004/33) lays out technical requirements in support of these standards. Together, the two directives were transposed into UK law as the Blood Safety and Quality Regulations 2005 [2], which came into force on 8 February 2005. Two further 'daughter' Directives (2005/61 and 2005/62), which cover aspects of traceability, reporting of adverse reactions and events, and specifications for quality systems, came into force by separate amending legislation in 2006.

The regulations impose safety and quality requirements on human blood collection, testing, processing and storage. The requirements apply to all 'blood establishments', which include the blood transfusion services in England, Scotland, Wales and Northern Ireland. In addition, the collection and processing of blood components within hospital premises confers the status of 'blood establishment' upon the hospital, bringing such activities and premises under the control of the regulations. The regulations replace some of those (in relation to inspection, licensing and accreditation) previously covered under the Medicines Act. They lay down a requirement for inspection not less than every 2 years by the regulatory authority (MHRA). Failure to comply with the licensing regulations can lead to the imposition of a fine or closure

225

of an organization, and, in the worst cases, a fine or imprisonment for the designated 'responsible person' of the blood establishment.

Many of the provisions of the regulations, such as traceability, reporting of adverse events and specifications for quality systems, apply to hospital blood transfusion laboratories as well as to blood establishments. The regulations have had wide-reaching implications for both blood services and hospital blood transfusion laboratories.

Quality guidelines

Uniformity and process control within blood services can be achieved by compliance with detailed quality guidelines. The *Guidelines for the Blood Transfusion Services* [3] in the United Kingdom and the *American Association of Blood Banks Technical Manual* [4] are two examples of such documents. Although such guidelines do not possess legal status, they set out the requirements to be met for good manufacturing practice. Deliberate noncompliance would be regarded very seriously. Unavoidable noncompliance should be carefully documented and should include a clear explanation of the reasons for noncompliance.

Duty of care

Putting aside the ethical principles, quality guidelines and regulatory frameworks described above, there remains the clear duty of care that must be at the heart of the provision of blood transfusion. This duty must be according to an accepted standard. At present, the standard is determined according to the Bolam principle: 'The test is the standard of the ordinary skilled man exercising and professing to have that special skill' [5]. This defines the standard as that of a responsible body of doctors skilled in the same specialty. The standard of care can be supported by the application of professional guidelines, although currently the latter have no legal standing. The duty of care of blood services, according to the defined standard, is both to the blood donor and to the recipient patient.

Duty to the donor

The two general principles that underpin blood donation are that there should be every effort to ensure no harm to the health of the donor and no risk to the health of the recipient patient. The duty to the donor includes compliance with strict medical selection procedures. The donor should be informed about the screening tests performed on the donation and should provide a written consent to testing. Information should be provided on situations that could potentially pose risk to the donor, e.g. the administration of growth factors prior to stem cell donation or the use of general anaesthetic during bone marrow donation. In these instances, a donor would need to consent formally to the procedure. The blood services in the UK make leaflets available at all routine blood donation sessions, to inform prospective blood donors of relevant issues. Additionally, the blood service has a duty to maintain the confidentiality of a donor, particularly in the event of a recipient patient being harmed by blood obtained from a single donor. The duty of care to the donor also extends to the clinician prescribing the blood, to ensure appropriate use, particularly as that donation is provided on a voluntary basis with no expectation of monetary gain.

Duty to the recipient patient

In the UK the standard of care for patients receiving blood transfusion is addressed under the legislation referred to above. It is suggested that, as a minimum, this standard of care should include the provision of adequate information to the recipient patient and ensuring appropriate clinical use of individual blood components.

Consent to transfusion

Any patient being asked to consent to a medical treatment or investigation has the right to be informed of the aims, benefits and risks of the treatment, and to be given details of any alternatives. Without such information, consent is not valid. The standard NHS 'Patient agreement to investigation or treatment' form includes a section completed by the health professional who has the discussion with the patient. This section documents that an explanation has been given to the patient about the proposed investigation or treatment, including the possibility of extra procedures that may be found necessary, and blood transfusion is specifically mentioned at this point. The patient signs a general consent to the procedure/investigation described, embracing the possibility of additional procedures, but has the opportunity to list any procedures for which he or she withholds consent without further discussion. The UK Advisory Committee on the Safety of Blood, Tissues and Organs (SaBTO) held a public consultation on the issue of consent for blood transfusion during 2010, leading to a number of recommendations, including the use of standardized patient information, improved staff training and ensuring best practice is followed, but not recommending that an individual signed patient consent is obtained for transfusion [6].

The patient must have the capacity to consent. No doctor should force a competent adult to accept any treatment even if that adult's decision appears to be irrational. An adult could be incapacitated and therefore unable to give consent because of loss of consciousness or mental retardation. In general, no other person can give consent on behalf of an incapacitated adult. (In some countries, e.g. Scotland, the power of *parens patriae* applies, where another adult can take responsibility as a parent for an incapacitated individual.) Prior wishes may be taken into consideration where the adult has previously been competent and the treatment is regarded as noncontroversial. Treatment may be given to an adult incapable of consenting if the treatment is urgent and in the patient's best interests. In an elective situation, however, it would be best to seek a ruling from a court of law. The General Medical Council has published a comprehensive guide to consent and this is recommended for more detailed reading [7] (Table 22.2).

In the case of children, the Family Law Reform Act 1969 makes it lawful for a minor to consent to, or refuse, treatment when he or she reaches the age of 16 years. In the case of a child below 16 years of age, the parents usually give consent, although such children are able to give valid consent in their own right if they are capable of understanding clearly the nature of the proposed treatment [8]. Here, a difficulty could be where parents have specific religious beliefs that prevent them from consenting to blood transfusion for their child. In this instance, a doctor can decide to provide a treatment, including blood transfusion, in the child's best interests. The treatment must be carried out in order to save life or to ensure improvement of or to prevent deterioration in the physical or mental health of the child. This would form the basis of a doctor's individual decision during an emergency situation, but in the case of a planned blood transfusion it would be appropriate to seek a ruling from a court of law. In these circumstances it is recommended that the doctor's medical defence body is consulted for advice on how to proceed.

For consent to be informed and valid, it must be based on adequate information. Attempts have been made to define what constitutes adequate information and it is legally acceptable that the explanation need not include all the potential adverse consequences if the risk of them occurring is small or immaterial. Minor insignificant reactions to transfusion occur relatively commonly, whereas the risk of complications with serious or fatal long-term consequences, e.g. transmission of HIV, is extremely low. However, there is heightened public awareness of such low risk, and it is therefore appropriate for these events to be included in a preliminary explanation. Again, the standard that applies in the UK is that of a responsible body of skilled doctors, the Bolam principle. In the USA, however, a different rule applies, the standard being judged according to that which a prudent patient would think relevant to receive, a situation that is likely to develop within the UK in the next few years.

There must be no coercion in obtaining consent. A competent adult is able to accept or refuse treatment even if that decision could lead to harm or indeed death. If an individual doctor decides to treat an adult without consent, then that doctor should be prepared to explain and justify the decision.

Jehovah's Witnesses

Jehovah's Witnesses, because of their religious beliefs, will never accept normal blood transfusion therapy, although in appropriate circumstances could find cell salvage in continuous circulation acceptable. Many Jehovah's Witnesses carry an Advance Medical Directive, which states the individual's views and requirements to be followed in the event that the individual is

Table 22.2 Informed consent must include these elements.

Capacity to understand
Should be based on adequate information
Should be obtained without coercion

unconscious or otherwise unable to express his or her views. Where the situation is one relating to a competent adult, as long as it is clear that there is no coercion, the decision to refuse treatment must be respected, even if it would lead to harm or indeed death of the patient. In an emergency situation, if the patient is unconscious and therefore incapacitated, then prior previously held beliefs must be taken into account and blood transfusion should not be prescribed if those beliefs made it clear that it was unacceptable. In the situation of a child, where the parents' religious beliefs could prevent the child from being given a necessary blood transfusion, it would be advisable to seek a proper legal ruling, which would usually mean the child becoming a ward of court and therefore decisions on the treatment being taken by the court.

Patient recourse

Despite compliance with standards and appropriate care, things do, and will, go wrong. In some countries, e.g. New Zealand and the Scandinavian countries (Sweden, Norway, Finland and Denmark), compensation for medical accidents is provided under a 'no-fault' system. However, in most countries there is a need to prove liability. In these circumstances, liability will rest either with the individual doctor or with the health employer if vicarious liability applies (this is the current position in the UK for all NHS work). There have been examples of no-fault compensation awarded in the UK in specific circumstances, e.g. the Vaccine Damage Payment Scheme, which provides payment of a fixed lump sum where serious mental or physical damage has been caused by the administration of specified vaccines. A vCJD compensation scheme, administered by the vCJD Trust, was set up to provide payments for people infected with vCJD through exposure to bovine products or otherwise through exposure to BSE or vCJD within the UK. This scheme therefore covers individuals believed to have been infected through UK blood transfusions. Specifically in relation to blood transfusion, there are schemes (the MacFarlane Trust and the Eileen Trust) for recipients infected with HIV through the use of plasma products and through blood transfusion both before and after the introduction of mandatory screening of the blood supply in the UK. These were ex gratia payments to those affected, with the government

emphasizing that they should not be regarded as an admission of liability or as compensation, but as a response to a particular and tragic situation. Requests for similar treatment for individuals infected with other agents, such as hepatitis B and C, were, at first, refused. However, a scheme known as the Skipton Fund was subsequently set up for recipients who had been infected with hepatitis C through treatment with NHS blood components/products, although only those transfused prior to the introduction of testing of blood donations in September 1991 qualify for such payments. Similar treatment does not apply to recipients infected with other agents through blood transfusion, although such cases are small in number. It becomes difficult to explain the different treatments of patients who have suffered apparently similar unfortunate and unexpected adverse effects through treatment with blood transfusion.

A patient who has suffered harm can bring an action either in medical negligence or under product liability. If brought in negligence, there would be a need to prove a breach in the duty of care and that the breach directly caused harm to the patient. If brought under product liability, negligence need not be present; a defective product must have directly caused the harm (Table 22.3).

An example of an action that could be brought under medical negligence would be that of the transfusion of a unit of red cells to the wrong recipient patient because of failure to check patient identification. Here, there would be a clear breach of the duty of care, which is in checking the patient identification against the red cell unit, and it would also be simple to demonstrate that harm, in the form of an acute haemolytic transfusion reaction, had occurred as a direct result of the breach. The recipient patient would be able to seek damages for the injury and compensation for any consequent financial loss. A further

Table 22.3 Comparison of medical negligence versus product liability.

Medical negligence	Product liability
Duty of care	Defective product
Breach of the duty	Harm caused directly by the defect
Harm caused directly by the breach	

example would be where a blood transfusion recipient acquired an infection from the blood transfusion and where the blood transfusion only became necessary because of negligent treatment of the underlying medical condition.

Cases of product liability in relation to blood transfusion in Europe are few. The most notable case was that of a number of recipients (114) in England and Wales who brought a claim under the Consumer Protection Act in 2000–2002 [9]. In his judgement, Burton found that the Blood Service was liable for the damage because the product (i.e. the blood) did not provide the safety that the consumer (patient) was 'generally entitled to expect'. The claimants were awarded damages on a provisional basis according to the damage (extent of hepatitis C disease) present at the time of the action. Provisional damages allow for the claimants to return with a future claim should their medical condition deteriorate. The judgement in the hepatitis C litigation was not appealed. Similar claims in relation to transfusion-transmitted infection have been settled in the absence of any successful challenge to the ruling. The case attracted much attention within Europe and has been the precedent for claims for other types of 'defective product', such as blood bearing white cell antibodies which were the cause of Transfusion Related Acute Lung Injury (TRALI). Other case law within Europe is scarce, although some European countries (e.g. France and the Scandinavian countries) provide for no-fault compensation in relation to infection acquired through medical treatment.

Key points

1 All those involved in the provision of blood and blood components must be aware of the relevant regulatory framework(s).
2 Those prescribing blood transfusion must be aware of consent issues.
3 Valid consent is based on having relevant information.
4 A competent adult can choose to refuse blood transfusion, despite the likely consequences, and that choice must be respected.
5 No-fault compensation/payment schemes apply for some transfusion complications in the UK, but not for all.

6 The Consumer Protection Act has opened the door for claims from blood transfusion recipients without the need to prove negligence.

References

1 Directive 2002/ 98/ EC of the European Parliament and of the Council (2003). Available at: http://ec.europa.eu/he alth/blood_tissues_organs/key_documents/index_en.htm# anchor0_more (accessed December 2011).
2 UK Blood Safety and Quality Regulations (BSQR). Available at: http://www.legislation.gov.uk/uksi/2005/50/ contents/made#top (accessed December 2011).
3 Guidelines for the Blood Transfusion Services in the United Kingdom, 7th edn; 2005 and addendum 2007. Available at: http://www.transfusionguidelines.org.uk/in dex.aspx?Publication=RB&Section=25 (accessed December 2011).
4 American Association of Blood Banks. Technical Manual, 17th edn. Bethesda, MA: AABB, 2011.
5 Bolam v Friern Barnet Hospital Management Committee. 2 All ER 118; 1957.
6 General Medical Council. Consent Guidance; Patients and Doctors Making Decisions Together. London: GMC; 2008.
7 Advisory Committee on the Safety of Blood, Tissues and Organs (SaBTO). Patient Consent for Blood Transfusion; 2011. Available at: http://www.dh.gov.uk/en/Publications andstatistics/Publications/PublicationsPolicyAndGuidance /DH_130716?ssSourceSiteId=ab (accessed December 2011).
8 Gillick v West Norfolk and Wisbech Area Health Authority. 3 All ER 402; 1984.
9 A and others v National Blood Authority. 3 All ER 289; 2002.

Further reading

Braithwaite M & Beresford N. Law for Doctors: Principles and Practicalities. London: Royal Society of Medicine Press; 2002.
Goldberg R. Paying for bad blood. Strict product liability after the hepatitis C litigation. Med Law Rev 2002; 10: 165–200.
Grubb A & Pearl DA. Blood Testing, Aids and DNA Profiling. Bristol: Family Law (Jordan and Sons Ltd); 1990.
The Consumer Protection Act 1987. In: Halsbury's Statute of England. London: HMSO.
Warden J. HIV infected haemophiliacs: 90 million more. Br Med J 1989; 299: 1358.

Blood transfusion in hospitals

Erica M. Wood[1], Mark H. Yazer[2] & Michael F. Murphy[3]

[1]Monash Medical Centre, Departments of Clinical Haematology and Epidemiology and Preventive Medicine, Monash University, Melbourne, Victoria, Australia
[2]The Institute for Transfusion Medicine, Pittsburgh and Department of Pathology, University of Pittsburgh, Pittsburgh, Pennsylvania, USA
[3]University of Oxford and NHS Blood and Transplant and Department of Haematology, John Radcliffe Hospital, Oxford, UK

The aim of transfusion practice is to provide 'the right blood to the right patient at the right time for the right reason'. It focuses on ensuring that, when it is clinically indicated, patients receive the correct transfusion support, in a safe, timely and cost-efficient manner, with incidents and adverse reactions recognized and managed effectively. Specialists in all branches of medicine and surgery are involved in prescribing blood, and engagement, cooperation and coordination is required by staff, and with patients, to manage the complex, interacting sequences of the process.

In many countries, blood for transfusion is neither safe, sufficient, nor reliably available. In these settings, haemorrhage is a major direct cause of mortality. However, even in modern healthcare settings with adequate blood supplies, patients die from transfusion complications [1, 2] or from lack of adequate transfusion support: for example, massive haemorrhage is still one of the most common direct causes of maternal death worldwide. Some instances of undertransfusion are due to patient refusal to accept transfusion support or failure by physicians to recognize and respond to clinical manifestations of bleeding. However, others can be attributed to either lack of knowledge of transfusion protocols or failures of communication within, and between, clinical teams. At the other extreme, patients are frequently overtransfused and transfusion-associated circulatory overload (TACO) is increasingly recognized as a common serious adverse event [3].

Mistransfusion, or 'wrong blood' events, i.e. administering an incorrect unit of blood, which either does not meet the patient's needs or is intended for another recipient, can also have serious consequences, including severe haemolysis due to ABO incompatibility, and is another well-recognized cause of mortality and morbidity. Human errors leading to mistransfusion can occur at any step in the process and usually result from failures to comply with clerical or technical procedures, or systems that are either poorly constructed or not understood. Multiple errors are frequently involved in these cases. Some can be detected during the bedside check at the time of administering blood, and this remains a final opportunity to prevent mistransfusion. It has been observed that as many as 1 in 19 000 red cells are given erroneously and 1 in 33 000 will involve ABO-incompatible units [4]. Estimates of mortality due to mistransfusion range from 1 in 600 000 units to 1 in 1.8 million.

Enormous investments have been made to reduce the risks of transfusion-transmitted infections, but to date generally there has been much less investment in improving hospital systems required for clinical practice. Consequently, evidence of progress in reducing procedural risks and improving the safety of hospital transfusion practice is slower to accumulate. Some interventions, such as the practice of a bedside ABO group check before transfusion or the use of physical barriers to transfusion, such as a code to link the patient's wristband, pretransfusion sample and unlock

Practical Transfusion Medicine, Fourth Edition. Edited by Michael F. Murphy, Derwood H. Pamphilon and Nancy M. Heddle.
© 2013 John Wiley & Sons, Ltd. Published 2013 by John Wiley & Sons, Ltd.

the designated unit of blood from secure storage, are intrinsically attractive. For a variety of reasons they have been difficult to implement fully and are not yet widely used [5]. Data to support the effectiveness of many procedural interventions are still limited and many serious (and often preventable) adverse events continue to be reported. However, where haemovigilance programmes have been able to highlight these issues and their causes, and action has been taken to address them, progress has been demonstrated in at least some of these areas [1].

Effective quality frameworks are required to minimize transfusion risks and to ensure that the supply of donated blood is managed effectively. These in turn require a patient-centred approach to transfusion, committed leadership and adequate resources.

Key features of hospital transfusion governance

Many countries have established requirements that blood centres or services (termed 'blood establishments' in Europe) and hospital transfusion laboratories maintain robust quality systems to ensure good practice – which may include meeting national or regional standards for good manufacturing, laboratory and/or clinical practice (also see Chapter 17). These requirements are typically overseen by national regulatory authorities and/or professional authorities to ensure compliance. For example, to meet EU Directives, the UK Blood Safety and Quality Regulations [6] outline requirements for quality management in transfusion laboratories, including staff training, process validation, documentation, storage and handling, traceability and reporting of adverse events.

However, this regulation has typically not yet extended to the practice in clinical areas and other measures are needed to ensure that processes and systems that influence the quality and governance of clinical transfusion practice at the hospital level are optimized and working as expected. Recommendations for the practice are derived from clinical experience and the peer-reviewed evidence base, along with lessons from haemovigilance and external quality assessment (EQA) schemes. These are translated into policies, standards and guidelines by government agencies and professional groups, who in

turn assess implementation and compliance and promote best practice through training, education and communication.

In England, the Care Quality Commission regulates healthcare providers. Many of the national standards for governance and risk assessment are applicable to blood transfusion, including those relating to patient engagement, informed consent, staff training and competency assessment, participation in audit and other quality improvement activities, and reporting of incidents. Specifically, the National Patient Safety Agency in England in 2006 issued a safety notice requiring competency-based training and assessment for all staff involved in blood transfusion, a bedside identity check for administering blood that matches the blood pack with the patient wristband (excluding compatibility form or case notes) and a formal risk assessment of the alternative means of confirming patient identity. The National Health Service Litigation Authority also inspects acute care English hospitals against risk management standards that include blood transfusion. Hospitals are expected to have transfusion policies and provide evidence of implementation and monitoring for effectiveness.

Similar expectations apply in other countries. For example, the Australian Commission on Safety and Quality in Healthcare recently released a standard on clinical transfusion practice as part of new national safety and quality standards [7] that outline requirements against which hospitals will be assessed for accreditation. In the USA, authorities from state health departments through to national regulators like the Joint Commission on Accreditation of Healthcare Organizations (JCAHO) and the Food and Drug Authority are involved in assessing and regulating transfusion practice.

At an institutional level, executive management is responsible for implementation of standards and policies, including through initial and ongoing staff training and appraisal, and for monitoring through clinical audit and other quality system activities.

Hospital transfusion committees

Hospital transfusion committees (HTC) are focal points for overseeing transfusion practice at the institutional level. Their roles are outlined in documents such as the UK NHS *Better Blood Transfusion* health circulars and statements from regulatory bodies like the US JCAHO.

To be effective and to deliver on their objectives, HTCs require support from dedicated hospital transfusion teams, at a minimum consisting of a medical specialist, transfusion practitioner(s) and blood bank scientist/manager. Other necessary resources include IT and clerical support to facilitate regular meetings, data retrieval and audit. HTCs are essential components of institutional clinical governance, so they must be incorporated into hospital frameworks for clinical governance, performance and risk management, and report findings and activities in a timely and meaningful way, accompanied by recommendations for action. HTCs have the remit to promote best practice, review clinical transfusion practice, monitor performance of the hospital transfusion service, participate in regional or national initiatives and communicate with local patient representative groups as appropriate (Table 23.1).

Composition

A chairperson with understanding and experience of transfusion practice should be appointed by hospital senior management. Ideally, the chairperson should

Table 23.1 Activities of the hospital transfusion committee.

Area or activity	Example
Policies and procedures	Develop and promulgate policies and procedures, including for: • Clinical indication and decision to transfuse • Establishing and enforcing transfusion thresholds • Informed consent process • Collection of samples for compatibility testing, including patient identification and specimen labelling requirements • Transfusion administration and monitoring • Indications for specialized components (e.g. irradiated, CMV seronegative, phenotype-matched) • Maximum surgical blood ordering schedule (MSBOS) • Blood conservation strategies including use of cell salvage and pharmacological agents • Management of patients who decline transfusion • Management of adverse reactions
Education, training and assessment	Develop strategies for education, training and assessment of all staff involved in transfusion Monitor implementation and results of education and training activities Develop and/or promulgate information/materials for patients
Audit, monitoring and review	Develop annual audit plans and monitor performance Review adverse event reports Conduct incident, 'near miss' and sentinel event reviews Oversee traceability and record-keeping obligations
System performance	Review: • Blood component availability, utilization and wastage rates • Activation of massive transfusion protocol, use of uncrossmatched emergency red cell stocks • Performance of institutional transfusion laboratory and blood service ('blood establishment') • Participation in regional and national audit, transfusion practice improvement and haemovigilance programme activities • Participation in EQA activities Oversee hospital and laboratory accreditation activities relating to transfusion Contingency and disaster planning Function and performance of HTC

not be the medical specialist responsible for the hospital transfusion service, who could be perceived to have a vested interest.

The following membership is suggested:
• representatives of all major clinical blood users, including junior medical staff;
• specialist haematologist/pathologist with responsibility for transfusion;
• hospital blood bank senior scientist/manager;
• specialist practitioner(s) of transfusion;
• senior nursing representative;
• representatives from hospital management and clinical risk management;
• local blood centre medical specialist (*ex officio*); and
• other co-opted representatives as required, e.g. from medical records, portering staff, clinical audit, training or pharmacy.

Administration of blood and blood components and management of the transfused patient

This process involves multiple steps:
• counselling patients regarding the need for blood transfusion, when alternative approaches (salvaged blood, iron and/or erythropoietic stimulating agents) are predicted to be insufficient or inappropriate for their circumstances;
• prescription;
• requests for blood components;
• sampling for pretransfusion compatibility testing;
• collection and delivery from approved storage facility (e.g. monitored blood refrigerator) to clinical area;
• pretransfusion checking process;
• administration;
• patient monitoring; and
• documentation of all steps.

Errors occurring at blood sampling, collection and administration can lead to patient misidentification and mistransfusion. Prescription errors, however, lead either to failure to provide special components to meet recipient special needs or to transfusions that are unnecessary or inappropriate and carry the potential for complications. For example, TACO has occurred when transfusions have been given on the basis of a spuriously low haemoglobin value resulting from samples taken from IV ('drip') arms or measured by gas analysers, or as a result of a clerical error where the decision was based incorrectly on another patient's results. Fatal errors have also occurred in prescribing the volume or rate of transfusion. Failure to monitor transfused patients, particularly in the first 15 minutes of receiving each unit, can lead to life-threatening reactions being overlooked and delays in resuscitation.

Hospitals should have written procedures to cover all these steps, against which relevant staff are trained and assessed, and which are readily available for quick reference at the bedside. Clinical responsibilities, actions, documents, potential errors and some of their consequences are outlined in Tables 23.2 to 23.8. Prescription charts, donation numbers of components and batch/lot numbers of fractionated plasma products issued and transfused, nursing observations and recipient vital signs related to the transfusion should be kept in the medical case notes as permanent records. Regulatory and accreditation authorities require a complete audit trail of blood to the patient's bedside. Many hospitals comply with this requirement by returning signed and dated compatibility forms or compatibility labels to the transfusion laboratory.

Technologies to reduce patient misidentification errors in administering blood

Additional manual systems of patient identification
Sets of distinctive (e.g. coloured) labels with the same unique number can be allocated to each pretransfusion blood sample. A transfusion label can be incorporated into an additional patient wristband at the time of phlebotomy, affixed to the request form, sample tube and into the current medical notes, and the unique number can also be printed on to the compatibility labels and compatibility report form. At the time of administration, the additional unique number provides a supplementary means of cross-checking.

Electronic bedside processes for safe transfusion practice
The use of bedside hand-held computers, barcoded staff identity badges, barcoded printed wristbands for patients and portable printers for sample tube labels provide the means for improving patient identity and safety [8]. For example, at sample collection, phlebotomist and patient identity can be scanned and barcoded labels generated at the bedside to attach to the

Table 23.2 Examples of some errors and other problems in the transfusion process, and their potential outcomes.

Problem	Potential outcome
Unnecessary prescription	Patient subjected to unnecessary risks, including transfusion-associated circulatory overload Blood component wastage
Prescribed components do not meet patient special requirements	Transfusion complications, e.g. transfusion-associated graft-versus-host disease
Blood not stored in controlled environment	Blood component wastage Transfusion complications (e.g. risk of bacterial growth)
Pretransfusion samples taken from incorrect patient Sample transposition or other laboratory errors Incorrect unit of blood collected and/or administered	Mistransfusion and potential for ABO- or RhD-incompatible transfusion
Insensitive techniques in pretransfusion testing	Potential for acute and delayed haemolytic transfusion reactions
Poor laboratory stock control	Blood component wastage Inappropriate overuse of group O red cells and potential for consequent shortages of that group
Delay in emergency provision of blood components	Patient morbidity/mortality due to hypoxia or coagulopathy

sample tube at the time and place where it is collected. In the laboratory, allocated units are labelled to incorporate the patient's unique identification barcode and the unit number. At administration, staff are prompted by a hand-held computer to scan their own identification barcode, the barcoded patient wristband, the compatibility label and the unit number on the blood component. The computer prompts the staff to check the identity of the (conscious) patient verbally and the barcode scans confirm that the unit is correct for the patient. The user and transfusion laboratory are alerted if there is a mismatch. It also provides prompts to check for special requirements, pretransfusion observations and the unit expiry date. Documentation of each step is transmitted to the laboratory information system to confirm traceability of

Table 23.3 Prescription of blood components.

Responsibility	Action	Documentation	Examples of potential problems and errors
Medical staff	Ensure patient is aware of need for transfusion and has received, read and understood information related to risks and benefits	Patient information materials Hospital consent form	Staff and patient insufficiently informed about risks/hazards Failure to take account of patient religious beliefs or other views
	Prescribe component, any special requirements, quantity/volume and rate/duration of transfusion	Prescription form or chart	Unnecessary prescription, failure to follow hospital guidelines or as result of error in laboratory test results Lack of awareness of, or failure to prescribe, special components
	Document rationale for transfusion	Patient medical record	

Related national and hospital procedures and documents
Guidelines for the use of blood and blood components, including special requirements
Practice guidelines/procedures for individual diseases/treatments

Table 23.4 Requests for blood and blood components.

Responsibility	Action	Documentation	Examples of potential problems and errors
Medical and registered nursing staff	Provide full patient identification, location, diagnosis, details of type and quantity of component and time required Provide previous obstetric and transfusion history when requesting red cells	Written/electronic request form or laboratory telephone log in an emergency	Incomplete or incorrect patient information leading to failure to recognize historical laboratory record Failure to record requirement for special components or phenotyped units Failure to request special components Failure to comply with hospital MSBOS
Hospital transfusion laboratory staff	Review historical record and whether further sample for pretransfusion testing required	Previous laboratory record	Patient identification error in transcribing telephone request Failure to locate/heed information contained in historical record Failure to request new sample in recently transfused patient with potential to overlook newly developed red cell antibodies

Related hospital procedures and documents
Pretransfusion sampling and testing protocols
Maximum surgical blood ordering schedules (MSBOS)

Table 23.5 Sampling for pretransfusion compatibility testing.

Responsibility	Action	Documentation	Examples of potential problems and errors
Medical, nursing and phlebotomy staff	Direct questioning of patient to provide surname, first name and date of birth when judged capable Check that details given match those on patient wristband and on request form		Patient misidentification due to failure to positively identify patient, or wristband missing or with incomplete information
	Take blood sample and immediately label at bedside with required patient information	Sample correctly labelled and signed	Patient misidentification as a result of: Sample tube pre-labelled or labelled away from bedside with another patient's ID Addressograph label affixed from incorrect patient
Hospital blood transfusion laboratory staff	Determine that sample labelling meets requirements for pretransfusion testing; if unacceptable, inform requester of need for another sample	If unacceptable, document reasons	Potential to issue inappropriate unit Failure to provide blood in a timely manner if clinicians unaware of need for another sample

Related hospital procedures and documents
Hospital sample labelling policy
Hospital policies for allocation and maintenance of unique patient identifiers and for resiting wristbands

Table 23.6 Collection and delivery of blood components from transfusion storage facility to clinical area.

Responsibility	Action	Documentation	Examples of potential problems and errors
Authorized and trained staff	Take documentation bearing patient identification to issue refrigerator	Completed prescription form or collection slip	Incorrect unit collected if no documentation bearing patient ID
	Check that unit removed and accompanying transfusion compatibility form bear identical patient identification details		Incorrect unit removed
	Record time and sign that correct unit has been collected		Lack of audit trail from failure to sign out unit from issue refrigerator

Related hospital procedures and documents
Hospital blood collection policy

Table 23.7 Administration of blood components.

Responsibility	Action	Documentation	Examples of potential problems and errors
Medical and registered nursing staff	At bedside, direct questioning of patient to provide surname, first name and date of birth when judged capable	Prescription form Compatibility form (if used) Compatibility label Patient wristband	Unit transfused to wrong patient if checked away from bedside or no verification of patient identity
	Check that patient identity is identical with documents		
	Check blood group is compatible	Compatibility form (if used) Compatibility label Base label on blood pack	Incorrect ABO/RhD group transfused if failure to detect laboratory grouping or labelling error
	Check special requirements fulfilled	Prescription chart Blood pack	Inappropriate component transfused if failure to note laboratory issuing error
	Check unit not past expiry date is intact with no visual evidence of deterioration		Transfusion of time-expired component
			Transfusion of potentially bacterially contaminated unit
	Document and sign date and time of commencement and completion	Compatibility form and/or prescription chart	
	Retain donation number in patient record	Label/sticker on prescription chart or in patient record	Failure to complete audit trail

Related hospital procedures and documents
Hospital blood administration policy

Table 23.8 Monitoring of transfused patients.

Responsibility	Action	Documentation	Examples of potential problems and errors
Authorized and trained staff	Measure and record clinical observations prior to each unit	Observation chart, recording date and time	Without baseline observations, cannot detect changes warning of transfusion reaction
	Explain to patient possible adverse effects to be reported and keep patient under close visual observation in first 15–20 min of each unit		Patient not aware of symptoms that can warn of transfusion reaction
	Measure temperature and pulse 15 min after start of each unit	Observation chart, recording time	Potential to miss early signs of serious transfusion reaction
	Measure and record clinical observation at end of each unit	Observation chart, recording time	Cannot know whether subsequent changes in patient's condition are temporally related to ongoing transfusion

Related hospital procedures and documents
Hospital policies on monitoring transfused patients and management of transfusion reactions

the unit and the competency of staff in safe transfusion practice.

Electronic bedside systems can be linked to similar systems controlling release of blood from remote blood refrigerators to provide full electronic process control and to facilitate electronically controlled remote issue (see later in this chapter and Reference [9]).

Electronic systems for blood transfusion are increasingly being implemented, although further studies are needed to confirm cost-effectiveness. The rationale for their use would be even greater if they were integrated with other processes requiring patient identification, such as medication administration.

Influencing clinical practice

Potential factors influencing transfusion practice and decision making include:
• physician knowledge and perception based on clinical experience;
• peer pressure and feedback;
• effectiveness of hospital governance frameworks;
• educational prompts at the time of decision making;
• patient knowledge and preferences [10];
• financial pressures or incentives;
• public and political perceptions; and
• fear of litigation.

Improving transfusion practice within a hospital community requires a planned, consistent approach, endorsed and implemented through clinical governance frameworks, supported over time and monitored for effect.

Guidelines, algorithms and protocols

Guidelines are systematically developed statements to assist practitioner and patient decision making about appropriate healthcare for specific clinical circumstances. A list of websites with some examples of guidelines is included at the end of this chapter. Data from randomized controlled trials are generally not available to assess the impact of professional guidelines, but even national guidelines rarely lead to change without local implementation and dissemination strategies, and these require time and resources.

Developing an institutional strategy to implement guidelines is a useful opportunity to gain ownership and participation. For example, educational opportunities arise from examining the evidence basis for the guidelines, and dissent and other local barriers to implementation, such as limited staff or IT resources, or effects on laboratory turnaround times, can be identified.

Institutions should adopt recommendations from authoritative professional guidelines and carefully review their content to consider whether any customization is required for local use. This may involve separating guidelines into sections and/or incorporating some recommendations into other local protocols for specific conditions, e.g. a fresh frozen plasma guideline incorporated into protocols for management of disseminated intravascular coagulation and massive haemorrhage. These local documents should be incorporated into transfusion policies and disseminated, with training, for all involved staff.

Experience in other medical fields has demonstrated that embedding guideline recommendations into materials used during transfusion decision making and administration processes can significantly improve compliance. Examples include:
• listing indications for special blood components on transfusion request forms or electronic request screens;
• using electronic warning systems to alert prescribers when, based on laboratory values, planned transfusions do not meet guidelines (see below);
• listing, on specific transfusion observation charts, actions to be taken in the event of reactions; and
• detailing checks to be made on the compatibility form prior to administering blood.

Intraoperative algorithms for the use of platelets and plasma to correct microvascular bleeding during and after cardiac bypass surgery have also proved to be successful in reducing inappropriate use of these components, especially when combined with near-patient testing and rapid availability of results.

Clinical audit

Clinical audit is a quality improvement process that seeks to improve patient care and clinical outcomes, through systematic review of care against explicit criteria or standards, followed by the implementation of change. Analysis of audit findings can lead to recommendations for improvements when deficiencies or non-guideline-based practices are identified, in turn generating cycles where feedback and clarification of hospital policies lead to improved practice.

Audits can be conducted retrospectively or concurrently. Retrospective transfusion audits are often performed under the auspices of the HTC. Some regulatory agencies require a certain percentage of all transfusions to be reviewed by the HTC and those felt to have been administered without reasonable

justification brought to the committee's attention. If, from available data, a transfusion is felt to be egregious, further information should be requested from the responsible physician. If the explanation is inadequate, or if the physician fails to reply, other steps, such as letters to department chairs, can also be taken. Advantages of this type of review are that communications from the HTC carry additional weight and they can be educational tools to inform physicians of institutional protocols. The main disadvantages are the limited number of transfusion episodes that can be audited and, because audits are performed after the event, educational opportunities are lost if the staff who ordered the transfusion cannot be located or cannot recall the event. Retrospective audits also cannot influence clinical practice for the episodes being audited.

Audits performed concurrently with blood component ordering, but before product issue, can take several forms. A simple example involves transfusion laboratory staff comparing component orders with hospital guidelines; if criteria are not met, the ordering physician is contacted, the reasons for ordering the transfusion discussed and plans established. Intervention by transfusion medicine physicians has been demonstrated to be effective in reducing unnecessary transfusions [11]. Audits of this type have been criticized for potentially causing delay in providing necessary products (although they would also prevent unnecessary transfusions before they were administered). Significant time, effort and good communication are required to make these audits effective.

Another approach to concurrent audit involves automation to warn clinicians at the time of ordering that the transfusion might not be necessary. Where a hospital uses computerized order entry and institutional guidelines are in place, warnings can appear on the screen when physicians try to order blood for patients whose laboratory values suggest that transfusion is not indicated. Figure 23.1 demonstrates the response where a physician attempts to order red cells for a patient whose latest haemoglobin value is above the threshold set by the HTC. The warning appears, giving the physician the option of either cancelling the order or proceeding, depending on the patient's current clinical situation (which might not be accurately reflected in a historical laboratory value). In the first few months after these warnings were instituted at hospitals of the University of Pittsburgh Medical

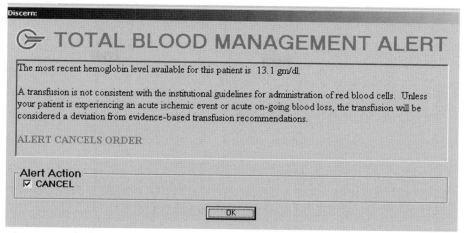

Fig 23.1 Warning message displayed when a physician at a University of Pittsburgh Medical Center (UPMC, Pittsburgh, PA) hospital attempts to order red cells using the computerized order entry system on a patient whose most recent haemoglobin value is in excess of the institutional guidelines.

Center (Pittsburgh, USA), cancellation was observed for 12% and over 25% of non-guideline-based red cell and plasma orders, respectively. The ability to track individual physicians and hospital locations that generate the greatest number of warnings also supports provision of focused education.

Many countries have regional or national clinical audit programmes, with participation being either voluntary or, increasingly, mandated by accreditation or governmental agencies. Participation provides opportunities to compare performance between similar institutions for the purposes of benchmarking and to promote engagement in practice improvement activities more broadly. The UK national audit programme and several of the practice improvement collaboratives in Australia have made their audit tools available to invite collaboration, comparisons of practice and sharing of resources.

Surveys

Many activities that fall under an 'audit' banner are not comparing practice with a standard, but are monitoring or surveying practice. These activities, many of which can be quantified, often provide information and baseline data that can lead to the development of quality or performance indicators. Trend analysis, or comparison of organizations or blood users with each other, is a powerful means of exerting peer pressure and influencing practice (benchmarking, as above).

Performance indicators can be applied to:
• clinical and laboratory practice issues: e.g. percentage of primary arthroplasties requiring allogeneic transfusion; proportion of patients receiving platelets after coronary artery bypass grafting; red cell use by surgical procedure (by surgeon or unit); or percentage of anaemic patients being investigated, correctly diagnosed and managed appropriately to minimize unnecessary transfusions; and
• process issues: e.g. percentage of mislabelled samples received in the laboratory, patient wristband errors; numbers of units crossmatched to units transfused (C : T) ratio; hospital blood wastage; percentage of group O red cells used.

National schemes

Many countries now have national schemes to monitor transfusion practice and promote practice improvement. These may be voluntary or mandatory, and institutions may be anonymous or identified. The programmes can be used to influence policy at national and local level, and to educate clinicians. Examples include:
• Haemovigilance programmes. The UK SHOT scheme is a voluntary system for collecting data on

serious transfusion adverse events and near misses. It produces annual reports with recommendations. Many other regional and national examples exist and experiences presented in these reports have been very valuable in identifying areas for improvement. A national haemovigilance programme in the USA with voluntary hospital participation was launched in 2010 as a joint effort between the AABB and the Centers for Disease Control (Chapter 18).

• EQA schemes. These programmes periodically provide clinical material to be tested by transfusion laboratories. Results are returned for analysis and collated reports disseminated to participants.

• Utilization and wastage schemes, such as the UK Blood Stocks Management Scheme, collate and publish details of blood stock inventory and wastage, and allow participants to benchmark against comparable hospitals.

Patient knowledge and preferences, public and political perceptions and fear of litigation

Many patients, and indeed the general public, have a very limited understanding of the true benefits and risks of transfusion and may consequently have considerable anxieties about transfusion. Patients who have received a transfusion often do not recall the consent process, either because they were not given full information or because they rapidly forgot it. Communication with both transfusion recipients and the general public needs to be improved. Involvement of patients in decision making about transfusion and the safety of transfusion procedures such as blood sample collection and the administration of blood are potential important interventions to improve the quality and safety of blood transfusion [10]. However, it is as yet unclear how willing patients and healthcare staff would be for patients to undertake a more active role. Furthermore, the use of advance directives and the clinical team's recognition that some patients have a religious or moral objection to the receipt of some or all blood components will allow patients to receive care that is consistent with their wishes and beliefs.

Transfusion-transmitted human immunodeficiency virus (HIV) led to substantial reductions in allogeneic red cell use in many countries after 1982. These declines are even more significant considering population growth and ageing during this period. Over the same interval, autologous donations increased greatly.

Some physicians were sued when transfused patients contracted HIV and the transfusions had not been clinically indicated (also see Chapter 22).

The potential for transfusion-transmitted variant Creutzfeldt–Jakob disease (vCJD) was one of the concerns that led the UK Department of Health in 1998 to require that all hospitals should have HTCs, implement good transfusion practice and explore the feasibility of cell salvage. Universal leucocyte reduction of blood was introduced in the UK in 1999 as a further preventive measure for vCJD. This resulted in a significant increase in the price of blood, which was an additional encouragement for hospitals to implement more judicious approaches to transfusion and use of alternatives to transfusion. As a consequence, red cell use in the UK has decreased by about 20% over the last 10 years, despite an increase in the volume and complexity of clinical care over this period.

Local investigation and feedback following 'near misses' and serious adverse events

SHOT defines a 'near miss' as any error that, if undetected, could result in the determination of a wrong blood group or the issue, collection or administration of an incorrect, inappropriate or unsuitable component but which was recognized before transfusion took place [1]. In Europe, 'serious adverse events' must also be reported to the competent authority. These events are defined as any untoward occurrences associated with the collection, testing, processing, storage and distribution of blood or blood components that might lead to death or life-threatening, disabling or incapacitating conditions for patients, or that result in, or prolong, hospitalization or morbidity. Systematic root cause analyses of these incidents provide opportunities to detect and understand system and process weaknesses and take corrective action to minimize recurrence. Typical weaknesses identified through root cause analyses include: inadequate training; human factors such as fatigue, misconceptions, ignorance of relevant policies; environmental factors such as distractions or interruptions, time pressures or access to equipment and IT support; and defective or risky processes.

Sample errors, most importantly those where the tube is labelled with the intended patient's details but contains blood from another patient, 'wrong blood in tube' (WBIT) events, are some of the most common detectable errors reported to haemovigilance programmes. These inevitably arise as a result of failures to identify systematically and positively the patient at the bedside. However, investigations almost always uncover other contributing factors, which need to be understood and addressed, for example:

• Failure to positively identify the patient. Healthcare workers have often not been trained in and are unfamiliar with hospital policies and procedures, or perceive this activity as unimportant or suggesting an inadequate knowledge of patients under their care.
• Reduced junior doctors' hours and shift patterns of those involved in direct patient management, and inadequate communication and documentation, leading to unfamiliarity with patients.
• Admission and discharge practices, which frequently lead to patients having samples taken for pretransfusion testing before case notes are available or wristbands applied, leading to the potential for misidentification.

Exposure to avoidable patient morbidity or fatality often triggers clinical awareness of transfusion hazards and can instigate procedural changes. Corrective action should involve counselling and educating individuals who failed to comply with procedures, but focusing on addressing important, underlying system issues identified above and supporting staff in often traumatic situations [12].

Education and continuing professional development

Education of all individuals in the transfusion process has traditionally been difficult, but UK experience shows it to be achievable when made an integral part of mandatory hospital training programmes and subjected to external inspection. However, it requires considerable dedicated resources, a flexible and pragmatic approach to accommodate shift patterns and availability of staff, including temporary staff. Observational competency assessment is more readily achieved with the help of clinical 'champions'. Training and knowledge-based assessments can be facilitated by web-based programmes (such as the e-learning modules of the Australian BloodSafe program, which have been completed by over 80 000 staff nationally and internationally), which also permit management oversight of participation.

Education is an essential component of strategies to gain clinician compliance with procedures and guidelines and to modify practice. Educational interventions are more successful when they are interactive, focused on a specific objective and directed at groups of individuals with reflections on their own practice. Continuing professional development schemes for the various craft groups encourage knowledge acquisition with documentation (typically via participant portfolios) of accredited activity in educational, professional and vocational areas.

Centralization of transfusion services

The medical and patient safety benefits of a centralized transfusion service (CTS) vary depending on its organisation [13]. The CTS in Pittsburgh, USA (city population 306 000; catchment population 2.1 million), operates as follows. The main blood supplier, the Central Blood Bank (CBB) delivers blood components to a central laboratory. This stand-alone central facility also houses the red cell reference laboratory and performs most of the automated, batched pretransfusion testing. The laboratory then distributes products to 19 CTS-networked hospitals in a 'hub and spoke' manner. Each hospital has an on-site transfusion laboratory, staffed and stocked with products in accordance with the acuity of patients treated and volume of transfusions performed. Each hospital laboratory performs routine pretransfusion testing and basic immunohaematology, thawing of plasma and cryoprecipitate, and some platelet pooling and leucocyte reduction (most is performed centrally).

Perhaps the most important patient safety benefit of a CTS is the ability to access patient records at different hospital sites. Since patients can visit different hospitals within the network, recipient immunohaematology and component modification requirements are available electronically at each hospital's blood bank, reducing the need for re-investigation and ensuring that any special component modifications are fulfilled for each patient whenever and wherever transfusion is required. Having records of recipient historical ABO groups provides additional opportunities to detect WBIT errors. In 16 cases where recipient historical ABO groups on file at the Pittsburgh CTS did not match the ABO group of specimens submitted for pretransfusion testing, 6/16 were detected based on an historical ABO group collected previously at a different hospital [14]. Requiring a second ABO group to be performed on a separate specimen before ABO-specific RBCs are issued on recipients without an historical ABO group on file would achieve the same end.

Other advantages of a CTS include availability of transfusion medicine expertise for community hospitals without experts on the staff. CTS transfusion physicians participate on HTCs of all networked hospitals, supporting rapid implementation of evidence-based practice and benchmarking. Consolidating technical expertise into one reference immuno-haematology laboratory permits rapid and expert service provision. There are also numerous opportunities for cost savings, through greater efficiency from technical and nontechnical employees, economies of scale and use of automation. Blood supplier logistics are greatly simplified by delivery to one central location and lower inventory levels can be supported due to the ability to circulate blood components between hospitals to reduce wastage.

Pretransfusion compatibility testing

This typically comprises:
- determination of the recipient ABO and RhD group;
- a screen for red cell alloantibodies reactive at 37°C in recipient plasma;
- a check for previous records or duplicate records, and comparison of current with historical findings (these three elements comprise a 'group and screen');
- identification of the specificity of any alloantibody detected in the antibody screen;
- selection of appropriate component(s), bearing in mind blood group compatibility (and extended red cell phenotype, where relevant), and any modifications, such as irradiation or washing, to meet individual requirements;
- a serological or electronic crossmatch; and
- labelling of the blood with recipient identifying information.

Detection of red cell antigen–antibody reactions

Detection and identification of blood group antigens and auto- and alloantibodies depends on interpretations of serological reactions. Various test systems

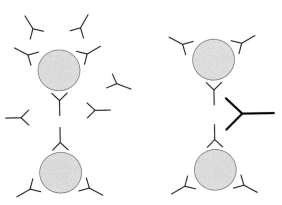

Red cells incubated with serum containing IgG antibody

Unbound antibody washed away. Anti-human globulin added to precipitate cells

Fig 23.2 Indirect antiglobulin test.

are available to demonstrate these interactions and methods must be optimized in order to obtain the necessary sensitivity and specificity for their intended clinical use. Failure to follow the instructions provided by reagent manufacturers can lead to incorrect conclusions.

Test methods have been developed to allow detection of antibodies of different isotypes. Antibodies with specificities for red cell antigens are usually IgG or IgM. Pentameric IgM antibodies can cross-link antigens on adjacent cells, causing direct agglutination of red cells. Conversely, IgG antibodies are monomeric and, although divalent, the distance between the Fab regions on a single IgG molecule is generally insufficient to allow direct agglutination. Methods such as the indirect antiglobulin test (IAT) (which uses a secondary anti-isotype antibody; see Figure 23.2) or the enzyme method (which uses proteolytic enzymes such as papain or ficin to cleave negatively charged, hydrophilic residues from red cell membranes) must therefore be used to detect most IgG red cell antibodies.

Test systems for detection of serological reactions can be classified into three broad categories.

Liquid-phase ('tube') systems
Liquid-phase systems rely on visualization of haemagglutination reactions in individual glass/plastic tubes or 96-well microplates. The presence or absence of

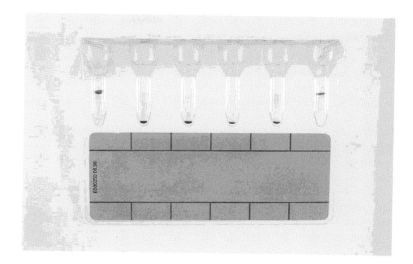

Fig 23.3 Column-agglutination technology for blood grouping and antibody screening. Samples may consist of patient cells and reagent antisera or reagent red cells and patient serum/plasma. Positive results are seen in the first and last columns, the other columns show negative reactions.

agglutinated red cells distinguishes positive and negative reactions, allowing grading of reaction avidity according to the strength of haemagglutination. While not the most sensitive methods available today, IAT methods using red cells suspended in low-ionic-strength solution remain the gold standard for detection of clinically significant red cell alloantibodies. These methods require meticulous procedural attention, in particular during washing to remove unbound IgG.

Column-agglutination systems

Introduction of column-agglutination systems has resulted in very significant changes to routine laboratory practice. Synthetic gel mixtures or glass microbeads configured into vertical columns on small cards form density barriers, retaining agglutinates and allowing the passage of unagglutinated cells. Positive reactions (antibody/antigen interactions) are distinguished by agglutinates at or near the top of the gel column and negative reactions appear as buttons of red cells at the bottom (Figure 23.3).

Reagent (IgM) antibody can be incorporated into the columns, allowing phenotyping simply by addition of test cells to the top of the column. Similarly, the IAT can be performed in columns containing antiglobulin reagent to which plasma and reagent red cells are added. Because plasma proteins are less dense than the gel, washing is not needed. This property, and the relative stability of reaction endpoints, gives column agglutination methods a simplicity and reliability not

achieved by other methods. Manual and automated methods for performing and interpreting these tests are now widely available.

Solid-phase systems

These techniques are performed in microplates and provide another alternative to tube or column IAT. Positive reaction endpoints are characterized by red cell monolayers in the wells while discrete buttons of red cells at the bottom of the well indicate negative reactions (Figure 23.4). Solid-phase systems require carefully standardized centrifugation and washing steps; however, unlike liquid-phase test systems, fully automated equipment allows these steps to be performed safely and consistently without operator intervention.

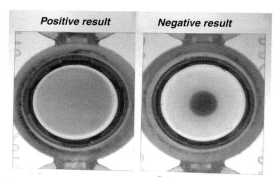

Fig 23.4 Solid-phase blood grouping technology. See text for an explanation of results.

243

Reduction of error in pretransfusion compatibility testing

Analysis of mistransfusion cases from SHOT in 2011 showed that laboratory errors were implicated in up to 55% of incidents [1]. Many of these were due to human error in sample transposition or in test setup or interpretation. Provided that correct laboratory identifiers (such as barcodes) are placed on patient samples, these events can be avoided by using fully automated systems interfaced to transfusion laboratory computer systems.

Basic features of fully automated ('walk away') systems should include:

- trays or carousels to stack samples;
- automated liquid handling and other robotic operations;
- devices to ensure that positive sample identification is maintained;
- clot sensor and liquid level alarms;
- an optical device to record reaction patterns; and
- comprehensive system management software that interprets reaction patterns and flags discrepant results.

When automation cannot be used for the whole process (i.e. antibody identification), steps must be taken to minimize the occurrence of error and its impact. High standards of training, participation in internal and external quality assessment schemes, and strict adherence to validated documented procedures are among the measures that reduce errors.

The most important procedure in the transfusion laboratory is the recipient ABO group determination. Different practices are in place in different countries, but this critical procedure should be performed independently by two people (except in urgent situations where uncrossmatched group O red cells will be issued) if there is no record of a grouping result from a historical sample. Obtaining a second sample from the patient drawn by a different phlebotomist separate from the first sample collection (often called an 'ABO check type sample') serves as the preferred means of verifying the results of the first ABO grouping. Similarly, determination of an RhD group should be performed in duplicate, in the absence of full automation.

ABO and RhD grouping

Patient red cells should be tested against monoclonal anti-A and anti-B grouping reagents and patient

Table 23.9 ABO grouping patterns.

	Forward type (recipient RBCs)		Reverse type (recipient plasma/serum)		
Group	Anti-A	Anti-B	A cells	B cells	O cells*
A	+++	–	–	+++	–
B	–	+++	+++	–	–
O	–	–	+++	+++	–
AB	+++	+++	–	–	–

*Positive in some patients with cold agglutinins.

serum/plasma should be tested against A_1 and B reagent red cells, except in neonates. The expected reaction patterns in ABO grouping are illustrated in Table 23.9. Patient red cells should be tested with an IgM monoclonal anti-D reagent, which does not detect the common DVI variant (because individuals with this phenotype can become alloimmunized if transfused with RhD positive RBCs; thus as recipients they should be typed as RhD negative and transfused with RhD negative RBCs). ABO and RhD groups must be repeated when discrepancies are found and these should be performed using a fresh suspension of washed cells, ideally from a new sample.

Antibody screening

The IAT performed at 37°C is the best method available for detection of clinically significant red cell antibodies. It is simple (especially when using a column-agglutination system), sensitive and has a high degree of specificity.

Patient serum/plasma should be tested against two or more 'screening cells' using the IAT. The reagent red cells used for screening should between them express antigens reactive with all clinically significant antibodies; ideally the phenotypes R_1R_1, rr and R_2R_2 should be represented in the screening cell set. Different national standards and guidelines are in place, but in many countries it is recommended that the screening cells express the Jka, Jkb, S, s, Fya, Fyb antigens and incorporate the following phenotypes: Jk(a+b–), Jk(a–b+), S+s–, S–s+, Fy(a+b–), Fy(a–b+), since stronger reactions may be obtained with cells having double-dose antigen expression.

Antibody screening performed in advance of the requirement for transfusion also provides the laboratory with time to identify the specificity of any antibody detected and, when clinically significant, to select antigen-negative units for crossmatching.

Antibody identification

When an antibody has been detected in screening tests, the specificity should be determined by testing patient serum/plasma against a panel of reagent red cells of known phenotypes. In addition to the IAT, other methods (e.g. using enzyme-treated red cells) may be helpful, particularly when mixtures of antibodies are present. Antibody specificity can be determined when the serum/plasma is reactive with at least two examples of red cells bearing the antigen and nonreactive with at least two examples of red cells lacking the antigen. When a single antibody specificity has been determined, it is essential that additional clinically significant antibodies are also detected, if present. Multiple antibodies can be confirmed only by testing against red cells that are antigen negative for the recognized specificity, but that express other antigens to which clinically significant antibodies may arise.

Autoantibodies

These may be suspected when patient serum/plasma reacts with all cells used in the reverse ABO group (in the case of cold autoantibodies) or with all cells in the antibody identification panel, including the patient's own red cells. Autoantibodies are common, but not all autoantibodies give rise to clinically significant haemolysis. Serological investigations should focus on obtaining the correct ABO and RhD group of the patient and excluding the presence of underlying alloantibodies.

Cold-type autoimmune haemolytic anaemia
These autoantibodies tend not to cause problems in alloantibody identification unless they react at 37°C. Red cells should be washed at 37°C before performing the direct antiglobulin test (DAT), which will usually be strongly positive due to coating with C3d.

Warm-type autoimmune haemolytic anaemia
Red cells will usually have a positive DAT due to coating with IgG with or without complement and an eluate prepared from these cells typically reacts with all panel cells. Rarely, red cells may be coated with IgA or IgM and IgG. Underlying alloantibodies may be detected following removal of autoantibodies from patient serum. This may be achieved either by absorbing the patient's serum with the patient's own red cells (treated with a combination of papain and dithiothreitol, or 'ZZAP') or, if the patient has been recently transfused, performing absorption and elution studies with reagent red cells of specific phenotypes.

These processes can be very time-consuming and the treating clinical unit should be advised that investigations may take some time before any underlying alloantibodies can be identified and antigen-negative RBC units can be available; hence, the urgency of transfusion support requirements must be determined. Chapter 29 has more information on immune-mediated haemolysis.

Selection of red cells for transfusion

Red cell units that are compatible with the recipient's ABO and RhD groups are routinely issued. As group O red cells are the 'universal donor' type they can be safely administered to recipients of any blood group; otherwise group A and B (and O) recipients can only receive ABO-identical red cells due to the presence of naturally occurring antibodies to the A and B antigen(s) lacking on their RBCs. Group AB recipients lack naturally occurring anti-A and anti-B antibodies and can thus receive RBCs of any blood group. Group O RBCs may be issued in life-threatening situations where blood is required before the patient has been grouped. In these emergency situations, if the patient is a premenopausal female, group O, RhD-negative uncrossmatched RBCs should be used (see below). Group-specific units can be provided as soon as the patient's group is known. Care should be taken to establish the recipient's ABO group before a large number of group O red cells are transfused, as a massive transfusion with group O units could obscure the recipient's actual ABO group and complicate the further selection of both RBCs and other components.

Premenopausal females should ideally receive RhD- and K-matched red cells and in some countries this is a requirement to prevent alloimmunization, which could lead to severe haemolytic disease of the fetus and newborn (HDFN). RhD positive patients can always safely receive RhD negative units. Patients with anticipated long-term red cell transfusion requirements (see Chapters 28 and 29) should also ideally receive red cells matched at least for Rh and K antigens. Red cells for fetal or neonatal exchange transfusions should also be selected to be compatible with the maternal serum/plasma and any known maternal antibodies.

A recipient of an ABO-incompatible allogeneic haemopoietic stem cell graft will need to be transfused with red cells of the donor's group in the case of a minor ABO mismatch or group O in the case of a combined (bidirectional) ABO mismatch. RhD-negative red cells should also be selected for an RhD-positive recipient of an RhD-negative stem cell donation (see Chapter 28).

Selection of blood for patients with red cell alloantibodies is summarized in Table 23.10. However, in life-threatening situations, the immediate need for red cell transfusion may necessitate the use of potentially incompatible units. Discussions between the treating clinical unit and transfusion service about risks of haemolysis when using uncrossmatched red cells for a patient with a positive antibody screen are essential.

The laboratory also has responsibility for ensuring that requests for irradiated, CMV seronegative or other requirements are fulfilled in accordance with institutional policies and that patient records are 'flagged' for these needs.

Crossmatching

Red cell crossmatching techniques have been simplified in recent years and only the immediate spin (IS) and IAT crossmatches remain in common use.

The IAT crossmatch can be abolished in favour of an electronic, or IS only, crossmatch when antibody screening is performed with screening cells that express the most common antigens capable of stimulating clinically significant antibodies and the patient's serum/plasma has never been found to contain clinically significant antibodies. Studies have shown that there is negligible risk in omitting the IAT crossmatch. Although up to 0.2% IAT crossmatches may reveal an unpredicted incompatibility, few of these transfusions result in haemolysis. Antibodies directed against low frequency antigens may be missed, but the majority of these are clinically insignificant.

Table 23.10 Recommendations for selection of blood for patients with red cell alloantibodies.

	Typical examples	Procedure
Antibodies considered clinically significant	Anti-RhD, -C, -c, -E, -e Anti-K, -k Anti-Jk^a, -Jk^b Anti-S, -s, -U Anti-Fy^a, -Fy^b	Select ABO-compatible, antigen-negative blood for serological crossmatching
Antibodies directed against antigens with an incidence of <5% and where the antibody is often not clinically significant	Anti-C^w Anti-Kp^a Anti-Lu^a Anti-Wr^a (anti-Di3)	Select ABO-compatible blood for serological crossmatching
Antibodies primarily reactive below 37°C and never or only very rarely clinically significant	Anti-A$_1$ Anti-N Anti-P$_1$ Anti-Le^a, -Le^b, -Le^{a+b} Anti-HI (in A$_1$ and A$_1$B patients)	Select ABO-compatible blood for serological crossmatching, performed strictly at 37°C
Antibodies sometimes reactive at 37°C and clinically significant	Anti-M	If reactive at 37°C, select ABO-compatible, antigen-negative blood for serological crossmatching If unreactive at 37°C, select ABO-compatible blood for serological crossmatching performed strictly at 37°C
Other antibodies active by IAT at 37°C	Many specificities	Seek advice from blood centre

If the IAT crossmatch is omitted, there must be some check included to detect ABO incompatibility. The IS crossmatch (i.e. agglutination in saline following centrifugation) is a serological check that can be used. However, this technique is fallible when the patient has low levels of anti-A or anti-B antibodies and, unless ethylenediamine tetra-acetic acid (EDTA) saline is used, false-negative results may also arise as a result of steric hindrance of agglutination by complement. False-positive IS results arising from rouleaux or cold agglutinins can also cause ABO discrepancies. Limitations of the IS crossmatch have heralded the acceptance of electronic issue as an alternative method of preventing the release of ABO-incompatible units of blood.

Electronic crossmatch and issue

Electronic crossmatch can only be used for detecting ABO incompatibility between the donor unit and recipient. There are several essential requirements for adopting this approach, which are common to the various professional standards.
• The computer contains logic to prevent assignment and release of ABO-incompatible blood.
• No clinically significant antibodies are detected in the current patient plasma/serum sample and there is no record of previous detection of such antibodies.
• There are concordant results of at least two determinations of patient ABO and RhD groups on file, at least one of which is from a current sample.
• Critical system elements (application software, readers and interfaces) have been validated on-site and there are mechanisms to verify the correct entry of data prior to release of blood, such as barcode identifiers to enter information when it cannot be automatically transferred. Fully automated blood grouping and antibody screening, although not a requirement in some national guidelines, is strongly recommended.

Electronic issue has been widely used for over a decade and is now routine practice in many countries. It has several potential advantages over serological crossmatching:
• reduced technical workload;
• rapid availability of blood;
• improved blood stock management through reduced numbers of crossmatched red cells and reduced wastage;
• less handling of biohazardous material;

• elimination of unwanted false-positive results in the IS; and
• ability to issue blood electronically at remote sites, using trained nonlaboratory staff.

This last characteristic has allowed development of systems for electronic remote blood issue. When patient details are entered, the system checks that criteria for electronic issue are fulfilled and either allows access to ABO and RhD compatible units in the remote blood refrigerator or dispenses compatible units. A compatibility label is printed and attached to the unit and rescanned to ensure it is the correct one for the unit. Such systems reduce the time taken for the issue of blood, particularly in small hospitals without transfusion laboratories.

Maximum surgical blood ordering schedule (MSBOS)

This consists of a table of elective surgical procedures that lists the extent of pretransfusion testing that is routinely required before the case begins (see Table 23.11). The MSBOS is prepared taking into account the likelihood of transfusion and the response time for having blood available, following an immediate spin crossmatch or electronic issue. An MSBOS reduces the workload of unnecessary crossmatching and issuing of blood and can improve stock management and reduce wastage.

The successful implementation of an MSBOS depends on all parties agreeing to the schedule, education of blood prescribers, confidence of senior staff that there is a robust system for accessing blood promptly when there is unexpected blood loss and ability to override the schedule when there are reasons to suggest that indicate that greater blood loss will occur. The schedule is constructed by:
• analysing each surgical procedure in terms of the crossmatch : transfusion (C : T) ratio;
• routinely managing procedures with a C : T ratio greater than 2 (i.e. a low probability of transfusion) with a group and screen, and issuing blood only when there is a need for transfusion; and
• allocating an agreed number of units for procedures with a C : T ratio of less than 2.

An overall C : T ratio of 1.5 for elective surgery is achievable when the laboratory is centrally issuing blood in accordance with the MSBOS. However,

Table 23.11 Example of maximum surgical blood order schedule (MSBOS, general surgery).

Operation	Red cells crossmatched or group & screen (G&S)
Lumbar spine disc replacement	No pretransfusion testing required
Caesarean section	No pretransfusion testing required
Colonoscopy with polypectomy	No pretransfusion testing required
Tonsillectomy	No pretransfusion testing required
Spinal laminectomy and decompression	G&S
Carotid endarterectomy	G&S
Lung biopsy	G&S
Mammoplasty reduction	G&S
Splenectomy	2
Coronary artery bypass graft	2
Total hip arthroplasty	2
Resection/repair ascending aortic aneurysm	4
Heart transplant	6
Liver transplant	10

lower ratios are possible with use of electronic crossmatch (see above) and/or remote electronic issue from blood refrigerators in theatre suites. In addition to reducing the number of allocated, crossmatched red cells for specific surgical patients, which increases the number of available units in the general inventory, another benefit of adhering to recommendations of the MSBOS is that fewer patients with unexpected antibodies will be taken to surgery without appropriate transfusion support. As the MSBOS indicates the extent of pretransfusion testing that should be performed before surgery, adherence to its recommendations will lead to antibody screening being performed on patients with a reasonable chance of requiring intraoperative transfusion, thereby allowing the transfusion service to locate and crossmatch compatible units before the case begins, should unexpected antibodies be detected.

In recipients with red cell alloantibodies who require transfusion, consideration should be given to the time taken to acquire and crossmatch

antigen-negative units, and the treating clinical team should be informed.

Selection of platelets and plasma components

Platelets are collected by apheresis or separated from whole blood donations using either the 'platelet-rich plasma' or buffy coat methods. ABO and RhD compatible platelets are preferable, but when these are not available, ABO incompatible platelets may be used. Many countries provide platelets suspended in additive solution, to reduce recipient exposure to plasma and to support platelet viability and function.

Plasma for transfusion is collected by apheresis or separated from whole blood donations. Plasma should be ABO compatible with the recipient, but where the recipient's blood type is not known, such as in an emergency, AB plasma can be used. Plasma depleted of cryoprecipitate (cryodepleted or cryopoor plasma) may be used in the treatment of thrombotic thrombocytopenic purpura. Other preparations, such as pooled, solvent-detergent plasma, are also available in some regions.

Cryoprecipitate is prepared from whole blood donations or apheresis plasma collections. Cryoprecipitate should ideally be of the same ABO group as the recipient, but this is not essential. Cryoprecipitate is mainly used as a source of fibrinogen, where a virally inactivated fibrinogen concentrate is not available.

Frozen products must always be thawed using an approved device and method.

Key points

1 The transfusion process is unique as it links blood donors with patients in an altruistic, potentially life-saving activity. For many patients, there is still no substitute for donated blood components.
2 Prescribers of blood components have a duty of care to their patients to ensure that the benefits of the transfusion outweigh the risks, and a moral obligation to donors to ensure that their donations are used appropriately.
3 The transfusion process is multistep and complex, involving many different staff across the broad spectrum of clinical practice and settings, often working under challenging conditions. In this context there are many opportunities for human error to occur.

4 Investments in quality infrastructure, computerization and automation and training in the clinical and laboratory aspects of transfusion practice are essential to minimize or, ultimately, prevent errors in the transfusion process.

Acknowledgement

This chapter updates the material in the previous edition by Sue Knowles and Geoff Poole.

References

1 PHB Bolton-Maggs (ed.) & H Cohen on behalf of the Serious Hazards of Transfusion (SHOT) Steering Group. The 2011 Annual SHOT Report; 2012.
2 US Food and Drug Administration. Fatalities reported to FDA following blood collection and transfusion: Annual Summary for Fiscal Year 2010. Available at: http://www.fda.gov/BiologicsBloodVaccines.
3 Narick C, Triulzi D & Yazer MH. Transfusion-associated circulatory overload after plasma transfusion. *Transfusion* 2011, 18 July. Epub ahead of print.
4 Linden JV, Wagner K, Voytovich AE & Sheehan J. Transfusion errors in New York State: an analysis of 10 years' experience. *Transfusion* 2000; 40: 1207–1213.
5 Murphy MF, Stanworth SJ & Yazer M. Transfusion practice and safety: current status and possibilities for improvement. *Vox Sanguinis* 2011; 100: 46–59.
6 UK Blood Safety and Quality Regulations. Available at: www.transfusionguidelines.org.uk.
7 Australian Commission on Safety and Quality in Health Care. *National Safety and Quality Health Service Standards*. Sydney: ACSQHC; 2011.
8 Turner CL, Casbard AC & Murphy MF. Barcode technology: its role in increasing the safety of blood transfusion. *Transfusion* 2003; 43: 1200–1209.
9 Staves, J, Davies A, Kay J et al. Electronic remote blood issue: a combination of remote blood issue with a system for end-to-end electronic control of transfusion to provide a 'total solution' for a safe and timely hospital blood transfusion service. *Transfusion* 2008; 48, 415–424.
10 Davis RE, Vincent CA & Murphy MF. Blood transfusion safety: the potential role of the patient. *Transfus Med Rev* 2011; 25(1): 12–23.
11 Tavares M, DiQuattro P, Nolette N et al. Reduction in plasma transfusion after enforcement of transfusion guidelines. *Transfusion* 2011; 51: 754–761.
12 Stainsby D, Russell J, Cohen H & Lilleyman J. Reducing adverse events in blood transfusion. *Br J Haematol* 2005; 131(1): 8–12.
13 Simpson M. *Strategies for Centralized Blood Services*. Bethesda, MD: AABB Press; 2006.
14 MacIvor D, Triulzi DJ & Yazer MH. Enhanced detection of blood bank sample collection errors with a centralized patient database. *Transfusion* 2009; 49: 40–43.

Further reading

Department of Health. *Better Blood Transfusion*, HSC 2007/001. London: HMSO; 2007.
Dzik WH, Corwin H, Goodnough LT et al. Patient safety and blood transfusion: new solutions. *Transfus Med Rev* 2003; 17: 169–180.
Eisenstaedt RS. Modifying physicians' transfusion practice. *Transfus Med Rev* 1997; 11: 27–37.
Judd WJ. Requirements for the electronic crossmatch. *Vox Sanguinis* 1998; 74 (Suppl. 2): 409–417.
Klein HG & Anstee D (eds). *Mollison's Blood Transfusion in Clinical Medicine*, 11th edn. Oxford: Blackwell Publishing; 2005.
McClelland DBL (ed.). *Handbook of Transfusion Medicine*, 4th edn. Norwich: TSO; 2007. Available at: www.transfusionguidelines.org.
Saxena S & Shulman I (eds). *The Transfusion Committee: Putting Patient Safety First*. Bethesda, MD: AABB Press; 2006.

Guidelines and other resources

For a range of guidelines and other resources on laboratory and clinical hospital transfusion practice:

AABB: www.aabb.org/resources

Australian and New Zealand Society of Blood Transfusion: www.anzsbt.org.au

British Committee for Standards in Haematology: www.bcshguidelines.com

Canadian resources: www.transfusion.ca, www.transfusionontario.org and www.transfusionmedicine.ca

International Society of Blood Transfusion: www.isbtweb.org

Joint Commission on Accreditation of Healthcare Organizations: www.jointcommission.org

Network for Advancement of Transfusion Alternatives: www.nataonline.com

World Health Organization: www.who.int/bloodsafety

24 Blood transfusion in a global context

David J. Roberts[1], Alan D. Kitchen[2], Stephen Field[3], Imelda Bates[4] & Jean Pierre Allain[5]

[1]University of Oxford and NHS Blood and Transplant and Department of Haematology, John Radcliffe Hospital, Oxford, UK
[2]National Transfusion Microbiology Laboratory and NHS Blood and Transplant, Colindale, London, UK
[3]Welsh Blood Service, Cardiff, Wales, UK
[4]Liverpool School of Tropical Medicine, Liverpool, UK
[5]NHS Blood and Transplant and Division of Transfusion Medicine, Department of Haematology, University of Cambridge, Cambridge, UK

Introduction

'17% of the world's population has access to 60% of the global blood supply'

Inequality in the provision of 'safe blood' round the world mirrors the unequal distribution of almost all other resources crucial for effective health services or indeed for health itself. Unfortunately, in many countries, providing safe blood is made more difficult by lack of donors and the high frequency of transfusion-transmissible infections. At the same time, the problems posed by the poor supply of blood are compounded by the frequent need for urgent life-saving transfusions in childbirth, in children with malaria and the increased demand for HIV/AIDS patients.

The purpose of this chapter is not to guide those developing transfusion services in less affluent countries but to inform a wider audience of the problems faced in the development of effective transfusion services in these countries. A secondary aim is to stimulate some debate and analysis of the problems faced by transfusion services globally. Finally, a short chapter must be selective and our choice of topics and examples, and their solutions, reflect our own experience in Southeast Asia and sub-Saharan Africa.

Blood safety or blood supply?

A safe and rapid supply of blood is an essential part of medical services. An unsafe blood supply is costly in both human and economic terms. Transfusion of infected blood not only causes direct morbidity and mortality in the recipients but also has an economic and emotional impact on their families and communities and undermines confidence in modern healthcare. Those who become infected through blood transfusion are often infectious to others and contribute a significant secondary wave of iatrogenic infections. Investment in safe supplies of blood is cost-effective for every country, even those with few resources. At the same time, an insufficient supply costs lives; in developing countries, transfusion does save lives because, unless transfused, severely anaemic patients do not survive. This has been shown in 26% of haemorrhages in pregnant women when not transfused and in infants with acute malaria [1, 2]. Where should the priority be? The shockwave of the HIV epidemics put overwhelming emphasis on blood safety but now that >80% of HIV infected patients survive >10 years, the supply of blood should take back its legitimate place as a priority.

Practical Transfusion Medicine, Fourth Edition. Edited by Michael F. Murphy, Derwood H. Pamphilon and Nancy M. Heddle.
© 2013 John Wiley & Sons, Ltd. Published 2013 by John Wiley & Sons, Ltd.

The World Health Organization (WHO) has identified four key objectives for blood services to ensure that blood is safe for transfusion.
• Establish a coordinated national blood transfusion service that can provide adequate and timely supplies of safe blood for all patients in need.
• Collect blood only from voluntary nonremunerated blood donors from low risk populations and use stringent donor selection procedures.
• Screen all blood for transfusion-transmissible infections and have standardized procedures in place for grouping and compatibility testing.
• Reduce unnecessary transfusions through the appropriate clinical use of blood, including the use of intravenous replacement fluids and other simple alternatives to transfusion, wherever possible.

The WHO also emphasizes that effective quality assurance should be in place for all aspects of the transfusion process, from donor recruitment and selection, through infection screening, blood grouping and blood storage, to administration to patients and clinical monitoring for adverse events.

It is axiomatic that transfusion medicine is a distinct and multidisciplinary sector of the health service and should be incorporated into national health plans. It is the responsibility of governments to develop policies and legislation that will facilitate the development of a national transfusion service and ensure that the blood transfusion process and its associated quality assurance programmes are of a high standard. However, it must be realized that in some areas such as sub-Saharan Africa, transfusion is almost exclusively an emergency measure to treat patients with extreme, life-threatening anaemia. This situation has two important consequences.
• Blood is considered a therapeutic commodity with little more regard from the medical community and government than drugs delivered by the pharmacy.
• Whole blood is an appropriate choice, helping to reduce the cost of transfusion (sparing component preparation expenses).

The WHO has provided a recommended structure of national blood transfusion services. They suggest that at the national level the transfusion service should have a medical director, an advisory committee and clear national transfusion policies and strategies with the appropriate statutory instruments to ensure the national coordination and standardization of blood testing, processing and distribution. Notwithstanding these recommendations, transfusion activities must be integrated with other services at local and national levels.

There has been some progress to realize WHO's recommendations for a national blood programme. In Africa, in 2002 the WHO estimated that among the 46 member states in the African continent, only 14 had a national blood policy and just six had a policy to specifically encourage and develop a system of voluntary nonremunerated donation. In the most recent survey, in 2007, 40/41 of African states surveyed had a national blood policy, but only 56% (23/41) countries were able to implement their policies.

It is worthwhile reflecting on why the development of national transfusion services has not been achieved. A key reason is that it is logistically complex. Management skills to run such services are lacking. There has been an understandable emphasis on primary healthcare over the last 25 years and this may have diffused interest in hospital-based curative medicine. A second reason may be the high cost of blood transfusion in relation to disposable income and healthcare budgets. The average annual income in sub-Saharan Africa is in the range of $400–1000, and a unit of blood costs $10–20 in a hospital service and $60–100 in a centralized service. Blood is therefore an expensive commodity in relation to the annual per capita budget for healthcare in these countries and it remains to be seen if blood costing more than $50 per unit when produced in centralized, externally funded units is sustainable. Precise cost–benefit analyses for the use of blood have not been done. Nevertheless, blood transfusion for severe malarial anaemia and severe haemorrhage can be life saving, and it seems plausible that the cost of transfusion probably approaches the generally accepted cost–benefit range of $1 per year of life saved for health interventions in the poorest countries.

The WHO 'volunteer only' policy has had considerable negative side effects in sub-Saharan African countries that implemented it on the basis that it increased blood safety. This was based on the assumption that volunteer nonremunerated donors (VNRD) were safer than the traditional family-replacement donors (FRD). Recent data from multiple sources showed clearly that there was no difference in prevalence of confirmed viral markers between first time VNRD (60–90% of VNRD) and genuine FRD [3]. Blood shortage was maintained if not worsened by

---

Box 24.1 Case studies: examples of blood transfusion systems in sub-Saharan Africa

Integrated National Blood Service – Ivory Coast

The Côte d'Ivoire blood service was created in 1992 with substantial subsidies from the European Union. A National Blood Transfusion Centre is located in Abidjan, the capital, with three smaller provincial centres. In addition, blood depots are located in hospitals of five other main cities. For a population of 18 million, approximately 80 000 units of blood were collected in 2002, mostly from volunteer blood donors recruited amongst secondary school students (>60%), although 24% of them were first-time donors.

Any hospital in the country can access the blood supply free of charge to the hospital and the patients. The government allocates funding. Less than 20% of the blood is processed into blood components that are mostly used in the capital. Antibodies to HIV, HCV as well as HBsAg are tested by EIA in the capital. The recurrent cost per unit produced is estimated at $40.

Regional hospital – Ghana

In a 1200-bed hospital, the current demand for blood components is, in adults, whole blood for acute anaemia or massive haemorrhage and in children 200 ml plasma-depleted red cells for anaemia related to malaria, sickle cell disease or thalassaemia. Approximately 10 000 candidate donors are screened per year and 7000 blood units are available for clinical use. Patients' families are asked to pay $14 for a unit of blood and $7 if the blood is replaced. Volunteer blood is primarily collected in secondary schools (80% of total volunteer donations). Anti-HIV, HBsAg and anti-HCV are screened pre-donation with high performance rapid tests so that blood bags (representing one-third of the total consumable budget) are not wasted. Furthermore, deferred donors can be identified, informed and counselled, and contribute to a decreasing prevalence of viral markers in volunteer donors.

Rural community hospital – Zimbabwe

This 40-bed hospital is too isolated to conveniently order and receive blood from the regional hospital centre and has to rely on its own resources to produce the 100–200 blood units per year they need. They have procured the blood bags and the anti-HIV and HBsAg rapid tests from the regional blood centre. Because of the small demand, collecting and keeping a refrigerated blood stock is neither feasible nor economical. The staff have designed an alternative strategy called 'blood club'. The local population was informed about transfusion through village meetings and sketches presented by the local drama group, which illustrated situations involving the need for blood and blood donors. Volunteers who agreed to join the club were registered and tested for blood group and HBsAg. HBsAg negative volunteers (80%) are called upon if blood is needed in the hospital. When a patient needs blood, the blood group is determined and two blood group-matched volunteers are brought to the hospital and tested for anti-HIV. Blood is then collected from an HIV-negative donor. The patient's family are charged $9 for each unit of blood.

---

excluding a perfectly acceptable source of blood and costs were kept unnecessarily high.

To prepare enough safe blood in a sustainable fashion, African countries need to develop their own ways to produce it. Uncritical adoption of external advice and models may lead to unsustainable and inappropriate solutions. What then are the models of transfusion services in Africa and what are the consequences for the timely supply of safe blood?

Organization of transfusion services in sub-Saharan Africa

African countries have developed a variety of systems to try to achieve a sustainable safe blood supply. These vary from large, modern, national blood centres to locally organized donor programmes for individual district healthcare facilities [4].

A minority of countries have invested significant resources in transfusion services, often with financial support and advisers from European governments, the United States Agency for International Development (USAID) or nongovernmental organizations (NGOs), including Red Cross, Red Crescent, Family Health International and the Safe Blood for Africa Foundation. In these countries, there has been a commitment to establishing centralized systems based on the example of wealthy nations (Box 24.1). These centres typically collect over 10 000 units a year, use automated equipment and produce some blood components. Blood donor recruitment, screening and processing of donated blood are carried out in specifically designed premises away from the hospitals where blood is transfused. However, the majority of countries in sub-Saharan Africa do not operate a centralized transfusion service. Each hospital recruits blood donors and processes blood for transfusion. These hospitals often handle less than 1000 units a year and experience difficulties in standardization, quality assurance and in maintaining supplies of high quality reagents [5].

Recruiting voluntary donors from the community is complex and expensive and depends on regular education programmes, collection teams, vehicles and cold storage. It is proving very difficult to expand the number of volunteer donors [5]. Indeed, over the last 15 years, there has been increasing difficulty in persuading donors to donate, as fear of knowing one's HIV test result has become more widespread. There are also cultural beliefs surrounding blood donation that inhibit donors coming forward. Some of these appear to be misinformation about donating blood (e.g. 'men will become impotent if they donate blood'; 'HIV can be caught from the blood bag needle'). It is worth noting that similar problems faced widespread acceptance of blood donation when Percy Oliver and Geoffrey Keynes began to establish the first blood banks of volunteer donors in London over 70 years ago.

There are, however, other cultural beliefs that are much more complex and related donors' to deepseated and ethnographically diverse understanding of the value of blood to the individual and to society, e.g. blood is related to kinship or personal health. Understanding local beliefs surrounding blood and blood donation is likely to be important in developing effective services.

As volunteer donors are in short supply, family members are frequently used to provide blood for their relatives in hospital. In 2002, in Africa as a whole, WHO estimated that over 60% of blood originated from replacement/family donors. In sub-Saharan Africa the proportion of blood derived from replacement donors is certainly higher. These replacement donors should be family members, but relatives may not only be reluctant to donate for the reasons discussed above but are also open to exploitation by 'professional donors' who charge relatives a fee to donate in their place. Most viral infections such as HIV, HBV and HCV have similar prevalence in replacement and volunteer donors. There are therefore no objective reasons to reduce replacement donors in sub-Saharan Africa (and elsewhere); being both volunteer and nonremunerated, they share with volunteer nonremunerated donors in Sub-Saharan Africa the difficulties of becoming regular donors. Local transfusion systems allow many patients to survive serious illness and are often maintained by dedicated staff in difficult circumstances. However, even with the best input from local staff, these district services experience problems of supply and safety.

The supply of blood

Patients in poorer countries usually present late in the course of their disease, and the delays and lack of stored blood inherent in the replacement donor system mean that patients may die before a blood transfusion can be organized. By the time a donor has been found, screened and venesected, and the blood is transfused into the patient, several hours or even days can elapse. A survey of the blood supplied by a dedicated district service in East Africa showed that the average delay in sourcing blood for children with severe malaria anaemia was 6 hours. Anecdotal evidence suggests that in some areas and at some times in many areas blood may not be available at all. Finally, locally based services at regional or national centres have difficulty in separating blood, even into simple fractions such as red cells, platelets and plasma, to provide specific components if needed.

Testing and storage of donor blood

Local blood transfusion services encounter many problems, including lack of funding, insufficient training, poor management, frequent failure to supply reagents and consumables, and breakdown of the cold chain mostly related to frequent power cuts. Blood frequently has to be collected in small hospital-based units often with no dedicated staff and no specifically allocated budget. In the year 2000, the WHO review estimated that 25% of the blood in sub-Saharan Africa was not tested for anti-HIV and that blood transfusion was the origin of 5–10% of new HIV infections. Since then, a lot of investment has gone into providing HIV, HBsAg and to some extent HCV tests. The latest survey shows that >98% of blood is tested for HIV. The residual risk of HBV infection remains substantial because of donations containing undetected low levels of HBsAg or occult HBV DNA. Recent estimates of the residual risk of HIV transmission are 1:2600–6000, hepatitis C 1:400–1500 and hepatitis B 1:300–500, when using enzyme immunoassay (EIA) screening [6, 7].

253

The cost of local blood supply

When a transfusion service is provided by individual hospitals, it places an enormous burden on laboratory resources. There has been almost no research into the cost of setting up and running transfusion services in resource-poor countries. One survey showed that in a typical district hospital in southern Africa, the overall cost of the transfusion service, including consumables, proportional amounts for capital equipment, staff time and overheads, was 36% of total laboratory costs. Each unit of whole blood cost the laboratory approximately $20 to collect and process.

The cost of a national service is even greater because of the additional costs of quality assurance, local education programmes, dedicated collection team(s), vehicles and cold storage. In addition, a national service has to solve the very real practical problems of maintaining regular distributions of sufficient quantities of blood to remote facilities. It is also frequently observed that the creation of a national service creates internal migration of technical staff from hospitals to national or regional centres. One solution to this would be to train staff specifically for the processing, testing and issue of blood and so release the time of valuable, skilled hospital staff.

Clinical use of blood

In contrast to Europe, most transfusions in sub-Saharan Africa are given for life-threatening emergencies, most often anaemia in children or pregnant women and haemorrhage following childbirth or trauma. Transfusions are administered to children predominantly for malaria-related anaemia and can undoubtedly reduce the mortality of children with severe anaemia. In these clinical circumstances, whole blood is indicated and should remain the main and cheapest blood component while packed red cells are indicated for nonhaemorrhagic indications, particularly in paediatrics and medicine. Many clinical guidelines, albeit based on consensus opinion rather than well-defined evidence, suggest transfusions are indicated if Hb < 4 or 5 g/dL with symptoms of decompensation [1, 8]. Even in areas of high HIV prevalence, young children generally have a relatively low risk of becoming naturally infected with HIV and potentially have a long life expectancy. Pregnant women are the second most common recipients of blood, particularly for haemorrhagic emergencies. Significant quantities of blood are also used in trauma, surgery and general medicine. There are neither systematic reviews nor international guidelines covering the use of blood in these specific contexts, and few audits of blood use. The scope for improving clinical practice and reducing unnecessary transfusion through education and the use of guidelines is probably substantial.

The problems surrounding the rapid supply of a safe supply of blood have led to the use of autologous blood transfusion. There are logistical and training problems to be overcome. However, small programmes have been established for autologous transfusion of elective surgery patients at district hospitals.

Putting the WHO objectives into practice: improving the supply, safety and use of blood in sub-Saharan Africa

Some countries have used external funds to establish an integrated national service, but few have been able to make the transition to a sustainable, national transfusion service in the absence of external funding and even fewer have been able to reach an adequate blood supply. Moreover, in several countries, external funding for ten or more years has failed to develop a functioning national transfusion service, and these failures have led some funders to withdraw grants to national transfusion services. However, some recent success has been achieved in developing a transfusion service in several centres in Nigeria (see Box 24.2). The alternative is that, in many areas, transfusion services have to be optimized within the existing general hospital budget. Whatever sums are available the specific, often interconnected problems, surrounding the supply, safety, cost and use of blood must be addressed. There has to be a balance between providing an ideal integrated national service and the more pragmatic solutions afforded by local services.

Improving the blood supply and the safety of the donor pool

Careful donor selection is crucial not only to improve the supply of blood but also to reduce transfusion-transmitted infection risk (see Box 24.3 and

---

Box 24.2 Towards development of a National Transfusion Service in Nigeria

Nigeria, the most populous country in Africa, had in 2004 a highly fragmented hospital-based transfusion system. There was little coordination from the central government and most of the blood came from replacement and paid donors. Testing for transmissible disease markers was inconsistent and poorly controlled. The current practice of family replacement donors in a hospital-based blood service is the most economical option, but in the face of high child and maternal mortality rates the blood supply has proved to be insufficient. There was therefore the need to change practice.

The Safe Blood for Africa Foundation with a grant from USAID established a demonstration blood service in capital Abuja. This service collected its blood from voluntary unremunerated donors in the local community. The blood was tested for HIV, hepatitis B and C, labelled with ISBT 128 compliant labels and distributed to the local hospitals. A simple but effective quality management system was established with standard operating procedures written and followed. A validated transfusion computer system was installed which only allowed release of validated units of blood to hospitals. The objective of this project was to be the model for other centres throughout the country. The Federal Ministry of Health soon established regional centres in Kaduna, Owerri, Port Harcourt, Ibadan, Maiduguri and Jos, and has a long-term plan to roll out further centres in future. The Minister of Health also established an expert committee which drafted a national blood policy and national guidelines for the standards for the practice of transfusion in Nigeria. The Safe Blood for Africa Foundation provided technical assistance for the establishment of these centres and provided training to the staff in all elements of transfusion.

The major problem was to recruit blood donors. The youth were encouraged to donate with the establishment of a Club 25 programme. There was active promotion through the media and was highlighted by a televised donation by the President on the occasion of the official opening of the Abuja centre. A problem encountered was the high number of donors presenting with haemoglobin levels below the required standard of 12.5 g/dL. This is probably a reflection of the poor health status within the community.

Table 24.1). The selection of volunteer donors from lower risk populations is considered the most effective approach and considerable effort has been devoted to promoting voluntary, repeat donations. However, in most parts of Africa, replacement donors are the main resource. They are typically males 25–35 years old. As the availability of replacement donors is limited, the most effective way to improve the availability and safety of blood is to recruit volunteer donors. In practice these are often secondary school students with median age ranging between 16 and 20 years. They are younger and have a greater proportion of females than replacement donors. Experience has shown that while recruiting volunteer donors in schools can be relatively inexpensive, making them into repeat donors is difficult and expensive. Since only repeat donation has been proven to increase blood safety, encouraging both volunteer nonremunerated and family-replacement donors to donate blood repeatedly is the challenge for sub-Saharan African blood services in order to provide safer blood [3, 9].

Several strategies have been devised to encourage repeat donors and thus reduce the risk of virus carriage. In Zimbabwe, Pledge 25 Club, a programme using education and incentives to attract school students to give blood 25 times, has been successful. Similar, less ambitious schemes, for example a 'Club 5', could also be effective. The WHO slogan of 'Safe blood starts with me' has also resulted in educational programmes around the world. These schemes can be complemented by strategies to recruit donors from faith-based organizations or collaborating with radio stations to organize and promote blood donations. The success of well-organized requests for blood donors has been proven in some campaigns but remains to be tested in many countries where national calls for donors have not been made in the absence of centralized blood transfusion services. Specific strategies intending to encourage family-replacement donors to become repeat donors are being developed, shifting from donating blood for someone they know to someone they do not know.

The best use of fluid replacement regimes for severe haemorrhage requires further study. At the same time, other novel solutions are being sought to alleviate the shortage of blood. It may be feasible to use placental blood as an accessory source of blood to transfuse small children in malarious areas. The placenta containing this blood is normally discarded after delivery. However, the high haematocrit and easy availability may make it suitable for small-volume emergency transfusions if blood can be collected free of bacterial contamination, which appears to be a major obstacle to implementation of such programmes.

255

Box 24.3 Epidemiology of bloodborne infections in sub-Saharan Africa

HIV
The overall prevalence of HIV antibody in sub-Saharan Africa ranges between 0.5 and 16%. In donors, it tends to remain below 5% in West Africa, below 10% in East and Central Africa and above 10% in southern Africa [4, 10, 11, 18].

Hepatitis B
Chronic hepatitis B prevalence, indicated by the presence of circulating HBsAg, ranges between 5 and 25% of the population including blood donors. This high prevalence is due to (vertical) transmission at birth or (horizontal) infection in infancy and the virtual absence of national vaccination programmes. Infection after the age of 10 is uncommon. HBsAg is more prevalent in West Africa (10–25%) than in East or Central Africa (5–10%); the lowest prevalence is found in southern Africa (5% or less).

Hepatitis C
Antibody to HCV is not routinely screened for in many parts of Africa, but the prevalence of this infection ranges between 0.5 and 3% and reaches 10–15% in Egypt. The prevalence may be high locally, suggesting the importance of specific factors such as various types of injections and past diagnostic or vaccination campaigns contributing to spread the infection.

Other infections
Most countries in sub-Saharan Africa do not screen for *HTLV* since the prevalence is low (<2%).
  Although the risk of acquiring syphilis from infected blood is low, most blood banks in sub-Saharan Africa do screen for *Treponema pallidum*. Fresh blood is potentially infectious for syphilis, but storage at 4°C can inactivate the bacterium.
  Malaria can be transmitted by transfusion. In areas of low or no malaria transmission, screening for the parasite is important, as recipients are likely to have no immunity. In countries where malaria is highly endemic, the prevalence of *Plasmodium* in donor blood is often very high (16–55%) [19] and excluding donors with low-grade parasitaemia is often impracticable and pre-emptive treatment of patients receiving transfusion with antimalarial drugs often an unfortunate necessity [20].
  Bacterial contamination of blood components is underrecognized and may reach 10% of products at the time of issue [15, 16].

Residual risk of transfusion transmission of bloodborne viruses
Improving the size and reliability of the donor pool affects not only the supply but also the safety of blood. In particular, a previously screened donor pool would reduce the substantial residual risks of transfusion-transmitted infection due to the window period for HIV and HCV and occult chronic carriage for HBV (HBsAg negative/DNA positive).
  The present residual risk of viral transmission by transfusion has been assessed for HIV. In studies conducted in Kenya, Zambia and the Democratic Republic of the Congo, the risk of HIV transmission by transfusion was estimated to be between 1 and 3%, related in part to prevalence, but also to test performance, storage conditions and staff training. The residual risk of HBV infection remains substantial because of donations containing undetected low levels of HBsAg or occult HBV DNA. This risk remains high for children below the age of 10 but the problem is at least in part mitigated by the very high prevalence of adult recipients carrying HBV markers (60–90%). Precise estimates of the residual risk of HIV transmission in Ivory Coast in 2002–2004 were 1:2600–6000, HCV 1:400–1500 and HBV 1:300–500, when using EIA screening.
  These figures represent the risk of the respective infection even when using the best EIAs. This residual risk emphasizes the pressing need to improve the safety of the donor pool, to develop cheap and reliable nucleic acid testing and to optimize the use of blood.

Improving screening for blood-transmitted infections

Test sensitivity is critical in the face of high prevalence rates for HIV, HBV and HCV (Box 24.3 and Table 24.1) [4, 10, 11]. These high prevalence rates pose a very substantial danger and a major logistic and technical challenge to those trying to provide safe blood. Even with the best available testing procedures using antigen or antibody detection there remains a substantial residual risk of HIV transmission in the order of 1 in 3000 though the failure to detect seronegative early HIV infection in the pre-seroconversion window period (see above). In these situations, the prevalence rate may be reduced by 90% in repeat donors, reinforcing the value of a stable donor pool.

  The techniques used for screening must be considered carefully to ensure effective screening of the particular donor population and the skills of the staff involved. Nucleic acid testing is highly effective and has been introduced in South Africa and a few centres elsewhere [12]. However, widespread use of NAT remains neither affordable nor practical for most centres and countries. Cheaper and/or simplified methods to perform NAT testing would be useful.

Table 24.1 Prevalence of transfusion-transmissible agents in sub-Saharan African blood donors.

Country	Year collected	Prevalence (%)					
		Anti-HIV	HBsAg	Anti-HCV	HTLV	Syphilis	Malaria
Benin	1998	0.5–3	12	1.4–2.3	0.3–5.4		33.5
Botswana	2000	10	5	1			
Cameroon	1994–1998	4.1–5.8	10–16	1.6			
Ghana	1998–2002	1.7–3.8	15	1.7–8.4	0.5	13.5	
Kenya	1995–1998	4.5–3.0	4.2–3.9	1.5–1.8			
Malawi	2000	10.7	8.1	6.8	2.5		
Mozambique	2007	13.8	7.5	1.1	1.1		
Nigeria	2004–2005	2.0	9.9	1.9		0.5	55.0
RDC	1998	6.4	9.2	4.3			
Republic of South Africa*	2001	4.5	5	0.5			
Tanzania	1998	8.7	11	8–10.3	0	12.7	
Togo	1995–2000			3.3	1.8		
Uganda	2000	3.9–5.4					
Zambia	1991–1995	8–16	6.5				
Zimbabwe	1997	8.8	2.5–15.4		0.1		

*Donors of African origin.

New approaches adapted to local situations appear promising. In small blood banks, the expensive microtitre plate systems used post donation can be replaced by cheaper, more cost-effective, high-performance rapid tests performed pre- or post-donation. Pre-donation testing provides the advantages of reducing material waste and easy, on-site communication with deferred donors who, otherwise, could not be reached [13]. There are fears that pre-donation testing may reduce the willingness of donors to come forward, although published data did not find evidence of this. At present, WHO does not recommend pre-donation testing. There is a diversity of opinion and some consider that WHO and aid agencies need to show flexibility and consider the benefits of multiple strategies adapted to local needs rather than recommending rigid models designed for totally different populations, staff and resources.

Without good quality assurance in collection, processing and testing of blood, the risk of HIV transmission by blood transfusion in high prevalence areas is very substantial [14]. There are encouraging reports that the application of stringent blood donor selection and universal screening with fourth-generation p24 antigen and HIV antibody assays when well monitored and controlled may be able to reduce the risk of HIV transmission to <1 in 3000 [7].

Some new technology is on the horizon. Rapid immunochemical and nucleic acid dipsticks are being developed for bloodborne pathogens and may cut the cost of pre- and post-donation testing to a tenth of present costs. Clearly, these and other inexpensive and effective testing technologies, as well as pathogen inactivation techniques, directed towards the needs of developing countries should become a major target of external support.

The WHO has established systematic evaluations of both EIA and rapid tests to guide developing countries in their choice of tests. These evaluations include test costs. Many rapid tests for anti-HIV and HBsAg and fewer for anti-HCV are available, but sensitivity and specificity, ease of use and cost vary greatly. Some of these tests are performed in one single step with results obtained in 10–20 minutes using whole blood, plasma or serum samples. The best assays have sensitivity similar to EIA for anti-HIV, detect 0.2 ng/mL of HBsAg and have >99% sensitivity for anti-HCV and >99% specificity.

Blood safety has often focused on the risk of viral infection in donors but bacterial contamination of units is a substantial problem. Two recent studies have highlighted the considerable risk of bacterial infection in nearly 10% of whole blood units [15, 16]. Contamination appears to be of environmental rather than of donor origin and clearly may pose a substantial risk to patient safety. Quantifying and reducing these hazards will be an important challenge in the future.

Reducing the cost of transfusion services

The challenge for Africa is that enough safe blood should be available for health services and individuals even when resources are extremely limited. The majority of a blood unit cost originates from imported goods such as equipment, blood bags, grouping and screening assays. Staff costs are a relatively small proportion of the overall costs because salaries are low and because negligible resources are put into staff training, supervision and auditing mechanisms. According to published studies, a unit of blood from a hospital-based service may cost between $10 and 40, but even $10 is not affordable by most families in sub-Saharan Africa. Staff and logistic support for collecting volunteer nonremunerated donor blood account for 100–300% of additional costs compared to family-replacement donor blood collection. In any event, the relative high cost of providing blood makes it impossible to recoup the cost of blood by user fees alone and blood services will require internal or external public funding for the foreseeable future [17].

Because transfusion is such an expensive service, the costs often have to be subsidized by aid packages, external agencies or governments. Resources for transfusion services are often vulnerable to fickle, political and nonsustainable fluctuations. Developing systems that rely more on local resources means that in the long term they may be more dynamic, productive and sustainable. Certainly, much more research is needed comparing the cost-effectiveness of various strategies to supply safe blood to patients in poor countries.

Improving the clinical use of blood: guidelines for transfusion practice

The use of simple guidelines can reduce unnecessary transfusions and many institutions in sub-Saharan Africa and Asia have developed guidelines to promote rational use of blood transfusions and blood components. The scope for improvement in clinical practice is great. For example, strict enforcement of a transfusion protocol in a Malawian hospital reduced the number of transfusions by 75% without any adverse effect on mortality.

The principles underlying most transfusion guidelines are similar and combine a clinical assessment of whether the patient is developing complications of inadequate oxygenation, with measurement of their haemoglobin (as a marker of intracellular oxygen concentration). In sub-Saharan countries, the recommended haemoglobin threshold for transfusions is often well below that which would be accepted in more wealthy countries. In the USA, anaesthetists suggest that transfusions are almost always indicated when the haemoglobin concentration is less than 6 g/dL whereas in many African countries transfusions are recommended for children at haemoglobin concentrations less than 4 g/dL, provided there are no other clinical complications.

Ensuring that the transfusion guidelines are implemented is extremely difficult for poorer countries without formal monitoring and auditing systems. This is particularly problematic if the quality of haemoglobin measurements is not assured. Studies have shown that if clinicians do not have confidence in haemoglobin results, they will rely entirely on clinical judgement to guide transfusion practice and this can lead to significant numbers of inappropriate transfusions. In a typical district hospital in Africa the cost of providing a unit of blood is approximately 40 times the cost of a quality-assured haemoglobin test. Investment in improving the haemoglobin testing therefore has the potential for significant cost-saving downstream in the much more expensive transfusion process, as well as reducing the risk of transfusion-related infections.

Conclusion: the future of blood transfusion in a global context

Fulfilling the first WHO objective of establishing 'a coordinated national blood transfusion service that can provide adequate and timely supplies of safe blood for all patients in need' has proved to be very difficult in many countries, even given substantial external funding. Nevertheless, some countries have made progress and have recently established national transfusion services. On the other hand, progress has been made by developing local services and there has to be a balance between providing an ideal integrated national service and the more pragmatic solutions afforded by local services. Such a system does not necessarily imply centralization but hybrid systems including both purpose-built off-site large blood centres as well as hospital-based smaller units implementing adequate methods and quality assurance might serve patients optimally. There remains considerable scope to optimize fluid management regimens and to reduce unnecessary transfusions through the appropriate clinical use of blood and products.

Increased blood supply depends on the recruitment of all types of nonremunerated donors, whether volunteer nonremunerated donors or family-replacement donors, and the development of innovative strategies to make both groups of donors to give blood regularly. The examples and discussions in this chapter have centred on Africa, but the same considerations apply to many of the poorer countries in Asia and Latin America. In Brazil, both volunteer nonremunerated donors and family-replacement donors are considered under the same term of 'voluntary' donors. Here, there are wide variations in resources available for healthcare, not only between but also within countries.

In all countries, increased blood supply depends on the recruitment of volunteer donors and this should become the priority for policy development and resource allocation. A reliable and expanded donor pool will not only provide a life-saving therapy but also improve safety. Resources must be made available by governments to ensure that the essential supplies are available, such as blood bags, grouping reagents and test kits, and laboratory and blood bank management systems also need to be improved to ensure effective testing and processing, and the maintenance of the cold chain. Hospitals and other health facilities could cooperate to directly purchase cheap, high quality tests adapted to their needs.

There is currently a feeling of guarded optimism about the future of blood supply and safety in developing countries. The recent increase in allocation of resources for the prevention of HIV across the world, including the investment by governments of wealthy countries and contributions from international and private agencies, have begun to recognize the importance of reducing HIV transmission through blood but run the risk of neglecting other basic laboratory services, e.g. blood grouping and haemoglobin measurements. Parallel to the price reduction for antiviral drugs, the cost of screening tests supplied to developing countries has also decreased. The high cost of anti-HCV testing should now be reduced as the patent has expired in Europe. Also possible methods of pathogen inactivation applicable to whole blood are being developed that could, in one step, reduce or eliminate the risks of viral, bacterial and parasitic infections. More effective and efficient methods for testing blood are to be welcomed and pathogen reduction methods applicable to whole blood would be an enormous relief if affordable. The real challenge will be to integrate improvements in the supply and safety of blood in sustainable, coordinated national transfusion services.

Key points

1 In the last 5 years, nearly all African states had a national blood policy, but just over half have been able to implement their policies.
2 The main obstacles to implementation are a lack of trained staff, the high cost of blood in relation to the healthcare budgets and recruitment of donors.
3 In the absence of centralized services, facilities rely on blood collected by hospitals from family or replacement donors.
4 The high rate of chronic viral infections in the populations implies that the residual risk of infection of HIV and hepatitis B infection remains substantial with EIA testing.
5 Several initiatives are being trialled to improve the supply and/or safety of blood by encouraging repeat voluntary donors, reviewing donor testing strategies, developing systems that rely more on local resources, using umbilical cord blood and researching methods for low cost NAT testing.
6 There are few guidelines covering the use of blood and few audits of blood use so the scope for improving clinical practice and reducing unnecessary transfusion is probably substantial.

References

1 Lackritz EM, Campbell CC, Ruebush 2nd TK, Hightower AW, Wakube W, Steketee RW *et al*. Effect of blood transfusion on survival among children in a Kenyan hospital. *Lancet* 1992; 340: 524–528.

2 Bates I, Chapotera GK, McKew S & van den Broek N. Maternal mortality in sub-Saharan Africa: the contribution of ineffective blood transfusion services. *BJOG* 2008; 115: 1331–1339.

3 Allain JP. Moving on from voluntary non-remunerated donors: who is the best donor? *Br J Haematol* 2011; 154: 763–769.

4 Tagny CT, Diarra A, Yahaya R, Hakizimana M, Nguessan A, Mbensa G, Nébié Y, Dahourou H, Mbanya D, Shiboski C, Murphy E & Lefrère JJ. Characteristics of blood donors and donated blood in sub-Saharan Francophone Africa. *Transfusion* 2009; 49: 1592–1599.

5 Bates I, Manyasi G & Medina Lara A. Reducing replacement donors in sub-Saharan Africa: challenges and affordability. *Transfus Med* 2007, December; 17(6): 434–442.

6 Chaudhuri V, Nanu A, Panda SK & Chand P. Evaluation of serologic screening of blood donors in India reveals a lack of correlation between anti-HBc titer and PCR-amplified HBV DNA. *Transfusion* 2003; 43: 1442–1448.

7 Basavaraju SV, Mwangi J, Nyamongo J, Zeh C, Kimani D, Shiraishi RW, Madoda R, Okonji JA, Sugut W, Ongwae S, Pitman JP & Marum LH. Reduced risk of transfusion-transmitted HIV in Kenya through centrally co-ordinated blood centres, stringent donor selection and effective p24 antigen-HIV antibody screening. *Vox Sanguinis* 2010; 99: 212–219.

8 Akech SO, Hassall O, Pamba A, Idro R, Williams TN, Newton CR & Maitland K. Survival and haematological recovery of children with severe malaria transfused in accordance to WHO guidelines in Kilifi, Kenya. *Malar J* 2008; 7: 256.

9 Allain JP, Sarkodie F, Boateng P, Asenso K, Kyeremateng E & Owusu-Ofori S. A pool of repeat blood donors can be generated with little expense to the blood center in sub-Saharan Africa. *Transfusion* 2008; 48: 735–741.

10 Tapko JB, Sam O & Diarra-Nama A. Report on the status of blood safety in the WHO African region for 2004. WHO, AFRO; 2007.

11 Tagny CT, Owusu-Ofori S, Mbanya D & Deneys V. The blood donor in sub-Saharan Africa: a review. *Transfus Med* 2010; 20: 1–10.

12 Vermeulen M, Lelie N, Sykes W, Crookes R, Swanevelder J, Gaggia L, Le Roux M, Kuun E, Gulube S & Reddy R. Impact of individual donation nucleic acid testing on risk of human immunodeficiency virus, hepatitis B virus and hepatitis C virus transmission in South Africa. *Transfusion* 2009; 49: 1115–1125.

13 Owusu-Ofori S, Temple J, Sarkodie F, Candotti D *et al.* Pre-donation screening of blood donors with rapid tests: implementation and efficacy of a novel approach to blood safety in resource-poor settings. *Transfusion* 2005; 45: 133–140.

14 Moore A, Herrera G, Nyamongo J, Lackritz E, Granade T, Nahlen B, Oloo A, Opondo G, Muga R & Janssen R. Estimated risk of HIV transmission by blood transfusion in Kenya. *Lancet* 2001; 358: 657–660.

15 Adjei AA, Kuma GK, Tettey Y, Ayeh-Kumi PF, Opintan J, Apeagyei F, Ankrah JO, Adiku TK & Nater-Olaga EG. Bacterial contamination of blood and blood components in three major blood transfusion centers, Accra, Ghana. *Jpn J Infect Dis* 2009; 62: 265–269.

16 Hassall O, Maitland K, Pole L, Mwarumba S, Denje D, Wambua K, Lowe B, Parry C, Mandaliya K & Bates I. Bacterial contamination of pediatric whole blood transfusions in a Kenyan hospital. *Transfusion* 2009; 49: 2594–2598.

17 Hensher M & Jefferys E. Financing blood transfusion services in sub-Saharan Africa: a role for user fees? *Health Policy Plan* 2000; 15: 287–295.

18 Cunha L, Plouzeau C, Ingrand P, Gudo JP, Ingrand I, Mondlane J, Beauchant M & Agius G. Use of replacement blood donors to study the epidemiology of major blood-borne viruses in the general population of Maputo, Mozambique. *J Med Virol* 2007; 79: 1832–1840.

19 Owusu-Ofori AK, Parry C & Bates I. Transfusion-transmitted malaria in countries where malaria is endemic: a review of the literature from sub-Saharan Africa. *Clin Infect Dis* 2010; 51: 1192–1198.

20 Rajab JA, Waithaka PM, Orinda DA & Scott CS. Analysis of cost and effectiveness of pre-transfusion screening of donor blood and anti-malarial prophylaxis for recipients. *East Afr Med J* 2005; 82: 565–571.

Further reading

African Society of Blood Transfusion. Available at: http://www.afsbt.org/ (accessed 7 June 2012).

Bates I, Mundy C, Pendame R *et al.* Use of clinical judgement to guide administration of blood transfusions in Malawi. *Trans R Soc Trop Med Hyg* 2001; 95: 510–512.

English M, Ahmed M, Ngando C, Berkley J & Ross A. Blood transfusion for severe anaemia in children in a Kenyan hospital. *Lancet* 2002; 359: 494–495.

Fairhead J, Leach M & Small M. Where techno-science meets poverty: medical research and the economy of blood in The Gambia, West Africa. *Soc Sci Med* 2006; 65: 1109–1120.

Hassall O, Ngina L, Kongo W *et al.* The acceptability to women in Mombasa, Kenya, of the donation and transfusion of umbilical cord blood for severe anaemia in young children. *Vox Sanguinis* 2007; 94(2): 125–131.

World Health Organization. Blood Transfusion Safety. Available at: http://www.who.int/bloodsafety/en/ (accessed 7 June 2012).

PART FOUR
Clinical Transfusion Practice

25 Inherited and acquired coagulation disorders

Vickie McDonald[1] *& Samuel J. Machin*[2]

[1]University College London Hospitals NHS Foundation Trust, London, UK
[2]Haemostasis Research Unit, Department of Haematology, University College London, London, UK

Normal haemostasis

Haemostasis is a complex process involving the interaction of many components – blood vessels, platelets, coagulation factors, coagulation factor inhibitors and fibrinolytic enzymes – that ultimately leads to clot formation followed by resolution. In a normal individual there is a constant balance between procoagulant and anticoagulant activities.

The generation of thrombin is key to successful haemostasis (Figure 25.1). Historically it was thought that two initiating coagulation cascades, the intrinsic and extrinsic pathways, ultimately led to generation of thrombin, which in turn converted fibrinogen to fibrin. We now know that the coagulation process is a complex network of positive and negative feedback loops that are explained better by the 'cell based' model of coagulation [1]. This describes three overlapping phases: *initiation*, *amplification* and *propagation*. Initiation of coagulation occurs when exposure of tissue factor (TF) on damaged endothelial cells/activated monocytes leads to the generation of activated factor VII (FVIIa) and formation of TF-VIIa complex (under normal circumstances, approximately 1–2% of circulating plasma factor VII circulates in the activated form). The TF-VIIa complex activates factors IX (FIXa) and X (FXa) and trace amounts of thrombin are subsequently generated by FXa. Concurrent to this, platelets adhere to the subendothelial matrix and are activated, providing a phospholipid surface for coagulation factor activity. VWF is bound to and released from endothelial cells leading to further platelet recruitment and activation.

During amplification and propagation, the small amounts of thrombin generated activate factors V, VIII and XI. This allows formation of the 'tenase' complex (FIXa/FVIIIa) to generate further FXa and the 'prothrombinase' complex (FXa/FVa), which leads to the explosive generation of thrombin from prothrombin and, ultimately, by activation of fibrin and factor XIII, production of a crosslinked stable clot.

The initial TF-VIIa complex is quickly inhibited by tissue factor pathway inhibitor (TFPI); however, by this time, positive feedback loops between thrombin and factors XI, V and VIII are sufficient to amplify the signal and propagate the clot formation. Factor XI is also activated by factor XIIa formed from the HMWK-prekallikrein complex on endothelial cells, but this contribution to physiological haemostasis is not significant.

There are inbuilt mechanisms to control the procoagulant response. These include TFPI, which inactivates the TF-FVIIa complex, antithrombin, which complexes with and inactivates FIXa, FXa, FXIa and thrombin, the protein C and S pathways, which inactivate FVa and FVIIIa, and thrombomodulin, which binds to thrombin and alters its substrate specificity for factors V, VIII and fibrinogen. Fibrinolysis is also part of the normal haemostatic response. Circulating plasminogen is activated to form the serine

Practical Transfusion Medicine, Fourth Edition. Edited by Michael F. Murphy, Derwood H. Pamphilon and Nancy M. Heddle.
© 2013 John Wiley & Sons, Ltd. Published 2013 by John Wiley & Sons, Ltd.

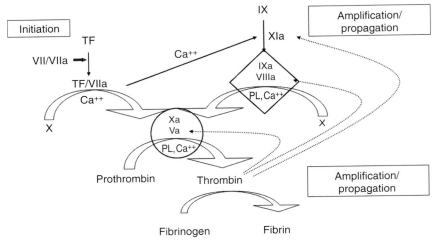

Fig 25.1 The procoagulant pathway. The diamond represents the tenase complex and the circle represents the prothrombinase complex.

protease plasmin, which digests crosslinked fibrin to form D-dimers and other fibrinogen fragments.

Investigation of abnormal haemostasis

Abnormalities in the haemostatic system may be congenital or acquired and clinical presentation can vary from asymptomatic to life-threatening haemorrhage. A careful history should be taken focusing on personal or family bleeding history, bleeding following dental work, surgery or childbirth and objective evidence of excess bleeding such as development of anaemia, requirement for transfusion or surgical intervention.

The initial laboratory investigation of patients with abnormal haemostasis should include a platelet count, prothrombin time (PT), activated partial thromboplastin time (APTT) and Clauss fibrinogen. Additional screening tests that can also be performed are listed in Table 25.1. If one/more of these tests are abnormal, further specialized investigations should be performed in order to define precisely the defect and its severity.

In high dependency units, the availability of near patient testing devices to rapidly assess coagulation (PT and APTT) and overall global haemostasis (thromboelastogram, TEG®) potentially allows rapid treatment decisions to be made without sending a citrated sample to the laboratory. TEG® measures

the changes in elastic shear stresses seen during clot formation and subsequent fibrinolysis. A stationary pin attached to a torsion wire is immersed in a

Table 25.1 Simple laboratory haemostasis screening tests.

System	Test	Factor implicated
Coagulation	PT	II, V, VII, X
	APTT	VIII, IX, XI, XII
	INR – only in patients receiving oral anticoagulation	
	TT	Fibrinogen, heparin
	Clauss fibrinogen	Fibrinogen
Platelets	Platelet count	
	Blood film inspection	
	Platelet function (using PFA-100™ which measures *in vitro* 'high shear' bleeding time)	
Fibrinolysis	D-dimers	
	Euglobulin clot lysis time	
Global haemostasis	Thromboelastogram	

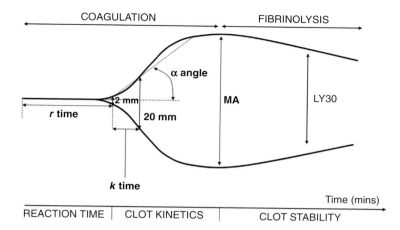

Fig 25.2 Schematic representation of thromboelastography (TEG®).

rotating cup that contains whole blood and as clot forms the pin and cup rotate together. The magnitude of pin movement (in mm) is proportional to the strength of the clot. Five major parameters are measured (Figure 25.2):

1 Reaction time (*r*), which is the time from adding the sample to first measurable clot (predetermined as 2 mm). It is shortened by hypercoagulable states and increased by coagulation factor deficiencies/heparin effect.

2 Time *k*, which is the time to achieve a predesignated clot strength (designated as 20 mm amplitude). This parameter is most reflective of fibrinogen function.

3 Alpha (α) angle, which is the slope of the trace between R and K and reflects the speed of fibrin accumulation and polymerization.

4 Maximum amplitude (MA) is the highest vertical amplitude of the TEG® tracing and is an indication of platelet function. Affected by thrombocytopenia, abnormal platelet function and problems with the interaction between fibrinogen and platelets.

5 LY30 is the rate of amplitude reduction 30 minutes after the MA is reached. This is reflective of clot stability, in particular the degree of fibrinolysis and breakdown of the clot.

Schematic representations of abnormal traces and the causes are shown in Figure 25.3. In a modified version of TEG® called ROTEM®, it is the pin rather than the cup that oscillates but similar measurements are given.

It is important to note that in some disorders (e.g. mild haemophilia or von Willebrand disease, or

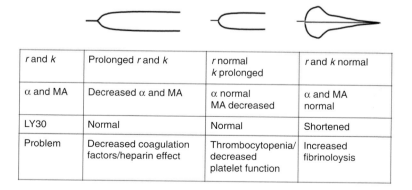

r and *k*	Prolonged *r* and *k*	*r* normal *k* prolonged	*r* and *k* normal
α and MA	Decreased α and MA	α normal MA decreased	α and MA normal
LY30	Normal	Normal	Shortened
Problem	Decreased coagulation factors/heparin effect	Thrombocytopenia/decreased platelet function	Increased fibrinoloysis

Fig 25.3 Schematic representation of common abnormalities seen in TEG®.

VWD), tests such as the APTT may not be overly prolonged, so if a bleeding disorder is strongly suspected from the patient's history and the clinical picture, specific factor assays and/or immunological tests should be performed regardless of the 'screening' test result.

Inherited haemostatic defects

Haemophilia A

This disorder results in reduced or absent activity of factor VIII. The factor VIII gene is on the long arm of the X-chromosome and there is often a family history of haemophilia. However, up to one-third of cases are as a result of new mutations. Some female carriers may be symptomatic.

Haemophilia A is classified into mild, moderate or severe according to factor VIII activity (FVIII:C) (Table 25.2). The minimal effective level for haemostasis is generally about 25–30%.

Investigations
Laboratory abnormalities seen in haemophilia A include:
• prolonged APTT;
• reduction of FVIII:C;
• normal VWF activity (it is important to measure VWF activity in order to exclude VWD, which will also give low factor VIII levels).

Management
The mainstay of treatment is to raise the FVIII:C sufficiently to prevent or arrest spontaneous and traumatic bleeds or to cover surgery. There are a number of products currently available, including:
• recombinant factor VIII preparations;
• plasma-derived factor VIII concentrates (which vary in degree of purity);
• DDAVP (for mild disease only – baseline factor VIII above 15%);
• tranexamic acid.

Table 25.2 Clinical manifestations and treatment of haemophilia A and B.

Factor level (% normal)	Clinical manifestation	Treatment
<1% (severe disease)	Usual age of onset <1 year Spontaneous bleeding common (haemarthrosis, muscle haematoma, haematuria) Bleeding post-surgery and dental extraction Post-traumatic bleeding Crippling joint deformity if inadequate treatment	Regular FVIII or IX prophylaxis in children and some adults Factor VIII or IX to treat bleeds Factor VIII or IX for surgery or invasive procedures +/− tranexamic acid
1–5% (moderate disease)	Usual age of onset <2 year Occasional spontaneous bleeding Bleeding post-surgery and dental extraction Post-traumatic bleeding	Some patients may need regular factor VIII or IX prophylaxis Factor VIII or IX to treat bleeds Factor VIII or IX for surgery or invasive procedures +/− tranexamic acid
6–40% (mild disease)	Usual age of onset >2 year Bleeding post-surgery and dental extraction Post-traumatic bleeding	Regular prophylaxis usually not required Treatment of bleeds or cover for surgery/ invasive procedures: Haemophilia A: DDAVP, tranexamic acid, factor concentrate Haemophilia B: Tranexamic acid, factor concentrate

Recombinant products are the initial product of choice to prevent spontaneous joint bleeds in children with severe haemophilia (prophylaxis), as well as treatment of bleeds in previously untreated patients because of the lack of risk of transmission of infection [2]. Plasma-derived factor concentrates undergo donor screening and specific double viral inactivation procedures, but transmission of some viruses, such as human parvovirus B19, and new emerging infections, such as prion disease, remain a theoretical risk.

There has been concern that patients treated with recombinant factor VIII products have a higher incidence of inhibitor development than those treated with plasma-derived factor concentrates. However, the evidence is conflicting and at present recombinant products are the recommended first line for previously untreated patients. The choice of product for previously treated patients will depend on factors such as previous response to treatment, a history of inhibitor development and whether they have been previously exposed to plasma products.

Patients with moderate/severe haemophilia will require factor VIII concentrates for bleeding, prior to invasive procedures, surgery, etc. One unit factor VIII/kg body weight will result in an increase in plasma factor VIII level by 2%. The amount of factor VIII concentrate required is calculated according to the formula:

Units of factor VIII required = weight (kg) × desired FVIII:C level (%) × 0.5

The plasma half-life of factor VIII is 8–12 hours, and thus repeated doses at 12-hourly intervals are usually needed. Alternatively, a continuous infusion of factor VIII can be given for surgery. For major soft tissue bleeds, levels above 50% are generally sufficient; however, for major surgery, a preoperative level of 100% is necessary and thereafter levels of 50–100% are sufficient for adequate wound healing. Factor VIII:C can be measured before and after doses of concentrate to ensure appropriate levels have been achieved.

Mild haemophilia A should be treated with DDAVP (with or without tranexamic acid) where possible [2]. DDAVP (0.3 µg/kg body weight) is given intravenously, subcutaneously or alternatively a 300 µg dose (for adults) can be administered via intranasal spray. This dose typically increases the levels of factor VIII and VWF 3–5 times above baseline. Hyponatraemia and water intoxication are side effects of this drug, and hence it is not recommended for patients with cardiac failure or children under 2 years of age. It is also thought to have thrombogenic potential and should be used with caution in the elderly or those with known vascular disease. The response to DDAVP should be assessed in all patients prior to its use to treat bleeding or cover invasive procedures to ensure that an adequate increase in factor VIII levels is achieved.

Tranexamic acid reduces fibrinolysis and is of particular use in patients with bleeding from mucosal surfaces, such as epistaxis, oral bleeding or menorrhagia. It is given as an adjunct to DDAVP to reduce bleeding. It should be avoided in patients with haematuria to avoid the complication of clot retention. It is usually given for 7–10 days to allow adequate healing.

Haemophilia B

This X-linked recessive disorder results in a deficiency of factor IX. The clinical features are identical to those of haemophilia A (Table 25.2).

Investigations
Laboratory abnormalities seen in haemophilia B include:
• prolonged APTT;
• reduction of factor IX coagulant activity.

Management
The main types of products that are currently used for treatment include:
• recombinant factor IX products;
• high purity plasma-derived factor IX concentrates.

The product of choice for prophylaxis, treatment of bleeding or cover for surgical procedures in previously untreated patients is recombinant factor IX [2]. If unavailable, then high purity plasma-derived factor IX concentrates should be used. Prothrombin complex concentrates (PCC), containing factors II, VII, IX and X, have been used in the past but are not recommended now due to their prothrombotic effects.

The dosage of factor IX required can be calculated according to the formula:

$$\text{Units of factor IX required} = \text{weight (kg)} \times \text{desired level (\%)} \times 1.0$$

The plasma half-life of factor IX is 18–30 hours and therefore if repeated doses are needed, they should be given every 12–24 hours or by continuous infusion.

The choice of product for patients who have required previous treatment with factor concentrates depends on the history of inhibitor development and response to treatment. There is some evidence to suggest that plasma-derived products have different pharmacokinetic properties to recombinant products; therefore, the response to treatment should be monitored closely if switching from one product to another.

Treatment of patients with inhibitors

Patients with haemophilia can develop inhibitory antibodies to factors VIII or IX. Inhibitor development is often heralded by increased frequency of bleeding or loss of response to factor VIII. It is diagnosed by measuring factor VIII levels before and after a dose of factor VIII concentrate and by a Bethesda inhibitor assay.

For patients with haemophilia A, if the inhibitor is of low titre (i.e. <5 Bethesda units), then bleeding episodes can be treated with higher than normal doses of human factor VIII [3]. If the inhibitor is of high titre (i.e. >10 Bethesda units), human factor VIII is ineffective to control bleeding and the use of recombinant FVIIa or FEIBA® (Baxter) is recommended. For major haemorrhage, recombinant FVIIa (dose of 70–90 μg/kg initially every 2 hours) is generally recommended as first-line therapy (if available). Eradication of inhibitors with 'immune tolerance induction' using factor VIII concentrates alone or together with immunosuppression is considered the best long-term treatment option for these patients [3].

For patients with haemophilia B, recombinant factor VIIa is used for bleeding [3]. Immune tolerance using factor IX concentrates can be attempted, although this is more difficult than in haemophilia A. Up to 50% of haemophilia B patients who develop an inhibitor have anaphylaxis or severe allergic reactions to factor IX concentrates.

Table 25.3 Variants of von Willebrand disease.

Type 1	Autosomal dominant inheritance
	Partial quantitative deficiency of VWF
	Normal VWF multimers
	Mild bleeding disorder which decreases during pregnancy, elderly
Type 2	Autosomal dominant inheritance
	Qualitative deficiency of VWF
	Numerous subtypes
	Abnormal VWF multimers
	Generally mild bleeding disorder
Type 3	Autosomal recessive inheritance
	Severe quantitative deficiency of VWF
	Severe haemophilia-like bleeding disorder

Von Willebrand disease (VWD)

This is the most common of the inherited bleeding disorders and is due to a quantitative and/or qualitative defect in the VWF protein. VWF has two main functions: it promotes the adhesion of platelets to the subendothelium by binding to the platelet receptor glycoprotein Ib and it protects factor VIII:C from proteolytic degradation by forming a noncovalent association. Patients who are blood group O have lower levels of VWF than other blood groups.

VWD is classified into three different types (Table 25.3) [4]. Clinical symptoms vary; some patients may be asymptomatic whereas others will have haemophilia-like bleeding. Laboratory abnormalities seen in VWD include (variably):
• prolonged PFA-100™ closure time;
• reduction of VWF antigen (VWF:Ag);
• reduction of VWF ristocetin cofactor activity (VWF:RiCoF);
• reduction of FVIII:C (which can cause prolonged APTT);
• abnormal VWF multimers in some subtypes.

The goal of therapy in patients with VWD is to correct the dual defect of haemostasis, i.e. the abnormal platelet adhesion and the abnormal coagulation due to low FVIII levels. Treatment differs for the various types of VWD [5]:
• Type 1. To reduce exposure to blood components, DDAVP is the treatment of choice and a dose of 0.3 μg/kg body weight is usually given intravenously or subcutaneously. Intranasal doses (300 μg for adults or 150 μg for children) can also be given. These doses

give a two- to fivefold increase in endogenous VWF and FVIII:C levels. The choice of route of administration depends on the patient and the nature of the bleeding or surgery. It is important to test an individual's response to DDAVP prior to using it to 'cover' procedures. Tranexamic acid is often also given either alone for minor bleeding/procedures or in conjunction with DDAVP.

• Types 2 and 3. VWF 'replacement therapy' is generally required. At present there are no recombinant VWF concentrates available so either a factor VIII concentrate rich in VWF or a purified VWF concentrate is the treatment of choice, preferably those with double viral inactivation steps.

In the past, cryoprecipitate was used to treat patients with VWD; however, it is now unacceptable to use such untreated plasma derivatives when there are 'safer' alternatives available.

Other inherited disorders

Hereditary deficiencies of other coagulation factors are rare. Factor XI deficiency is particularly common amongst Ashkenazi Jews and is transmitted as an autosomal recessive trait. There is a poor correlation between factor XI levels and bleeding tendency, which usually presents following surgery or dental procedures. If available, factor XI concentrates should be given to treat bleeding; if not, then FFP should be administered. There have been concerns about the potential thrombogenicity of factor XI concentrates, so peak levels should ideally not exceed 70 IU/dL [6].

Cryoprecipitate can be used for fibrinogen deficiency/dysfibrinogenaemias, but fibrinogen concentrates should be used in preference if they are available because they undergo additional viral inactivation steps [2]. Deficiencies of factors II, V, VII, X and XIII can all be treated with FFP, but if more specific therapies are available they should be used in preference. Currently, there are specific factor concentrates for factors VII and XIII. Prothrombin complex concentrates (PCCs) contain factors II, IX and X with variable amounts of VII and are used in conditions associated with deficiencies of one/more of these factors (e.g. treatment of overdosage with warfarin). They can be given to patients with factors II or X deficiency (although thromboembolic risks should be considered). Factor V-deficient patients are treated with

FFP and it is recommended that virally inactivated plasma is used.

Patients with deficiencies of 'contact factors' (factor XII, prekallikrein and high-molecular-weight kininogen) do not bleed excessively and do not require any treatment.

Acquired haemostatic defects

Disseminated intravascular coagulation (DIC)

This is a complex disorder resulting from inappropriate and excessive activation of the haemostatic system that can be manifested by both thrombotic and haemorrhagic pathology. DIC may be acute (uncompensated) with decreased levels of haemostatic components or chronic (compensated) with normal or sometimes elevated levels of coagulation factors.

The main triggering mechanism for DIC is the exposure of blood to a source of tissue factor that initiates coagulation, e.g. on the surface of endothelial cells or monocytes stimulated by endotoxins/cytokines as a result of sepsis, on the surface of damaged cells (placental abruption, cerebral trauma) or from malignant cells.

The final consequence of coagulation activation is thrombin generation and fibrin formation, which may result in microthrombus formation (e.g. gangrene of fingers, toes and renal failure). Secondary activation of the fibrinolytic pathway occurs with subsequent lysis of fibrin and the formation of crosslinked complexes such as D-dimers. Raised levels of these fibrin degradation products (FDP) further add to the bleeding diathesis as they inhibit the action of thrombin and also inhibit platelet function by binding to the platelet membrane.

Hepatic synthesis of coagulation factors is unable to compensate fully for the ongoing consumption of clotting factors, so there is a reduction in levels of particularly factors V, VIII, XIII and fibrinogen. In addition, a consumptive thrombocytopenia develops. This combination of coagulation factor deficiency, thrombocytopenia and the inhibitory actions of raised FDPs causes the generalized and continued bleeding tendency characteristic of DIC. The main causes of DIC are listed in Table 25.4.

In order of frequency the following laboratory abnormalities are seen in DIC [7]:
• fall in platelet count/thrombocytopenia: ~50% of patients have a platelet count $\leq 50 \times 10^9$/L;

Table 25.4 Main causes of DIC.

Condition	Examples
Infection	Septicaemia, viraemia
Malignancy	Leukaemia (especially acute promyelocytic)
	Metastatic carcinomas
Obstetric disorders	Septic abortion
	Placenta praevia and abruptio placentae
	Eclampsia
	Amniotic fluid embolism
Trauma	Extensive surgical trauma
	Fat embolism
Shock	Burns
	Heat stroke
Liver disease	Acute hepatic necrosis
Transplantation	Tissue rejection
Extracorporeal circulation	Cardiac bypass surgery
Extensive intravascular haemolysis	ABO-incompatible transfusion
Certain snake bites	
Vascular abnormalities	Kasabach–Merrit syndrome

Table 25.5 International Society of Thrombosis and Haemostasis Diagnostic Scoring system for overt DIC.

Risk assessment:
Does the patient have an underlying disorder known to be associated with overt DIC?
If **yes**: proceed
If **no: do not use this algorithm**
Order global coagulation tests (PT, platelet count, fibrinogen, fibrin-related marker)
Score the test results
- Platelet count: $>100 \times 10^9/L = 0$, $<100 \times 10^9/L = 1$, $<50 \times 10^9/L = 2$
- Elevated fibrin marker (e.g. D-dimer, fibrin degradation products): no increase = 0, moderate increase = 2, strong increase = 3
- Prolonged PT: <3 s = 0, >3 but <6 s = 1, >6 s = 2
- Fibrinogen level: >1 g/L = 0, <1 g/L = 1

Calculate score:
≥ 5 compatible with overt DIC: repeat score daily
<5 suggestive for nonovert DIC: repeat next 1–2 d

- increased FDPs: raised D-dimers, increased fibrin monomers;
- prolonged PT and APTT: in 50–60% cases of DIC;
- reduced fibrinogen levels;
- anaemia, fragmented red cells, raised reticulocyte count.

In order to help with the diagnosis of DIC in the clinical setting, scoring systems such as that from the International Society for Thrombosis and Haemostasis (ISTH) have been devised [8] (Table 25.5). The most important aspect of management is removal/alleviation of the underlying trigger as well as treatment of any associated infection, hypovolaemia, etc. Obstetric emergencies should be attended to immediately. Abnormalities of laboratory tests in the absence of bleeding are not a reason to treat with plasma products. The current BCSH guidelines suggest the following therapies if the patient is bleeding, at high risk of bleeding or requires surgical intervention [7].
- Platelet concentrates if the platelet count is $\leq 50 \times 10^9/L$.
- FFP if the PT or APTT are prolonged. Almost all procoagulant factors and inhibitors are contained within FFP. Standard doses of 15 mL/kg should be given, but patients often need up to 30 mL/kg. PCCs can be considered if the patient is at risk of fluid overload but they do not contain all clotting factors, e.g. no factor V.
- Fibrinogen replacement with either cryprecipitate or fibrinogen concentrates if plasma levels are <1.0 g/L. Cryoprecipitate contains fibrinogen in a 'concentrated' form and two pooled packs (adult therapeutic doses) are the standard dose. Fibrinogen concentrates are virally inactivated plasma-derived preparations that also have the advantage of being highly concentrated; 3–4 g of concentrate will raise the fibrinogen level by 1 g/L.

Following initial replacement therapy, any further treatment should be guided by the clinical and laboratory response with suggested threshold values: platelets $>50 \times 10^9/L$, fibrinogen >1.0 g/L and the maintenance of the PT and APTT <1.5 times the mean control.

Heparin anticoagulation may also be useful in situations where initial replacement therapy has failed to control excessive bleeding or when DIC is complicated by microvascular thrombosis or large vessel thrombosis. Low dose continuous intravenous therapy (500–1000 IU/h) is one suggested regimen.

Critically ill patients with DIC who are not bleeding should receive heparin thromboprophylaxis.

Specific clotting factor inhibitor concentrates (e.g. activated protein C or antithrombin) may have a role in the management of certain groups of patients (e.g. those who do not respond to simple replacement therapy, overwhelming sepsis and meningococcaemia).

Purpura fulminans is the condition of DIC associated with skin ecchymoses and necrosis. Primary disease is usually associated with varicella zoster infection whereas secondary disease is precipitated by overwhelming bacterial sepsis (e.g. meningococcal). It is more common in children and primary purpural fulminans often has associated low protein S levels. Therapy is controversial; however, in primary disease associated with low protein S levels, plasma exchange or plasma infusions to keep the protein S levels >25% have been used [9]. Other treatment modalities such as steroids or intravenous immunoglobulin have also been used but the efficacy is unclear. Heparin has been reported to reduce the skin necrosis.

Trauma

It is estimated that approximately 10 000 people per year die following trauma in England and Wales and 30–40% do so due to uncontrolled haemorrhage. By the time the patient reaches hospital, a coagulopathy has often already set in and needs to be corrected promptly to prevent further haemorrhage and allow treatment of injuries. The coagulopathy is multifactorial with the leading causes being:
- consumption of clotting factors and platelets;
- dilution of clotting factors due to fluid resuscitation/massive transfusion;
- acidosis leading to clotting factor dysfunction;
- hypothermia leading to clotting factor dysfunction;
- DIC, particularly in those with brain injuries.

The combination of acidosis, hypothermia and coagulopathy is referred to as the 'lethal triad'. Early recognition of the condition is imperative using standard coagulation testing, but there are limitations in this setting and the value of newer tests of global haemostasis, such as TEG® and ROTEM®, is being explored. Blood component replacement remains the cornerstone of management. The target for red cell replacement is usually Hb >8 g/dL and for platelets is >50–75 × 10^9/L. FFP transfusion is likely to be needed once one blood volume has been transfused and is usually given at a dose of 15 mL/kg. In addition, if the fibrinogen level is <1 g/L then fibrinogen concentrates or cryoprecipitate can be given. Recombinant FVIIa has also been used in the trauma setting. There is only evidence for its benefit in blunt trauma in clinical studies [10]. In addition the results of the CRASH-2 trial have showed that early administration of tranexamic acid to trauma patients significantly reduces mortality from bleeding [11].

Massive transfusion

The management of massive blood loss and transfusion is discussed in Chapter 26.

Liver disease

All coagulation factors (except VWF) and protease inhibitors are synthesized by hepatocytes. The liver also removes activated intermediates of coagulation from the bloodstream. In liver disease a hypocoagulable state may result from a number of mechanisms – reduced synthesis of coagulation factors; cholestasis and subsequent malabsorption resulting in vitamin K deficiency; and an acquired 'dysfibrinogenaemia'. The platelet count is often reduced due to hypersplenism.

Laboratory abnormalities seen in liver disease include prolonged PT, APTT and thrombin time (TT); the latter may result from low fibrinogen concentration or dysfibrinogenaemia. A prolonged reptilase time in spite of a normal fibrinogen concentration implies a dysfibrinogenaemia and elevated D-dimers.

Coagulation abnormalities occur quite frequently in patients with severe liver disease but they are not always associated with bleeding. Bleeding is often precipitated by an event such as surgery or liver biopsy and is rarely attributable to the haemostatic defect alone. If there is bleeding (or a very strong possibility that bleeding will occur), then FFP is indicated. Large volumes of FFP are often required to control the bleeding/correct the defect, and this can be problematic in patients who may already have an expanded plasma volume. Complete normalization of a prolonged PT is often not possible and the use of PCCs may be considered. However, one must be aware of the potential risks of inducing thrombosis or DIC in these patients, particularly since they already suffer from impaired clearance of activated clotting factors and reduced levels of antithrombin. Vitamin K in doses of 10–20 mg may produce some improvement in the coagulation abnormalities. Since thrombocytopenia and platelet function defects are also a feature of hepatic disease, platelet concentrates may also need to be given to maintain a platelet count above 50×10^9/L. For patients undergoing liver biopsies, the prothrombin time should be corrected to within 2–3 seconds of the upper limit of normal.

Uraemia

The haemostatic defect is mainly due to platelet dysfunction and a defect in platelet–vessel wall interactions. Many qualitative platelet defects can be demonstrated *in vitro*, including impaired aggregation in response to agonists as well as storage pool defects. However, these abnormalities do not appear to correlate well with clinical bleeding. It is also thought that plasma from uraemic patients contains an inhibitor that interferes with normal VWF–platelet interaction.

Dialysis is useful in reversing the haemostatic defects in uraemia – although this may not correct them entirely. Anaemia (particularly when the haematocrit is <20%) should be corrected by either blood transfusion or erythropoietin as this improves platelet function and shortens bleeding time. Infusions of DDAVP (0.3–0.4 µg/kg) have been used successfully to provide short-term correction of the bleeding time and decreased symptoms of bleeding.

Complications of anticoagulant and thrombolytic drugs

Vitamin K antagonists

Coumarin and phenindione derivatives act by blocking the γ-carboxylation of glutamic acid residues of vitamin K-dependent coagulation factors, resulting in decreased biological activity of factors II, VII, IX and X, as well as proteins C and S. The INR monitors their effect on the haemostatic system. Some clinical situations may be associated with an increased risk of bleeding during anticoagulation and these are listed in Table 25.6.

Management of excessive anticoagulation depends on the INR level and whether there is minor or major bleeding [12]. It should be noted that the risk of major bleeding from warfarin is around 2% per year, with a

Table 25.6 Conditions associated with increased risk of bleeding during anticoagulation with vitamin K antagonists.

Age (possible)
Uncontrolled hypertension
Alcoholism
Liver disease
Vitamin K deficiency
Poor drug or clinic visit compliance
Active major bleeding
Previous intracranial bleeding
Potential bleeding lesion (e.g. aneurysm, internal ulcer)
Thrombocytopenia
Platelet dysfunction (e.g. use of aspirin)

case fatality of 20%. Therefore, in the event of major bleeding, prompt appropriate action is required. In the absence of haemorrhage, warfarin should be stopped for a few days and recommenced when the INR falls into the desired range. Small doses of vitamin K (1–2.5 mg) may be given intravenously/orally if the INR >5.0, as there is a significantly greater risk of serious haemorrhage at this level.

If the patient is bleeding, then the anticoagulant effect should be reversed. Vitamin K 5–10 mg should be given intravenously and will have an initial onset of action after 4–6 hours. The action of vitamin K is, however, not maximal for at least 24 hours and therefore additional measures are required.

• Prothrombin complex concentrates (PCCs) – Beriplex®, CSL Behring, Octaplex®, Octapharma – which contain factors II, VII, IX and XI, are now recommended as the first line for warfarin reversal when available. Ideal dosing is unclear. Two regimens are currently in use: either dosing calculated on 50 IU FIX/kg body weight or alternatively fixed dosing regimens giving either 500 IU or 1000 IU. Whilst a dose of 50 IU FIX/kg will effectively reverse anticoagulation, it should be remembered that clinical assessment still remains paramount as INR correction is quickly achieved by the correction of FVII levels alone. The disadvantage of these concentrates is that they carry the potential risk of inducing thromboembolism as they often contain activated coagulation components. Therefore, when using these products, caution should be exercised, especially in high risk groups.
• In the absence of PCCs, FFP (12–15 mL/kg) will immediately supply the necessary coagulation factors.

However, there are some potential problems with this type of therapy. Very large amounts of plasma (1–2 L) may need to be infused in order to correct the coagulopathy, and even though the INR may correct into the normal range, this is misleading since it is not sensitive to factor IX – the concentration of which is only minimally increased by treatment with FFP. The levels of individual clotting factors will typically remain <20% after FFP infusion.

Haemorrhage occurring in a warfarinized patient with an INR in the therapeutic range should be managed as above and repeat dosing may be required due to the short duration of action of both PCC and FFP. Red cell and platelet transfusion may become necessary if major bleeding occurs. Additional investigations to exclude any underlying local lesions should also be remembered.

New oral anticoagulants

The last few years has seen the development and introduction of new oral anticoagulants that have the advantage of not requiring routine monitoring. The drugs that are currently in use or advanced stages of development are the direct thrombin inhibitor dabigatran and the FXa inhibitors Rivaroxaban and Apixaban [13]. They have fewer drug interactions than warfarin, but the increased bleeding risk with nonsteroidal anti-inflammatory drugs still applies. There are no ideal tests for overanticoagulation; the dilute thrombin time, ecarin clotting time or anti-Xa assay using the relevant drug can be used. There are no specific reversal agents for these drugs and PCCs have been used to treat bleeding with Xa inhibitors while rVIIa has been used to treat bleeding with both IIa and Xa inhibitors. Dialysis will also remove the drug from the body in cases of intractable, severe haemorrhage.

Thrombolytic agents

These agents generally cause a state of systemic lysis. However, the degree to which this is affected varies according to the particular drug used. Streptokinase has a greater effect on the laboratory markers of systemic lysis than does tissue plasminogen activator, but this does not appear to correlate with the incidence of bleeding.

Laboratory tests such as the thrombin time and fibrinogen levels will detect the presence of a systemic lytic state, but they do not predict the likelihood of haemorrhage, and nowadays most protocols use fixed-dose schedules.

Haemorrhage complicating these agents is most commonly local (e.g. at the site of catheterization in the groin); however, intracranial or gastrointestinal bleeding may occur. Measures such as pressure packs will often control local bleeding; more serious bleeding usually necessitates discontinuing thrombolysis. Most agents have a short half-life (minutes) and so the fibrinolytic state will reverse within a few hours of drug cessation. The exception to this is APSAC (acylated plasminogen-streptokinase activator complex), which has a half-life of 90 minutes. In the case of life-threatening haemorrhage, infusions of cryoprecipitate or FFP can be given to reverse the hypocoagulable state. Antifibrinolytic drugs such as epsilon-aminocaproic acid may/may not provide some additional benefit.

Vitamin K deficiency

Conditions that impair vitamin K absorption (e.g. biliary tract obstruction) as well as haemorrhagic disease of the newborn can result in a coagulopathy similar to that seen with warfarin overdosage. Any serious/life-threatening bleeding should be treated in the same manner.

Cardiopulmonary bypass

Haemostatic disturbances that occur during cardiopulmonary bypass are usually due to platelet dysfunction. If there is persistent bleeding (despite adequate platelet transfusion) and a coagulopathy other than that caused by heparin has been demonstrated, then FFP should be used.

Acquired prothrombotic conditions treated with plasma products

Thrombotic thrombocytopenic purpura

Patients with acute thrombotic thrombocytopenic purpura (TTP) require plasma exchange with FFP to achieve remission. Large daily doses of FFP are needed, usually in the order of 3 L/day. Solvent–detergent plasma should be used if available to reduce the risk of virus transmission. FFP contains ADAMTS13, the metalloproteinase enzyme that is deficient or inhibited in TTP. ADAMTS13 degrades ultralarge multimers of VWF that cause the excessive platelet activation and consumption in this condition. The reduced activity of protein S in SD-treated

FFP has been associated with the development of venous thromboembolism in patients with TTP; this risk is small and SD plasma should still be used in preference to standard FFP. Methylene blue-treated plasma is not recommended because it has been shown to be less effective than solvent–detergent plasma in these patients. Patients with acute idiopathic TTP often require immunosuppression to maintain remission. Rituximab is increasingly being used in TTP and reduces the total amount of plasma received by patients by reducing the number of relapses [14].

Inherited deficiencies of inhibitors of coagulation

Previously, FFP has been used as a source of antithrombin, protein C and protein S for patients with inherited deficiencies of these inhibitors who may be receiving heparin therapy for spontaneous thrombosis or who are undergoing surgery. Now that specific concentrates are being manufactured (antithrombin and protein C), FFP should be used only when these are not available.

Key points

1 Basic initial screening tests for haemostasis include the platelet count, prothrombin time, activated partial thromboplastin time and fibrinogen level.

2 In inherited bleeding disorders, recombinant products should be used where available.

3 The mainstay of treatment of DIC remains management of the underlying cause. In bleeding patients, prompt administration of FFP and cryoprecipitate with regular laboratory monitoring is required.

4 Appropriate guidelines (e.g. those provided by the BCSH) should be followed when managing major haemorrhage, aiming for the following parameters: Hb >8 g/dL; platelets >50 × 10^9/L; PT and APTT <1.5 × mean control; fibrinogen >1.0 g/L.

5 PCCs should be the first choice for urgent reversal of vitamin K antagonists along with vitamin K. FFP may be used if PCCs are contraindicated or unavailable.

6 Patients with TTP should receive plasma exchange with solvent–detergent plasma or standard FFP if not available. Methylene blue treated plasma should not be used.

References

1 Hoffman M. A cell-based model of coagulation and the role of factor VIIa. *Blood Rev* 2003; 17 (Suppl. 1): S1–S5.

2 Keeling D, Tait C & Makris M. Guideline on the selection and use of therapeutic products to treat haemophilia and other hereditary bleeding disorders. A United Kingdom Haemophilia Center Doctors' Organisation (UKHCDO) guideline approved by the British Committee for Standards in Haematology. *Haemophilia* 2008; 14: 671–684.

3 Hay CR, Brown S, Collins PW, Keeling DM & Liesner R. The diagnosis and management of factor VIII and IX inhibitors: a guideline from the United Kingdom Haemophilia Centre Doctors' Organisation. *Br J Haematol* 2006; 133: 591–605.

4 Laffan M, Brown SA, Collins PW et al. The diagnosis of von Willebrand disease: a guideline from the UK Haemophilia Centre Doctors' Organization. *Haemophilia* 2004; 10: 199–217.

5 Pasi KJ, Collins PW, Keeling DM et al. Management of von Willebrand disease: a guideline from the UK Haemophilia Centre Doctors' Organization. *Haemophilia* 2004; 10: 218–231.

6 Bolton-Maggs PH, Perry DJ, Chalmers EA et al. The rare coagulation disorders – review with guidelines for management from the United Kingdom Haemophilia Centre Doctors' Organisation. *Haemophilia* 2004; 10: 593–628.

7 Levi M, Toh CH, Thachil J & Watson HG. Guidelines for the diagnosis and management of disseminated intravascular coagulation. British Committee for Standards in Haematology. *Br J Haematol* 2009; 145: 24–33.

8 Toh CH & Hoots WK. The scoring system of the Scientific and Standardisation Committee on Disseminated Intravascular Coagulation of the International Society on Thrombosis and Haemostasis: a 5-year overview. *J Thromb Haemost* 2007; 5: 604–606.

9 Chalmers E, Cooper P, Forman K et al. Purpura fulminans: recognition, diagnosis and management. *Arch Dis Child* 2011; 96: 1066–1071.

10 Hauser CJ, Boffard K, Dutton R et al. Results of the CONTROL trial: efficacy and safety of recombinant activated Factor VII in the management of refractory traumatic hemorrhage. *J Trauma* 2010; 69: 489–500.

11 Shakur H, Roberts I, Bautista R et al. Effects of tranexamic acid on death, vascular occlusive events, and blood transfusion in trauma patients with significant haemorrhage (CRASH-2): a randomised, placebo-controlled trial. *Lancet* 2010; 376: 23–32.

12 Keeling D, Baglin T, Tait C et al. Guidelines on oral anticoagulation with warfarin – fourth edition. *Br J Haematol* 2011; 154: 311–324.

13 Garcia D, Libby E & Crowther MA. The new oral anticoagulants. *Blood* 2010; 115: 15–20.

14 Scully M, McDonald V, Cavenagh J *et al.* A phase 2 study of the safety and efficacy of rituximab with plasma exchange in acute acquired thrombotic thrombocytopenic purpura. *Blood* 2011; 118: 1746–1753.

Further reading

British Committee for Standards in Haematology. Guidelines for the use of fresh frozen plasma, cryoprecipitate and cryosupernatant. *Br J Haematol* 2004; 126: 11–28.

British Committee for Standards in Haematology. Guidelines on the assessment of bleeding risk prior to surgery or invasive procedures. *Br J Haematol* 2008; 140: 496–504.

Paediatric Working Party of the UK Haemophilia Doctors Organization. The management of haemophilia in the fetus and neonate. *Br J Haematol* 2011; 154: 208–215.

Richards M, Williams M, Chalmers E, Liesner R, Collins P, Vidler V & Hanley J on behalf of the Paediatric Working Party of the UK Haemophilia Doctors' Organization. Guideline on the use of prophylactic factor VIII concentrate in children and adults with severe haemophilia A. *Br J Haematol* 2010; 149: 498–507.

Tripodi A & Mannucci PM. Mechanisms of disease: the coagulopathy of chronic liver disease. *N Engl J Med* 2001; 365: 147–156.

26 Massive blood loss

Beverley J. Hunt[1] *& John R. Hess*[2]

[1]Kings College, London, UK and Departments of Haematology, Pathology and Rheumatology, Guy's and St Thomas' NHS Foundation Trust, London, UK

[2]Departments of Pathology and Medicine, University of Maryland School of Medicine, Baltimore, MD, USA

Definition and burden of massive blood loss

Massive blood loss is defined either as the cause of acute haemorrhagic mortality or, arbitrarily, as replacement of the patient's blood volume in less than 24 hours. Uncontrolled haemorrhage is the major cause of death in the developing world through injury and obstetric bleeding. Worldwide, injury is the leading cause of death among those aged 5–44 years, leading to 5 million deaths annually [1]. About 1.6 million people die as a result of intentional acts of interpersonal, collective or self-directed violence every year. Road traffic injuries are the ninth leading cause of death globally and are predicted to rise to the third leading cause of death and disability by 2020. More than 90% of trauma deaths occur in low income and middle income countries. Uncontrolled haemorrhage causes about one-third of in-hospital trauma deaths and can contribute to deaths from later multiorgan failure.

In the USA, where most injured patients are treated in trauma centres, injury is the leading cause of death in the 1–44 year age group and the third leading cause of death overall. Haemorrhage is the cause of 30 to 40% of injury deaths and most such hospital deaths occur within hours of admission [2].

Obstetric haemorrhage remains the leading cause of maternal mortality worldwide [3].

• One woman dies from obstetric haemorrhage every 4 minutes, 140 000–160 000 each year.

• The latest Confidential Enquires into Maternal Deaths in the UK, 2006–2008, 'Saving Mothers' Lives', indicates that obstetric haemorrhage still accounts for maternal deaths every year, with 'early warning signs of impending maternal collapse … unrecognised' [4].

• The European Project and Haemorrhage Reduction (EUPHRATES) observed considerable variation between the 14 participant European countries in the medical policies for immediate management of obstetric haemorrhage.

Massive blood loss in situations such as liver transplantation can be predicted, and thus sophisticated monitoring and management protocols can be employed [5]. Best practice in managing massive blood loss as shown by 'Saving Mothers Lives' is not always followed [4]. This seems, in part, to be due to poor understanding of the appropriate use of monitoring, blood components and pharmacologic agents.

Management is aimed at limiting blood loss and the correction of tissue hypoxia and coagulation abnormalities. This requires a multidisciplinary approach including the control of pain, ventilation and temperature, rapid control of bleeding, and blood component or pharmacologic treatment of coagulation disorders. This chapter aims to describe the appropriate use of blood components. The use of pharmacologic agents is covered in Chapter 37. It is important to recognize that the evidence base to support current recommendations is modest and evolving rapidly.

Practical Transfusion Medicine, Fourth Edition. Edited by Michael F. Murphy, Derwood H. Pamphilon and Nancy M. Heddle.
© 2013 John Wiley & Sons, Ltd. Published 2013 by John Wiley & Sons, Ltd.

Physiological response of coagulation to blood loss

During traumatic, surgical and obstetric haemorrhage blood loss depletes blood coagulation factors and platelets [6]. It may also be associated with widespread tissue factor exposure leading to massive thrombin activation, with both early fibrin clot formation and increased tissue plasminogen activator production leading to simultaneous coagulation factor consumption and fibrinolytic activation [7]. This activation and loss of coagulation factors and fibrinolytic activation will consume and deplete haemostatic factors. Haemostasis is also strongly influenced by body temperature and acidosis. In hypothermia, a coagulation screen or thromboelastography performed at 37°C will underestimate the extent of any coagulopathy. Platelet function is profoundly disturbed at temperatures below 33°C. Metabolic acidosis from tissue hypoxia interferes with plasma coagulation reducing procoagulant activity by two-thirds at pH 7. Early abnormalities of coagulation in massive blood loss are independent predictors of mortality. Key factors in the development of coagulopathy include:

- injury severity;
- haemorrhagic shock;
- blood loss;
- haemodilution;
- acidosis;
- hypothermia;
- hypocalcaemia;
- coagulation factor and platelet consumption;
- fibrinolytic activation.

These factors can cause an acute coagulopathy of trauma and combine with further resuscitative haemodilution and heat loss to form a vicious cycle [8]. If the lethal triad of hypothermia, acidosis and coagulopathy is present, surgical control of bleeding alone is unlikely to be successful and is associated with high mortality.

Management of bleeding

The general principles are to achieve rapid control of bleeding and restoration of tissue perfusion (Table 26.1) [9]. Mild hypotension is well tolerated for short periods, whereas overly aggressive early resuscitation may move more blood through the vascular

Table 26.1 The changing principles of massive blood loss management.

Over the last 5 years there have been changing views about the haemostatic management of massive blood loss.

- Retrospective data from battle fields has suggested survival is improved if haemostatic blood components are given upfront; this is known as 'amage control resuscitation'.
- Fibrinogen is important. *In vitro* and mainland Europe anecdotal experience suggests the previous triggers for fibrinogen replacement were too low.
- The use of prothrombin complex concentrates (factors II, VII, IX and X) and factor XII concentrates has entered clinical practice without being properly trialled.
- Aprotinin has been withdrawn but tranexamic acid has been shown to reduce mortality and is safe.
- Analysis of rFVIIa off-licence use has shown a 5% risk of arterial thrombosis.

Unfortunately:

- The use of TEG/ROTEM still has not been adequately validated.
- It is the authors' experience that haemostatic management of bleeding is poorly taught and remains poorly managed in many areas.

deficits and worsen coagulopathy. Adequate analgesia is necessary to control pain and prevent tachycardia, which can be misinterpreted as a sign of hypovolaemia.

Heart rate, blood pressure and urine output are useful but nonreliable signs for the initial assessment of the degree of blood loss, especially in young people where blood pressure is usually preserved until very late. Combinations of clinical signs and measurements such as the shock index (heart rate divided by systolic blood pressure) are more useful, especially when measured repeatedly [7]. Peripheral pulses are lost before the femoral pulse, which is lost before the carotid.

The clinical signs of shock are the 'three windows on the microcirculation':

- mental status/level of consciousness (cerebral perfusion) – agitation, confusion, somnolence or lethargy;
- peripheral perfusion – cold and clammy skin, delayed capillary refill, tachycardia;
- renal perfusion – urine output (<0.5 mL/kg/h).

These clinical findings help to differentiate whether a patient is 'haemodynamically normal' or 'apparently haemodynamically stable' but in compensated shock. Arterial blood gas analysis can measure lactate or base deficit, which are highly sensitive measures of persistent shock. Clinical scores based on heart rate, systolic blood pressure, injury mechanism and base deficit, lactate, pH or haemoglobin concentration have high predictive power for the requirements for massive transfusion.

In the most seriously injured, attempts to correct all injuries at initial surgery leads to prolonged operations with hypothermia and coagulopathy complicating the process. 'Damage control' surgery aims to shunt major injured vessels, tie off other sources of active bleeding, pack oozing, tie off gut and drain biliary and urinary sources of contamination [9]. Such patients are taken to intensive care units with their wounds packed open for warming, resuscitation and preparation for their next surgery. Ultimately, severely injured patients treated with staged surgeries have lower mortality.

Fluid management

Traditional injury treatment guidelines generally employed early and aggressive fluid administration to restore blood volume and achieve a prompt restoration of blood pressure [10]. However, some studies have shown increased mortality rates with rapid infusion of fluids compared to more modest volumes and immediate compared with delayed administration. The concept of low volume fluid resuscitation or 'permissive hypotension' avoids the detrimental effects of early aggressive resuscitation while maintaining a level of tissue perfusion that, although decreased from normal, is adequate for short periods. This approach is contraindicated in brain and spinal cord injuries and its effectiveness still needs to be confirmed in randomized clinical trials.

Over the last decade, the fluids themselves have performed poorly in clinical trials. Saline and Ringer's lactate have been shown to be inflammatory [11]. Hypertonic saline was not better than equivalent volumes of normal saline in a large resuscitation trial. Dextrans and hydroxyethyl starch have been shown to interfere with platelet function and a large trial of albumin showed no benefit compared to cheaper crystalloid solutions. All of these fluids dilute the coagulation system and the colloids interfere with protein–protein interactions as well. Dextrans and starch can potentiate fibrinolysis and interfere with platelet function.

Crystalloid fluids are inexpensive and relatively safe and are probably the treatment of choice for patients with mild and many moderate injuries. They are the preferred fluids for keeping IV lines open for drug and blood administration.

Prevention of hypothermia and strategies for re-warming

In general, the greater the degree of hypothermia, the greater is the risk of uncontrolled bleeding. When hypothermia is associated with severe injury, mortality rates up to 100% have been reported [12]. The effects of hypothermia include altered platelet function, impaired coagulation factor function (as a rule of thumb, a 1°C drop in temperature is associated with a 10% drop in function), enzyme inhibition and fibrinolysis. Preventive measures include covering the patient to avoid additional heat loss, increasing ambient temperature, forced air re-warming, giving warm fluid therapy and, in extreme cases, extracorporeal re-warming devices.

Blood component use

In the Maryland Shock-Trauma Center, only 9% of the patients used blood components and only 1.7% were massively transfused [13]. Most patients do well receiving blood following conventional transfusion triggers based on laboratory tests. For a small fraction of the most seriously bleeding treatment must be started quickly and in ways that ensure adequate amounts of all components [14].

For the majority of moderately or more severely injured patients, a coagulation screen and full blood count should be performed as soon as possible to guide the use of blood components with frequent repeat testing determined by the rate of blood loss. The results may be misleading if the patient is hypothermic. Near-patient haemostatic testing with thromboelastography is a possible alternative in high use centres, where the recognition of platelet dysfunction and severe fibrinolysis can be hastened.

For severely injured patients needing immediate blood transfusion, giving all components simultaneously in unit ratios approaching 1 unit of plasma and

1 unit of platelets for each unit of red cells (1:1:1) can maximally deliver a haemoglobin of 10 g/dL, a platelet concentration of 90×10^9/L and coagulation factor levels at least two thirds of normal (a PT ratio less than 1.4) [8]. Storage-related decreases *in vivo* red cell and platelet survival reduce these values further. In patients bleeding and being transfused so rapidly that it is impossible to obtain concurrent laboratory measures, giving blood components at a 1:1:1 ratio assures at least adequate amounts of all components [8]. Using this initial approach, several groups have reported marked reductions in massive transfusion and improved survival, although there is no high quality evidence base to support this practice and other groups advocate giving red cells and plasma in a lower ratio such as 1:2 [15].

Use of red cell transfusion in trauma

Red cell transfusion is recommended to maintain Hb above 8 g/dL. No prospective randomized trial comparing restrictive and liberal transfusion regimens in massive transfusion exists. As noted above, the composition of currently available blood components and products may preclude such a trial in the acutely injured [8]. Among 203 trauma patients who survived 24 hours and were haemodynamically stable, a reanalysis of the Transfusion Requirements in Critical Care (TRICC) trial showed no benefit of trying to obtain a higher haemoglobin concentration [16].

Stored red cells have reduced 2,3-diphosphoglycerate, reduced membrane flexibility, fail to secrete ATP to modulate capillary diameter, and contain lipid and protein breakdown products that can reduce their effectiveness [17]. For all of these reasons, achieving haemorrhage control quickly and limiting transfusion in the postresuscitation period seem excellent practices.

There are no evidence-based guidelines for using red cell transfusion in obstetric haemorrhage, but full blood count monitoring to limit both haemorrhage and transfusion appears justified.

Platelets

Platelets are recommended by all guidelines in the management of massive blood loss when the platelet counts fall below 50×10^9/L. A higher target concentration of $\geq 100 \times 10^9$/L is for those with neurologic injury or polytrauma. One platelet apheresis concentrate will increase the platelet count by $30–50 \times 10^9$/L in normal-sized adults, depending on the platelet dose provided by the blood supplier. The platelet count should be checked 10–15 minutes after platelet infusion to ensure the adequacy of therapy. A poor increment of less than 20×10^9/L after 15 minutes may be indicative of antiplatelet antibodies, usually human leukocyte antigen (HLA Class I) antibodies, or a transfusion from the occasional donors whose platelets store poorly (Chapter 28).

Fresh frozen plasma (FFP)

The indication for use of FFP in massive transfusion and disseminated intravascular coagulation with significant bleeding is an INR or ATTT ratio >1.5. There is no evidence base for the dose that should be used. However, 15 mL/kg is widely accepted for the initial dose. For the acute reversal of the effects of warfarin, the best practice is to use prothrombin complex concentrate (PCC). However, if this is not available, a similar effect can be produced with an FFP dose of 15 mL/kg.

Fibrinogen and cryoprecipitate

Cryoprecipitate or fibrinogen is indicated when fibrinogen concentrations are <1.5 g/L. The trigger for giving supplementary fibrinogen has been set at a higher value than previously in view of the international recognition of the importance of fibrinogen as both the final point of the coagulation cascade and ligand for platelet aggregation. Ten units of cryoprecipitate increase the fibrinogen concentration by approximately 1.0 g/L. ABO blood group compatibility is not required with cryoprecipitate. Indications for the use of fibrinogen concentrate are the same as for cryoprecipitate, but this product is not licensed for this indication in the USA or the UK.

Other coagulation factors

Coagulation factor concentrates, specifically fibrinogen and PCCs, are used in mainland Europe in the place of FFP and cryoprecipitate [18]. These products allow the reconstitution of the extrinsic coagulation system when used with platelets as a source of factor V. Early data from small poor-quality studies suggest that rapid reconstitution of plasma coagulation and platelet counts leads to rapid haemorrhage control with improved survival and reduced blood use. However, larger studies are required to fully assess efficacy and posthaemorrhage thrombotic risk and cost effectiveness.

Summary of practical haematological management of a bleeding patient [19] (also see Figure 26.1)

- Send a blood sample to the blood transfusion laboratory for ABO group and RhD group and phone the laboratory indicating the need for blood. If possible, wait for ABO and RhD compatible blood. In emergency cases use group O RhD-negative red cells until patients' ABO and RhD groups are known. Switch to blood of the same ABO and RhD groups as the patient as soon as possible to avoid inappropriate use of group O RhD-negative red cells.
- Send the baseline sample for FBC, coagulation screen, urea and electrolytes.
- When a fast rate of transfusion is required, a vasopressor or infuser or pump and blood warmer should be used.
- Haemostasis. An early coagulation screen and platelet count or thromboelastography will provide a guide to the use of blood components. It is important to appreciate that at least 1.5 blood volumes (i.e. 7–8 litres in adults) must be transfused before the platelet count falls below 50×10^9/L in an average healthy individual, but counts may be lower following massive injury. After initial resuscitation with 1:1:1 or 1:2:2 ratios of plasma, platelets and red cells, transfusion of replacement blood components should be given as necessary according to the results of screening coagulation tests, aiming to keep:
- Platelet count $>50 \times 10^9$/L;
- PT and APTT ratio less than 1.5 times the control value by giving FFP 15 mL/kg;
- Fibrinogen >1.5 g/L.
- Be mindful of the other possible complications of blood transfusion:
  (a) Hypocalcemia. Calcium gluconate (2 mL of 10% solution per unit of blood) when calcium concentration is low or there are clinical signs or electrocardiographic changes.

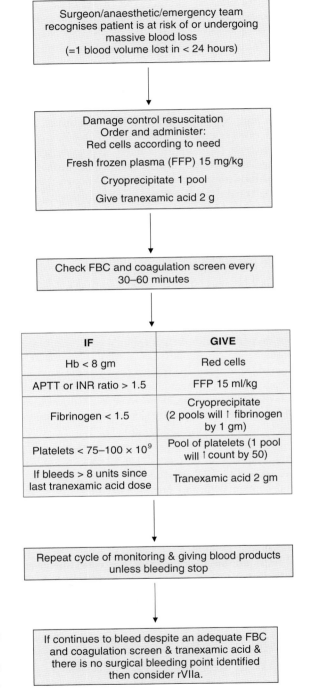

Fig 26.1 Algorithm for the management of massive blood loss.

(b) Hyperkalaemia may occur due to its high concentration (40 mmol/L) in stored blood. This is only a problem in those with hepatic or renal disease.

(c) Acid–base disturbances. Despite the presence of lactic acid in transfused red cells, this usually improves acidosis in shocked patients. Furthermore, transfused citrate produces an alkalosis once it is metabolized.

(d) Hypothermia. Warm the patient and the red cell component.

Organization of transfusion of patients with trauma and for major accidents

In a major accident, large numbers of people may be injured within a short space of time. This requires a coordinated approach from the rescue services and the hospital. A 'major accident procedure' is a necessity within every hospital and should be tested periodically by holding a 'major accident exercise'.

The following must be incorporated into the procedure:

• The telephone numbers of those who 'need to know' is held by the hospital switchboard.
• Suspend the issue of blood for nonemergency cases.
• Increase the stocks to a predefined level by arranging deliveries from the nearest blood centre and maintain stocks throughout the emergency. The blood transfusion laboratory must have a dedicated telephone line to arrange this, as the main hospital switchboard may be blocked with other calls.
• The risk of clinical clerical errors can be high in this emergency situation so special care must be taken in the identification of casualties and labelling blood samples. In the emergency department, every attempt to maintain good clinical practice should be made. Full identification details of each patient should be given on blood request forms and sample vials, wherever possible, and at least the hospital record number of the patient and their sex.
• The practice of issuing blood in a major disaster is best not changed from routine practice, i.e. compatibility testing should be carried out whenever possible. If this is not possible, every effort should be made to ensure that blood is ABO and RhD group matched. When the recipients blood group is not known group O RhD-negative blood should be given to girls and women in the reproductive age, unless there is life-threatening bleeding and O RhD-negative blood is not available. O RhD-positive blood can be given to males with unknown blood groups.

• Blood components such as FFP and platelets need to be available quickly for those who are receiving massive transfusion.
• Dealing with requests to donate blood. Following a major accident, there may be calls from the public, offering to donate blood. These potential donors should be given the telephone number of the nearest blood centre so that they can attend one of the routine donor clinics.

The future

Resuscitation of massively bleeding patient with initial 1:1:1 ratios of plasma, platelets and red cells is rapidly becoming the norm with demonstrated improved survival and reduced blood use. The efficacy, safety and cost effectiveness of fibrinogen concentrates and 6-factor PCCs need to be assessed to see whether they will replace initial FFP and platelet therapy because of their more rapid availability than thawed plasma, better virological safety and reduced reactions.

Conclusions

The management of bleeding and coagulopathy in massive blood loss has been an area of major research activity in the last five years and is the subject of major ongoing research. The priority of initial treatment is to maintain tissue perfusion while improving haemostasis. Attention to patient characteristics such as hypothermia is critical to good clinical outcomes.

Key points

1 Massive blood transfusion is the administration of one or more blood volumes in 24 hours.
2 The aim of resuscitation is to maintain adequate tissue oxygenation through adequate numbers of red cells and control hemorrhage.
3 Initially use 'damage control resuscitation'.
4 Check the full blood count and coagulation screen at presentation and then regularly.

5 After initial 'damage control resuscitation' carry out the following.

6 Maintain haemoglobin >8 g/dL.

7 Maintain INR and APPT ratio <1.5 with FFP at 15 mL/kg.

8 Maintain platelet counts > 50×10^9/L.

9 Maintain fibrinogen >1.5 g/L.

10 In those bleeding or at risk of bleeding after trauma, give 1 gm tranexamic acid at presentation and then 1 gm in an infusion over 8 hours. Consider tranexamic acid in other major bleeding scenarios.

References

1 Peden M, Scurfield R, Sleet D, Mohan D, Hyder AA, Jarawan E et al. (eds). World Report on road traffic injury prevention. Geneva: World Health Organization; 2004.

2 Dutton RP, Stansbury LG, Leone S, Kramer B, Hess JR & Scalea TM. Trauma mortality in mature trauma systems: are we doing better? An analysis of trauma mortality patterns, 1997–2008. J Trauma 2010; 69: 620–626.

3 World Health Organization. Trends in Maternal Mortality: 1990 to 2008. Geneva: World Health Organization; 2010.

4 Special Issue: Saving Mothers' Lives: Reviewing maternal deaths to make motherhood safer: 2006–2008. The Eighth Report of the Confidential Enquiries into Maternal Deaths in the United Kingdom. Br J Obstet Gynaecol 2011; 118 (Issue Suppl. s1): 1–203.

5 Roullet S, Biais M, Millas E, Revel P, Quinart A & Sztark F. Risk factors for bleeding and transfusion during orthotopic liver transplantation. Ann Fr Anesth Reanim 2011, April; 30(4): 349–352.

6 Fouche Y, Sikorski R & Dutton RP. Changing paradigms in surgical resuscitation. Crit Care Med 2010, September; 38(9 Suppl.): S411–S420.

7 Murthi SB, Stansbury LG, Dutton RP, Edelman BB, Scalea TM & Hess JR. Transfusion medicine in trauma patients: an update. Expert Rev Hematol 2011; 4(5): 527–537.

8 Armand R & Hess JR. Treating coagulopathy in trauma patients. Transfus Med Rev 2003, July; 17: 223–231.

9 Duchesne JC, McSwain Jr NE, Cotton BA, Hunt JP, Dellavolpe J, Lafaro K, Marr AB, Gonzalez EA, Phelan HA, Bilski T, Greiffenstein P, Barbeau JM, Rennie KV, Baker CC, Brohi K, Jenkins DH & Rotondo M. Damage control resuscitation: the new face of damage control. J Trauma 2010, October; 69(4): 976–990.

10 American College of Surgeons Committee on Trauma. Advanced Trauma Life Support Program for Doctors, seventh edn. Chicago, IL: American College of Surgeons; 2004.

11 Koustova E, Stanton K, Gushchin V, Alam HB, Stegalkina S & Rhee PM. Effects of lactated Ringer's solutions on human leukocytes. J Trauma 2002, May; 52(5): 872–878.

12 Jurkovich GJ, Greiser, Luterman A & Curreri PW. Hypothermia in trauma victims: an ominous predictor of survival. J Trauma 1987; 27(9): 1019–1124.

13 Como JJ, Dutton RP, Scalea TJ, Edelman BB & Hess JR. Blood transfusion rates in the care of acute trauma. Transfusion 2004; 44: 809–813.

14 Levi M, Fries D, Gombotz H, van der Linden P, Nascimento B, Callum JL, Bélisle S, Rizoli S, Hardy J-F, Johansson PI, Samama CM, Grottke O, Rossaint R, Henny CP, Goslings JC, Theusinger OM, Spahn DR, Ganter MT, Hess JR, Dutton RP, Scalea TM, Levy JH, Spinella PC, Panzer S & Reesink WH. Prevention and treatment of coagulopathy in patients receiving massive transfusions. Vox Sanguinus 2011; 101: 154–174.

15 Johansson PI, Stensballe J, Rosenberg I, Hilsløv TL, Jørgensen L, Secher NH. Proactive administration of platelets and plasma for patients with a ruptured abdominal aortic aneurysm: evaluating a change in transfusion practice. Transfusion 2007; 47(4): 593–598.

16 McIntyre L, Hebert PC, Wells G, Fergusson D, Marshall J, Yetisir E & Blajchman MJ; Canadian Critical Care Trials Group. Is a restrictive transfusion strategy safe for resuscitated and critically ill trauma patients? J Trauma 2004, September; 57(3): 563–568.

17 Hess JR. Red cell changes during storage. Transfus Apher Sci 2010; 43(1): 51–59.

18 Nienaber U, Innerhofer P, Westermann I et al. The impact of fresh frozen plasma vs coagulation factor concentrates on morbidity and mortality in trauma-associated haemorrhage and massive transfusion. Injury 2011; 42(7): 697–701.

19 Rossaint R, Bouillon B, Cerny V, Coats TJ, Duranteau J, Fernández-Mondéjar E, Hunt BJ, Komadina R, Nardi G, Neugebauer E, Ozier Y, Riddez L, Schultz A, Stahel PF, Vincent JL & Spahn DR; Task Force for Advanced Bleeding Care in Trauma. Management of bleeding following major trauma: an updated European guideline. Crit Care 2010; 14(2): R52.

Further reading

Cotton BA, Reddy N, Hatch QM et al. Damage control resuscitation is associated with a reduction in resuscitation volumes and improvement in survival in 390 damage control laparotomy patients. Ann Surg 2011, October; 254(4): 598–605.

CRASH-2 collaborators, Roberts I, Shakur H, Afolabi A *et al.* The importance of early treatment with tranexamic acid in bleeding trauma patients: an exploratory analysis of the CRASH-2 randomised controlled trial. *Lancet* 2011, 26 March; 377(9771): 1096–1101.

Hess JR, Brohi K, Dutton RP *et al.* The coagulopathy of trauma: a review of mechanisms. *J Trauma* 2008, October; 65(4): 748–754.

Hess JR, Lindell AL, Stansbury LG, Dutton RP & Scalea TM. The prevalence of abnormal results of conventional coagulation tests on admission to a trauma center. *Transfusion* 2009; 49: 34–39.

Holcomb JB, Wade CE, Michalek JE *et al.* Increased plasma and platelet to red blood cell ratios improves outcome in 466 massively transfused civilian trauma patients. *Ann Surg* 2008; 248(3), 447–458.

Khan KS, Wojdyla D, Say L, Gülmezoglu AM & Van Look PFA. WHO analysis of causes of maternal death: a systematic review. *Lancet* 2006; 367: 1066–1074.

Klug EG, Sharma GK & Lozano R. The global burden of injuries. *Am J Public Health* 2000; 90(4): 523–526.

Napolitano LM, Kurek S, Luchette FA *et al.* Clinical practice guideline: red blood cell transfusion in adult trauma and critical care. *Crit Care Med* 2009, December; 37(12): 3124–3157.

Rossaint R, Cerny V, Coats TJ, Duranteau J, Fernández-Mondéjar E, Gordini G, Stahel PF, Hunt BJ, Neugebauer E & Spahn DR. Key issues in advanced bleeding care in trauma. *Shock* 2006, October; 26(4): 322–331.

Winter C, Macfarlane A, Deneux-Tharaux C *et al.* The European project on haemorrhage reduction: attitudes, trial and early warning system (EUPHRATES). *BJOG* 2007; 114(7): 845–854.

27 Good blood management in acute haemorrhage and critical care

Gavin J. Murphy[1], *Nicola Curry*[2], *Nishith Patel*[3] *& Timothy S. Walsh*[4]

[1]School of Cardiovascular Sciences, University of Leicester, Leicester, UK
[2]John Radcliffe Hospital, Oxford, UK
[3]School of Clinical Sciences, University of Bristol, Bristol, UK
[4]Edinburgh University and Edinburgh Royal Infirmary, Edinburgh, Scotland, UK

Introduction

Good blood management emphasizes the importance of utilizing blood components as part of an overall treatment strategy that is focused on improving patient outcome. Acute haemorrhage and acute anaemia are common in surgical, obstetric and critical care patients. They are also prevalent in nonsurgical patients with upper gastrointestinal haemorrhage. These often critically ill patients are characterized by:
1 A high red cell transfusion requirement.
2 An association with urgent or emergency procedures or clinical events. Patients are usually cared for in highly monitored environments in which cointerventions with therapeutic adjuncts and the use of evidence-based protocols can reduce the use of conventional blood components.
3 Coagulopathy that requires management to assist correction of cardiovascular instability and anaemia.
This chapter reviews the evidence to guide blood management strategies in patients with critical illness or who are undergoing major surgery with an emphasis on those that have been shown to improve clinical outcomes. It also specifically considers changes in the management of massive haemorrhage/blood transfusion that have occurred in recent years, chiefly as a result of the lessons learned from recent armed conflicts, as this represents a clinical situation where appropriate blood management is a key determinant of patient outcomes, including survival.

Red cell transfusion

Anaemia and acute haemorrhage

In surgical and critically ill patients this accounts for almost 50% of all red cell utilization. In a UK study [1] the main users of allogeneic red cells were upper GI haemorrhage (13.8%), orthopaedic surgery (6.3%), trauma (5.9%), liver/GI surgery (5.5%) and cardiac surgery (5.2%). Over 10% of all red cell transfusions are administered in the intensive care unit (ICU) setting.

In acute haemorrhage, the therapeutic priority is to achieve source control; during this period the aim is to maintain adequate oxygen delivery to prevent tissue hypoxia and organ dysfunction using fluids, red cells and interventions to prevent or correct coagulopathy. Once haemorrhage has been stopped management is similar to that for the acutely anaemic patient. This is supported by prospective epidemiological studies in critical care patients where transfusion indicators, i.e. haemoglobin thresholds, are similar in bleeding and nonbleeding patients [2]. Anaemia in the absence of haemorrhage occurs in surgical patients as a result of low preoperative red cell mass or haemodilution and this may account for the greater proportion of all red cell transfusions. For example, in cardiac surgery severe haemorrhage occurs in up to 15% of patients but red cell transfusion occurs in 50–95% of patients, depending on institutional transfusion practice [3].

Practical Transfusion Medicine, Fourth Edition. Edited by Michael F. Murphy, Derwood H. Pamphilon and Nancy M. Heddle.
© 2013 John Wiley & Sons, Ltd. Published 2013 by John Wiley & Sons, Ltd.

Acute anaemia is also common in critical care where the aetiology is multifactorial and includes haemodilution, occult blood loss, therapeutic blood sampling and/or impaired haemopoiesis, which may be acute as a result of sepsis, for example, or chronic as a result of chronic renal or other systemic disease. Anaemia is strongly associated with adverse outcomes in the critically ill and despite the use of multiple interventions and therapeutic adjuncts such as avoidance of haemodilution, excessive therapeutic blood sampling or other modalities, as listed below, red cell transfusion is common. Up to 35–45% of patients receive a blood transfusion within 5 days of ICU admission, of which as many as 90% are administered to reverse anaemia [2].

Indications for red cell transfusion

Whereas red cell transfusion for acute haemorrhage in patients with incipient hypovolaemic shock is clearly life-saving the indications for red cell transfusion to reverse severe anaemia in the critically ill are poorly defined. Observational studies suggest a high likelihood of harm including infection, ischaemic and pulmonary morbidity and mortality (Figure 27.1) from excessive red cell transfusion. However, this evidence is subject to numerous biases including residual confounding from unmeasured variables, treatment and regression bias that arises due to more liberal administration of red cells to sicker patients and publication bias. Determining whether there is a causal effect of transfusion on adverse outcomes from these types of study is impossible.

Higher levels of evidence such as RCTs comparing restrictive versus liberal transfusion thresholds that result in equally matched patient groups exposed to different transfusion volumes do not show an increase in adverse effects attributable to red cell transfusions, although a recent meta-analysis of these RCTs performed in adult patients suggests that more restrictive transfusion practice may be associated with modest benefits in terms of reduced infection, although with no benefits in terms of reduced cardiac or other complications [4]. This meta-analysis included mainly small, poorly reported studies, with lack of blinding and allocation concealment in many cases raising the possibility of detection and performance bias. The results of the analysis were also heavily influenced by a single large RCT, the Transfusion Requirements in Critical Care Study that was undertaken over a decade ago, and administered nonleucocyte-reduced red cells to patients with a relatively low incidence of cardiovascular disease, a principal determinant of both tolerance of anaemia and the risk of ischaemic complications. The difference in transfusion volume between treatment groups in these RCTs was often less than 2 units of blood, an amount that observational data suggests as having only very modest effects on clinical outcomes; even large RCTs may be inadequately powered to detect such an effect. However, the important finding of this analysis was that restrictive transfusion practice in patients with acute anaemia and without cardiovascular disease is safe using transfusion thresholds of 7 g/dL. Moreover, the use of more liberal transfusion thresholds have no clinical benefit, and in fact may have adverse effects. Safe restrictive thresholds in patients with cardiovascular disease remain to be defined.

Treatment adjuncts that reduce transfusion (also see Chapters 34 and 35)

The safety and efficacy of commonly used techniques or interventions that reduce transfusion exposure as summarized in a series of recent systematic reviews [5–12] are summarized in Figures 27.2 and 27.3.

Autologous transfusion techniques

Preoperative autologous donation (PAD)
PAD involves the patient donating one or more units of his/her own blood preoperatively, often in conjunction with the administration of erythropoietin. This blood is held within the blood transfusion laboratory, where it is administered as required during the perioperative stay, as an alternative to allogeneic red cells. PAD is effective at reducing exposure to allogenic blood (Figure 27.2), but overall exposure to transfused red cells (both autologous and allogeneic) is increased, and PAD is not associated with improved clinical outcomes (Figure 27.3). Autologous red cells are presumably as susceptible as allogeneic red cells to storage-related changes that have been linked to transfusion-related morbidity, and where the local allogeneic blood supply is safe from infectious diseases PAD may not confer any overall clinical benefit.

Interventions that Reduce the Risk of Acute Anaemia & Haemorrhage: Risk of Transfusion

Intervention	Author	Sample size	RR (95% CI)	P value
Preoperative Autologous Donation	Henry	1506	0.32 (0.22; 0.47)	<0.01
Acute Normovolaemic Haemodilution	Davies	1423	0.36 (0.25; 0.51)	<0.01
Mechanical Cell salvage	Carless	6025	0.62 (0.55; 0.70)	<0.01
EPO and Iron (critical care)	Zarychanski	3144	0.85 (0.80; 0.91)	<0.01
EPO and Iron (cardiac surgery)	Alghamdi	227	0.36 (0.16; 0.81)	0.01
Tranexamic Acid versus Placebo	Henry	4842	0.61 (0.53; 0.70)	<0.01
Aprotinin versus Placebo	Henry	11172	0.66 (0.60; 0.72)	<0.01
Aprotinin versus Tranexamic Acid/ EACA	Henry	4185	0.90 (0.81; 1.00)	0.06
Desmopressin	Carless	1387	0.96 (0.87; 1.06)	0.42

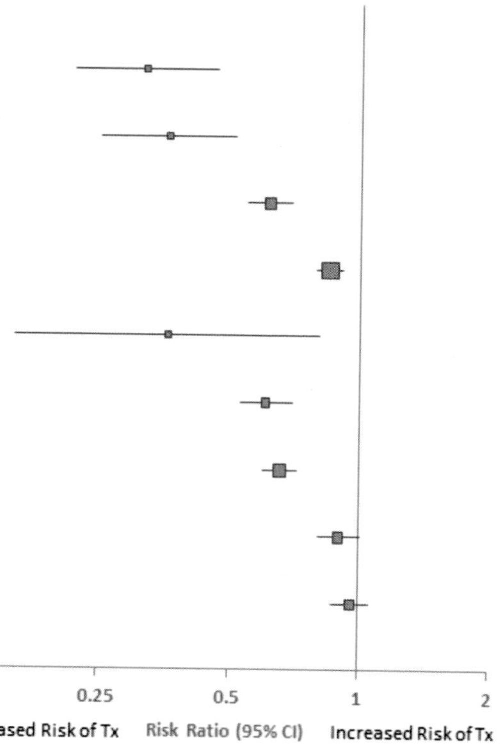

Fig 27.2 Forest plot summarizing the effects of commonly used therapeutic adjuncts aimed at reducing bleeding and transfusion on allogeneic red cell exposure. Data derived from recently published meta-analyses [5–11] as indicated. Box size represents relative precision of the estimate as derived from the sample size and variance.

287

Interventions that Reduce the Risk of Acute Anaemia & Haemorrhage: Clinical Outcomes

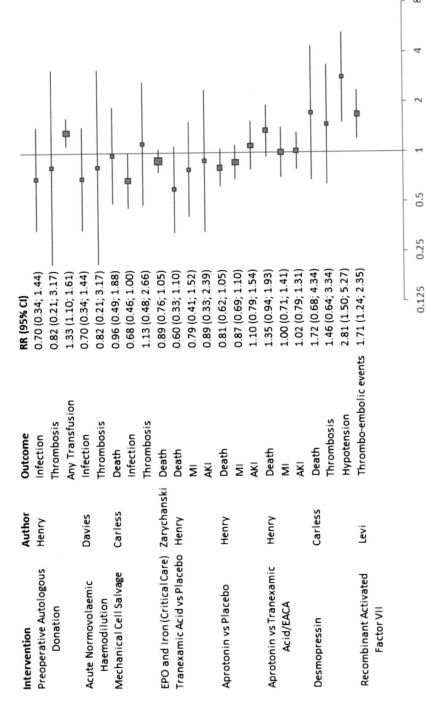

Intervention	Author	Outcome	RR (95% CI)
Preoperative Autologous Donation	Henry	Infection	0.70 (0.34; 1.44)
		Thrombosis	0.82 (0.21; 3.17)
		Any Transfusion	1.33 (1.10; 1.61)
Acute Normovolaemic Haemodilution	Davies	Infection	0.70 (0.34; 1.44)
		Thrombosis	0.82 (0.21; 3.17)
Mechanical Cell Salvage	Carless	Death	0.96 (0.49; 1.88)
		Infection	0.68 (0.46; 1.00)
		Thrombosis	1.13 (0.48; 2.66)
EPO and Iron (Critical Care)	Zarychanski	Death	0.89 (0.76; 1.05)
Tranexamic Acid vs Placebo	Henry	Death	0.60 (0.33; 1.10)
		MI	0.79 (0.41; 1.52)
		AKI	0.89 (0.33; 2.39)
Aprotonin vs Placebo	Henry	Death	0.81 (0.62; 1.05)
		MI	0.87 (0.69; 1.10)
		AKI	1.10 (0.79; 1.54)
Aprotonin vs Tranexamic Acid/EACA	Henry	Death	1.35 (0.94; 1.93)
		MI	1.00 (0.71; 1.41)
		AKI	1.02 (0.79; 1.31)
Desmopressin	Carless	Death	1.72 (0.68; 4.34)
		Thrombosis	1.46 (0.64; 3.34)
		Hypotension	2.81 (1.50; 5.27)
Recombinant Activated Factor VII	Levi	Thrombo-embolic events	1.71 (1.24; 2.35)

0.125   0.25   0.5   1   2   4   8

Intervention Beneficial   Risk Ratio (95% CI)   Intervention Harmful

Fig 27.3 Forest plot summarizing the effects of commonly used therapeutic adjuncts aimed at reducing bleeding and transfusion on important clinical outcomes. Data derived from recently published meta-analyses [5–12] as indicated. Box size represents relative precision of the estimate as derived from the sample size and variance.

PAD may be advantageous in less developed health-care systems where transmission of infection by transfusion remains an issue. However, PAD is restricted to patients scheduled for elective surgery, requires significant investment in infrastructure for the harvesting, testing and storage of autologous red cells in parallel to the systems in place for allogeneic blood and its adoption has not been widespread.

Acute normovolaemic haemodilution (ANH)
ANH involves removing blood from a patient, usually during induction of anaesthesia, replacing it with crystalloid or colloid fluid to maintain circulating volume and storing the blood for reinfusion during surgery as a response to blood loss, or at the end of surgery. Significant haemodilution reduces the red cell mass lost during surgery and replacement of losses with autologous blood has better homeostatic properties than colloid or crystalloid. ANH may also improve haemostasis by preventing consumption or loss of clotting factors during prolonged procedures or as a result of cardiopulmonary bypass and ANH has been shown to reduce bleeding rates. ANH also significantly reduces allogeneic red cell exposure and is inexpensive (Figure 27.2). ANH has not been shown to result in specific clinical benefits to patients beyond reducing transfusion exposure (Figure 27.3). The disadvantages of ANH relate principally to the safety of low haematocrits during surgery, which may increase the risk of neurological, myocardial and renal injury.

Mechanical cell salvage
Blood lost as a result of acute haemorrhage during major surgery can be collected (salvaged) using commercially available and widely used devices that wash the blood, removing plasma proteins, cell fragments and other contaminants of the surgical field and allowing reinfusion of washed autologous cells. A systematic review of 75 RCTs in orthopaedic (36 studies), cardiac (33 studies), and vascular (6 studies) surgery has demonstrated that this technique significantly reduces red cell exposure (Figure 27.2) and more importantly improves clinical outcomes including the risk of perioperative infection (Figure 27.3). The net cost benefit of cell salvage has been estimated to be between £112 and £359 per person [6]. The administration of unwashed blood or blood harvested from postoperative losses was not found to be harmful overall. However, published guidelines do not recommend the use of unwashed (risk of excessive bleeding) or postoperative shed mediastinal fluid (risk of infection) in the setting of cardiac surgery [13].

Pharmacological interventions

Recombinant human erythropoietin (RhEpo)
RhEpo is commonly administered along with iron supplementation to reverse chronic anaemia preoperatively in surgical patients, where it has been shown to reduce transfusion exposure without apparent adverse effects (Figures 27.2 and 27.3). A meta-analysis of RCTs evaluating the use of RhEpo and iron + RhEpo in critical care patients also shows a reduction in red cell exposure (odds ratio of transfusion 0.73, 95% confidence intervals (CI) 0.64–0.84) without apparent detriment (odds ratio of death 0.86, 95% CI 0.71–1.05) [8]. The studies included in this meta-analysis were generally of poor quality and underpowered to detect important clinical outcomes. A more recent high quality RCT has shown an increased risk of developing thromboembolic complications attributable to RhEpo administration [14], although overall survival was improved in a subset of trauma patients in this study. The increase in thromboembolic complications is attributable to increased viscosity as well as a direct effect of RhEpo on platelet aggregation and is most evident in patients with existing renal and cardiovascular disease.

Antifibrinolytics
The lysine analogues tranexamic acid and epsilon-amino caproic acid (EACA) act by irreversibly binding to the active site of plasminogen, thereby inhibiting clot lysis. Tranexamic acid reduces transfusion exposure in a wide range of acute settings including cardiac, orthopaedic and liver surgery [10]. More recently it has been shown to improve outcomes including survival if administered early in the management of acute blunt trauma [15]. There is little consensus as to the most effective dose of these agents. Few adverse effects have been reported, but systematic reviews indicate that tranexamic acid does not improve clinical outcomes in cardiovascular surgery, unlike other clinical settings, suggesting a possible safety signal in patients at greatest risk of thromboembolic complications. Such an effect appears to be more pronounced with the serine protease inhibitor aprotinin, which acts

289

as an antifibrinolytic as well as having a range of other anti-inflammatory and anti-apoptotic actions. Aprotinin has greater efficacy at reducing bleeding relative to tranexamic acid but data from RCTs suggests that this is also associated with an increased risk of adverse outcomes including mortality (Figure 27.3).

Desmopressin

Desmopressin is a synthetic analogue of arginine vasopressin that induces the release of the contents of endothelial cell-associated Weibel–Palade bodies, including the von Willebrand factor. Its use is indicated in the management of patients with mild haemophilia and von Willebrand disease undergoing minor surgical procedures. The increase in Factor VIII and von Willebrand factor concentrations, as well as evidence of increased platelet aggregation in response to desmopressin, has led to its evaluation as a haemostatic agent in major surgery. A recent Cochrane review failed to demonstrate any significant reduction in transfusion exposure or improvement in clinical outcomes (Figures 27.2 and 27.3). There were reductions in blood loss and the volume of red cells administered attributable to desmopressin use, but these were not deemed to be of clinical significance.

Recombinant activated Factor VII (rFVIIa)

This is a potent pharmacological prohaemostatic agent licensed for use in patients with haemophilia. This has led to the off-label use of rFVIIa for the treatment of severe coagulopathic bleeding in trauma and surgical settings as an adjunct to conventional non-RBC blood components. Its use is associated with a significant (68%) increased risk of major thrombotic complications, especially arterial thrombosis (Figure 27.3).

Coagulopathy

Coagulopathy is a poorly defined term; it may refer to severe impairment of blood coagulation in the setting of trauma or, alternatively, to the laboratory finding of abnormal screening tests of coagulation in a critical care patient. The lack of a clear definition of coagulopathy complicates epidemiological analyses and the development of accurate diagnostic tests and treatments. However, it remains a significant clinical problem and, depending on the definition, affects up to 30% of critically ill patients, 30% of trauma patients, 15% of cardiac surgery patients and 6% of those with acute upper GI haemorrhage. More detailed information on the underlying pathogenesis of acquired coagulopathy can be found in Chapter 25. Coagulopathic patients, whether or not they are actively bleeding, have a worse overall prognosis than similar patients without coagulopathy. This is attributable to the severity of the underlying illness and prior or ongoing significant haemorrhage and shock. It may also be attributable in part, however, to the adverse effects of prohaemostatic therapies; FFP and platelets are recognized causes of transfusion complications such as transfusion-related acute lung injury (TRALI), transfusion-associated circulatory overload (TACO), transfusion-associated dyspnoea (TAD) and transfusion-transmitted infection (TTI) [16] (see Chapters 6 to 16 for more details). Platelets have also been shown in some studies to increase the risk of stroke in patients with cardiovascular disease. These risks, although offset by the risks of ongoing bleeding in coagulopathic patients, may be clinically significant in those without coagulopathy, or when administered to those who are not actively bleeding.

Diagnosis

Effective treatment of coagulopathy, particularly in a bleeding patient, requires accurate and timely diagnosis. The nature of coagulopathy is heterogeneous and is influenced by the patient group, e.g. severe trauma, liver surgery or cardiac surgery, the type of intervention, e.g. cardiopulmonary bypass or transplant surgery, and also by the blood management strategy adopted, e.g. the use of antifibrinolytics and non-red-cell blood components. Specific defects in the coagulation pathway are commonly not detected by standard coagulation screening tests that by taking as long as 65 minutes are often considered impractical in the setting of ongoing blood loss. Near patient testing is increasingly advocated in this setting.

The most widely used near patient testing devices include the Thromboelastogram (TEG®) or ROTEM® (also see Chapter 25). These are whole blood viscoelastic tests that evaluate the effects of coagulation factors, platelets and red cells on overall

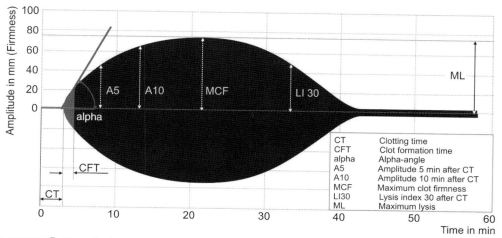

Fig 27.4 ROTEM® Thromboelstograph trace and interpretation. Reproduced with permission from TEM International GmbH.

clotting potential. Both work along similar principles, whereby progressive clot formation in the presence of an activator is measured as impedance to a rotating pin within the clot. The resultant trace can then be used to infer information as to the activity of separate components of the clotting pathway, including the coagulation cascade, platelet function and lysis (Figure 27.4). These platforms, although user friendly and widely used, have limited sensitivity and specificity, and a recent systematic review has highlighted the lack of evidence of clinical benefit associated with their use [17]. Near patient platelet function analysers and alternative laboratory assays such as thrombin generation testing have been shown to predict bleeding accurately and target therapy in small single-centre studies, but wider validation of these techniques is awaited.

Treatment

Without accurate diagnostic tests to identify specific defects in the coagulation pathway that are associated with adverse clinical outcomes, the management of coagulopathy is often empiric, nonspecific and based on the assumption that reversal of coagulopathy is beneficial. The clinical efficacy, safety and cost effectiveness of this approach is questionable, and this remains an important and underresourced area of research.

Platelet transfusion

Acute haemorrhage during surgery is a common indication for therapeutic platelet use. For example, cardiac surgery utilizes over 17% of all platelet transfusions in the UK [1]. Indications for and effective doses of platelets in the setting of acute haemorrhage are unclear and not supported by evidence. Observational studies report lower mortality rates in trauma patients receiving high dose platelet transfusion for major blood loss (Table 27.1), but there are no RCT data outside the haemato-oncology setting that can be used to guide practice (see Chapter 28 for further details).

Thrombocytopenia in critically ill patients is a risk factor for major bleeding and death, and the prevalence of mild ($<150 \times 10^9$/L) and moderate ($<50 \times 10^9$/L) thrombocytopenia in adult ITU patients is reported at 40% and 8% respectively [18]. There is little evidence from critical care studies that prophylactic correction of thrombocytopenia translates into a survival advantage, or indeed reproducibly raises platelet counts in critically ill patients. Thrombocytopenia increases the risk of haemorrhage during invasive procedures such as central line or spinal catheter insertion, and these are often performed using platelet transfusion 'cover'. Consensus recommendations [19, 20] for platelet administration during haemorrhage and in the critically ill are summarized in Table 27.2. These thresholds for platelet transfusions

Table 27.1 Efficacy of high dose platelet use in massive traumatic haemorrhage.

Patient group	Study type	Patient number	Comparator groups	Outcome
Trauma received MT	Retrospective cohort	466	High (≥1:2) versus low (<1:2) platelet: RBC ratio	↑ survival with high platelet ratio (60% versus 40%) at 30 days
Trauma received MT	Retrospective cohort	657	Low ratio (<1:18), medium ratio (≥1:18 and <1:12), high ratio (≥1:12 and <1:6) and highest ratio (≥1:6)	A high platelet: red cell ratio (adjusted $p < 0.001$) independently associated with ↑ survival at 24 hours
Trauma received MT	Retrospective cohort	214	High (≥1:20) versus low (<1:20) platelet: red cell ratio	↑ survival with high platelet ratio (63% versus 33%) at 30 days

MT, massive transfusion; all studies defined MT as ≥10 units red cells within 24 hours.

are empirical, have been derived largely from studies in haemato-oncology patients and do not account for alterations in platelet function or clinical status, which limits their utility.

FFP transfusion

Nearly half of all FFP administered in the UK is to critically ill patients; 12% cardiac, 9% liver disease and

Table 27.2 Platelet thresholds for prophylactic and therapeutic platelet transfusion. Adapted from References [19] and [20].

Clinical indication	Treatment value (10^9/L)
Therapeutic	
Massive transfusion	>50
Massive transfusion and multiple trauma or TBI	>100
DIC and bleeding	>50
Intracerebral bleeding	>100
Prophylactic	
Pre-invasive procedure, i.e. LP, CVC, epidural	>50
Pre-surgery	>50
Pre-surgery at high risk sites: i.e. brain/eye	>100

TBI, traumatic brain injury; DIC, disseminated intravascular coagulation; LP, lumbar puncture; CVC, central venous catheter.

liver transplant, 7% GI haemorrhage, 6% vascular surgery, 6% haematology, 3% trauma and 2% obstetrics [1]. A recent UK study reported 13% of critically ill adult patients received FFP during an ITU admission [21]. Half of these transfusions (48%) were for bleeding, while the remainder were for preprocedural prophylaxis (15%) or prophylaxis alone (36%). One-third were given to patients with normal PT values. Clinical efficacy of FFP has not been clearly demonstrated, however, either for treatment or prophylaxis. Indeed, it has been reported that standard FFP doses (12–15 mL/kg) are insufficient to significantly increase individual coagulation factor levels. A recent systematic review examining 80 RCTs highlighted that there are few well-supported indications for FFP administration [22] (see Table 27.3), but, despite this, numbers of FFP transfusions are increasing.

Fibrinogen replacement

Traditionally, fibrinogen is replaced during major blood loss or as part of the management for disseminated intravascular coagulation (DIC) once the Clauss fibrinogen value falls below 1 g/L. Fibrinogen is one of the earliest coagulation factors to fall in major bleeding and adequate, timely replacement of fibrinogen is hypothesized to result in improved haemorrhage control. New European trauma guidelines reflect this shift in practice and recommend 1.5 g/L as the transfusion trigger [20], although this recommendation is based on weak evidence. Cryoprecipitate is the first-line treatment in the UK for acquired hypofibrinogenaemia, and a standard adult dose (2 pools) raises

Table 27.3 Summary of FFP RCTs in critically ill patient groups. Adapted from Yang *et al.* [22].

Patient group	Total number of RCTs	Total number of patients	Therapeutic RCTs	Prophylactic RCTs	Findings
Cardiac surgery	19	948	4	15	No significant benefit from FFP
Liver disease	10	381	3	7	No significant benefit from FFP
Liver failure	1	118	1*	0	↑ survival with plasma exchange and haemofiltration
Thrombotic thrombocytopenic purpura	7	317	7	0	2 RCTs found ↑ response rates/survival
Severe closed head injury	1	44	0	1	↑mortality, ↑ AEs, ↑ delayed IC haematoma with FFP arm
Massive haemorrhage	1	41	1	0	No significant difference in clinical bleeding
Haemato-oncology	0				

*This trial evaluated plasma exchange in patients with liver failure.
RCT, randomized controlled trial; AE, adverse events; IC, intracranial.

the plasma fibrinogen level by 1 g/L. There are no clinical data to confirm effectiveness of cryoprecipitate in active bleeding and there is increasing interest in the use of fibrinogen concentrates. These are currently not licensed in the UK but have obvious advantages in light of their reduced infection risk and standardized fibrinogen concentration (Table 27.4). Case studies in trauma and RCTs in cardiac and urology surgery have reported positive outcomes following administration of fibrinogen concentrate (Table 27.5), but

Table 27.4 Comparison of FFP and PCC, cryoprecipitate and fibrinogen concentrate.

Coagulation factor replacement		Fibrinogen replacement	
FFP	PCC	Cryoprecipitate	FgC
Pooled product – nonstandardized	Pooled product – standardised	Pooled product – nonstandardized	Pooled product – standardized
All coagulation factors	Factors II, VII, IX, X, proteins C and S	FVIII, FXIII, vWF, FN, Fg	Fg
Frozen –30°C Requires thawing	Room temperature (<25°C)	Frozen –30°C Requires thawing	Room temperature (<25°C)
Large volume (often 800–1200 mL)	Small volume – 2000 IU in 80 mL	2 pools ∼ 350 mL	Small volume – 2 g in 100 mL
Standard FFP – no viral inactivation	Yes – pasteurization and a nanofiltration step for virus removal	No viral inactivation	Yes – pasteurization 60°C for 20 hr; Fg adsorption/precipitation removes virus
TRALI, TACO, TTI TAD	Thrombosis, DIC	TRALI, TTI	TTI, thrombosis
£400 for 1 litre	£700 for 2000 IU	£380 for 2 pools	£800 for 2 g

Fg, fibrinogen; FgC, fibrinogen concentrate; FVIII, factor VIII; FXIII, factor XIII; FN, fibrinonectin; IU, international units.

Table 27.5 Studies evaluating the safety and efficacy of fibrinogen concentrate in trauma and major surgery.

Patient group	Study type	Intervention	Comparator	Outcome
Cystectomy	RCT	FgC 45 mg/kg ($n = 10$)	Placebo ($n = 10$)	Significant increased MCF ↓ postoperative red cell use at 48 h
Cardiac surgery	RCT	FgC 2 g ($n = 10$)	No FgC ($n = 10$)	1 MI and 1 PE in intervention group No significant difference in transfusion need
Cardiac surgery	RCT	FgC median 8 g (dose directed by ROTEM) ($n = 29$)	Placebo ($n = 31$)	Significant reduction in transfusion No difference in AE
Cardiac surgery	Controlled comparative	FgC mean 5.7 g ($n = 10$)	FFP mean 4.2 U ($n = 5$)	Significant reduction in red cell, FFP and platelet need
Cardiac surgery	Prospective cohort, historical control	FgC mean 7.2 g ($n = 6$)	FFP mean 9.1 U ($n = 12$)	Significant reduction in red cell, FFP and platelet need
Trauma	Retrospective cohorts, 2 databases	FgC +/− PCC Median 4 g FgC, 1200 IU PCC ($n = 18$)	10 U FFP ($n = 18$)	No difference in mortality ↓ MOF
Trauma	Retrospective cohorts, 2 databases	FgC +/− PCC Median 6 g FgC, 1200 IU PCC ($n = 80$)	FFP median 6 U ($n = 601$)	Significant reduction of red cell and platelet use No difference in mortality
Mixed	Retrospective cohort	FgC median 4 g ($n = 69$)	–	FgC may be life saving No severe AE reported
Bleeding	Retrospective cohort	FgC 2 g ($n = 43$)	–	RBC, FFP and platelet requirements were reduced with FgC
Trauma	Retrospective Single centre	7 g FgC median 2400 IU PCC 10 U FFP ($n = 131$)	–	↓ mortality compared to TRISS
Cardiac surgery	Retrospective cohort	FgC mean 6.5 g ($n = 39$)	–	FgC increased Fg level and contributed to bleeding control
Surgery	Retrospective cohort	FgC median 2 g ($n = 37$)	–	FgC increased Fg level and reduced RBC use
Mixed	Retrospective cohort	FgC median 4 g ($n = 30$)	–	FgC is safe

RCT, randomized controlled trial; FgC, fibrinogen concentrate; MCF, maximal clot firmness; MI, myocardial infarction; PE, pulmonary embolism; AE, adverse events; FFP, fresh frozen plasma; PCC, prothrombin complex concentrate; MOF, multiorgan failure; TRISS, trauma score–injury severity score.

Table 27.6 Summary of observational trauma studies examining the effects of FFP : RBC ratios on outcomes.

Massive transfusion cohort size	% with blunt injury	Massive transfusion definition used	Coagulation status pre-intervention	Coagulation status post-intervention	Mortality reported to improve with increased FFP?	Specific ratio recommended by study
246	6	≥10 U/24 h	INR: 1.5–1.8*	NR	Y	1:1.4
135	42	≥10 U/24 h	NR	NR	Y	1:1
259	46	>10 U/24 h	NR	NR	Y	≥2:3
466	65	≥10 U/24 h	INR: 1.6	NR	Y	1:2
133	NR	>10 U/6 h	INR: 1.4	INR: 1.2–2* Maximum reduction at 1:1 and 1:2 ratios	Y	1:2–1:3
713	92	>10 U before ITU	APTT 53 s	NR	Y	1:1
250	85	≥10 U/24 h	NR	NR	N	N/A
415	100	≥8 U/12 h	INR: 1.8–1.9*	NR	Y	≥1:1.5
134	40	≥10 U/24 h	INR: 1.6 survivors, 1.9 nonsurvivors	NR	N‡	N/A
383	NR	≥10 U/24 h	NR	NR	Y	≥1:3
466	65	≥10 U/24 h	INR: 1.3–1.5*	NR	Y	≥1:1 at 6 h
214	54	≥10 U/24 h	NR	NR	Y	≥1:2
50†	88	≥10 U/24 h	PT 12	Maximum reduction of PT at 1:2–3:4 ratio	NR	N/A
103	63	≥10 U/24 h	INR: 1.6 survivors, 2.4 nonsurvivors	NR	N‡	N/A

*INR varied in patient groups allocated to intervention with different FFP : RBC ratios.
†This cohort received ≥4U/24 hour.
‡After adjustment for survival bias.
FFP, fresh frozen plasma; RBC, red blood cell; U, units; INR, international normalized ratio; NR, not reported; APTT, activated partial thromboplastin time; N/A, not applicable; PT, prothrombin time.

more evidence is needed as the studies are small and few are RCTs, and in no study has cryoprecipitate been directly compared to fibrinogen concentrate.

Prothrombin complex concentrates (PCCs)
PCCs are plasma-derived coagulation factor concentrates that contain 3 or 4 vitamin K dependent factors at high concentration. PCCs contain 4 coagulation factors – II, VII, IX and X – as well as variable amounts of anticoagulants and heparin.

PCCs are recommended for the treatment of serious or life-threatening bleeding related to oral anticoagulant therapy. Studies have shown that PCCs are safe and effective and normalize INR values rapidly when compared to FFP. Outcome data examining the effect of PCC on bleeding rates and mortality are not yet available. PCCs are currently licensed for treatment and perioperative prophylaxis of haemorrhage in patients with congenital and acquired deficiency of factors II, VII, IX or X, if purified specific coagulation factors

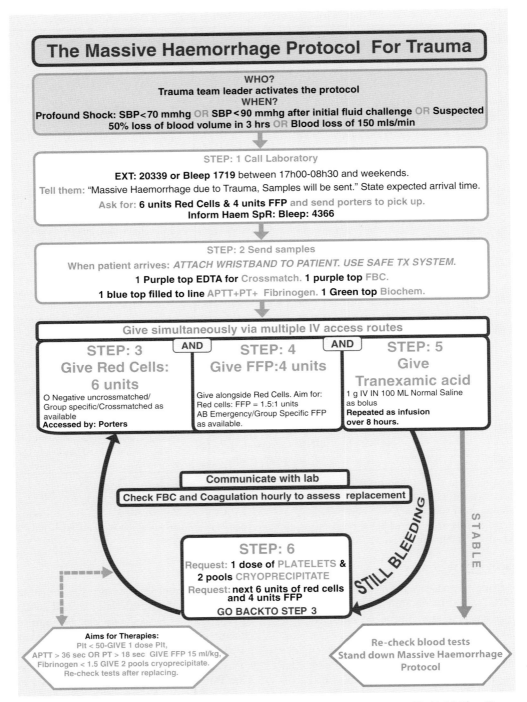

Fig 27.5 Example of a Massive Transfusion Protocol used in the setting of trauma. Courtesy of Dr R. Naidoo, Department of Haematology, John Radcliffe Hospital, Oxford.

are unavailable. PCCs are increasingly being considered as a substitute for FFP (Table 27.4 summarizes the differences between products) for use in coagulopathy associated with hepatic failure and traumatic haemorrhage. There is currently insufficient evidence to support these indications.

Massive blood transfusion (see also Chapter 26)

Strategies to manage massive blood transfusion have undergone major changes over the last few years, driven primarily by dismal outcomes observed in these patients using current treatment algorithms and evidence emerging from studies in battle casualties that higher volumes of FFP and platelets (approaching ratios of 1:1:1) lead to increased survival in massively transfused patients (Table 27.6). Some of these studies have demonstrated that early transfusion of FFP is key to favourable outcome rather than a high ratio per se. Importantly, there is no single FFP : RBC ratio that appears to be superior.

These results have led to development of empirical early delivery of FFP and platelets in major haemorrhage protocols, with guidance of transfusion by coagulation testing later in the process. Major haemorrhage is, of course, not limited to trauma patients, but there is very little evidence to inform practice in other clinical settings. There are, however, clear differences between patient groups; many gastrointestinal haemorrhage patients are elderly, have limited cardiovascular reserve and may be susceptible to fluid overload. Massive haemorrhage protocols for trauma should not be applied to other clinical areas without significant consideration of patient comorbidities.

Major haemorrhage protocols

Between October 2006 and September 2010 delays in the provision of blood in UK hospitals led to 11 deaths and 83 incidents of harm being reposted to the National Patient Safety Agency. In light of this, a Rapid Response Report concerning the transfusion of blood in an emergency was produced, which recommended the adoption of major haemorrhage protocols in every hospital [23]. Furthermore, the use of 'drills' to test local policies and ongoing education of all staff likely to be involved in massive haemorrhage

protocols are advised. An example of a hospital protocol for major haemorrhage in trauma is given in Figure 27.5. Following data from the CRASH-2 study [15], tranexamic acid should be given to all adult trauma patients at risk of bleeding, so long as administration can be given within 3 hours of injury.

Summary

The timely administration of blood components to patients with acute haemorrhage and in the critically ill is often life-saving; however, the clinical status of these patients also means that they are highly susceptible to organ dysfunction, and inappropriate transfusion with its associated risks may also have important adverse effects on clinical outcomes. Recent systematic reviews have identified important aspects of blood management that improve outcome as well as identifying gaps in knowledge that need to be addressed by future research. Restrictive transfusion practice is safe in critically ill patients without cardiovascular disease, and the safety of the approach in high risk groups is currently being evaluated in RCTs. Therapeutic adjuncts that reduce transfusion and improve outcomes are well defined and the wider application of these techniques will drive quality improvement. Coagulopathy associated with acute haemorrhage remains underresearched with no clear understanding of the underlying pathogenesis, accurate diagnostic tests or evidence-based treatments. The significant proportion of blood components utilized by these patients, their poor outcomes and significant utilization of healthcare resources are arguments for greater investment in this field.

Key points

1 Blood management focuses on improving patient outcomes in the setting of acute haemorrhage and acute anaemia in critically ill patients.
2 Restrictive use of allogeneic red cell transfusion is safe in patients without cardiovascular disease.
3 The use of techniques that enable autologous transfusion will reduce red cell transfusion and in the case of cell salvage will improve clinical outcomes and be cost effective.

4 Pharmacological blood conservation strategies effectively reduce transfusion exposure and in the setting of trauma improve survival.

5 Utilization of blood-conserving pharmacological strategies must consider the apparent increased risk of thromboembolic and other adverse clinical outcomes associated with greater efficacy in terms of reducing transfusion exposure, particularly in those at risk of cardiovascular complications.

6 Critically ill and acute surgical patients often develop coagulopathy. This is poorly defined and there are currently no validated sensitive and specific diagnostic tests that have been validated clinically or shown to improve clinical outcome.

7 The current evidence to support the prophylactic use of FFP and platelets in the critically ill is poor.

8 Massive transfusion protocols that place emphasis on communication, pre-emptive treatment and the use of higher platelet/FFP : RBC ratios appear to improve outcomes.

References

1 Wells AW, Llewelyn CA, Casbard A, Johnson AJ, Amin M, Ballard S, Buck J, Malfroy M, Murphy MF & Williamson LM. The EASTR Study: indications for transfusion and estimates of transfusion recipient numbers in hospitals supplied by the National Blood Service. *Transfus Med* 2009; 19: 315–327.

2 Corwin HL, Gettinger A, Pearl RG, Fink MP, Levy MM, Abraham E, MacIntyre NR, Shabot MM, Duh MS & Shapiro MJ. The CRIT Study: anemia and blood transfusion in the critically ill – current clinical practice in the United States. *Crit Care Med* 2004; 32: 39–52.

3 Bennett-Guerrero E, Zhao Y, O'Brien SM, Ferguson Jr TB, Peterson ED, Gammie JS & Song HK. Variation in use of blood transfusion in coronary artery bypass graft surgery. *J Am Med Assoc* 2010; 304: 1568–1575.

4 Carless PA, Henry DA, Carson JL, Hebert PP, McClelland B & Ker K. Transfusion thresholds and other strategies for guiding allogeneic red blood cell transfusion. *Cochrane Database Syst Rev* 2010; (10): CD002042.

5 Henry DA, Carless PA, Moxey AJ, O'Connell D, Forgie MA, Wells PS & Fergusson D. Pre-operative autologous donation for minimising perioperative allogeneic blood transfusion. *Cochrane Database Syst Rev* 2002; (2): CD003602.

6 Davies L, Brown TJ, Haynes S, Payne K, Elliott RA & McCollum C. Cost-effectiveness of cell salvage and alternative methods of minimising perioperative allogeneic blood transfusion: a systematic review and economic model. *Health Technol Assess* 2006; 10: iii–iv, ix–x, 1–210.

7 Carless PA, Henry DA, Moxey AJ, O'Connell D, Brown T & Fergusson DA. Cell salvage for minimising perioperative allogeneic blood transfusion. *Cochrane Database Syst Rev* 2010; (4): CD001888.

8 Zarychanski R, Turgeon AF, McIntyre L & Fergusson DA. Erythropoietin-receptor agonists in critically ill patients: a meta-analysis of randomized controlled trials. *CMAJ* 2007; 177: 725–734.

9 Alghamdi AA, Albanna MJ, Guru V & Brister SJ. Does the use of erythropoietin reduce the risk of exposure to allogeneic blood transfusion in cardiac surgery? A systematic review and meta-analysis. *J Card Surg* 2006; 21: 320–326.

10 Henry DA, Carless PA, Moxey AJ, O'Connell D, Stokes BJ, Fergusson DA & Ker K. Anti-fibrinolytic use for minimising perioperative allogeneic blood transfusion. *Cochrane Database Syst Rev* 2011; (3): CD001886.

11 Carless PA, Henry DA, Moxey AJ, O'Connell D, McClelland B, Henderson KM, Sly K, Laupacis A & Fergusson D. Desmopressin for minimising perioperative allogeneic blood transfusion. *Cochrane Database Syst Rev* 2004; (1): CD001884.

12 Levi M, Levy JH, Andersen HF & Truloff D. Safety of recombinant activated factor VII in randomized clinical trials. *N Engl J Med* 2010; 363: 1791–1800.

13 Ferraris VA, Brown JR, Despotis GJ, Hammon JW, Reece TB, Saha SP, Song HK, Clough ER, Shore-Lesserson LJ, Goodnough LT, Mazer CD, Shander A, Stafford-Smith M, Waters J, Baker RA, Dickinson TA, Fitzgerald DJ, Likosky DS & Shann KG. 2011 update to the society of thoracic surgeons and the society of cardiovascular anesthesiologists blood conservation clinical practice guidelines. *Ann Thorac Surg* 2011; 91: 944–982.

14 Corwin HL, Gettinger A, Fabian TC, May A, Pearl RG, Heard S, An R, Bowers PJ, Burton P, Klausner MA & Corwin MJ; EPO Critical Care Trials Group. Efficacy and safety of epoetin alfa in critically ill patients. *N Engl J Med* 2007; 357: 965–976.

15 CRASH-2 Trial collaborators, Shakur H, Roberts I, Bautista R *et al.* Effects of tranexamic acid on death, vascular occlusive events, and blood transfusion in trauma patients with significant haemorrhage (CRASH-2): a randomised, placebo-controlled trial. *Lancet* 2010; 376(9734): 23–32.

16 SHOT (Serious Hazards of Transfusion), Annual Report; 2010. Available at: http://www.shotuk.org/wp-content/uploads/2011/07/SHOT-2010-Report.pdf.

17 Afshari A, Wikkelsø A, Brok J, Møller AM & Wetterslev J. Thrombelastography (TEG) or thromboelastometry (ROTEM) to monitor haemotherapy versus usual care

in patients with massive transfusion. *Cochrane Database Syst Rev* 2011; (3): CD007871.

18 Arnold DM, Crowther MA, Cook RJ, Sigouin C, Heddle NM, Molnar L & Cook DJ. Utilization of platelet transfusions in the intensive care unit: indications, transfusion triggers, and platelet count responses. *Transfusion* 2006; 46: 1286–1291.

19 Stainsby D, MacLennan S, Thomas D, Isaac J & Hamilton PJ. British Committee for Standards in Haematology Guidelines on the management of massive blood loss. *Br J Haem* 2006; 135: 634–641.

20 Rossaint R, Bouillon B, Cerny V, Coats TJ, Duranteau J & Fernández-Mondéjar E. Task Force for Advanced Bleeding Care in Trauma. Management of bleeding for major trauma: an updated European guideline. *Crit Care* 2010; 14: R52.

21 Stanworth SJ, Walsh TS, Prescott RJ, Lee RJ, Watson DM & Wyncoll D; Intensive Care Study of Coagulopathy (ISOC) investigators. A national study of plasma use in critical care: clinical indications, dose and effect on prothrombin time. *Crit Care* 2011; 15: R108.

22 Yang L, Stanworth S, Hopewell S, Doree C & Murphy M. Is fresh frozen plasma clinically effective? An updated systematic review of randomised controlled trials. *Transfusion* 2012, 18 January. DOI: 10.1111/j.1537-2995.2011.03515.x. Epub ahead of print.

23 National Patient Safety Agency. The transfusion of blood and blood products in an emergency. Rapid Response Report, NPSA/2010/RRR017; 2010. Available at: http://www.nrls.npsa.nhs.uk/alerts/?entryid45=83659.

Further reading

Blajchman MA, Glynn SA, Josephson CD & Kleinman SH; State-of-the-Science Symposium Transfusion Medicine Committee. Clinical trial opportunities in Transfusion Medicine: Proceedings of a National Heart, Lung, and Blood Institute State-of-the-Science Symposium. *Transfus Med Rev* 2010; 24: 259–285.

http://www.nba.gov.au/guidelines/review.html. Website of the state-wide blood management programme currently being implemented by the Department of Health of the Government of Western Australia.

Napolitano LM, Kurek S, Luchette FA, Corwin HL, Barie PS, Tisherman SA *et al.* American College of Critical Care Medicine of the Society of Critical Care Medicine; Eastern Association for the Surgery of Trauma Practice Management Workgroup. Clinical practice guideline: red blood cell transfusion in adult trauma and critical care. *Crit Care Med* 2009; 37: 3124–3157.

28 Haematological disease

Lise J. Estcourt[1], Simon J. Stanworth[1] & Michael F. Murphy[2]

[1]NHS Blood and Transplant, John Radcliffe Hospital, Oxford, UK
[2]University of Oxford and NHS Blood and Transplant and Department of Haematology, John Radcliffe Hospital, Oxford, UK

Background

Patients with haematological diseases are major users of blood components. Haematological diseases requiring transfusion support cover a whole spectrum of clinical disorders: fetal, neonatal and paediatric practice (Chapter 32), haemoglobinopathies (Chapter 29), haemophilia (Chapter 25), immune disorders (Chapter 31) and bone marrow failure syndromes, in addition to haematological malignancies.

The haemopoietic system has a dramatic capacity for increasing the production of blood cells, but this capability varies between different diseases. The scenario of anaemia related to marrow ablation following chemotherapy is very different to anaemia in an individual with a well-compensated chronic haemolytic process. Although over 15% of all red cell units are transfused to patients with haematological disease, most are to patients with malignant disorders [1]. The requirement for blood transfusions in this group is related to both the underlying condition itself and the myelosuppressive/myeloablative effects of the specific treatments used.

This chapter considers the following topics:
• the *indications* for red cell, platelet and granulocyte transfusions in haematology patients and
• the approaches to the management and prevention of *complications* associated with transfusions in haematology patients, including the use of special types of blood components.

Red cell transfusions

The ready availability of red cell components means that anaemia can be easily treated. There are some special considerations in the management of anaemia that are applicable to haematology patients, as well as other clinical groups.
• The cause should be established and treatment other than blood transfusion should be used where appropriate, e.g. in patients with iron deficiency or megaloblastic or autoimmune haemolytic anaemia (AIHA). Anaemia of malignancy may be due to the effects of marrow infiltration or therapy, 'inhibitory' cytokine-mediated influences leading to the secondary anaemias (of chronic disorders) or low levels of erythropoietin.
• There is no universal 'trigger' for red cell transfusions, i.e. a given level of haemoglobin concentration (Hb) at which red cell transfusion is appropriate for all patients. Clinical judgement balancing factors such as quality-of-life indices play an important role in the decision to transfuse red cells or not [2].

Patients receiving intensive myelosuppressive/myeloablative treatment

There are specific considerations relating to the use of red cell transfusions in patients receiving intensive myelosuppressive/myeloablative treatment, including the need to provide a 'reserve' in case of severe infection or haemorrhage, and the convenience of having

Practical Transfusion Medicine, Fourth Edition. Edited by Michael F. Murphy, Derwood H. Pamphilon and Nancy M. Heddle.
© 2013 John Wiley & Sons, Ltd. Published 2013 by John Wiley & Sons, Ltd.

a standard policy for red cell transfusion in the setting of an acute haematology service, even if this may result in some patients being overtransfused.

The level of Hb used as the 'trigger' for transfusion varies from centre to centre but is usually in the range 8–10 g/dL. A restrictive policy is generally advocated because of the data from trials in other patient groups indicating the safety of this approach and the well-recognized risks of transfusion. There are no definite data to support the use of a higher level, although studies in animal models of thrombocytopenia and in uraemic patients suggest that correction of anaemia also results in correction of prolonged bleeding times [3].

Red cell transfusions and chronic anaemias

In patients with chronic anaemia requiring regular transfusions, red cell transfusions should be used to maintain the Hb just above the lowest level not associated with symptoms of anaemia [2]. There is considerable variation in this level depending on the patient's age, level of activity and coexisting medical problems, such as cardiovascular and respiratory disease; for example, some young patients are asymptomatic with an Hb below 7 g/dL, while some elderly patients are symptomatic even at an Hb above 10 g/dL. Special considerations apply to patients with haemoglobinopathies, and these are considered in Chapter 29.

The use of recombinant erythropoietin (RhEpo) in haematological disease

The clinical use of recombinant RhEpo might be considered in several situations in haematology patients, e.g. delayed erythroid engraftment after allogeneic bone marrow/peripheral blood progenitor cell transplantation, the treatment of anaemia in patients with myeloma or myelodysplasia, and in the management of Jehovah's Witnesses with haematological disorders. Evidence supports an association between increases in Hb, reduced red cell transfusion requirements and possibly improvement in quality-of-life indices with RhEpo therapy, although the findings concerning quality-of-life measures are more difficult to compare between studies. Uncertainties also remain about the factors predicting responsiveness, since a number of individuals fail to show adequate responses to

RhEpo. However, as discussed in Chapter 46, recent systematic reviews have raised concerns about adverse events (increased morbidity and mortality) in patients treated with RhEpo [4, 5]. The most recent American guidelines [4] now only recommend using RhEpo in patients with haematological malignancies who are being treated with palliative intent.

Red cell transfusions and immune blood disorders

In immune haemolytic anaemia, antibodies bind to red blood cell surface antigens and initiate destruction via the complement system and/or the macrophage system. Immune haemolytic anaemia may be alloimmune, autoimmune or drug induced (Table 28.1).

AIHAs are uncommon (incidence 1 to 3 per 100 000 per year). They are characterized by the production of antibodies directed against high frequency red cell antigens and often exhibit reactivity against donor red cells. The degree of haemolysis depends on a number of factors, including the characteristics of the bound antibody (e.g. class, quantity, specificity, thermal amplitude), the target antigen (e.g. density, expression) and other host-related genetic factors (e.g. markers of macrophage activity). The antibody class in turn will affect the degree of classical complement activation (IgM) or binding to splenic and other tissue macrophages via Fc receptors (IgG1 and IgG3 antibodies). The direct antiglobulin test (DAT) is usually positive but can be negative. The threshold of cell bound antibody detection, using the antiglobulin test, is 200 to 500 antibody molecules per cell, but fewer than 100 molecules of IgG per cell may significantly reduce RBC survival *in vivo*. In warm antibody AIHA, IgG antibodies predominate and the DAT is positive with IgG alone (20%), IgG and complement (detected as C3d) (67%) or C3d only (13%). In cold antibody AIHA, the antibodies (usually IgM) easily elute off red cells, leaving complement on the red cell surface (DAT is positive with C3d alone).

Warm antibody AIHA (Table 28.1)

Therapy of warm antibody AIHA depends on the severity of the haemolysis. Treatment is usually required once symptomatic anaemia develops. Steroids are the first-line treatment (e.g. prednisolone in doses of 1 mg/kg daily) and are effective in inducing a remission in about 80% of patients. Steroids reduce both production of the red cell autoantibody

Table 28.1 Causes of immune haemolytic anaemia.

Alloimmune
Haemolytic disease of the newborn (Chapter 32)
Haemolytic transfusion reactions
After allogeneic stem cell, renal, liver or cardiac
   transplantation when donor lymphocytes transferred in
   the allograft ('passenger lymphocytes') may produce red
   cell antibodies against the recipient and cause haemolytic
   anaemia (Chapter 7)

Autoimmune
Warm-autoantibody (antibody maximally active at 37°C;
   usually IgG with anti-Rh specificity)
   Idiopathic (> 30% of cases)
   Secondary to lymphoproliferative disease (e.g. chronic
      lymphocytic leukaemia, lymphoma)
   Secondary to autoimmune disease (e.g. SLE)
Cold-autoantibody (antibody maximally active at less than
   37°C; usually IgM)
   Idiopathic
   Chronic cold haemagglutinin disease (monoclonal usually
      with anti-I specificity)
   Secondary to infections (polyclonal)
      Mycoplasma (anti-I specificity)
      Infectious mononucleosis (anti-i specificity)
   Secondary to lymphoproliferative disease
   Secondary to autoimmune disease
Paroxysmal cold haemoglobinuria (usually polyclonal IgG
   with anti-P specificity)
   Secondary to viral infections, e.g. measles, mumps,
      chickenpox
   Congenital or tertiary syphilis

Drug-induced
Hapten mechanism, e.g. high dose penicillins (greater
   than 10 million units/day), cephalosporins
Autoantibody mechanism. e.g. α-methyldopa
Immune-complex mechanism, e.g. quinine

and destruction of antibody-coated cells. Splenectomy may be necessary if there is no response to steroids or if remission is not maintained when the dose of prednisolone is reduced. Other immunosuppressive drugs, such as azathioprine and cyclophosphamide, may be effective in patients who fail to respond to steroids and splenectomy. Ciclosporin and rituximab may also be effective in patients who are refractory to all treatment.

Blood transfusion may be required if there is fulminant haemolytic anaemia or severe anaemia not responding to steroids or other therapy. The presence of red cell autoantibodies on the patient's red cells and in the plasma can cause problems in the identification of compatible blood. It is important to exclude the presence of red cell alloantibodies and autoabsorption of autoantibodies in the plasma using enzyme treatment of the patient's red cells may be necessary to permit the investigation of the plasma for alloantibodies (Chapter 23).

Cold antibody AIHA (Table 28.1)

In cold autoantibody AIHA the IgM antibodies attach to red cells and cause their agglutination in the cold peripheries/extremities of the body; activation of complement can cause intravascular haemolysis when the cells return to the higher temperatures in the core of the body. This can occur after certain infections (Table 28.1), producing a mild-to-moderate transient haemolysis, or can be associated with chronic disease.

Chronic cold haemagglutinin disease usually occurs in the elderly, with a gradual onset of haemolytic anaemia. After exposure to cold the patient develops an acrocyanosis similar to Raynaud's disease as a result of red cell autoagglutination. If possible, the underlying cause of the antibody production should be treated (associated with clonal B-cell lymphocyte proliferation) and patients should avoid exposure to cold. Treatment with steroids, alkylating agents and splenectomy is usually ineffective. Rituximab is increasingly used as a well-tolerated and effective treatment, producing remission in about 50% of patients. Regular blood transfusion is occasionally required to prevent symptoms of anaemia. The laboratory can usually find compatible blood by using prewarmed techniques when performing compatibility testing.

Paroxysmal cold haemoglobinuria (Table 28.1)

Paroxysmal cold haemoglobinuria is a rare condition that is typically seen in children following a viral illness. It is associated with complement-fixing IgG antibodies that are biphasic (typically anti-P specificity), adhering to the red cell membrane in the cold peripheries, with lysis occurring due to complement activation when the cells return to the central circulation. The lytic reaction is demonstrated *in vitro* by incubating the patient's red cells and serum at 0°C and then warming the mixture to 37°C (direct Donath–Landsteiner test). This test can be falsely negative due

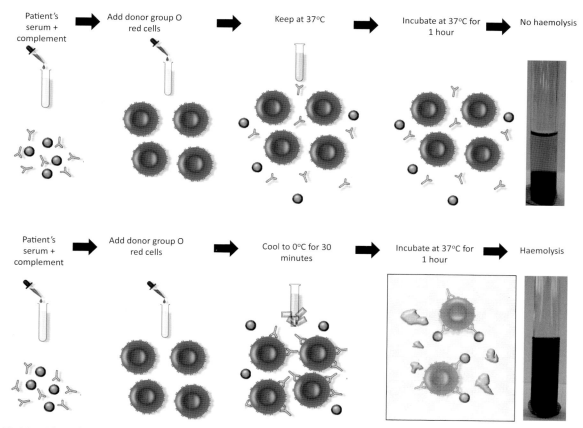

Fig 28.1 The indirect Donath–Landsteiner test for paroxysmal cold haemoglobinuria.

to a lack of complement; hence, a more accurate test is the indirect Donath–Landsteiner test (Figure 28.1). Haemolysis is self-limiting, but supportive transfusions may be necessary. P-negative blood should be considered if there is no sustained response to transfusion of P-positive crossmatch compatible blood.

The issue of whether it is necessary to use an in-line blood warmer when transfusing patients with cold antibody AIHA is controversial. It is logical to keep the patient warm and a common practice to use a blood warmer if the patient has florid haemolytic anaemia.

Drug-induced AIHA (Table 28.1)

There are three basic mechanisms of drug-induced immune RBC injury. In the hapten mechanism, the drug binds strongly to RBC proteins. IgG antibodies are directed against drug epitopes and only react with drug-coated RBCs. Antibody production usually occurs 7 to 10 days after starting the drug and the patient typically is receiving high doses of the drug. Many patients will have a positive DAT but do not have haemolysis. When haemolysis occurs it usually results in a gradual drop in haemoglobin. In the autoantibody mechanism the drug induces formation of IgG autoantibodies via unknown mechanisms. α-Methyldopa can cause a positive DAT 6 to 12 weeks after starting the drug; however, most patients do not have clinical and laboratory signs of haemolysis. In the immune-complex mechanism the drug forms immune complexes with antibody (usually IgM), which then attach to RBC membrane, causing complement mediated lysis. Classically it occurs on second or subsequent exposure to the drug and the patient may present with severe intravascular haemolysis occurring within minutes to hours of drug ingestion.

Platelet transfusions

In general, platelet transfusions are indicated for the prevention and treatment of haemorrhage in patients with thrombocytopenia or platelet function defects. The cause of the thrombocytopenia should be established before platelet transfusions are used because they are not always appropriate treatment for thrombocytopenic patients, and in some instances are contraindicated, e.g. in thrombotic thrombocytopenic purpura, haemolytic–uraemic syndrome and heparin-induced thrombocytopenia (Chapter 30).

Bone marrow failure

Therapeutic platelet transfusions are established as an effective treatment for patients who are bleeding. However, *prophylactic* platelet transfusion therapy for the prevention of haemorrhage in chronically thrombocytopenic patients with bone marrow failure remains more controversial. Guidelines for platelet transfusion in many countries recommend that the platelet transfusion trigger for prophylaxis is 10×10^9/L [6], and most local departmental policies would follow this recommendation, with an acceptance that selected patients with additional risk factors, such as sepsis or invasive infections, might benefit from higher thresholds.

Unfortunately, many audits continue to document that compliance with these general recommendations is poor, and a recent national comparative audit in the UK [7] showed that a large proportion (28%) of platelet transfusions were given inappropriately. One critical question is whether the evidence from published trials, when combined, demonstrates equivalence in terms of the safety of a platelet count threshold of 10×10^9/L rather than 20×10^9/L. A recent systematic review [8] has suggested that there is insufficient evidence to answer this question. However, many of the bleeding events in these studies were relatively minor and platelet transfusions are associated with well-described risks. Hence, there is no evidence to change from the current practice of a platelet transfusion threshold of 10×10^9/L unless there are other risk factors for haemorrhage.

Much of the recent research interest has focused on the optimal dose of platelets. A large randomized controlled trial [9] showed there was no significant difference in the number of patients who bled between the low dose (1.1×10^{11} platelets/m²), medium dose (2.2×10^{11} platelets/m²) and high dose (4.4×10^{11}/m²) treatment arms. Overall, a low dose transfusion policy reduced patients' total platelet requirements, but at the expense of a higher number of platelet transfusions. In the UK the standard adult dose is approximately 2.4×10^{11} platelets, which is close to the low dose used in the recently published large platelet dose trial [9].

A question remains as to whether a prophylactic platelet transfusion strategy is appropriate and safe in all subgroups of patients with haematological malignancies, but this awaits the publication of randomized controlled trials in progress [10, 11]. A strategy of transfusing platelets only for therapeutic indications in the context of clinical bleeding may be appropriate for some patients with *chronic* persisting thrombocytopenia due to bone marrow failure syndromes, e.g. myelodyplasia.

Prophylactic platelet transfusions for invasive procedures depends on the type of procedure.
- No increase in platelet count required: bone marrow aspiration and biopsy.
- Platelet count should be raised to 50×10^9/L: lumbar puncture, insertion of intravascular lines, transbronchial and liver biopsy, and laparotomy.
- Platelet count should be raised to more than 100×10^9/L: surgery in critical sites such as the brain or the eyes.

Immune thrombocytopenias

- Autoimmune thrombocytopenias: platelet transfusions should be used only in patients with major haemorrhage [3, 12].
- Posttransfusion purpura: platelet transfusions are usually ineffective in raising the platelet count, but may be needed in large doses to control severe bleeding in the acute phase (Chapter 12).
- Neonatal alloimmune thrombocytopenia: human platelet antigen (HPA)-matched platelet concentrates are the most appropriate treatment for this condition (Chapter 32).

Massive blood transfusion

- Clinically significant dilutional thrombocytopenia only occurs with the transfusion of more than 1.5 times the blood volume of the recipient.

• The platelet count should be maintained above 50×10^9/L in patients receiving transfusions for massive acute blood loss (Chapter 26).

Disseminated intravascular coagulation

• In acute disseminated intravascular coagulation (DIC), where there is bleeding associated with severe thrombocytopenia, platelet transfusions should be given in addition to coagulation factor replacement (Chapter 25).
• In chronic DIC, or in the absence of bleeding, platelet transfusions are not indicated.

Cardiopulmonary bypass surgery

• Platelet function defects and some degree of thrombocytopenia frequently occur after cardiac bypass surgery, but prophylactic platelet transfusions are not indicated (Chapter 27).
• Platelet transfusions should be reserved for patients with bleeding not due to surgically correctable causes.

Granulocyte transfusions

Severe persisting neutropenia is the principal limiting factor in the use of intensive treatment of patients with haematological malignancies. It may last for 2 weeks or more after chemotherapy or stem-cell transplantation, and during this period the patient is at risk of life-threatening bacterial and fungal infections. The use of haemopoietic growth factors, such as granulocyte colony-stimulating factor (G-CSF), may reduce the duration and severity of severe neutropenia, but they are only effective if the patient has sufficient numbers of haemopoietic precursors. Moreover, the time to response may be several days. Supportive treatment with granulocyte transfusions is a logical approach, although a number of factors have limited its application:
• difficulties in the collection of neutrophils, which are present in low numbers in normal individuals and which are difficult to separate from red cells because of their similar densities (commercially available long-chain starch solutions now facilitate this separation);

• the short half-life of neutrophils after transfusion, coupled with short storage times and negative effects on function of prolonged storage;
• The frequent occurrence of adverse effects such as febrile reactions, including occasional severe pulmonary reactions and human leucocyte antigen (HLA) alloimmunization causing platelet refractoriness.

Various methods have been used in the past to increase the number of neutrophils collected, including obtaining granulocytes from patients with chronic myeloid leukaemia, treating donors with steroids and using hydroxyethyl starch to promote sedimentation of red cells. However, a number of clinical trials of granulocyte transfusions in the 1970s and 1980s suggested they had limited efficacy in adults, and interest in their usage declined. Some centres continued to use granulocyte transfusions for small children and neonates because concentrates collected from adult donors produced a relatively much greater dose per recipient weight, and sometimes appeared to be clinically effective.

There has recently been a resurgence of interest in granulocyte transfusions because of the accumulating evidence that G-CSFs can be safely administered to normal individuals [13]. Much larger doses of granulocytes can be collected from donors using regimens including G-CSF administered 12–16 hours prior to apheresis, together with oral steroids such as dexamethasone to further improve the yields. Further evidence of the safety of this approach for donors and the efficacy of granulocyte transfusions collected in this way are required before granulocyte transfusion therapy becomes accepted in the care of patients with severe neutropenia and fungal infection, in conjunction with other potential approaches such as improved diagnostic strategies and organism-targeted antimicrobials. Evidence of survival benefit following granulocyte transfusions are clearly needed and a trial to evaluate this is currently ongoing (resolving infections in neutropenia with granulocytes, or RING). High dose granulocyte transfusions collected using donors treated with G-CSFs might therefore be considered as indicated in patients of any age with severe neutropenia due to bone marrow failure under the following circumstances:
• proven bacterial or fungal infection unresponsive to antimicrobial therapy or probable bacterial or fungal infection unresponsive to appropriate blind antimicrobial therapy;

305

- neutrophil recovery not expected for 5–7 days;
- children and lighter adults might be expected to show better incremental responses to granulocyte transfusions.

Granulocyte transfusions might be considered inappropriate for:

- patients with haematological disease resistant to treatment;
- ventilated patients; and
- patients with known HLA alloimmunization.

Approach to complications associated with blood transfusion in haematology patients

Transfusion-transmitted CMV infection

Clinical features and risk factors

CMV infection may cause significant morbidity and mortality in immunocompromised patients, mainly due to pneumonia. Patients who have never been exposed to CMV are at risk for primary infection transmitted by blood components prepared from blood donors who have previously had CMV infection and still carry the virus.

Patients who have been previously exposed to CMV and are CMV seropositive are at risk of reactivation of CMV during a period of immunosuppression. The extent to which CMV-seropositive patients are at risk from reinfection with different strains of CMV remains unknown, but this risk is generally considered to be low. The patients at risk of transfusion-transmitted CMV infection are shown in Table 28.2 [14], and the generally accepted indications for the use of CMV-seronegative or 'CMV-safe' blood components are shown in Table 28.3.

Prevention

The use of CMV-seronegative blood components has been shown to reduce the incidence of CMV infection in groups at risk for transfusion-transmitted CMV infection to 1–3%. This incomplete prevention may be due to:

- occasional failure to detect low level CMV antibodies;
- loss of antibodies in previously infected blood donors; and
- transfusion of blood components prepared from recently infected donors.

Table 28.2 Patients at risk for transfusion-transmitted cytomegalovirus (CMV) infection. Reproduced from Clark & Miller [6].

Risk well established

CMV-seronegative recipients of allogeneic bone marrow/ peripheral blood progenitor cell transplants from CMV-seronegative donors

CMV-seronegative pregnant women

Premature infants (<1.2 kg) born to CMV-seronegative women

CMV-seronegative patients with HIV infection

Risk less well established

CMV-seronegative patients receiving autologous bone marrow/peripheral blood progenitor cell transplants

CMV-seronegative patients who are potential recipients of allogeneic or autologous bone marrow/peripheral blood progenitor cell transplants

CMV-seronegative patients receiving solid organ (kidney, heart, lung, liver) transplants from CMV-seronegative donors

Risk not established

CMV-seronegative recipients of allogeneic bone marrow/ peripheral blood progenitor cell transplants from CMV-seropositive donors

CMV-seropositive recipients of bone marrow/peripheral blood progenitor cell transplants

CMV-seropositive recipients of solid organ transplants

Table 28.3 Indications for the use of cytomegalovirus (CMV)-seronegative or CMV-safe blood components.

Transfusions in pregnancy

Intrauterine transfusions

Transfusions to neonates and to infants in the first year of life

Transfusions to the following groups of CMV-seronegative patients:

After allogeneic bone marrow/peripheral blood progenitor cell transplants where the donor is also CMV-seronegative

After autologous bone marrow/peripheral blood progenitor cell transplants

Potential recipients of allogeneic bone marrow/peripheral blood progenitor cell transplants

Patients with HIV infection

CMV is transmitted by leucocytes, and a number of studies have found that pre-storage leucocyte reduction of blood components is as effective as the use of CMV-seronegative blood components in the prevention of transfusion-transmitted CMV infection in neonates, patients undergoing remission induction therapy for acute leukaemia and after bone marrow transplantation (the only prospective randomized trial was conducted in transplant recipients using bedside leucocyte-reduction filters, which cannot be adequately quality controlled for leucocyte reduction). These data suggest that pre-storage leucocyte-reduced blood components can be accepted as a substitute for CMV-seronegative blood components for patients at risk of transfusion-transmitted CMV infection when CMV-seronegative blood components are not available, i.e. that leucocyte-reduced blood components are 'CMV-safe'. A consensus conference in Canada recommended that where universal leucocyte reduction had been implemented, both leucocyte-reduced and CMV-seronegative blood should be used for CMV-seronegative pregnant women, intrauterine transfusions and CMV-seronegative allogeneic haemopoietic cell transplant recipients [15]. Further information about the effectiveness of leucocyte reduction of blood components in the prevention of transfusion-transmitted infections is unlikely to become available, and some haematology centres have decided to abandon the use of CMV-seronegative blood components where pre-storage leucocyte-reduced blood components are used routinely [16].

Transfusion-associated graft-versus-host disease

Pathogenesis and clinical features

Transfusion-associated graft-versus-host disease (TA-GVHD) is a rare but serious complication of blood transfusion. As discussed in Chapter 11, there is engraftment and proliferation of donor T-lymphocytes and interaction with recipient cells expressing HLA antigens causing cellular damage particularly to the skin, gastrointestinal tract, liver and spleen, and the bone marrow. Clinical manifestations usually occur 1–2 weeks after blood transfusion, and early features include fever, maculopapular skin rash, diarrhoea and hepatitis. Haematology patients at risk are those who are undergoing transplantation, have Hodgkin's lymphoma or have received therapy with certain drugs, e.g. purine analogues.

Prevention

The dose of donor lymphocytes sufficient to cause TA-GVHD is unknown, but may be lower than is achievable by current techniques for leucocyte reduction of blood components. However, there have been no case reports of TA-GVHD in the UK since 2001 following the implementation of universal leucocyte reduction of blood in the UK in 1999. Gamma-irradiation to destroy the proliferative capability of donor lymphocytes remains the usual method of choice to prevent TA-GVHD (see Chapter 11), although it is a radioactive source and requires regular recalibration. An alternative to gamma-irradiation is X-ray irradiation, which is used in several European countries. Key considerations in the assessment of methods for the prevention of TA-GVHD are their effectiveness and the avoidance of excessive damage to red cells and platelets. The currently recommended indications for the use of irradiated blood for haematology patients are shown in Table 28.4 [17]. Although gamma-irradiation is currently the accepted method of preventing TA-GVHD, pathogen-reduction technologies have been shown to be as effective at inactivating lymphocytes. Pathogen-reduced platelet components are accepted as safe from the risk of TA-GVHD in some countries without the need for further processing such as gamma-irradiation.

How to ensure that patients receive the correct 'special' blood?

An important issue for haematology departments and hospital blood banks is how to ensure that patients receive special blood components (e.g. CMV-seronegative, gamma-irradiated) when these products are indicated and that standard blood components are not transfused, as this may have devastating consequences.

Each hospital needs to establish its own procedures so that patients receive the correct special blood components, where they are indicated. These should include the following:
• Education of ward medical and nursing staff about the indications for special blood components and the importance of receiving the correct type of blood component.
• Requests for blood components to include the patient's diagnosis and any requirement for special blood components.

Table 28.4 Indications for irradiation of blood components in haematology patients. Reproduced from British Committee for Standards in Haematology [17].

Indications

Except for stem cell infusions, all donations from first- or second-degree relatives, even if the patient is immunocompetent

Except for stem cell infusions all HLA-matched components, even if the patient is immunocompetent

All granulocyte components

Allogeneic bone marrow/peripheral blood progenitor cell transplantation: from the time of initiation of conditioning therapy and continuing while the patient remains on GVHD prophylaxis (usually 6 months) or until lymphocytes are $>1 \times 10^9$/L. If chronic GVHD is present or if continued immunosuppressive treatment is required, irradiated blood components should be given indefinitely

Allogeneic blood transfused to bone marrow and peripheral blood stem cell donors 7 days prior to or during the harvest must be irradiated

Autologous bone marrow/peripheral blood progenitor cell transplantation: during and 7 days before the harvest of haemopoietic cells, and then from the initiation of conditioning therapy until 3 months posttransplant (6 months if total body irradiation is used)

All adults and children with Hodgkin's lymphoma should have irradiated red cells and platelets for life

Severe T-lymphocyte immunodeficiency syndromes

Patients treated with purine analogues such as fludarabine, cladribine and deoxycoformycin and newer drugs such as bendamustine and clofarabine

Patients receiving alemtuzumab (anti-CD52)

Patients with aplastic anaemia receiving treatment with antithymocyte globulin (ATG)

Nonindications

Patients receiving rituximab (anti-CD20).

Non-Hodgkin's lymphoma (although this may be reviewed following some recent reports of TA-GVHD in patients with B-cell non-Hodgkin's lymphoma)

HIV infection

TA-GVHD, transfusion-associated graft-versus-host disease.

- Storing of individual patient's requirements for special blood components in the blood bank computer.
- The prescription for blood components should include any requirement for special blood components, enabling the ward staff to check that the blood component to be transfused complies with these requirements.
- Providing patients with cards indicating their special blood requirements, particularly for those patients receiving shared care between two hospitals and those with a long-term requirement for gamma-irradiated blood, e.g. patients with Hodgkin's lymphoma.

HLA alloimmunization and refractoriness to platelet transfusions [6]

Platelet refractoriness is the repeated failure to obtain satisfactory responses to platelet transfusions and occurs in more than 50% of patients receiving multiple transfusions.

Various methods are used to assess response to platelet transfusions. If the patient is bleeding, the clinical response is an important indication of the effectiveness of the transfusion. The response to a prophylactic platelet transfusion is assessed by measuring the increase in platelet count after the transfusion. Various formulas have been used to correct for the variation in response dependent on the patient's size and the number of platelets transfused; these include platelet recovery and corrected count increment. However, in practice, a (nonsustained) increase in the patient's platelet count of less than 5×10^9/L at 20–24 hours after the transfusion can be used as a simple measure of a poor response.

Causes

Many causes of platelet refractoriness have been described and can be subdivided into immune mechanisms, most importantly HLA alloimmunization and

Table 28.5 Causes of platelet refractoriness.

Immune
Platelet alloantibodies
  HLA
  HPA
  ABO
Other antibodies
  Platelet autoantibodies
  Drug-dependent platelet antibodies
Immune complexes
Nonimmune
Infection and its treatment, especially amphotericin B
Splenomegaly
Disseminated intravascular coagulation
Fever
Bleeding

nonimmune mechanisms involving platelet consumption (Table 28.5). Platelet consumption is the most frequent mechanism of platelet refractoriness, usually associated with sepsis. However, immune-mediated platelet destruction remains an important cause of platelet refractoriness; HLA antibodies are the commonest immune cause and the other immune causes are rare.

The precise mechanism of HLA alloimmunization remains uncertain, but primary HLA alloimmunization appears to be initiated by intact cells expressing both HLA class I and class II antigens such as lymphocytes and antigen-presenting cells. Platelets only express HLA class I antigens and hence leucocyte-reduced blood components cause primary HLA alloimmunization in fewer than 3% of recipients. Use of pre-storage leucocyte-reduced blood components has therefore led to a significant reduction in the incidence of HLA alloimmunization. However, secondary HLA alloimmunization does not require the presence of HLA class II antigens, and may occur in patients who have been pregnant or previously transfused with non-leucocyte-reduced blood components.

Investigation and management
If platelet refractoriness occurs, the following algorithm can be used for investigation and management (Figure 28.2 [18]).
1 A clinical assessment should be made for clinical factors likely to be associated with nonimmune platelet consumption.
2 If nonimmune platelet consumption appears likely, an attempt should be made to correct the clinical factors responsible, where possible, and platelet transfusions from random donors should be continued. If a poor response to random donor platelet transfusions persists, the patient should be tested for HLA antibodies.
3 If nonimmune platelet consumption appears to be unlikely, an immune mechanism should be suspected

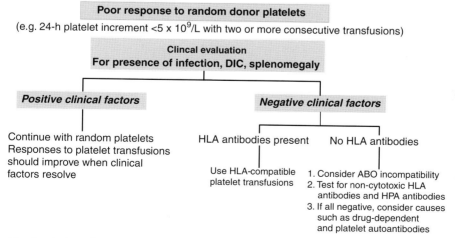

Fig 28.2 Algorithm for the investigation and management of patients with platelet refractoriness. DIC, disseminated intravascular coagulation.

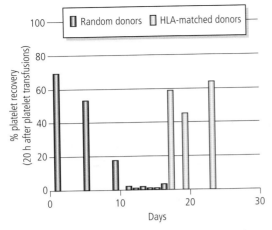

Fig 28.3 Responses to platelet transfusions in a female patient with acute myeloblastic leukaemia undergoing remission induction therapy. There were poor responses to the initial platelet transfusions and the patient was found to have HLA antibodies. There were improved responses to platelet transfusions from HLA-matched donors.

and the patient's serum should be tested for HLA antibodies. If HLA antibodies are present, the specificity of the antibodies should be determined as this may help in the selection of HLA-compatible donors. However, HLA antibodies stimulated by repeated transfusions are often 'multispecific' and it is not possible to determine their specificity.

4 Platelet transfusions from HLA-matched donors (matched for the HLA-A, -B antigens of the patient) should be used for patients with apparent immune refractoriness and the response to further transfusions should be observed carefully. Figure 28.3 shows improved responses to HLA-matched platelet transfusions in a patient with platelet refractoriness due to HLA alloimmunization. If responses to HLA-matched transfusions are not improved, the reason should be sought, and platelet cross-matching of the patient's serum against the lymphocytes and platelets of HLA-matched donors may be helpful in determining the cause and the selection of compatible donors for future transfusions. These matching strategies are based on counting the number of HLA-A and HLA-B mismatches between the patient and donor; this requires a large HLA typed donor panel and at times no suitable matches can be found. An alternative approach is HLA epitope matching; this only considers the epitopes on the HLA antigen, whereas standard HLA-matching considers the whole HLA antigen.

5 If there are no factors for nonimmune platelet consumption and HLA antibodies are not detected, consideration should be given to less frequent causes of immune platelet refractoriness.

(a) High titre ABO antibodies in the recipient. This is an unusual cause of platelet refractoriness and can be excluded by switching to ABO-compatible platelet transfusions if ABO-incompatible transfusions have been used for previous transfusions.

(b) HPA antibodies, which usually occur in combination with HLA antibodies, but sometimes occur in isolation.

(c) Drug-dependent platelet antibodies, which may be underestimated as a cause for platelet refractoriness.

Alloimmunization to red cell antigens

Incidence

Alloimmunization to red cell antigens is another important consequence of repeated transfusions in haematology patients. The incidence of red cell alloimmunization in adult haematology patients is in the range of 10–15% and is similar to other groups of multitransfused patients, e.g. patients with renal failure. However, a higher proportion of children requiring long-term transfusion support develop red cell alloimmunization. In sickle cell disease, the incidence is in the range of 20–30% (see Chapter 29). The implications of these observations include the following.

• Patients with sickle cell disease should be phenotyped for Rh, Kell, Fy, Jk and MNS antigens before the first transfusion and patients with thalassaemia and other children requiring chronic transfusion support should be phenotyped for Rh and Kell antigens.

• Blood for transfusion to children requiring long-term transfusion support, including patients with haemoglobinopathies, should be matched for Rh and Kell antigens to prevent alloimmunization.

• Phenotyping and antigen matching to prevent red cell alloimmunization is not required for other groups of patients requiring repeated transfusions.

Timing of sample collection for compatibility testing [19]

In patients with haematological disorders receiving repeated transfusions, an important issue is the timing of blood sample collection in relation to the previous transfusion.

• Where the patient is receiving very frequent transfusion, e.g. daily, it is only necessary to request a new sample every 3 days.

• In the UK, if the previous transfusion was 3–14 days earlier, the sample should ideally be taken within 24 hours of the start of the transfusion, although some laboratories stretch this to 48 hours for patients who have been repeatedly transfused without developing antibodies. Other countries, e.g. Canada, only require a sample within 3 days of the start of the transfusion.

• Where the previous transfusion was 14–28 days earlier, the sample should be taken within 3 days of the start of the transfusion.

• Where the previous transfusion was more than 28 days ago, the sample should be taken within 1 week of the planned transfusion.

Sample collection timeframe requirements do vary slightly from country to country.

ABO-incompatible bone marrow/peripheral blood progenitor cell transplants

ABO-incompatible bone marrow/peripheral blood progenitor cell transplants present particular problems (Table 28.6). The transplant may provide a new A and/or B antigen from the donor (major mismatch) or a new A and/or B antibody (minor mismatch). For *pretransplant,* blood component support should be with the patient's own ABO type. For *posttransplant,* selection of the appropriate group is more complicated (see Figure 28.4 [20]). The requirements for platelet and FFP support are also shown. These recommendations should be followed posttransplant until the patient has engrafted, ABO antibodies to the donor ABO group are undetectable and the direct antiglobulin test is negative.

• Major ABO incompatibility: the patient's own ABO group should be given. Plasma and platelets should be of the donor-type blood group. The European Group for Blood and Marrow Transplantation (EBMT) also advise that group O red cells can be used.

• Minor ABO incompatibility: red cells of the donor ABO group should be given. Plasma and platelets should be of a recipient-type blood group.

• Major and minor (bidirectional) ABO incompatibility: give group O red cells, group AB plasma and platelets of the recipient-type blood group.

Table 28.6 Problems associated with ABO-incompatible bone marrow/peripheral blood progenitor transplants.

Major ABO incompatibility (e.g. recipient O, donor A)

Failure of engraftment: risk not increased in ABO-incompatible transplants

Acute haemolysis at the time of reinfusion: avoided by processing donor bone marrow/peripheral blood progenitor cells

Haemolysis of donor-type red cells: avoid by using red cells of recipient type in the early posttransplant period

Delayed erythropoiesis: may be due to persistence of anti-A in the recipient, minimize transfusion of anti-A by using platelets and plasma from group A donors

Delayed haemolysis due to persistence of recipient anti-A: only switch to donor red cells when recipient anti-A undetectable and direct antiglobulin test undetectable

Minor ABO incompatibility (e.g. recipient A, donor O)

Acute haemolysis at the time of reinfusion: avoid by removing donor plasma if the donor anti-A titre is high

Delayed haemolysis of recipient cells due to anti-A produced by donor lymphocytes (passenger lymphocyte syndrome): maximum haemolysis usually occurs between days 9 and 16 posttransplant. Rare in T-cell-depleted grafts or when CD34+ cells selected in stem cell processing

Studies disagree on whether ABO incompatibility can also affect overall survival, disease-free survival or GVHD. A recent meta-analysis [21] found no difference in overall survival between recipients of ABO matched or mismatched grafts when the donor was related. However, in unrelated donor transplants there was a marginally reduced overall survival in patients who received bidirectional or minor-mismatched transplants.

• RhD-incompatible transplants can also cause difficulties. It is recommended that RhD-negative blood components should be used for RhD-positive recipients with RhD-negative donors. However, no cases of immunization have been reported when RhD-negative recipients have received RhD-positive transplants, and RhD-positive blood components may be used.

Iron overload

A major adverse consequence of repeated red cell transfusions over a long period in patients with haemoglobinopathies or myelodysplastic syndromes

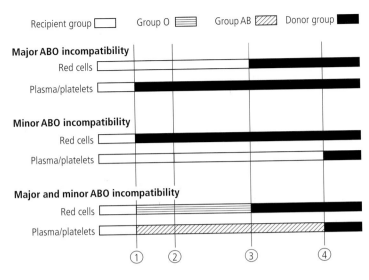

Recipient group ☐   Group O ☰   Group AB ▨   Donor group ■

Major ABO incompatibility
Red cells
Plasma/platelets

Minor ABO incompatibility
Red cells
Plasma/platelets

Major and minor ABO incompatibility
Red cells
Plasma/platelets

① ② ③ ④

① Begin pre-transplant chemotherapy
② Bone marrow transplant
③ ABO antibodies to donor RBC not detected. Direct antiglobulin test negative
④ RBC of recipient group no longer detected

Fig 28.4 Recommendations for ABO type of blood components in ABO-incompatible bone marrow/peripheral blood progenitor cell transplants. Adapted from Warkentin [20], with permission.

is iron overload. This important complication is described in detail in Chapter 29.

with haematological malignancies and the role of granulocyte transfusions.

Key points

1 Specialist transfusion support and advice is required for many patients with haematological disorders.
2 The need for transfusion, as in other groups of patients, is determined by assessment of individual patient's symptoms and blood counts and guided by national and local recommendations for the use of blood.
3 Special blood components are frequently needed to avoid complications such as TA-GVHD and transfusion transmission of CMV in haematology patients susceptible to these complications.
4 Responses to platelet transfusions should be carefully monitored to identify patients having poor responses, which require clinical and laboratory investigation to determine the most likely cause and the best approach to management.
5 Further work is needed to define the optimal thresholds for red cell and platelet transfusion in patients

References

1 Wallis JP, Wells AW & Chapman CE, on behalf of the Northern Regional Transfusion Committee. Changing indications for red cell transfusion from 2000 to 2004 in the North of England. *Transfus Med* 2006; 16: 411–417.
2 British Committee for Standards in Haematology. Guidelines on the clinical use of red cell transfusions. *Br J Haematol* 2001; 113: 24–31.
3 Valeri CR, Khuri S & Ragno G. Nonsurgical bleeding diathesis in anemic thrombocytopenic patients: role of temperature, red blood cells, platelets, and plasma-clotting proteins. *Transfusion* 2007; 47: 206S–248S.
4 Rizzo JD, Brouwers M, Hurley P *et al*. American Society of Hematology/American Society of Clinical Oncology clinical practice guideline update on the use of epoetin and darbopoetin in adult patients with cancer. *Blood* 2010; 116(20): 4045–4059.
5 Wilson J, Yao GL, Raftery J *et al*. A systematic review and economic evaluation of epoetin alfa, epoetin beta

and darbepoetin alfa in anaemia associated with cancer, especially that attributable to cancer treatment. *Health Technol Assess* 2007; 11(13): 1–220.

6 British Committee for Standards in Haematology. Guidelines for platelet transfusions. *Br J Haematol* 2003; 122: 10–23.

7 Estcourt LJ, Birchall J, Lowe D *et al.* Platelet transfusions in haematology patients: are we using them appropriately? *Vox Sang* 2012; 103(4): 284–293.

8 Estcourt LJ, Stanworth SJ, Doree C *et al.* Prophylactic platelet transfusion for the prevention of haemorrhage after chemotherapy and stem cell transplantation. *Cochrane Database Syst Rev* 2012; Issue 5. DOI: 10.1002/14651858.CD004269.pub3.

9 Slichter SJ, Kaufman RM, Assmann SF *et al.* Dose of prophylactic platelet transfusions and prevention of haemorrhage. *N Engl J Med* 2010; 362: 600–613.

10 Stanworth SJ, Dyer C, Choo L *et al.* Do all patients with haematologic malignancies and severe thrombocytopenia need prophylactic platelet transfusions? Background, rationale and design of a clinical trial (trial of platelet prophylaxis) to assess the effectiveness of prophylactic platelet transfusions. *Transfus Med Rev* 2010; 24: 163–171.

11 Wandt H, Schäfer-Eckart K, Wendelin K *et al.* A therapeutic platelet transfusion strategy without routine prophylactic transfusion is feasible and safe and reduces platelet transfusion numbers significantly: final analysis of a randomised study after high-dose chemotherapy and PBSCT. *Bone Marrow Transplantat* 2009; 43(S1s): S23.

12 Neunert C, Lim W, Crowther M *et al.* The American Society of Hematology 2011 evidence-based practice guideline for immune thrombocytopenia. *Blood* 2011; 117: 4190–4207.

13 Price TH. Granulocyte transfusion: current status. *Semin Hematol* 2007; 44: 15–23.

14 Sayers M, Anderson KC, Goodnough LT *et al.* Reducing the risk for transfusion-transmitted cytomegalovirus infection. *Ann Int Med* 1992; 116: 55–62.

15 Laupacis A, Brown J, Costello B *et al.* Prevention of post-transfusion CMV in the era of universal WBC reduction: a consensus statement. *Transfusion* 2001; 41: 560–569.

16 Clark P & Miller JP. Leucocyte-reduced and cytomegalovirus-reduced-risk blood components. In: PD Mintz (ed.), *Transfusion Therapy: Clinical Principles and Practice*, 3rd edn. Bethesda, MD: AABB Press; 2010.

17 British Committee for Standards in Haematology. Guidelines on irradiated blood components for the prevention of graft-versus-host disease. *Br J Haematol* 2010; 152: 35–51.

18 Dzik S. How I do it: platelet support for refractory patients. *Transfusion* 2007; 47(3): 374–378.

19 British Committee for Standards in Haematology. Guidelines for compatibility procedures in blood transfusion laboratories. *Transfus Med* 2004; 14: 59–73.

20 Warkentin PI. Transfusion of patients undergoing bone marrow transplantation. *Hum Pathol* 1983; 14: 261–266.

21 Kanda J, Ichinohe T, Matsuo K *et al.* Impact of ABO mismatching on the outcomes of allogeneic related and unrelated blood and marrow stem cell transplantations for hematologic malignances: IPD-based meta-analysis of cohort studies. *Transfusion* 2009; 49(4): 624–635.

Further reading

Campell-Lee SA. The future of red cell alloimmunisation. *Transfusion* 2007; 47: 1959–1960.

Cohen AR. New advances in iron chelation therapy. *Hematology Am Soc Hematol Educ Program* 2006: 42–47.

Drew WL & Roback JD. Prevention of transfusion-transmitted cytomegalovirus: reactivation of the debate? *Transfusion* 2007; 47: 1955–1958.

Estcourt LJ, Stanworth SJ & Murphy MF. Platelet transfusions for patients with haematological malignancies: who needs them? *Br J Haematol* 2011; 154(4): 425–440.

Heddle NM. Acute paroxysmal cold hemoglobinuria. *Transfus Med Rev* 1989, July; 3(3): 219–229.

Silberstein LE & Cunningham MJ. Autoimmune hemolytic anemias. In: CD Hillyer, LE Silberstein, PM Ness, KC Anderson & JD Roback (eds), *Blood Banking and Transfusion Medicine: Basic Principles and Practice*, 2nd edn. Philadelphia, PA: Churchill Livingstone; 2007.

Stanworth S, Massey E, Hyde C *et al.* Granulocyte transfusions for treating infections in patients with neutropenia or neutrophil dysfunction. *Cochrane Database Syst Rev* 2005; Issue 3. DOI: 10.1002/14651858/CD005339.

29

Blood transfusion in the management of patients with haemoglobinopathies

David C. Rees

Department of Haematological Medicine, King's College Hospital NHS Foundation Trust, London, UK

Introduction

Haemoglobinopathies are caused by mutations in the globin genes and are probably the commonest single gene disorders in the world. The α-globin and β-globin gene families are found on chromosome 16 and chromosome 11, respectively. Together with haem, they combine to form haemoglobin, which is a tetramer of two α-like and two β-like globins. Developmentally, two different α-globins and four different β-globins are produced, resulting in a variety of haemoglobins (Table 29.1). At birth there is a gradual switch from fetal to adult haemoglobin, which is largely complete in a year [1]. Quantitative defects in globin chain synthesis cause thalassaemia, whereas qualitative defects result in haemoglobin variants; the most important haemoglobin variant is haemoglobin S (HbS, β⁶ glutamic acid-valine), causing sickle cell disease (SCD). Blood transfusion is important in haemoglobinopathies, allowing correction of anaemia, suppression of abnormal erythropoiesis and replacement of abnormal erythrocytes.

α-Thalassaemia syndromes

Most people have four α-globin genes and the common types of α-thalassaemia are due to large deletions of one or more of these genes [2]. Deletion of both α-globin genes on a chromosome can occur, although this is only common in Southeast Asia and the eastern Mediterranean. There are three main α-thalassaemia syndromes.

α-Thalassaemia trait

This is usually due to the deletion of one or two α-globin genes. The haemoglobin is normal with mild hypochromia. Blood transfusion is never needed to treat the condition itself.

HbH disease

This occurs when there is only one functional α-globin gene. It is typically a mild condition, with haemoglobin of 7–10 g/dL and HbH (tetramers of β-globin) inclusion bodies in erythrocytes. The spleen is moderately enlarged. Blood transfusion is unusual, but may be necessary following Parvovirus B19 infection.

Hb Bart's hydrops fetalis

A complete or near-complete absence of functional α-globin genes results in progressive fetal anaemia from the 10th week of gestation. Without intervention this results in a hydropic fetus and miscarriage at 30–40 weeks, reflecting the importance of α-globin in forming HbF. Occasionally fetal anaemia has been detected and the pregnancy maintained until term with regular intrauterine transfusions. The resulting babies are transfusion dependent and usually seriously

Practical Transfusion Medicine, Fourth Edition. Edited by Michael F. Murphy, Derwood H. Pamphilon and Nancy M. Heddle.
© 2013 John Wiley & Sons, Ltd. Published 2013 by John Wiley & Sons, Ltd.

314

Table 29.1 Normal haemoglobins.

Structure	Name	Predominant expression
$\zeta_2\varepsilon_2$	Hb Gower 1	0–10th-week gestation
$\alpha_2\varepsilon_2$	Hb Gower 2	5th–10th-week gestation
$\zeta_2\gamma_2$	Hb Portland	5th–10th-week gestation
$\alpha_2{}^G\gamma_2$	HbF	12th-week gestation – 4th month
$\alpha_2{}^A\gamma_2$	HbF	12th-week gestation – 4th month
$\alpha_2\beta_2$	HbA	4th month – death
$\alpha_2\delta_2$	HbA$_2$	4th month – death

Table 29.2 Causes of β-thalassaemia intermedia.

Factors lessening severity of predicted β-thalassaemia major
Mild β-thalassaemia mutations, e.g. HbE/β-thalassaemia
Coinheritance of α-thalassaemia
Coinheritance of increased capacity to make HbF
Unexplained

Factors worsening severity of predicted β-thalassaemia trait
Coinheritance of triplicated α-globin gene
Dominant β-thalassaemia mutation
Unexplained

handicapped. This may either result from the effects of fetal anaemia or be caused by large deletions on chromosome 16. If fetal anaemia is found to be due to Hb Bart's hydrops fetalis, the likelihood of serious handicap should be discussed with the parents prior to starting intrauterine transfusions.

β-Thalassaemia syndromes

β-Thalassaemia results from a reduced rate of β-globin synthesis, but much of the pathology arises from the resulting excess of α-globin. β-globin is not part of fetal haemoglobin and there are no adverse fetal or neonatal effects. In contrast to α-thalassaemia, most cases of β-thalassaemia are caused by small mutations or deletions in the β-globin gene. More than 300 different mutations have been identified, and the many different combinations result in a phenotypic continuum from asymptomatic to transfusion dependence.

β-Thalassaemia trait

This results from the inheritance of one mutated β-globin gene. There is minimal anaemia, with hypochromia and microcytosis. Anaemia becomes more marked during pregnancy and occasionally blood transfusion is necessary, although regular or frequent blood transfusions have no role.

β-Thalassaemia intermedia

This is a clinical term referring to a range of conditions characterized by significant anaemia, splenomegaly and increased iron absorption. Patients typically grow and develop normally without the need for regular blood transfusions, at least for the first few years of life. Many different combinations of β-globin mutation cause thalassaemia intermedia [3] (Table 29.2). Anaemia may increase during infection or illness and intermittent transfusions may be necessary. The trigger for blood transfusion is based on clinical signs and symptoms rather than any specific haemoglobin concentration (Hb). Acute symptoms suggesting that transfusion may be beneficial include dyspnoea and fatigue. It can be difficult to decide if someone with severe thalassaemia intermedia would benefit from regular blood transfusions and treatment as for thalassaemia major. In children this is suggested by poor growth, recurrent illness, marked bony expansion, progressive splenomegaly or evidence of organ damage, such as pulmonary hypertension. Sometimes children require regular blood transfusions to progress through puberty; older adults, who previously managed without transfusion, may become transfusion dependent due to reduced cardiorespiratory function. The decision to start regular transfusions is clinical, not based on a particular genotype or Hb. Once regular transfusions start they should be continued long term. Iron overload can be a problem in thalassaemia intermedia, even in the absence of regular transfusions, and iron stores should be monitored regularly and chelation started as necessary [4].

β-Thalassaemia major

Thalassaemia major is the term used when a patient with β-thalassaemia is treated with regular blood transfusions from an early age. Without transfusions, the child either dies or is seriously ill, with failure

315

to thrive, bony deformity or a poor quality of life. It is usually due to the coinheritance of severe β-thalassaemia mutations (β° mutations) from both parents, but can be caused by combinations of less severe mutations (β⁺-thalassaemia) with exacerbation from epigenetic and environmental factors. The clinical problems result from excess α-globin chains, damaging the developing erythroid cells in the marrow such that they fail to mature into circulating red cells (ineffective erythropoiesis). The expanded erythroid component of the marrow produces large amounts of growth differentiation factor 15, which reduces hepcidin production by the liver; hepcidin inhibits gastrointestinal iron absorption and the inappropriately low levels result in increased iron absorption. The main clinical features of thalassaemia major are therefore:
- severe anaemia;
- bone marrow expansion with bony deformity and osteopenia;
- hypersplenism and hypermetabolism;
- iron overload.

Blood transfusion in β-thalassaemia major
The aim of regular, long-term blood transfusions in thalassaemia major is to:
- reduce or eliminate symptoms of anaemia;
- suppress ineffective erythropoiesis to prevent bony deformity;
- prevent the development of significant hypersplenism;
- suppress extramedullary haemopoiesis.

Studies measuring soluble transferrin receptor levels have shown that erythropoiesis is adequately suppressed by maintaining a pretransfusion Hb between 9 and 10 g/dL [5]. The posttransfusion Hb is usually kept below 15 g/dL to avoid problems with high blood viscosity and fluid overload. In practice these parameters are usually achieved by regular, simple transfusions given every 2–5 weeks, the frequency being determined by local resources and pretransfusion symptoms. Occasionally, more intensive transfusion is used to support cardiorespiratory problems or suppress extramedullary haemopoiesis. Automated exchange transfusions are also used, and typically patients have a full-volume exchange every 6 to 8 weeks. Exchange transfusion has the advantages of decreasing iron loading and less frequent hospital attendances, although it involves more donor exposure with increased risk of alloimmunization and infection; good vascular access is also important, and therefore the procedure is more difficult in young children (Table 29.3). It is more expensive than simple transfusion and unavailable in many parts of the world. The insertion of semi-permanent venous access devices is sometimes necessary if venous access is difficult. With adequate blood transfusion and iron chelation from an early age, the expectation is that children will grow and develop normally, with a good quality of life. Life expectancy should approach the normal range, although chelation failure means that median life expectancy is usually shortened; patients in developed countries born in the 1960s had a median survival of 30 years, but this has progressively increased [6].

Table 29.3 Advantages and disadvantages of different types of blood transfusion.

Simple transfusion	Manual exchange	Automated transfusion
Quick to organize	Slower to organize	Slower to organize and not always available
No special skills involved	Previous experience and training necessary	Specialist staff and equipment needed
Simple venous access only	Good venous access	Very good venous access at two sites
Quick to complete	Slow to complete	Quick to complete
Limited scope to reduce HbS percentage	Significant decrease in HbS percentage	Very significant decreases in HbS percentage
Fairly predictable final Hb levels and HbS percentage	Unpredictable final Hb and HbS percentage	Predictable final Hb and HbS percentage
Limited donor exposure	Moderate donor exposure	High donor exposure
Significant increase in iron stores	Minimal increase in iron stores	Minimal or no increase in iron stores

Sickle cell disease (SCD)

SCD refers to a group of conditions in which the patient is either homozygous for the mutated β^S allele or coinherits β^S with another β-globin mutation (Table 29.4). The primary pathological event is the polymerization of deoxygenated HbS, resulting in damage to the red cell membrane, cellular dehydration and increased cytoplasmic viscosity. These abnormal, rigid sickle cells cause vaso-occlusion, in which precapillary venules are blocked, resulting in both acute and chronic ischaemic damage. Clinical consequences of vaso-occlusion include hyposplenism, acute pain, acute chest syndrome, acute abdominal pain and chronic restrictive lung defects. Vaso-occlusion also leads to a further cascade of interlinked pathological events, including haemolytic anaemia, inflammation, oxidative stress, reperfusion injury, hypercoagulability, nitric oxide deficiency, hypoxaemia and vasculopathy. Vasculopathy and endothelial dysfunction seem to be particularly important for some chronic complications, including cerebrovascular disease and stroke, pulmonary hypertension, priapism and leg ulcers. Haemolyis is thought to contribute significantly to the vasculopathy by releasing free haemoglobin into the plasma, which inactivates nitric oxide resulting in vascular endothelial dysfunction [7].

Blood transfusion plays an important role in combating many of these pathological processes, including increasing Hb, reducing the number of circulating erythrocytes able to cause vaso-occlusion and reducing intravascular haemolysis. Increasing the Hb and haematocrit too much is potentially harmful as it

Table 29.4 Types of SCD.

Severe SCD
   HbSS (sickle cell anaemia)
   HbS β-thalassaemia
   HbS O^{Arab}
   HbS D^{Punjab}
Mild SCD
   HbSC
   HbS β$^+$-thalassaemia
   HbS Lepore
Very mild SCD
   HbSE
   HbS/hereditary persistence of fetal haemoglobin

increases blood viscosity, particularly in small blood vessels, and so can reduce oxygen delivery to tissues and precipitate acute ischaemic events, particularly in the brain. When planning a transfusion in SCD, it is important to decide what the target Hb and HbS percentage are, and then plan how best to achieve these. This can be through either a simple top-up transfusion or an exchange transfusion of some sort, in which blood is also removed. In SCD, there is not thought to be any benefit from exchange per se, and it is a way of decreasing the HbS percentage without increasing the haematocrit excessively. Exchange transfusions are performed most efficiently using automated apheresis, although this is not always available as an emergency and requires very good vascular access (Table 29.3).

Indications for transfusions in acute complications of SCD

- Acute anaemia. The need for transfusion is dependent on symptoms rather than on haemoglobin level, but is usually necessary when the Hb falls below 5 g/dL. A single, simple transfusion aiming to increase the Hb to 8–10 g/dL is typically used. Specific causes of acute anaemia include:
  - Parvovirus B19 infection – low reticulocyte count, viral symptoms.
  - Acute splenic sequestration – high reticulocyte count, enlarging spleen and rapidly falling Hb; potentially fatal without urgent transfusion; it is commonest in children under the age of 5 years and recurrent episodes usually require splenectomy.
  - Acute hepatic sequestration – rare complication with enlarging liver and reticulocytosis.
  - Acute pain – occasionally the Hb falls significantly (>2 g/dL) during an episode of acute pain and transfusion may be necessary to correct symptomatic anaemia.
- Acute chest syndrome. This is defined as new pulmonary shadowing on a chest X-ray in someone with SCD and is typically accompanied by chest pain, tachypnoea, hypoxia and increasing anaemia. Many cases recover with oxygen and antibiotics, although 5–10% of cases deteriorate and require respiratory support. Blood transfusion has an important role in managing severe cases. Severe cases are usually accompanied by progressive anaemia and observational evidence suggests that early top-up transfusion

317

to increase the Hb to about 10 g/dL can prevent deterioration; this also results in a significant reduction in HbS percentage. If deterioration is rapid or mechanical ventilation necessary, the HbS should be reduced to less than 30% with haemoglobin of about 10 g/dL, which will often involve an urgent exchange transfusion [8].

• Stroke. If acute neurological symptoms occur, urgent blood transfusion should be arranged whilst investigating the cause, which is likely to be cerebrovascular disease. The aim of transfusion is both to reduce HbS to less than 30% and increase the Hb to about 10 g/dL. This will usually require an exchange transfusion and a retrospective study suggested that outcome is better if an exchange transfusion is used initially rather than a top-up [9]. It is probably important to correct significant anaemia rapidly with a top-up transfusion before the exchange, to limit the area of brain ischaemia, if there is going to be a delay of more than a few hours before the exchange transfusion can be performed.

• Multiorgan failure. This can occur following severe sepsis or acute chest syndrome, and usually patients will have been fully exchanged as part of the prodrome to this often agonal event. Generally the HbS is kept at less than 30%.

• There is no evidence to support the use of blood transfusions in the treatment of acute pain, priapism or osteomyelitis. In some cases these may be accompanied by significant anaemia and so benefit from transfusion, or surgery may be necessary and transfusion used preoperatively.

Indications for regular transfusion in SCD

• Secondary stroke prevention. Following a first stroke there is a 20–90% chance of further strokes. Retrospective studies suggest that the risk of recurrence is reduced by up to 90% with regular blood transfusions to keep the HbS less than 30 or 50%. This requires regular exchange or top-up transfusions, with evidence suggesting that the high risk of stroke returns once the transfusions stop [10].

• Primary stroke prevention in children with abnormal transcranial Doppler (TCD) scans. Children with narrowed intracerebral blood vessels, as detected by TCD, are at high risk of acute stroke. A randomized

controlled trial showed that keeping HbS less than 30% with regular transfusions reduced stroke risk by 90% [11]. Transfusions are typically continued life-long, although the target HbS is often increased to 50% after about three years without any cerebrovascular deterioration.

• Recurrent acute chest syndrome. Hydroxyurea is effective at stopping recurrent acute chest syndrome in 80% cases; if hydroxyurea fails, regular blood transfusions may help prevent further episodes.

• Progressive organ failure. Hepatic, renal, cardiovascular and pulmonary failure are problems in older SCD patients, and regular transfusions can help support organ function or prevent further deterioration. As survival in SCD improves, there are increasing numbers of older patients and increasing amounts of blood used for this indication.

• Other indications. Regular transfusions may have a role in preventing frequent episodes of acute pain, chronic pain, avascular joint necrosis, leg ulcers, pulmonary hypertension, acute pain in pregnancy and recurrent splenic sequestration, depending on individual circumstances.

Preoperative blood transfusion in SCD

Perioperative complications are increased in SCD, including the development of pain and acute chest syndrome. In high-risk surgery, such as cardiac, brain and long operations, it is accepted that preoperatively the HbS should be less than 30% with minimal anaemia. This will usually involve an exchange transfusion before surgery. For other types of surgery, the need for transfusion is less clear. Studies suggest no advantage of exchange over top-up transfusion, unless the patient has significant organ damage, cerebrovascular disease or had previous severe complications [12]. The recently completed TAPS (transfusion alternatives preoperatively in sickle cell disease) randomized controlled trial suggested that simple preoperative transfusion reduces the risk of complications, such as acute chest syndrome, for some types of operation, particularly abdominal and throat surgery. In practice, most people with sickle cell anaemia and Hb less than 9 g/dL should probably be transfused to a target Hb of about 10 g/dL prior to general anaesthesia for moderate-risk surgery.

Complications of transfusions in haemoglobinopathies

All the routine complications of blood transfusion can occur. Particular problems include:
• Alloimmunization. Rates vary from 10 to 20% depending on the similarity between the ethnicities of donor and recipient populations, and the extent of blood group matching. In many countries, including northern Europe and the USA, the thalassaemic and SCD populations are mostly of a different ethnic origin to the majority of the blood donor population, increasing the risk of alloimmunization. An extended red cell phenotype should be performed before starting transfusion (C, c, D, E, e, K, k, Jka, Jkb, Fya, Fyb, Kpa, Kpb, MNS, Lewis). The risk of alloimmunization can be reduced by choosing blood matched for Rh and Kell groups in both thalassaemia [13] and SCD [14]. Leucocyte reduction reduces the risk of transfusion reactions, prion transmission and possibly alloimmunization.
• Autoantibody formation. This typically accompanies the development of alloantibodies and occurs in up to 25% of thalassaemia major patients and a smaller percentage with SCD. It is associated with non-leucocyte-reduced transfusions and splenectomy. This can result in significant autoimmune haemolysis, in which transfusion fails to increase the Hb significantly. Management includes avoiding unnecessary blood transfusion, with a possible role for corticosteroids, intravenous immunoglobulin and rituximab. Blood transfusion may be unavoidable in severe haemolysis and should be used to treat life-threatening anaemia.
• Infection. The prevalence of transfusion-transmitted infections varies widely but is rare in most developed countries. Prion infection is an increasing concern. Before starting a transfusion programme, children should be vaccinated against hepatitis B.
• Iron overload. This is predominantly due to the iron content of transfused blood, although increased absorption is important in thalassaemia intermedia.

Iron chelation

Regular blood transfusions inevitably cause iron overload. Each unit of transfused blood contains about 200 mg of iron, and typically iron chelation is started after 12 months of regular transfusions or when the ferritin exceeds 1000 μg/L. Without treatment, iron accumulates in and damages the liver, heart and endocrine organs. In thalassaemia, iron-related heart disease is the major cause of death. In SCD marked cardiac iron deposition is unusual, although significant morbidity results from hepatic siderosis.

It is important to assess iron stores accurately to monitor chelation therapy (Table 29.5). If there is evidence of progressive iron overload, intensive efforts should be made to improve iron chelation; these will usually focus on improving treatment adherence. Cardiac siderosis is a potentially fatal complication, suggested by the development of arrhythmias, heart failure and increasing iron stores on cardiac MRI, and necessitates intensive chelation therapy. Iron chelation techniques include:
• Venesection rapidly removes excess iron, although clearly this is not possible in transfusion-dependent patients. Venesection is often used in haemoglobinopathy patients post-bone-marrow transplantation.
• Desferrioxamine. This has been used for more than 30 years. Good compliance has been shown to improve survival. Side effects are few but include growth impairment, retinal and cochlear toxicity at higher doses. Side effects become increasingly common as iron stores approach normal. Negative iron balance is typically achieved in a transfusion-dependent patient at a dose of 40 mg/kg 5 nights per week. The main problem is that it has to be given parenterally, usually by overnight subcutaneous infusions. Adherence to desferrioxamine treatment is poor and this results in toxic iron accumulation. In heart failure secondary to iron overload, continuous intravenous desferrioxamine has been shown to be effective [15].
• Deferiprone (L1). This oral iron chelator was developed in the 1980s. Side effects include neutropenia and arthritis. The drug has been licensed as a second-line chelator in thalassaemia in Europe for more than 10 years, but was only licensed for use in North America in 2011 because of concern about toxicity and lack of efficacy. Recent studies suggest that it is particularly effective at removing cardiac iron and various regimes in combination with desferrioxamine have been devised. Because of the risk of agranulocytosis, it

Table 29.5 Assessment of iron overload.

	Description	Advantages	Disadvantages
Monitoring transfused volume	Annual review of volume of transfused blood	Accurate measure of iron input; cheap	Does not assess iron loss through chelation or other means
Serum ferritin	Simple blood test	Cheap, widely available; monitors trends in hepatic iron	Increased by inflammation. Variable correlation with liver iron
Liver biopsy	Chemical measurement of liver iron in tissue sample	Accurate quantitation. Also shows liver histology	Invasive. Only small sample of liver analysed
Magnetic susceptrometry	Magnetic assessment of liver iron	Noninvasive. Accurate	Very few calibrated machines in world
T2* MRI	Assessment of liver and heart iron using MRI	Technology widely available. Assesses heart iron. Accurate	Variable results from different scanners. Young children need anaesthesia
R2 MRI	Assessment of liver iron using MRI	Widely available. Approved in USA and EU. Results similar between scanners	Cannot assess cardiac iron. Young children need anaesthesia

is recommended that weekly blood tests are performed on those taking deferiprone [16].

• Deferasirox. This oral iron chelator is licensed as a first-line treatment for transfusional iron overload around the world. It seems to be as effective as desferrioxamine with relatively few side effects. The main toxicity involves increases in serum creatinine, which in general have been nonprogressive and reversible. There is emerging evidence that it also removes cardiac iron [17].

Key points

1 Regular intrauterine transfusions should not be used in fetuses with Hb Bart's hydrops fetalis until the risk of severe handicap has been discussed with the parents.
2 Transfusions should be started in severe β-thalassaemia syndromes on the basis of symptoms rather than a particular Hb or genotype.
3 Blood transfused to haemoglobinopathy patients should be fully matched for Rh and Kell blood groups.
4 Urgent blood transfusion is indicated in SCD in acute anaemia, severe acute chest syndrome, multi-organ failure and acute neurological problems.

5 Regular transfusions are mainly used in SCD for primary and secondary stroke prevention.
6 Iron chelation should be actively considered after 10–12 blood transfusions.
7 Hepatic iron stores should be monitored in SCD and thalassaemia using a combination of transfusion history, serum ferritin and MRI.
8 In thalassaemia major and severe thalassaemia intermedia, cardiac iron should be monitored using MRI and intensive chelation started if there is evidence of significant or progressive cardiac iron overload.

References

1 Weatherall DJ. Pathophysiology of thalassaemia. *Bailliere's Clin Haematol* 1998; 11(1): 127–146.
2 Higgs DR, Engel JD & Stamatoyannopoulos G. Thalassaemia. *Lancet* 2012; 379: 373–383.
3 Danjou F, Anni F & Galanello R. Beta-thalassaemia: from genotype to phenotype. *Haematologica* 2011; 96(11): 1573–1575.
4 Taher AT et al. Optimal management of beta thalassaemia intermedia. *Br J Haematol* 2011; 152(5): 512–523.
5 Cazzola M et al. Relationship between transfusion regimen and suppression of erythropoiesis in

beta-thalassaemia major. *Br J Haematol* 1995; 89(3): 473–478.

6 Telfer P *et al*. Survival of medically treated thalassemia patients in Cyprus. Trends and risk factors over the period 1980–2004. *Haematologica* 2006; 91(9): 1187–1192.

7 Rees DC, Williams TN & Gladwin MT. Sickle-cell disease. *Lancet* 2010; 376(9757): 2018–2031.

8 Vichinsky EP *et al*. Causes and outcomes of the acute chest syndrome in sickle cell disease. National Acute Chest Syndrome Study Group. *N Engl J Med* 2000; 342(25): 1855–1865.

9 Hulbert ML *et al*. Exchange blood transfusion compared with simple transfusion for first overt stroke is associated with a lower risk of subsequent stroke: a retrospective cohort study of 137 children with sickle cell anemia. *J Pediat* 2006; 149(5): 710–712.

10 Ohene-Frempong K *et al*. Cerebrovascular accidents in sickle cell disease: rates and risk factors. *Blood* 1998; 91(1): 288–294.

11 Adams RJ *et al*. Prevention of a first stroke by transfusions in children with sickle cell anemia and abnormal results on transcranial Doppler ultrasonography. *N Engl J Med* 1998; 339(1): 5–11.

12 Vichinsky EP *et al*. A comparison of conservative and aggressive transfusion regimens in the perioperative management of sickle cell disease. The Preoperative Transfusion in Sickle Cell Disease Study Group. *N Engl J Med* 1995; 333(4): 206–213.

13 Thompson AA *et al*. Red cell alloimmunization in a diverse population of transfused patients with thalassaemia. *Br J Haematol* 2011; 153(1): 121–128.

14 Vichinsky EP *et al*. Alloimmunization in sickle cell anemia and transfusion of racially unmatched blood. *N Engl J Med* 1990; 322(23): 1617–1621.

15 Davis BA & Porter JB Long-term outcome of continuous 24-hour deferoxamine infusion via indwelling intravenous catheters in high-risk beta-thalassemia. *Blood* 2000; 95(4): 1229–1236.

16 Tanner MA *et al*. A randomized, placebo-controlled, double-blind trial of the effect of combined therapy with deferoxamine and deferiprone on myocardial iron in thalassemia major using cardiovascular magnetic resonance. *Circulation* 2007; 115(14): 1876–1884.

17 Pennell DJ *et al*. Efficacy of deferasirox in reducing and preventing cardiac iron overload in beta-thalassemia. *Blood* 2010; 115(12): 2364–2371.

Further reading

Guidelines for the Clinical Management of Thalassaemia, 2nd edn. Thalassaemia International Federation, 2007. Available at: www.thalassaemia.org.cy.

Olivieri NF & Brittenham GM. Iron-chelating therapy and the treatment of thalassemia. *Blood* 1997; 89: 739–761.

Serjeant GR & Serjeant BE. *Sickle Cell Disease*, 3rd edn. Oxford, UK: Oxford University Press; 2001.

Weatherall DJ & Clegg JB. *The Thalassaemia Syndromes*, 4th edn. Oxford, UK: Blackwell Scientific Publications; 2001.

30 Heparin-induced thrombocytopenia

Andreas Greinacher[1] & Theodore E. Warkentin[2]

[1]Department of Immunology and Transfusion Medicine, Universitätsmedizin Greifswald, Greifswald, Germany

[2]Department of Pathology and Molecular Medicine and Department of Medicine, Michael G. DeGroote School of Medicine, McMaster University, Transfusion Medicine, Hamilton Regional Laboratory Medicine Program and Service of Clinical Hematology, Hamilton Health Sciences, Hamilton, Ontario, Canada

Heparin-induced thrombocytopenia (HIT) is an antibody-mediated adverse effect of heparin. It is highly prothrombotic and treatment usually requires substitution of heparin with a rapidly acting nonheparin anticoagulant; vitamin K antagonists (warfarin) are contraindicated during the acute phase of HIT because their use can precipitate limb necrosis due to microthrombosis. Prophylactic platelet transfusions should be minimized. Given these special treatment considerations, the challenge is to distinguish HIT from non-HIT thrombocytopenia. Management of HIT requires knowledge in immunohaematology and haemostasis. Table 30.1 lists features of HIT with particular relevance to the transfusion medicine specialist.

Pathogenesis

Figure 30.1 illustrates the pathogenesis of HIT [1]. Key features include:

- Antigens form when platelet factor 4 (PF4) – a positively charged 31 kDa tetrameric member of the C-X-C subfamily of chemokines – forms multimolecular complexes with (negatively charged) heparin when both are present at stoichiometrically optimal concentrations (1:1 to 2:1 ratio of PF4 : heparin).
- Both PF4 and heparin bind to platelet surfaces; thus, *in situ* formation of PF4/heparin complexes on platelet membranes localizes subsequent formation of PF4/heparin/IgG immune complexes also to the platelet surfaces; i.e. there are no circulating immune complexes in HIT.

- The HIT antigen(s) reside(s) on PF4, rather than on heparin; indeed, nonheparin polyanions (e.g. polyvinyl sulfonate, or PVS) can substitute for heparin in forming HIT antigens.
- Ultralarge PF4/heparin complexes are more readily formed with unfractionated heparin (UFH) compared with low-molecular-weight heparin (LMWH), perhaps explaining the tenfold greater risk of HIT with UFH versus LMWH.
- Heparin causes platelet activation and release of PF4. However, immunization occurs most often post-surgery and major trauma (perhaps reflecting PF4 release from activated platelets and/or proinflammatory factors).
- Anti-PF4/heparin antibodies become detectable ~4 days (median) after an immunizing heparin exposure, with detection of platelet-activating antibodies 1 or 2 days later [2, 3].
- Anti-PF4/heparin antibodies of IgG and/or IgA and/or IgM can be formed (relative frequency, IgG > IgA > IgM); however, only IgG antibodies have the potential to cause HIT, because platelet activation occurs only when multimolecular complexes of PF4/heparin/IgG result in clustering of the platelet Fc receptors (FcγIIa), causing intravascular platelet activation.

Practical Transfusion Medicine, Fourth Edition. Edited by Michael F. Murphy, Derwood H. Pamphilon and Nancy M. Heddle.
© 2013 John Wiley & Sons, Ltd. Published 2013 by John Wiley & Sons, Ltd.

Table 30.1 HIT issues relevant to transfusion medicine.

HIT-related item	Transfusion medicine-related comment
PF4/heparin complexes form at optimal stoichiometric ratio	The Coombs test requires an optimal concentration of the antihuman immunoglobulin antibody to achieve agglutination of red cells
Acute HIT activates platelets, monocytes, endothelial cells and the coagulation cascade	Acute haemolytic transfusion reaction activates platelets, leucocytes, endothelial cells and the clotting cascade
Typical-onset HIT (day 5–14)	Timing resembles that of delayed haemolytic transfusion reaction
Rapid-onset HIT (<1 day)	Timing resembles that of acute haemolytic transfusion reaction (i.e. due to pre-existing anti-red-cell alloantibodies)
'Delayed-onset' HIT antibodies bind to and activate platelets even in the absence of heparin	In posttransfusion purpura, alloantibodies boosted by transfusing HPA-1a positive platelets bind to the patient's own (HPA-1a negative) platelets, causing severe thrombocytopenia (see Chapter 12)
Functional (platelet activation) assays are more predictive for HIT than immunoassays	HLA antibodies that test positive in lymphocytotoxicity tests are more clinically relevant compared to ELISA-only reactive HLA antibodies
Most ELISA-positive patients do not develop HIT	Most anti-red-blood-cell alloantibodies do not cause intravascular haemolysis
Particle gel immunoassay	Rapid assay utilizing gel card technology commonly used in transfusion medicine
Platelet transfusions (prophylactic)	Relatively contraindicated in HIT
PCCs contain heparin	PCCs are relatively contraindicated during acute HIT
High-dose intravenous IgG (IVIgG)	IVIgG is occasionally used as adjunctive treatment for severe HIT

ELISA, enzyme-linked immunosorbert assay; PCC, prothrombin complex concentrates; HLA, human leucocyte antigen; PF4, platelet factor 4.

- HIT does *not* exhibit features of a classic primary immune response: even when HIT occurs during a patient's very first exposure to heparin, IgG antibodies are readily detected after only 4 to 5 days, whereas IgM antibodies usually are not detected. If IgM antibodies are found, they become detectable at the same time as IgG (i.e. no IgM precedence).
- These atypical features of the HIT immune response could reflect presensitization due to exposure to bacteria, as negatively charged molecules on bacterial surfaces bind PF4 in a way that exposes HIT antigens [4].
- Platelet activation in HIT includes formation of procoagulant platelet-derived microparticles.
- Other procoagulant features of HIT include monocyte and endothelial cell activation, and neutralization of heparin by PF4.
- Sometimes, HIT antibodies strongly activate platelets in the absence of pharmacologic heparin (heparin-'independent' platelet activation): this is a feature of 'delayed-onset' HIT [5].

Epidemiology

- The overall frequency of HIT among heparin-exposed inpatients is ~0.2%.
- The frequency of HIT approaches 5–10% when there are multiple concurrent risk factors for HIT, e.g. (a) UFH use (versus LMWH or fondaparinux) for (b) at least 10–14 days (when antibodies peak), (c) postorthopedic surgery and (d) female sex (1.5–2.0×greater risk of HIT in females versus males) [6].
- HIT occurs more often in post-surgery patients than in medical patients [6]. HIT is rare in pregnancy and in paediatric patients, and probably does not occur in neonates.
- UFH is rarely administered nowadays to post-orthopaedic surgery patients. Thus, HIT nowadays occurs most often in postcardiac/postvascular surgery patients and general surgery patients who receive postoperative UFH thromboprophylaxis.
- Rarely, a transient HIT-mimicking syndrome with thrombocytopenia, thrombosis and high levels of

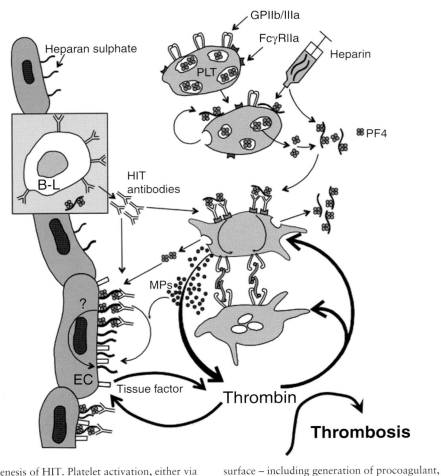

Fig 30.1 Pathogenesis of HIT. Platelet activation, either via binding of heparin to platelets (PLT) or by other mechanisms (e.g. surgery), leads to release of platelet factor 4 (PF4) from platelet α-granules. PF4/heparin complexes form, which in some patients triggers generation of platelet-activating anti-PF4/heparin antibodies ('HIT antibodies'), predominantly of the IgG class. Multimolecular complexes comprised of PF4, heparin and IgG are formed on platelet surfaces, leading to crosslinking of the platelet Fc receptors (FcγRIIa). This produces potent platelet activation, including: conformational changes in the platelet fibrinogen receptors (GPIIb/IIIa), resulting in platelet aggregation; procoagulant changes in the platelet surface – including generation of procoagulant, platelet-derived microparticles (MPs) – leading to thrombin generation; and further release of granule constituents such as PF4, triggering even more IgG-mediated platelet activation. Further, PF4 binds to endothelial cell (EC) heparan sulfate, resulting in HIT antibody binding to endothelial PF4/heparin complexes and, possibly, EC activation and expression of endothelial tissue factor (open rectangle), contributing further to thrombin generation. Thrombin activates platelets and endothelium, leading to thrombosis. Reprinted from Warkentin et al. [1], with modifications, with permission.

platelet-activating anti-PF4/heparin antibodies can occur without proximate exposure to heparin, but after infection or surgery ('spontaneous HIT') [7].

HIT: a 'clinicopathologic' syndrome

• Table 30.2 summarizes the major clinical and laboratory features of HIT [8].

Table 30.2 HIT viewed as a clinical–pathological syndrome.

Clinical	Pathological
At least one of: • **Thrombocytopenia** • **Thrombosis** (e.g. *venous*: DVT, pulmonary embolism, venous limb gangrene, adrenal haemorrhage, cerebral vein thrombosis, splanchnic vein thrombosis; *arterial*: limb artery thrombosis, stroke, myocardial infarction, mesenteric artery thrombosis, miscellaneous artery; *microvascular*) • Necrotizing skin lesions at heparin injection sites • Acute anaphylactoid reactions • Disseminated intravascular coagulation (DIC) **Timing:** above event(s) bear(s) temporal relation to a preceding immunizing heparin exposure Absence of another more compelling explanation	**Heparin-dependent, platelet-activating IgG** • Positive platelet activation assay (e.g. SRA, HIPA) • Positive anti-PF4/polyanion-IgG ELISA (infers possible presence of platelet-activating IgG)

DVT, deep-vein thrombosis; ELISA, enzyme-linked immunosorbent assay; HIPA, heparin-induced platelet activation (test); PF4, platelet factor 4; SRA, serotonin-release assay.

Iceberg model (Figure 30.2)

• HIT occurs in a minority of patients who form anti-PF4/heparin antibodies; e.g. anti-PF4/heparin antibodies are detectable in 50–80% of postcardiac surgery patients, yet HIT occurs in only 1–2% of these patients.

• According to the 'iceberg model', HIT occurs in the subset of patients who form strong heparin-dependent, platelet-activating antibodies of the IgG class; such antibodies are also readily detectable by PF4-dependent enzyme-linked immunosorbent assay (ELISA) [9, 10].

• Diagnostic sensitivity of the three major types of assays – ELISA-IgG/A/M, ELISA-IgG, washed platelet activation assay – are similarly high (>99%); however, their diagnostic specificity varies, as follows: platelet activation assays > ELISA-IgG > ELISA-IgG/A/M.

Clinical picture

Thrombocytopenia

• HIT usually results in mild-to-moderate thrombocytopenia (median platelet count nadir, 60×10^9/L (~90% have a nadir between 15 and 150×10^9/L) [11].

• In >90% of patients, the platelet count falls by >50% from the peak platelet count that immediately precedes the HIT-associated platelet count fall.

Timing

• 'Typical-onset' HIT indicates thrombocytopenia that begins 5–10 days after an immunizing heparin exposure [12].

• 'Rapid-onset' HIT refers to a platelet count fall that begins abruptly (<24 hours) after administration of heparin or a dose increase. Almost invariably, patients have been exposed to heparin within the recent past (past 5–100 days) [12].

• HIT antibodies are remarkably transient, becoming undetectable at a median of 50 to 85 days (depending on the assay performed) after an episode of HIT [12]. Antibodies have been reported to become substantially weaker within a week – with platelet count recovery – even if heparin is continued [2]. This indicates that a subclass of antibody-producing B cells is involved in HIT, which differs from classic immunohaematologic responses against alloantigens.

• 'Delayed-onset' HIT denotes thrombocytopenia that begins after the immunizing heparin exposure has been stopped or that worsens after stopping heparin; patient serum activates platelets *in vitro* even in the absence of pharmacologic heparin (heparin-'independent' platelet activation) and have strongly positive ELISAs [5]. Such patients often have disseminated intravascular coagulation (DIC). The disorder resembles a transient autoimmune reaction.

• 'Persisting' HIT refers to thrombocytopenia that is slow to recover (~1% of HIT patients take >1 month

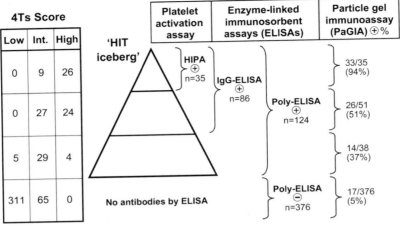

4Ts Score						
Low	Int.	High				
0	9	26				
0	27	24				
5	29	4				
311	65	0				

Fig 30.2 Iceberg model using published data [10]. The central 'iceberg' depicts three different antibody reaction profiles, as defined by a platelet activation test (HIPA) and two ELISAs (IgG-ELISA, poly-ELISA). The table on the far left shows the pretest probability scores (4Ts) for the three different antibody reaction profiles, as well as for patients who test negative in both ELISAs (bottom row of 4Ts table). On the far right, the corresponding results in the particle gel immunoassay (PaGIA) are shown. The data demonstrate that the sensitivity of the PaGIA for definite HIT (35 patients depicted as the 'tip of the iceberg') is only 94% (33/35). At the other extreme, ~5% of the patients who have no antibodies by ELISA will test positive in the PaGIA (17/376). ELISA (or EIA), enzyme-linked immunosorbent assay (or enzyme-immunoassay); HIT, heparin-induced thrombocytopenia; PaGIA, particle gel immunoassay. Reprinted, with permission, from Warkentin & Linkins [9].

for the platelet count to rise to $>150 \times 10^9$/L. In these patients, platelet numbers increase in parallel with gradually declining levels of heparin-independent platelet-activating antibodies.

Thrombosis and other sequelae

• HIT is strongly associated with venous and/or arterial thrombosis (relative risk, 10 to 15) [11].
• Thrombosis risk parallels the degree of thrombocytopenia, ranging from ~50% for patients with mild thrombocytopenia ($\sim150\times10^9$/L) to ~90% for patients with severe thrombocytopenia ($\sim20\times10^9$/L).
• Limb loss occurs in ~5% of patients with HIT: explanations include limb arterial thrombosis, warfarin-induced venous limb gangrene [13] and DIC-associated microvascular thrombosis.
• Venous limb gangrene is acral (distal extremity) necrosis in a limb with deep-vein thrombosis (DVT) that occurs despite palpable or Doppler-identifiable arterial pulses. Patients usually have a supratherapeutic INR (>3.5) as a result of anticoagulation with a vitamin K antagonist. A prodromal state is phlegmasia cerulea dolens, i.e. an inflamed, ischaemic, painful limb.

• Venous predominates over arterial thrombosis (~4:1 ratio) [11], except in patients with arteriopathy (~1:1 ratio in postcardiac/postvascular surgery patients).
• Venous thrombotic events include (listed in descending order of frequency): venous thromboembolism (DVT > pulmonary embolism) > adrenal vein thrombosis > cerebral venous (dural sinus) thrombosis > splanchnic vein thrombosis.
• Adrenal vein thrombosis presents as unilateral or bilateral adrenal haemorrhage; when bilateral, death due to acute adrenal failure can occur (special relevance for critically ill patients).
• Arterial thrombotic events include: limb artery thrombosis > cerebral artery thrombosis > myocardial infarction.
• Overt (decompensated) DIC occurs in 10–15% of patients with HIT, usually with platelet count nadirs $< 20\times10^9$/L; laboratory features include relative/absolute hypofibrinogenemia, elevated international normalized ratio (INR) and/or activated partial thromboplastin time (APTT) and (rarely) microangiopathy (red cell fragments, elevated lactate dehydrogenase, circulating normoblasts). Clinical features

Table 30.3 Anaphylactoid reactions associated with acute (rapid-onset) HIT.

Timing: onset 5–30 minutes after intravenous unfractionated heparin bolus (less commonly, following intravenous or subcutaneous low-molecular-weight heparin administration)

Clinical context: recent use of heparin (past 7–100 days)

Laboratory features: abrupt, sometimes rapidly reversible fall in the platelet count

Signs and symptoms:

Inflammatory: chills, rigors, fever and flushing

Cardiorespiratory: tachycardia, hypertension, tachypnoea, dyspnoea, bronchospasm, chest pain or tightness and cardiopulmonary arrest

Gastrointestinal: nausea, vomiting and large-volume diarrhoea

Neurological: pounding headache, transient global amnesia, transient ischaemic attack or stroke

include microvascular thrombosis (e.g. ischaemic limb necrosis despite palpable pulses) and increased risk of treatment failure due to APTT confounding (discussed subsequently).

• Anaphylactoid reactions occur in ~25% of HIT patients who receive an intravenous UFH bolus and occasionally in patients administered subcutaneous LMWH (Table 30.3). There is an associated abrupt decrease in platelet count that can recover quickly after stopping heparin.

Pretest probability scores

• The '4Ts' is a pretest probability score that estimates the likelihood of HIT based upon: *t*hrombocytopenia, *t*iming (of platelet count fall or thrombosis), *t*hrombosis (or other sequelae of HIT) and o*t*her causes for thrombocytopenia (Table 30.4) [14]. Low scores (3 or fewer points) are associated with <2% probability of HIT, whereas high scores (6 to 8 points) indicate ~50% frequency of HIT.

• A more recent scoring system is the HIT expert probability (HEP) score, which requires further validation; like the 4Ts system, the HEP score evaluates the extent and timing of thrombocytopenia, the presence of thrombosis (or other HIT sequelae) and other potential explanations for thrombocytopenia, but assigns different numerical scores.

• Pretest probability scores are especially useful if interpreted in combination with certain immunoassays so as to predict the posttest likelihood of HIT.

• Critically ill patients with low pretest probability scores may not have HIT even if they test positive [15].

Laboratory testing

Two general types of assays detect HIT antibodies: (a) platelet activation (or functional) assays and (b) PF4-dependent immunoassays.

• An unusual feature of HIT is that patient serum/plasma-based assays are very sensitive for detecting HIT antibodies, even at the earliest phase of the platelet count decline [3]. (In contrast, sensitivity is lower for detecting circulating alloantibodies in delayed haemolytic transfusion reactions if antigen-positive red cells remain in circulation; in this situation, the direct Coombs test is more sensitive.)

• A characteristic feature is *inhibition* of reactivity at very high concentrations of UFH (10–100 U/mL), due to disruption of antigenic PF4/heparin complexes.

• In the absence of new clinical events (e.g. new thrombosis, new platelet count fall), a negative assay for HIT antibodies should *not* be automatically repeated a few days later; this is because a subsequent positive test result is much more likely to indicate subclinical seroconversion than 'true' HIT [3].

Platelet activation assays

Washed platelet activation assays

• The best operating characteristics (highest sensitivity-specificity trade-off) are seen with the washed platelet activation assays, the ^{14}Cserotonin-release assay (SRA) and the heparin-induced platelet activation (HIPA) test.

• The SRA is performed in North America, using well-characterized (pedigree) donors, whereas the HIPA test is more widely used in Europe, and is usually performed with (random) donors at blood donation centres (four donors are tested separately to compensate for variable donor-dependent reactivity to HIT sera).

• Quality control manoeuvres include use of: (a) negative and graded (including weak-positive HIT serum) controls, (b) Fc receptor-blocking monoclonal antibodies (to confirm platelet activation occurs through platelet Fc receptors and (c) parallel testing in a

Table 30.4 The 4Ts pretest probability score. Reprinted, with permission, from Warkentin & Linkins [14].

	Score = 2	Score = 1	Score = 0
Thrombocytopenia Compare the highest platelet count within the sequence of declining platelet counts with the lowest count to determine the % of platelet fall **(Select only 1 option)**	• >50% platelet fall AND a nadir of ≥20 AND no surgery within preceding 3 days	• >50% platelet fall BUT surgery within preceding 3 days OR • Any combination of platelet fall and nadir that does not fit criteria for Score 2 or Score 0 (e.g. 30–50% platelet fall or nadir 10–19)	• <30% platelet fall • Any platelet fall with nadir <10
Timing (of platelet count fall or thrombosis*) Day 0 = first day of most recent heparin exposure **(Select only 1 option)**	• Platelet fall day 5–10 after start of heparin • Platelet fall within 1 day of start of heparin AND exposure to heparin within past 5–30 days	• Consistent with platelet fall day 5–10 but not clear (e.g. missing counts) • Platelet fall within 1 day of start of heparin AND exposure to heparin in past 31–100 days • Platelet fall after day 10	• Platelet fall ≤ day 4 without exposure to heparin in past 100 days
Thrombosis (or other clinical sequelae) (Select only 1 option)	• Confirmed new thrombosis (venous or arterial) • Skin necrosis at injection site • Anaphylactoid reaction to IV heparin bolus • Adrenal haemorrhage	• Recurrent venous thrombosis in a patient receiving therapeutic anticoagulants • Suspected thrombosis (awaiting confirmation with imaging) • Erythematous skin lesions at heparin injection sites	• Thrombosis not suspected
oTher cause for thrombocytopenia† **(Select only 1 option)**	• No alternative explanation for platelet fall is evident	**Possible other cause is evident:** • Sepsis without proven microbial source • Thrombocytopenia associated with initiation of ventilator • Other	**Probable other cause present:** • Within 72 hours of surgery • Confirmed bacteraemia/fungaemia • Chemotherapy or radiation within past 20 days • DIC due to non-HIT cause • Posttransfusion purpura (PTP) • Thrombotic thrombocytopenic purpura (TTP) • Platelet count < 20 AND given a drug implicated in causing D-ITP (see list) • Non-necrotizing skin lesions at LMWH injection sites (presumed DTH) • Other

Drugs implicated in drug-induced immune thrombocytopenia (D-ITP) Relatively common: glycoprotein IIb/IIIa antagonists (abciximab, eptifibatide, tirofiban): quinine, quinidine, sulfa antibiotics, carbamazepine, vancomycin.
Less common: actinomycin, amitriptyline, amoxicillin/piperacillin/nafcillin, cephalosporins (cefazolin, ceftazidime, ceftriaxone), celecoxib, ciprofloxacin, esomeprazole, fexofenadine, fentanyl, fucidic acid furosemide, gold salts, levofloxacin, metronidazole, naproxen, oxaliplatin, phenytoin, propranolol, propoxyphene, ranitidine, rifampin, suramin, trimethoprim.
Note: this is a partial list.

*In some circumstances, it may be appropriate to judge timing based upon clinical sequelae, such as timing of onset of heparin-induced skin lesions.
†Usually, oTher scores '0 points' if thrombocytopenia is not present. However, it may be appropriate to judge oTher based upon clinical sequelae, such as whether heparin-induced skin lesions are necrotizing (2 points, i.e. a non-HIT explanation is unlikely) or non-necrotizing (0 points, i.e. a non-HIT explanation is likely).

PF4-dependent ELISA (expected to be positive if the SRA or HIPA is positive – per iceberg model).

Other platelet aggregation assays
• Standard platelet aggregometry (using patient platelet-poor plasma tested against normal donor platelet-rich plasma) is not recommended, due to sub-optimal sensitivity and specificity and low test/control sample throughput.
• A whole blood aggregometry assay (Multiplate®) seems to have comparable sensitivity to washed platelet assays for detecting platelet-activating HIT antibodies if a highly reactive donor is used.

PF4-dependent immunoassays (antigen assays) (Table 30.5)

Enzyme-linked immunosorbent assays (solid-phase assays)
• Three commercial ELISAs are available to detect anti-PF4/heparin antibodies; reference centres also offer in-house assays. ELISAs are currently the most widely used tests for HIT.
• 'Polyspecific' ELISAs detect antibodies of the three major immunoglobulin classes (IgG/A/M).
• 'IgG-specific' ELISAs are preferred because their sensitivity is similarly high as the polyspecific assays, with substantially greater diagnostic specificity [9, 10].
• The magnitude of a positive ELISA result, expressed in optical density (OD) units, predicts for greater likelihood of a positive platelet activation test. For an ELISA with a positive OD range of 0.40 to 3.00 OD units, approximate frequencies of positive activation assays are [16]:

0.40 to 1.00, ~5%
1.00 to 1.50, ~20%
1.50 to 2.00, ~50%
>2.00, ~90%

• Diagnostic specificity is enhanced somewhat using a high heparin confirmatory step, especially at

Table 30.5 PF4-dependent antigen assays (immunoassays).

Manufacturer	PF4 (source)	Polyanion	Assay	Ab classes
Commercial immunoassays				
ELISAs				
Diagnostica Stago (Asnières-sur-Seine, France)	Recombinant	Heparin	1. Asserachrom HPIA	1. IgG/A/M
			2. Asserachrom HIPA-IgG	2. IgG
Hologic Gen-Probe (Waukesha, WI, USA)	Platelets (outdated)	Polyvinyl sulfonate (PVS)	1. PF4 Enhanced	1. IgG/A/M
			2. PF4 IgG	2. IgG
HYPHEN BioMed (Neuveille-sur-Oise, France)	Platelet lysate	Heparin bound to protamine	Zymutest HIA	IgG/A/M, IgG, IgA, IgM
Particle-based assays				
Milenia-Biotec (Giessen, Germany)	Platelets	Heparin	QuickLine HIT Test (lateral flow assay*)	IgG
DiaMed (Cressier, Switzerland)	Platelets	Heparin	PaGIA	IgG/A/M
Akers Biosciences (Thorofare, NJ, USA)	Platelets	None	PIFA Heparin/PF4	IgG/A/M
Instrumentation-based assay				
Instrumentation Laboratory (IL) (Bedford, MA, USA)	Platelets	PVS	1. HemosIL HIT-Ab$_{(PF4-H)}$	1. IgG/A/M
			2. HemosIL AcuStar HIT-IgG$_{(PF4-H)}$	2. IgG/A/M or IgG
'In-house' immunoassays (Laboratories of the Authors)				
Greifswald Laboratory	Platelets (outdated)	Heparin	PF4/heparin ELISA	IgG, IgA, IgM
McMaster Platelet Immunology Laboratory	Platelets (outdated)	Heparin	1. PF4/heparin ELISA	1. IgG, IgA, IgM
			2. Fluid-phase ELISA	2. IgG

*Also has features of a fluid-phase ELISA.

weak-positive OD values (0.40 to 1.00). However, at higher OD values, lack of high heparin inhibition does not necessarily rule out platelet-activating HIT antibodies.

Fluid-phase immunoassays
Two fluid-phase immunoassays have been described; these avoid denaturation of PF4-dependent antigens (as can occur in solid-phase ELISAs), potentially increasing diagnostic specificity.
• *Sepharose G fluid-phase (IgG-specific) ELISA (in-house assay).* After binding of antibodies to (5% biotinylated) PF4 in the fluid phase, IgG antibodies are captured using Sepharose G. After washing, the amount of biotin-PF4/heparin-antibody complexes immobilized to the beads is measured using peroxidase substrate after initial incubation with streptavidin-conjugated peroxidase.
• *Gold nanoparticle-based fluid-phase ELISA (rapid assay).* In this 'lateral-flow immunoassay', capillary action causes the test sample to interact sequentially with antigen (ligand-labelled PF4/polyanion complexes), then with (red-coloured) gold nanoparticles coated with antiligand and then with immobilized goat antihuman IgG. A positive reaction is a bold-coloured line, which can be read visually or quantitatively with an automated reader. The turnaround time is only 15 minutes after preparation of serum, and the single-assay design facilitates on-demand testing.

Particle-based solid-phase immunoassays (rapid assays)
• *Particle gel immunoassay (PaGIA).* This assay utilizes a gel centrifugation technology system widely used in transfusion medicine. The manufacturer has prepared red, high-density polystyrene beads to which PF4/heparin complexes have been bound. After addition of patient serum/plasma, anti-PF4/heparin antibodies (if present) bind to the antigen-coated beads; a secondary antihuman immunoglobulin antibody is added into the sephacryl gel. Upon centrifugation, agglutinated beads (indicating the presence of anti-PF4/heparin antibodies) do not migrate through the sephacryl gel, whereas nonagglutinated beads (indicating the absence of antibodies) pass through the gel, forming a red band at the bottom. Sensitivity is lower than with the ELISAs (~90–95% versus ~99%)

(Figure 30.2). The diagnostic specificity is intermediate between that of the (washed) platelet activation assay and ELISA. A positive reaction at 1/4 dilution of patient serum/plasma is more specific for HIT and a positive reaction at 1/32 dilution or greater predicts the presence of platelet-activating antibodies [17].
• *Particle immunofiltration assay (PIFA).* This assay utilizes a PIFA system, wherein patient serum is added to a reaction well containing dyed particles coated with PF4 (*not* PF4/heparin). Subsequently, nonagglutinated – but not agglutinated particles – will migrate through the membrane filter. Thus, a negative test is shown by a blue colour in the result well, whereas no colour indicates a positive test. The assay performed poorly in two reference laboratories and its use is not recommended.

Instrumentation-based immunoassays
Two automated assays that utilize proprietary instruments have recently been developed.
• HemosIL HIT-Ab(PF4-H). Using an analyser of the ACL TOP® family, this is a latex particle enhanced immunoturbidimetric assay that detects anti-PF4/heparin antibodies of all classes. In this competitive agglutination assay, the presence of anti-PF4/heparin antibodies within the patient sample will *inhibit* the binding of an HIT-mimicking monoclonal antibody (bound to latex particles) against PF4/PVS in solution. The degree of agglutination is inversely proportional to the level of anti-PF4/heparin antibodies (assessed by a decrease in light transmittance). A positive sample will therefore produce a *lower* OD than the negative control samples (the software automatically reports the results in U/mL as the inverse proportion). A positive test is a result ≥ 1.0 U/mL. The technology allows for rapid, on-demand single-patient testing.
• HemosIL AcuStar HIT-IgG(PF4-H). Using an ACL AcuStar® system instrument, this is a chemiluminescence assay that is also based upon binding of anti-PF4/heparin antibodies within patient serum/plasma to PF4/PVS. Magnetic particles coated with PF4/PVS capture anti-PF4/heparin antibodies present within a patient sample. After incubation, magnetic separation and a wash step, a tracer consisting of an isoluminol-labelled antihuman IgG antibody (or a mixture of three isoluminol-labelled monoclonal antibodies [anti-IgG/A/M]) is added, which binds to the

captured anti-PF4/heparin antibodies on the particles. After a second incubation, magnetic separation and a wash step, reagents that trigger the luminescent reaction are added and the emitted light is measured as relative light units (RLUs) by the instrument's optical system. The RLUs are directly proportional to anti-PF4/heparin antibody concentrations. Like the ELISAs, higher assay results indicate a greater likelihood of HIT.

Treatment

Treatment principles

The treatment principles of strongly suspected or confirmed HIT are [18]:
• Substitute heparin with a rapidly acting nonheparin anticoagulant, usually in therapeutic doses.
• Avoid/postpone warfarin pending platelet count recovery.
• Minimize prophylactic platelet transfusions.
• Test for HIT antibodies.
• Investigate for lower-limb DVT (e.g. ultrasound), even if not clinically apparent.

Rapidly acting, nonheparin anticoagulants

• Anticoagulants for treating HIT can be divided into: (a) long-acting, indirect (antithrombin-dependent) factor Xa inhibitors (danaparoid, fondaparinux) and (b) short-acting direct thrombin inhibitors (DTIs). (In theory, orally active direct factor Xa inhibitors, e.g. rivaroxaban, or DTIs, e.g. dabigatran, could be effective for treating HIT, but experience is not currently available.)
• Table 30.6 compares and contrasts the indirect factor Xa inhibitors versus the DTIs for the management of HIT and suspected HIT [8].
• The reader is referred elsewhere for dosing recommendations for the alternative nonheparin anticoagulants [18].
• HIT-associated consumptive coagulopathy can lead to treatment failure due to PTT-confounding [8, 19].
• Fondaparinux is a reasonable option for treating HIT [20]; further, its proven efficacy and safety in numerous (non-HIT) indications of antithrombotic prophylaxis and therapy are important considerations, given that ~90% of patients tested do not have HIT [19].

Prevention of warfarin-induced venous limb gangrene

• Warfarin and other vitamin K antagonists are *contraindicated* during the acute thrombocytopenic phase of HIT [18]. This is because their use is strongly associated with the risk of precipitating venous limb gangrene and (less often) central necrosis of skin and subcutaneous tissues ('classic' warfarin-induced skin necrosis) [13].
• Vitamin K should be given (5 to 10 mg by slow intravenous injection) if HIT is diagnosed in a patient who is receiving warfarin, especially if DTI therapy is planned (warfarin raises the APTT and thus risks APTT confounding of DTI therapy) [8, 18, 19].
• Prothrombin complex concentrates (PCCs) contain small amounts of heparin, and thus their use is relatively contraindicated during acute HIT.
• Argatroban–warfarin overlap is problematic because argatroban prolongs the INR. In a patient who bleeds while receiving argatroban, plasma or PCCs should not be given to reverse a very high INR because the coagulopathy is caused by argatroban rather than because of factor deficiency.

Management of isolated HIT

• 'Isolated HIT' is defined as HIT recognized because of thrombocytopenia, rather than because of a thrombotic event that draws attention to the possibility of HIT [11].
• Isolated HIT managed by simple discontinuation of heparin is associated with a ~50% risk of symptomatic thrombosis (most often VTE) and 5% risk of sudden death due to pulmonary embolism [11]; thus, a rapidly acting alternative anticoagulant is recommended when isolated HIT is strongly suspected or confirmed.
• Our practice is to continue therapeutic-dose alternative anticoagulation until there is recovery of the platelet count to a stable plateau within the normal range; we then repeat the venous ultrasound and, if it is still negative for DVT, we discontinue anticoagulation.

Adjunctive therapies

• *Thromboembolectomy* sometimes can salvage an ischaemic limb due to acute large-vessel artery occlusion by platelet-rich 'white clots'. Nonheparin

Table 30.6 A comparison of two classes of anticoagulant used to treat HIT.

	Indirect (AT-dependent) factor Xa inhibitors: danaparoid, fondaparinux	DTIs: argatroban, r-hirudin (lepirudin*, desirudin), bivalirudin
Half-life	√ Long (danaparoid, 25 h[†], fondaparinux, 17 h): reduces risk of rebound hypercoagulability	Short (<2 h): potential for rebound hypercoagulability
Dosing	√ Both prophylactic- and therapeutic-dose regimens[‡]	Prophylactic-dose regimens are not established (exception: subcutaneous desirudin)
Monitoring	√ direct (antifactor Xa levels); accurate drug levels obtained	Indirect (APTT): risk for DTI underdosing due to APTT elevation caused by non-DTI factors ('APTT confounding')
Effect on INR	√ No significant effect; simplifies overlap with warfarin	Increases INR: argatroban > bivalirudin > r-hirudin; complicates warfarin overlap
Protein C pathway	√ No significant effect	Thrombin inhibition could impair activation of protein C pathway
Reversibility of action	√ Irreversible inhibition: AT forms covalent bond with factor Xa	Irreversible inhibition only with r-hirudin
Efficacy and safety established for non-HIT indications	√ Treatment and prophylaxis of VTE (danaparoid, fondaparinux) and ACS (fondaparinux)	Not established for most non-HIT settings
Platelet activation	√ Danaparoid inhibits platelet activation by HIT antibodies (fondaparinux has no effect)	No effect
Major bleeding risk	√ Relatively low	Relatively high (~1% per treatment day)
Availability of antidote	No	No
Inhibition of clot-bound thrombin	No effect	√ Inhibits clot-bound thrombin
Regulatory approval to treat HIT	Danaparoid: yes (although not in the USA); fondaparinux: no	Argatroban: yes. Lepirudin: yes. Bivalirudin: no. Desirudin: no.
Drug clearance	Predominantly renal	Variable (predominantly hepatobiliary: argatroban; predominantly renal: r-hirudin)

Check mark (√) indicates favourable feature in comparison of drug classes.
*Lepirudin was discontinued in March 2012; however, it may continue to be available in some jurisdictions through another manufacturer.
[†]For danaparoid, half-lives of its anti-IIa (anti-thrombin) and its thrombin generation inhibition activities (2–4 h and 3–7 h, respectively) are shorter than for its antifactor Xa activity (~25 h).
[‡]Although therapeutic dosing is recommended for HIT, availability of prophylactic-dose regimens increases flexibility when managing potential non-HIT situations.
ACS, acute coronary syndrome; APTT, (activated) partial thromboplastin time; AT, antithrombin; DTI, direct thrombin inhibitor; VTE, venous thromboembolism.

anticoagulant protocols, however, are not well-established for vascular surgery.
• *High-dose intravenous immunoglobulin (IVIgG)* interferes with HIT antibody-induced platelet activation *in vitro* and reports indicate that its use can result in a platelet count increase in HIT. However, IVIgG is not an anticoagulant and its use should be considered adjunctive in special circumstances (e.g. severe, persisting HIT).

• *Thrombolytic therapy* may be considered in selected patients with limb- or organ-threatening thrombosis. Concomitant anticoagulation with a nonheparin anticoagulant should be administered if heparin is part of the standard thrombolysis protocol.
• *Inferior vena cava filters* should be *avoided* because their use contributes to local thrombus formation/extension and risks underutilization of anticoagulation, increasing chance of limb necrosis.

Repeat heparin exposure

- The immunology of HIT differs from the 'classic' immune response.
- Antibody titres decrease rapidly with cessation of HIT and in >60% of patients antibodies are no longer detectable after 100 days.
- In a patient with previous HIT who has become antibody-negative, re-exposure to heparin does not result in an anamnestic immune response. If repeat immunization occurs, at least 4–5 days are needed before antibodies are present in sufficient amounts to induce platelet activation.
- The low risk of triggering recurrent HIT allows for deliberate re-exposure to heparin for intraoperative anticoagulation during cardiac or vascular surgery [12, 18]. Usually, heparin is avoided before and after surgery (if antibodies are regenerated, HIT is unlikely to be retriggered in the absence of further postoperative heparin use).
- Preliminary data from Belgium and Japan indicate that patients who develop HIT in association with chronic dialysis can be re-exposed to long-term intermittent heparin safely and without an anamnestic response, once PF4/heparin antibodies are no longer detectable [19].

Key points

1 HIT is a highly prothrombotic, antibody-mediated adverse effect of heparin.
2 Venous thrombosis occurs most often, especially DVT and pulmonary embolism; unusual venous thrombotic events include adrenal haemorrhagic necrosis (secondary to adrenal vein thrombosis) and cerebral venous (dural sinus thrombosis). Arterial thrombosis most often involves large limb arteries, cerebral arteries and coronary arteries.
3 The frequency of HIT varies widely and occurs more often in patients who receive UFH (versus LMWH) and are postoperative (versus medical, obstetric or pediatric); there is minor female predominance.
4 HIT is caused by IgG class antibodies that strongly activate platelets, triggering a procoagulant platelet response; almost always, the antibodies recognize multimolecular PF4/heparin complexes (the antibodies recognize one or more

epitopes on PF4, as heparin can be substituted by certain other polyanions).
5 Washed platelet activation assays have the highest sensitivity-specificity trade-off for detecting HIT antibodies; although PF4-dependent ELISAs have high sensitivity for detecting HIT antibodies, they lack diagnostic specificity (except when strong positive ELISA results are observed, e.g. >2.00 optical density units in an IgG-specific ELISA).
6 HIT lacks features of a 'classic' immune response, i.e. antibodies of IgG class are detectable 4–5 days following an immunizing heparin exposure, without IgM precedence.
7 HIT antibodies are remarkably transient, accounting for why rapid-onset HIT only occurs in patients who have been exposed to heparin within the recent past. Also, it explains why heparin re-exposure is appropriate for patients with a previous history of HIT who require cardiac or vascular surgery, provided that platelet-activating antibodies are no longer detectable.
8 Vitamin K antagonists (e.g. warfarin) are contraindicated during the acute phase of HIT because their use can precipitate limb necrosis due to microthrombosis; vitamin K should be administered to a patient diagnosed with acute HIT who is receiving warfarin therapy.
9 Prophylactic platelet transfusions should be avoided during acute HIT, as thrombocytopenic bleeding (e.g. mucocutaneous hemorrhage) is not a feature of HIT and platelet transfusions in theory could increase thrombotic risk.
10 Treatment of HIT should focus on rapidly acting, nonheparin anticoagulants. There are two main classes of therapies: (a) long-acting indirect (antithrombin-dependent) factor Xa inhibitors (danaparoid, fondaparinux) and (b) direct thrombin inhibitors (argatroban, recombinant hirudin, bivalirudin).

References

1 Warkentin TE, Chong BH & Greinacher A. Heparin-induced thrombocytopenia: towards consensus. *Thromb Haemost* 1998; 79: 1–7.
2 Greinacher A, Kohlmann T, Strobel U, Sheppard JI & Warkentin TE. The temporal profile of the anti-PF4/heparin immune response. *Blood* 2009; 113: 4970–4976.

3 Warkentin TE, Sheppard JI, Moore JC, Cook RJ & Kelton JG. Studies of the immune response in heparin-induced thrombocytopenia. *Blood* 2009; 113: 4963–4969.

4 Krauel K, Pötschke C, Weber C, Kessler W, Fürll B, Ittermann T *et al.* Platelet factor 4 binds to bacteria, inducing antibodies cross-reacting with the major antigen in heparin-induced thrombocytopenia. *Blood* 2011; 117: 1370–1378.

5 Warkentin TE & Kelton JG. Delayed-onset heparin-induced thrombocytopenia and thrombosis. *Ann Int Med* 2001; 135: 502–506.

6 Warkentin TE, Sheppard JI, Sigouin CS, Kohlmann T, Eichler P & Greinacher A. Gender imbalance and risk factor interactions in heparin-induced thrombocytopenia. *Blood* 2006; 108: 2937–2941.

7 Warkentin TE, Makris M, Jay RM & Kelton JG. A spontaneous prothrombotic disorder resembling heparin-induced thrombocytopenia. *Am J Med* 2008; 121: 632–636.

8 Warkentin TE. Agents for the treatment of heparin-induced thrombocytopenia. *Hematol/Oncol Clin N Am* 2010; 24: 755–775.

9 Warkentin TE & Linkins LA. Immunoassays are not created equal. *J Thromb Haemost* 2009; 7: 1256–1259.

10 Bakchoul T, Giptner A, Bein G, Santoso S & Sachs UJH. Prospective evaluation of immunoassays for the diagnosis of heparin-induced thrombocytopenia. *J Thromb Haemost* 2009; 7: 1260–1265.

11 Warkentin TE & Kelton JG. A 14-year study of heparin-induced thrombocytopenia. *Am J Med* 1996; 101: 502–507.

12 Warkentin TE & Kelton JG. Temporal aspects of heparin-induced thrombocytopenia. *N Engl J Med* 2001; 344: 1286–1292.

13 Warkentin TE, Elavathil LJ, Hayward CPM, Johnston MA, Russett JI & Kelton JG. The pathogenesis of venous limb gangrene associated with heparin-induced thrombocytopenia. *Ann Int Med* 1997; 127: 804–812.

14 Warkentin TE & Linkins LA. Non-necrotizing heparin-induced skin lesions and the 4T's score. *J Thromb Haemost* 2010; 8: 1483–1485.

15 Selleng S, Malowsky B, Strobel U, Wessel A, Ittermann T, Wollert HG *et al.* Early-onset and persisting thrombocytopenia in post-cardiac surgery patients is rarely due to heparin-induced thrombocytopenia even when antibody tests are positive. *J Thromb Haemost* 2010; 8: 30–36.

16 Warkentin TE, Sheppard JI, Moore JC, Sigouin CS & Kelton JG. Quantitative interpretation of optical density measurements using PF4-dependent enzyme-immunoassays. *J Thromb Haemost* 2008; 6: 1304–1312.

17 Nellen V, Sulzer I, Barizzi G, Lämmle B & Alberio L. Rapid exclusion or confirmation of heparin-induced thrombocytopenia: a single-centre experience with 1291 patients. *Haematologica* 2012; 97: 89–97.

18 Warkentin TE, Greinacher A, Koster A & Lincoff AM. Treatment and prevention of heparin-induced thrombocytopenia. American College of Chest Physicians evidence-based clinical practice guidelines (8th edition). *Chest* 2008; 133(6 Suppl.): 340S–80S.

19 Warkentin TE. HIT paradigms and paradoxes. *J Thromb Haemost* 2011; 9(Suppl. 1): 105–117.

20 Warkentin TE, Pai M, Sheppard JI, Schulman S, Spyropoulos AC & Eikelboom JW. Fondaparinux treatment of acute heparin-induced thrombocytopenia confirmed by the serotonin-release assay: a 30-month, 16-patient case series. *J Thromb Haemost* 2011; 9: 2389–2396.

Further reading

Arepally GM & Ortel TL. Clinical practice. Heparin-induced thrombocytopenia. *N Engl J Med* 2006; 355: 809–817.

Cuker A & Cines DB. How I treat heparin-induced thrombocytopenia. *Blood* 2012; 119: 2209–2218.

Greinacher A. Heparin-induced thrombocytopenia. *J Thromb Haemost* 2009; 7(Suppl. 1): 9–12.

Greinacher A, Pötzsch B, Amiral J, Dummel V, Eichner A & Mueller-Eckhardt C. Heparin-associated thrombocytopenia: isolation of the antibody and characterization of a multimolecular PF4-heparin complex as the major antigen. *J Thromb Haemost* 1994; 71: 247–251.

Greinacher A, Holtfreter B, Krauel K, Gätke D, Weber C, Ittermann T *et al.* Association of natural anti-platelet factor 4/heparin antibodies with periodontal disease. *Blood* 2011; 118: 1395–1401.

Lubenow N, Hinz P, Thomaschewski S, Lietz T, Vogler M, Ladwig A *et al.* The severity of trauma determines the immune response to PF4/heparin and the frequency of heparin-induced thrombocytopenia. *Blood* 2010; 115: 1797–1803.

Warkentin TE & Greinacher A (eds). *Heparin-Induced Thrombocytopenia*, 5th edn. Boca Raton, Florida: CRC Press, 2013 (641 pages).

Warkentin TE & Greinacher A. Heparin-induced anaphylactic and anaphylactoid reactions: two distinct but overlapping syndromes. *Expert Opin Drug Saf* 2009; 8: 129–144.

Warkentin TE & Sheppard JI. Testing for heparin-induced thrombocytopenia antibodies. *Transfus Med Rev* 2006; 20: 259–272.

Warkentin TE, Cook RJ, Marder VJ, Sheppard JI, Moore JC, Eriksson BI *et al.* Anti-platelet factor 4/heparin antibodies in orthopedic surgery patients receiving antithrombotic prophylaxis with fondaparinux or enoxaparin. *Blood* 2005; 106: 3791–3796.

31 Immunodeficiency and immunoglobulin therapy

Siraj A. Misbah

Oxford University Hospitals, University of Oxford, Oxford, UK

Introduction

The increasing awareness of immunodeficiency and the rapid pace of genetic discovery have helped to ensure that immunodeficiency disorders are no longer viewed as arcane rarities by both clinical immunologists and nonimmunologists. In haematology, alongside the major changes in practice that have been driven by advances in fundamental immunology [1], haematologists are also likely to encounter patients with primary immunodeficiency disease because of the frequency of haematological complications associated with this group of disorders. Given that most haematologists will be familiar with the consequences of secondary immunodeficiency, either iatrogenic or associated with lymphoproliferative disease, this chapter will focus primarily on primary immunodeficiency disorders followed by a separate section on immunoglobulin therapy.

Primary immunodeficiency disorders

Many primary immunodeficiency disorders associated with single gene mutations have been aptly called experiments of nature in view of the unique insights that these diseases have provided in unravelling complex immunological functions. Currently, the World Health Organization – International Union of Immunological Societies (WHO/IUIS) committee on primary immunodeficiency diseases recognizes over 150 primary immunodeficiencies for which the underlying molecular basis has been elucidated [2]. As the genetic basis of old and new immunodeficiency disorders is unravelled, it has become clear that the same gene mutation may result in different phenotypes. In investigating and managing patients with primary immunodeficiencies, it is important to bear in mind this concept of genetic heterogeneity accompanied by equally significant clinical and immunological heterogeneity. For example, the same mutation in the gene encoding the Wiskott–Aldrich syndrome protein (WASP) may result in either full-blown Wiskott–Aldrich syndrome characterized by thrombocytopenia, infections and autoimmunity or a limted phenotype of X-linked thrombocytopenia [3]. Such examples have focused attention on the role of epigenetic changes in influencing disease phenotype.

Although primary immunodeficiencies can affect any part of the immune system, in practice patients with predominant defects of B-cell function and combined B- and T-cell defects constitute the bulk of a clinical immunologist's workload. The immunopathogenesis of antibody deficiency disorders and combined B- and T-lymphocyte deficiency is best understood within the context of B- and T-lymphocyte development. Whilst a detailed discussion of B- and T-cell development is outside the scope of this chapter, the schematic diagrams set out in Figures 31.1 and 31.2 summarize the major events in B- and T-cell

Practical Transfusion Medicine, Fourth Edition. Edited by Michael F. Murphy, Derwood H. Pamphilon and Nancy M. Heddle.
© 2013 John Wiley & Sons, Ltd. Published 2013 by John Wiley & Sons, Ltd.

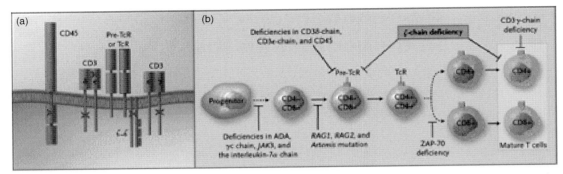

Fig 31.1 Mutations in multiple proteins, including the CD3 and ζ chains, that cause T-cell immunodeficiencies. The pre-T-cell receptor (pre-TcR) and mature TcR complexes consist of a receptor dimer associated with CD3 chains γ, δ and ε and a ζ-chain dimer (panel (a)). The pre-TcR complex differs from the mature complex owing to the presence of a surrogate chain (indicated by a dotted line) in the pre-TcR dimer. The CD3 and ζ chains facilitate the expression of the complex on the cell surface and send intracellular signals. Mutations in the receptor complexes that have been linked to T-cell immunodeficiencies are indicated with a bold X. T-cell differentiation (panel (b)) entails the progression from a progenitor cell to a CD4–CD8– thymocyte that expresses a pre-TcR, followed by differentiation into a CD4+CD8+ thymocyte expressing the mature TcR. This cell develops into a single CD4+CD– or CD4–CD+ thymocyte and, finally, into a CD4+CD8– or CD4–CD8+ mature T cell. Dashed lines indicate that intervening steps occur that are not shown. The stages of differentiation affected by mutations and deficiencies of different proteins are shown by T bars. Bold bars indicate a partial effect. ADA, adenosine deaminase; JAK3, Janus kinase 3; RAG, recombination-activating gene; and ZAP-70, zeta-chain-associated protein of 70 kDa. Reproduced with permission from Rudd CE. *N Engl J Med* 2006; 354: 1874. Copyright 2006 Massachusetts Medical Society. All rights reserved.

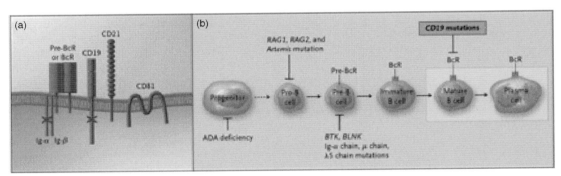

Fig 31.2 Mutations in multiple proteins, including pre-B-cell receptor (pre-BcR) and CD19, that cause B-cell immunodeficiencies. The pre-BcR and mature BcR complexes consist of an immunoglobulin dimer associated with the lg-α and lg-β subunits that generate intracellular signals (panel (a)). The pre-BcR differs from the mature complex owing to the presence of a surrogate light chain (indicated by a dotted line) in the pre-BcR dimer. Further associated with the BcR are CD19, CD21, CD81 (TAPA-1) and CD225 (Leu-13, not shown), which act as coreceptors to modulate the threshold of signalling. Mutations in the receptor complexes that have been linked to B-cell immunodeficiencies are indicated with a bold X. B-cell differentiation (panel (b)) entails a progression from a progenitor stem cell to a pro-B cell to a pre-B cell to an immature B cell and, finally, to a mature B cell. The dashed line indicates that intervening steps occur that are not shown. The pre-BcR provides signals for pre-B-cell differentiation. The stages of B-cell differentiation affected by mutations and deficiencies of different proteins are shown by T bars. ADA, adenosine deaminase; RAG, recombination-activating gene; BTK, Bruton's tyrosine kinase; and BLNK, mutated B-cell-linked protein. Reproduced with permission from Rudd CE. *N Engl J Med* 2006; 354: 1875. Copyright 2006 Massachusetts Medical Society. All rights reserved.

development and the points at which developmental arrest leads to immunodeficiency.

Predominant B-cell deficiency disorders

Common variable immunodeficiency

Of the 20 antibody deficiency disorders currently recognized, common variable immunodeficiency (CVID) is the commonest acquired primary immunodeficiency that is likely to be encountered by haematologists. As its name implies, CVID is characterized by a severe reduction in at least two serum immunoglobulin isotypes associated with low or normal B-cell numbers. In contrast, antibody deficiency disorders associated with severe reduction of all serum immunoglobulin isotypes with absent circulating B cells is a feature of diseases associated with mutations that interrupt B-cell development (Figure 31.2).

The term CVID embraces a heterogeneous group of disorders, all of which are characterized by late-onset hypogammaglobulinaemia as the unifying theme [4]. The commonest infective manifestation of antibody deficiency is recurrent infection with encapsulated bacteria, particularly *Streptococcus pneumoniae* and to a lesser extent with unencapsulated *Haemophilus influenzae*. Many patients develop frank bronchiectasis as a consequence of recurrent chest infections. Despite their inability to mount effective antibody responses to exogenous pathogens many patients with CVID mount paradoxical immune responses to self-antigens leading to autoimmune disease. In a haematological context, the most frequent of these autoimmune complications are immune thrombocytopenic purpura (ITP) and autoimmune haemolytic anaemia.

A whole host of other organ-specific and systemic autoimmune diseases may also occur, ranging from Addison's disease to systemic lupus erythematosus. Other noninfective complications associated with CVID include a curious predisposition to granulomatous disease, lymphoid interstitial pneumonitis and a 100-fold increase in the risk of lymphoma. Although the latter may occasionally be driven by Epstein–Barr virus (EBV), in the majority of cases no underlying infection is evident, raising the possibility that lymphoproliferative disease in these patients is a manifestation of defective immunoregulation.

Despite the inability of B cells in CVID to produce antibodies, recovery of antibody production has been

Table 31.1 Known molecular defects that present with a CVID-like clinical picture.

- Inducible costimulatory receptor (ICOS) deficiency
- CD19 deficiency
- Mutations in the transmembrane activator and calcium-modulator and cyclophilin ligand interactor (TACI) receptor
- Mutations in the receptor for B-cell activating factor of the TNF family (BAFF)

documented following infection with HCV and HIV, respectively [5]. This observation supports the concept that defective immunoregulation is contributing to poor B-cell function in these patients.

Given the range of infective and noninfective complications associated with CVID, many attempts have been made to produce a clinically useful disease classification based on immunological indices. Recent evidence suggests that a deficiency of switched IgM^- IgD^- $CD27^+$ memory B cells may well correlate with the development of bronchiectasis, autoimmunity and reactive splenomegaly in CVID. The molecular basis for some of the diseases previously included under the umbrella of CVID has recently been elucidated by the detection of mutations in a number of genes associated with B-cell function (Table 31.1). In addition to the molecular defects listed in Table 31.1, there are rare patients with mutations in certain X-linked genes (Bruton tyrosine kinase, CD40 ligand and signalling lymphocyte activation – associated protein) who may present with a clinical phenotype resembling CVID.

The management of CVID revolves around regular immunoglobulin replacement optimized to ensure a trough IgG level well within the normal range for effective prophylaxis against bacterial infections. Evidence from a longitudinal study of infection outcomes in 90 patients with CVID followed up over 20 years suggests that the dose of immunoglobulin required to reduce breakthrough infections is individual to a particular patient [6]. Achievement of this goal, therefore, is likely to be associated with a wide range of trough IgG levels. Early diagnosis and therapeutic intervention with immunoglobulin therapy significantly minimizes the risk of permanent bronchiectatic lung damage.

X-linked agammaglobulinaemia

X-linked agammaglobulinaemia (XLA) was one of the earliest primary immunodeficiencies to be clinically characterized in the 1950s. Its molecular basis was only elucidated in the 1990s with the discovery of mutations in a protein tyrosine kinase gene, named Bruton's tyrosine kinase (Btk).

The Btk gene is located on the long arm of the X-chromosome and encodes for a cytoplasmic tyrosine kinase, which is essential for B-cell signal transduction. Btk mutations are associated with B-cell developmental arrest in the bone marrow. The consequent disappearance of circulating B cells in association with severe panhypogammaglobulinaemia and poorly developed lymphoid tissue constitutes the cardinal immunological features of XLA. Over 400 different mutations in the Btk gene have been recorded to date but there are no significant correlations between genotype and clinical phenotype. The essential role of Btk in B-cell receptor signal transduction, as exemplified by B-cell failure in XLA, is currently being exploited by the development of Btk inhibitors for the treatment of B-cell lymphomas.

Most boys with XLA present with a history of recurrent sinopulmonary infections on a background of panhypogammaglobulinaemia after the age of 6 months, once the protective effect of transplacentally acquired maternal IgG has waned. As with CVID, delayed diagnosis of XLA and consequent failure to institute adequate immunoglobulin replacement is associated with a high risk of bronchiectasis [7].

In keeping with the absence of a T-cell defect in XLA, infection with intracellular pathogens is generally not a problem. The major exception to this rule is the predisposition to chronic enteroviral infections, including echovirus meningoencephalitis and vaccine-induced poliomyelitis. A clinical phenotype identical to XLA may be caused by mutations in the μ-immunoglobulin heavy-chain gene and other components of the B-cell receptor [8].

Severe combined immunodeficiency

Severe combined immunodeficiency (SCID) refers to a group of genetically determined disorders characterized by arrested T-cell development accompanied by impaired B-cell function [9]. The incidence of SCID is

Table 31.2 Classification of severe combined immunodeficiency.

Affected gene	Inheritance	Circulating lymphocyte phenotype
Adenosine deaminase (ADA)	AR	T− B− NK−
Common cytokine γ-chain (γc)	X-linked	T− B+ NK−
Jak-3	AR	T− B+ NK−
IL-7α	AR	T− B+ NK+
Recombination activating gene 1,2 (RAG1/RAG2)	AR	T− B− NK+
Artemis	AR	T− B− NK+
CD3 δ, ζ, ε	AR	T− B+ NK+
CD45	AR	T− B+ NK+

AR, autosomal recessive.

estimated to be between 1:50 000 and 1:100 000 live births.

Babies with SCID present with recurrent infections associated with lymphopenia. Among the range of pathogens responsible for infection in SCID, *Pneumocystis jiroveci* (*carinii*), aspergillus species and cytomegalovirus predominate in keeping with the profound T-cell deficiency seen in these babies.

To date, at least 11 distinct molecular defects that cause the SCID phenotype have been identified (Table 31.2). Whilst lymphopenia is characteristic of all forms of SCID (Figure 31.3), the circulating lymphocyte surface marker profile (Table 31.2) provides a useful clue as to the underlying genetic defect. For example, deficiency of adenosine deaminase, a key purine enzyme, results in severe lymphopenia affecting T, B and NK cells leading to its characterization as T–B–NK–SCID.

Given the profound impairment in T-cell immunity, babies with SCID are at risk of iatrogenic disease with live vaccines and transfusion-associated graft-versus-host disease. For these reasons, immunization with live vaccines should be regarded as absolutely contraindicated in these babies. Equally, any baby with SCID should only receive irradiated and cytomegalovirus-seronegative blood.

The severity of disease and the urgency with which curative haemopoietic stem cell transplantation

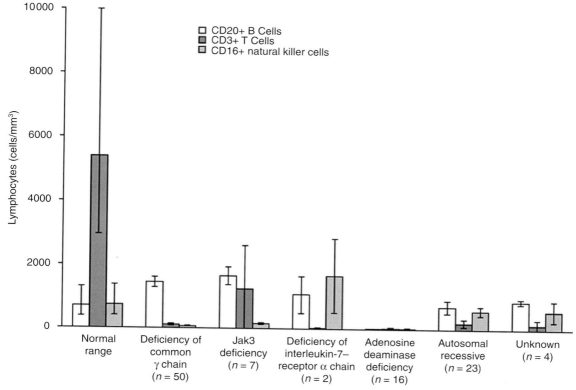

Fig 31.3 Mean (± SE) numbers of CD20+ B cells, CD3+ T cells and CD16+ natural killer cells at presentation in 102 patients with severe combined immunodeficiency, according to the cause of the disorder. The lymphopenia characteristic of all forms of severe combined immunodeficiency is apparent, as are the differences in the lymphocyte phenotypes in the various forms of the syndrome. The normal ranges at the author's institution are shown for comparison. Jak3 denotes Janus kinase 3. 'Autosomal recessive' refers to 23 patients with autosomal recessive severe combined immunodeficiency in whom the molecular defect has not been identified. Reproduced with permission from Buckley RH. *N Engl J Med* 2000; 343: 1314. Copyright 2000 Massachusetts Medical Society. All rights reserved.

(HSCT) should be undertaken has led SCID to be regarded as a paediatric emergency. The results of HSCT have improved significantly with early diagnosis and aggressive management of infections and nutritional problems seen in these babies at the time of diagnosis. At present, HSCT from an HLA-matched sibling donor offers an 80% chance of cure whilst a fully HLA-matched unrelated transplant offers a 70% chance of cure (Figure 31.4). Neonatal screening for SCID using polymerase chain reaction-based analysis of T-cell receptor excision circles (TRECs – a measure of thymic Tcell output) on Guthrie card blood samples has recently been introduced in parts of the USA [10].

In view of the single gene defects underlying SCID, gene therapy is an attractive option. Whilst offering great promise, the results of gene therapy to date have been mixed. Gene therapy has been successful in some children with ADA and common cytokine γ-chain deficiency, respectively, with evidence of T-, B- and NK-cell reconstitution in the former and T- and NK-cell reconstitution in the latter. However, the occurrence of insertional mutagenesis leading to T-cell lymphoproliferative disease in some children with common γ-chain SCID is an important reminder of the obstacles associated with this ground-breaking therapy [11].

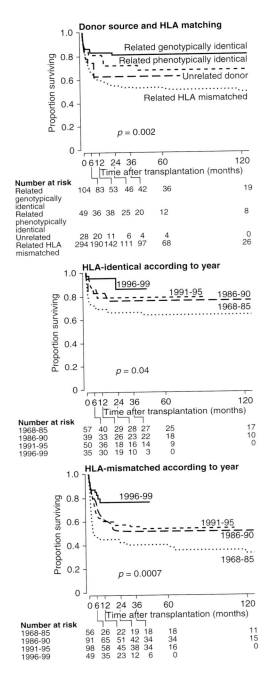

Donor source and HLA matching

Related genotypically identical
Related phenotypically identical
Unrelated donor
Related HLA mismatched

$p = 0.002$

Time after transplantation (months)

Number at risk

Related genotypically identical	104	83	53	46	42	36	19
Related phenotypically identical	49	36	38	25	20	12	8
Unrelated	28	20	11	6	4	4	0
Related HLA mismatched	294	190	142	111	97	68	26

HLA-identical according to year

1996-99
1991-95   1986-90
1968-85

$p = 0.04$

Time after transplantation (months)

Number at risk

1968-85	57	40	29	28	27	25	17
1986-90	39	33	26	23	22	18	10
1991-95	50	36	18	16	14	9	0
1996-99	35	30	19	10	3	0	

HLA-mismatched according to year

1996-99
1991-95
1986-90
1968-85

$p = 0.0007$

Time after transplantation (months)

Number at risk

1968-85	56	26	22	19	18	18	11
1986-90	91	65	51	42	34	34	15
1991-95	98	58	45	38	34	16	0
1996-99	49	35	23	12	6	0	

Fig 31.4 Cumulative probability of survival in SCID patients, according to donor source (related or unrelated donor) and HLA matching, and year of transplantation. Reproduced with permission from Antoine C *et al. Lancet* 2003; 361: 556.

Investigation of suspected immunodeficiency

Although a few patients may have distinctive clues on examination pointing towards an immunodeficiency, most patients have no physical signs that would specifically point to an immunodeficiency disorder. Conversely, it follows that a normal physical examination does not exclude immunodeficiency disease.

Immunodeficiency should be included in the differential diagnosis of any patient with severe, prolonged or recurrent infection with common pathogens or even a single episode of infection with an unusual pathogen. The type of pathogen involved provides important clues as to which component of the immune system may be defective and consequently guides the selection of relevant immunological tests (Table 31.3). Although this chapter is primarily devoted to primary immunodeficiency, it is essential to consider and exclude the possibility of HIV infection as a driver for immunodeficiency in many of these clinical scenarios [12].

In view of the complexity of many immunological tests it is essential that immunological investigations are performed under the guidance of a clinical immunologist to enable appropriate test selection, interpretation and advice on clinical management.

Management of immunodeficiency

Infections in any immunodeficient patient should be treated aggressively with appropriate antimicrobial therapy. In patients with antibody deficiency, lifelong immunoglobulin replacement remains the cornerstone of management. For children with SCID, HSCT remains the main curative option with the prospect of gene therapy for some forms of SCID. Patients with complement deficiency should be fully immunized with the full range of available vaccines against neisserial, pneumococcal and haemophilus infections. However, it is vital to avoid the use of live vaccines in any patient with immunodeficiency in view of the real risks of vaccine-associated disease, as exemplified by vaccine-induced poliomyelitis in XLA and BCG-induced mycobacterial disease in SCID.

Immunoglobulin therapy

Therapeutic immunoglobulin is a blood component prepared from the plasma of 10 000–15 000 donors.

Table 31.3 Patterns of infection as a guide to selection of immunological tests in suspected immune deficiency.

Type of pathogen	Consider	Relevant immunological tests
A – Encapsulated pathogens	Antibody deficiency Complement deficiency	Serum immunoglobulins, specific antibodies to polysaccharide and protein antigens Haemolytic complement activity
B – Viruses and intracellular pathogens	T-cell defect	Lymphocyte surface marker analysis Lymphocyte transformation
C – Combination of encapsulated pathogens and viruses and other intracellular pathogens	Combined B- + T-cell defect	As for A and B
D – Recurrent neisserial infection E – Recurrent staphylococcal abscesses and/or invasive fungal infections	Complement deficiency Phagocyte defect	Haemolytic complement activity Neutrophil respiratory burst Leucocyte adhesion molecule expression (selected cases)

The broad spectrum of antibody specificities contained in pooled plasma is an essential ingredient underpinning the success of intravenous (IVIg) and, more recently, subcutaneous immunoglobulin in infection prophylaxis in patients with antibody deficiency. Evidence from longitudinal studies in large cohorts of antibody-deficient patients and a meta-analysis of studies of IVIg replacement have highlighted the inverse correlation between trough IgG levels and the frequency of infection [13]. A similar inverse relationship between incidence of infections and steady-state IgG levels has recently been confirmed in studies of subcutaneous immunoglobulin in patients with primary immunodeficiency. In addition to its role in straightforward antibody replacement, the success of high dose IVIg in the treatment of ITP has led to a veritable explosion in its use as a therapeutic immunomodulator in many autoimmune diseases spanning multiple specialties (Table 31.4).

The mechanisms of action of high dose IVIg in autoimmune disease are complex and reflect the potent immunological actions of the different regions of an IgG molecule. It is helpful conceptually to consider the potential mechanisms of action in relation to the variable regions of IgG (F(ab')2), the Fc region and the presence in IVIg of other potent immunomodulatory substances other than antibody (Figure 31.5). In ITP, the traditional view of Fc-receptor blockade as the predominant mechanism by which IVIg is effective has recently been complemented by evidence from murine studies showing that IVIg-mediated amelioration of ITP is crucially dependent on interactions

with the inhibitory FcγRIIB as well as the activating receptor, FcγRIII. Evidence from murine studies indicates that upregulation of FcγRIIB expression occurs via the small sialylated immunoglobulin component of polyclonal IVIg (estimated at 1–3%). This observation has led to the hypothesis that the use of small doses of concentrated sialylated immunoglobulin might be as efficacious as the use of conventional high dose immunoglobulin for immunomodulation [14].

Immunoglobulin replacement in secondary antibody deficiency

IVIg replacement is beneficial in prophylaxis against infection in selected patients with secondary antibody deficiency associated with B-cell lymphoproliferative disease and myeloma. The predictors of response to IVIg are the presence of hypogammaglobulinaemia accompanied by low concentrations of pneumococcal antibodies and a failure to respond to test immunization with pneumococcal polysaccharide (Pneumovax). Whilst IVIg is clinically efficacious in patients fulfilling the above criteria, questions remain regarding its overall cost effectiveness [15]. For this reason, IVIg replacement should be reserved for those patients who have failed a trial of prolonged antibiotic prophylaxis. Despite evidence supporting the use of IVIg in secondary antibody deficiency, in practice its use has not been widespread due to the advent of more immunogenic pneumococcal conjugate vaccines coupled with improved overall management of these haematological malignancies.

Table 31.4 Use of IVIg as an immunomodulatory agent.

Disorder	Comments
Neurology	
Guillain–Barre syndrome	Treatment of choice and as efficacious as plasmapheresis (RCT, CR)
Multifocal motor neuropathy	Treatment of choice (RCT)
Chronic inflammatory demyelinating polyneuropathy	As an alternative to steroids (RCT)
Dermatomyositis	As an adjunct to immunosuppressive therapy (RCT)
Myasthenia gravis	For myasthenic crises (RCT)
Lambert–Eaton syndrome	For non-cancer-associated cases that have failed to respond to standard therapy (RCT)
Stiff-person syndrome	For severe cases unresponsive to standard therapy (RCT)
Haematology	
Immune thrombocytopenic purpura	Selected cases unresponsive to standard treatment (RCT)
Parvovirus-associated pure red cell aplasia	Selected cases
Paediatrics	
Kawasaki disease	Treatment of choice (RCT)
Dermatology	
Toxic epidermal necrolysis	Open studies/case series suggest benefit
Autoimmune blistering disorders	Open studies/case series suggest benefit
Streptococcal toxic shock syndrome	Open studies/case series suggest benefit

The list of indications is not exhaustive but covers those disorders where IVIg is frequently used. RCT – evidence from randomized controlled trials; CR – evidence from Cochrane review.

Adverse effects of intravenous immunoglobulin therapy

Immediate infusion-related adverse effects

Minor to moderate immediate infusion-related adverse effects in the form of headaches, chills, rigors and backache occur in approximately 1% of patients irrespective of the therapeutic dose of immunoglobulin. These adverse effects are largely related to the rate of infusion and/or the presence of underlying infection in the recipient and respond to a combination of a reduction in infusion rate coupled with simple analgesia. Very rarely, some patients with total IgA deficiency and pre-existing anti-IgA antibodies may develop anaphylaxis on exposure to IVIg preparations containing IgA. This risk is greatly minimized by the use of an IgA-depleted IVIg preparation in such patients.

Dose-related adverse effects

The increasing use of IVIg for therapeutic immunomodulation has been associated with the development of a range of haematological, neurological, nephrological and dermatological adverse effects that are directly linked to the high doses (2 g/kg) required for autoimmune disease in contrast to the low doses (0.4 g/kg) used for antibody replacement.

Haematological

High dose IVIg causes a dose-dependent increase in plasma viscosity [16], which is sufficient to precipitate serious arterial and venous thrombosis in patients with pre-existing thrombophilia, paraproteinaemia, severe polyclonal hypergammaglobulinaemia and atheromatous cardiovascular disease.

The risk of IVIg-associated acute haemolysis due to passive transmission of anti-blood-group antibodies has been greatly minimized by the institution of rigorous quality control measures designed to ensure that the titre of anti-blood-group antibodies in IVIg does not exceed 1:8.

Neurological

High dose IVIg is associated with the development of self-limiting acute aseptic meningitis in a minority

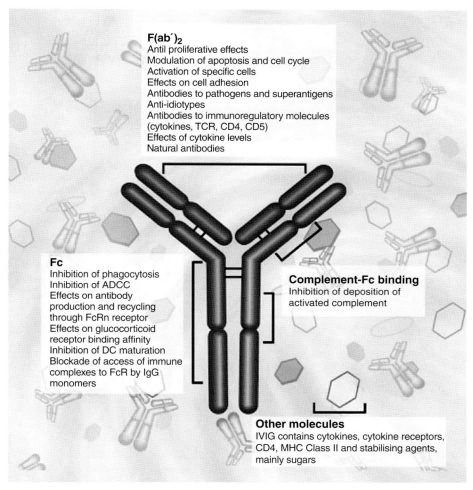

F(ab')₂
Antil proliferative effects
Modulation of apoptosis and cell cycle
Activation of specific cells
Effects on cell adhesion
Antibodies to pathogens and superantigens
Anti-idiotypes
Antibodies to immunoregulatory molecules
(cytokines, TCR, CD4, CD5)
Effects of cytokine levels
Natural antibodies

Fc
Inhibition of phagocytosis
Inhibition of ADCC
Effects on antibody
production and recycling
through FcRn receptor
Effects on glucocorticoid
receptor binding affinity
Inhibition of DC maturation
Blockade of access of immune
complexes to FcR by IgG
monomers

Complement-Fc binding
Inhibition of deposition of
activated complement

Other molecules
IVIG contains cytokines, cytokine receptors,
CD4, MHC Class II and stabilising agents,
mainly sugars

Fig 31.5 Immunomodulatory actions of intravenous immunoglobulin. Reproduced with permission from Jolles S, Sewell WAC & Misbah SA. *Clin Exp Immunol* 2005; 142: 3.

of patients (<5%). Patients with background migraine are at higher risk, raising the possibility that meningeal irritation may be due to the interaction of exogenous IgG with meningeal endothelium.

Renal

Nephrotoxicity due to high dose IVIg is a particular risk associated with sucrose-containing preparations, which trigger osmotic tubular injury leading to extensive vacuolar changes suggestive of historical cases of sucrose-induced nephropathy. The risk of renal damage is greatly minimized by avoiding the use of sucrose-containing IVIg preparations in patients with pre-existing diabetes and renal disease.

IVIg should also be avoided or used with caution in patients with mixed cryoglobulinaemia because of the real risk of the IgM component of cryoglobulin, containing rheumatoid factor reactivity complexing with infused exogenous IgG to cause acute immune-complex-mediated renal injury [17].

Dermatological

A variety of cutaneous adverse effects including eczema, erythema multiforme, urticaria and cutaneous

343

vasculitis may be triggered by high dose IVIg. The relatively small number of cases reported to date does not enable any useful analysis that might help in minimizing the development of dermatological adverse reactions.

Risks of viral transmission

Viral transmission is a risk with both low and high dose IVIg therapy. However, the increasingly stringent screening of donors coupled with the introduction of additional antiviral steps during plasma fractionation has greatly reduced but not eliminated the risk of HCV transmission with IVIg. For this reason, patients on maintenance IVIg should have their liver function monitored along with regular testing for HCV. The lack of any outbreaks of IVIg-associated HCV transmission since the last outbreak in 1993 [18] attests to the success of current viral safety measures. Unlike HCV, HIV and HBV have never been transmitted by IVIg since the process of Cohn-ethanol fractionation specifically inactivates both of these viruses.

Whilst recent reports of the development of new variant Creutzfeldt–Jakob disease in recipients of blood from donors with asymptomatic disease have raised concerns of the possibility of prion transmission by blood components, this risk remains largely theoretical with IVIg. Leucocyte reduction and the use of plasma from countries free of bovine spongiform

Table 31.5 Checklist for the use of high dose IVIg. Reproduced with permission from Association of British Neurologists. Guidelines on IVIg in neurological diseases. http://www.theabn.org/.

1 Prior to first infusion:

Check renal and liver function, full blood count, viscosity, serum C-reactive protein, serum immunoglobulins and electrophoresis. Take blood for hepatitis C serology (not necessary to delay treatment whilst awaiting result) and save aliquot of frozen serum.

Normal renal and liver function and serum IgA	Impaired renal function	Total IgA deficiency (<0.05 g/L)	Partial IgA deficiency	IgM/IgG paraprotein	Patients at risk of hyperviscosity: >4 cp (i.e. serum IgG >50 g/L or with serum IgM >30 g/L) or with background arterial disease
Proceed with any IVIg product	Avoid sucrose-containing IVIg and exercise caution; suggest using 0.4 g/kg/daily for 5 days and slower rate of infusion (suggest halving rate). Check creatinine daily before repeat dose is given	Use IVIg product containing low IgA content Check anti-IgA antibodies	Proceed with any IVIg product	Consider possibility of mixed cryoglobulinaemia Seek immunological advice before proceeding with IVIg	Exercise caution: use slower rate of infusion (suggest halving rate) and check viscosity at end of course

2 Adhere to the manufacturer's recommendations regarding reconstitution and rate of infusion.
3 Record batch number of product.

encephalopathy are measures designed to minimize this risk in the UK (see Chapter 15).

Practical aspects of immunoglobulin therapy – product selection and safe use

The availability of several different preparations of IVIg (at least six in the UK at present) has raised the question of whether IVIg should be considered to be a generic product. For the purposes of antibody replacement, it is reasonable to consider the different products equally efficacious since each product is required to fulfil the stringent criteria laid down by the World Health Organization for therapeutic immunoglobulin. With regard to the use of high dose IVIg as an immunomodulator, studies comparing the efficacy of different products in Kawasaki disease and chronic inflammatory demyelinating polyneuropathy (CIDP) have shown no difference in efficacy. Nonetheless, because differences in the manufacturing process affect opsonic activity, Fc-receptor function and complement fixation, it is best not to consider IVIg as a generic product. In view of this and the potential difficulty in tracking any future outbreak of IVIg-associated viral transmission, it is prudent to maintain patients requiring long-term treatment on the same IVIg product, irrespective of whether IVIg is being used for antibody deficiency or immunomodulation.

Table 31.5 provides a useful checklist for the safe use of high dose IVIg, including advice on product selection. Advice on individual products should be sought from a clinical immunologist.

Subcutaneous immunoglobulin

Following comparative trials, the subcutaneous route of immunoglobulin delivery has been shown to be as efficacious as IVIg in infection prophylaxis in patients with primary antibody deficiency [19]. In practice, SCIg has proven to be popular with both patients and clinicians in view of its ease of use in patients with poor venous access and minimal adverse effects, in comparison with IVIg (Table 31.6). Using a weekly infusion regimen, SCIg achieves steady-state IgG levels without the peaks and troughs associated with IVIg. When patients transfer from IVIg to SCIg, the achievement of equivalent or higher steady-state levels with the same dose of SCIg reflects the reduced catabolism with subcutaneous delivery.

Table 31.6 Adverse effects of intravenous versus subcutaneous immunoglobulin.

	SCIg	IVIg
Local reactions at site of infusion	Common (trivial)	Nil
Anaphylaxis	—	Very rare*
Viral transmission (HCV)	—	+†
Renal impairment	—	+
Aseptic meningitis	—	+
Thrombosis	—	+

*Possibly related to anti-IgA abs in some cases.
†Last outbreak in early 1990s.

The success of SCIg as replacement therapy in antibody deficiency has led to its increasing use for immunomodulation as in multifocal motor neuropathy [20]. The use of multiple infusion sites in a motivated patient has enabled the delivery of higher doses required for immunomodulation. Using currently available 16% SCIg preparations, patients with autoimmune neuropathies are able to self-treat themselves with volumes of 200 to 220 mL weekly (32–35.2 g). The recent licensing of a 20% SCIg preparation and the future development of hyaluronidase-based preparations will enable the delivery of even higher doses and drive expansion of the immunomodulatory use of SCIg.

Key points

1 Over 150 primary immunodeficiency disorders are currently recognized.
2 Common variable immunodeficiency is the commonest acquired treatable immunodeficiency.
3 IVIg or SCIg is the mainstay of treatment for patients with antibody deficiency.
4 Haemopoietic stem cell transplantation remains the main curative option for children with SCID.
5 High dose IVIg is widely used as a therapeutic immunomodulator in a range of autoimmune diseases.

References

1 Caligaris-Cappio F. How immunology is reshaping clinical disciplines: the example of haematology. *Lancet* 2001; 358: 49–55.

2 Herz-Al W, Bousfiha A, Casanova JL *et al.* Primary immunodeficiency diseases: an update on the classification from the International Union of Immunological Societies Expert Committee for Primary Immunodeficiency. *Frontiers in Immunology* 2011; 2: 1–26.

3 Buchbinder D, Nadeau K & Nugent D. Monozygotic twin pair showing discordant phenotype for X-linked thrombocytopenia and Wiskott–Aldrich syndrome: a role for epigenetics? *J Clin Immunol* 2011; 31: 773–777.

4 Cunningham-Rundles C. How I treat common variable immune deficiency. *Blood* 2010; 116: 7–15.

5 Jolles S, Tyrer M, Johnston M & Webster D. Long term recovery of IgG and IgM production during HIV infection in common variable immunodeficiency. *J Clin Path* 2001; 54: 713–715.

6 Lucas M, Lee M, Lortan J *et al.* Infection outcomes in patients with common variable immunodeficiency disorders: relationship to immunoglobulin therapy over 22 years. *J Allergy Clin Immunol* 2010; 125: 1354–1360.

7 Winkelstein JA, Marino MC, Lederman HM, Jones SM, Sullivan K, Burks AW, Conley ME, Cunningham-Rundles C & Ochs HD. X-linked agammaglobulinemia: report on a United States registry of 201 patients. *Medicine (Baltimore)* 2006; 85: 193–202.

8 Ferrari S, Zuntini R, Lougaris V *et al.* Molecular analysis of the pre-BCR complex in a large cohort of patients affected by autosomal recessive agammaglobulinaemia. *Genes Immunity* 2007; 8: 325–333.

9 van der Burg M & Gennery AR. The expanding clinical and immunological spectrum of severe combined immunodeficiency. *Eur J Paed* 2011; 170: 561–571.

10 Puck JM. Laboratory technology for population-based screening for severe combined immunodeficiency in neonates: the winner is T cell receptor excision circles. *J Allergy Clin Immunol* 2012; 129: 607–616.

11 Howe SJ, Mansour MR, Schwarzwaelder K *et al.* Insertional mutagenesis with acquired somatic mutations causes leukaemogenesis following gene therapy of SCID-X1 patients. *J Clin Invest* 2008; 118: 3143–3150.

12 Hanson IC & Shearer WT. Ruling out HIV infection when testing for severe combined immunodeficiencies and other T cell defects. *J Allergy Clin Immunol* 2012; 129: 875–876.

13 Orange JS, Grossman WJ, Navickis RJ *et al.* Impact of trough IgG on pneumonia incidence in primary immunodeficiency: a meta-analysis of clinical studies. *Clin Immunol* 2010;137: 21–30.

14 Anthony RM & Ravetch JV. A novel role for the IgG Fc glycan: the anti-inflammatory activity of sialylated IgG Fcs. *J Clin Immunol* 2010; 30: S9–S14.

15 Raanani P, Gaffer-Gvili A, Paul M *et al.* Immunoglobulin prophylaxis in chronic lymphocytic leukaemia and multiple myeloma: systematic review and meta-analysis. *Leuk Lymphoma* 2009; 50: 764–772.

16 Bentley P, Rosso M, Sadnicka A *et al.* Intravenous immunoglobulin increases plasma viscosity without parallel rise in blood pressure. *J Clin Pharm Ther* 2011, 18 July. DOI: 10.1111/j.1365-2710.2011.01287.x. Epub ahead of print.

17 Misbah SA. Rituximab-induced accelerated cryoprecipitation in HCV-associated mixed cryoglobulinaemia has parallels with intravenous immunoglobulin-induced immune complex deposition in mixed cryoglobulinaemia. *Arthritis Rheum* 2010; 62: 3122.

18 Schiff RI. Transmission of viral infections through intravenous immunoglobulin. *N Engl J Med* 1994; 15: 1649–1650.

19 Chapel HM, Spickett GP, Ericson D, Engl W, Eibl MM & Bjorkander J. The comparison of the efficacy and safety of intravenous versus subcutaneous immunoglobulin replacement therapy. *J Clin Immunol* 2000; 20: 94–100.

20 Misbah SA, Baumann A, Fazio R *et al.* A smooth transition protocol for patients with multifocal motor neuropathy going from intravenous to subcutaneous immunoglobulin therapy: an open label proof-of-concept study. *J Peripheral Nerv Syst* 2011; 16: 92–97.

Further reading

Castigli E & Geha RS. Molecular basis of common variable immunodeficiency. *J Allergy Clin Immunol* 2006; 117: 740–746.

Cavazzano-Calvo M & Fischer A. Gene therapy for severe combined immunodeficiency: are we there yet? *J Clin Invest* 2007; 117: 1456–1465.

Eibel H, Salzer U & Warnatz K. Common variable immunodeficiency at the end of a prospering decade: towards novel gene defects and beyond. *Curr Opin Allergy Clin Immunol* 2010; 10: 526–533.

Jolles S, Sewell WAC & Misbah SA. Clinical uses of intravenous immunoglobulin. *Clin Exp Immunol* 2005; 142: 1–11.

Misbah S, Kuijpers T, van der Heijden J *et al.* Bringing immunoglobulin knowledge up to date: how should we treat today? *Clin Exp Immunol* 2011; 166: 16–25.

Notarangelo LD, Fischer A, Geha RS *et al.* Primary immunodeficiency diseases: an update from the International Union of Immunological Societies Primary Immunodeficiency Diseases Classification Committee – 2009 update. *J Allergy Clin Immunol* 2009; 124:1161–1178.

32 Fetal, neonatal and childhood transfusions

Irene Roberts[1], Naomi Luban[2] & Helen V. New[3]

[1] Departments of Haematology and Paediatrics, Imperial College London, London, UK
[2] George Washington University School of Medicine and Health Sciences, Washington, DC, USA
[3] Department of Paediatrics, Imperial College Healthcare NHS Trust/NHS Blood and Transplant, London, UK

Introduction

Transfusion of children is a specialized area, particularly in the perinatal period, and requires close cooperation between experts in obstetrics and fetal medicine as well as neonatologists, paediatricians, haematologists, transfusion medicine specialists, nursing and laboratory staff. Recipients of fetal and neonatal transfusions are particularly vulnerable to potential side effects of transfusion, and a disproportionate number of errors occur during paediatric transfusion [1]. It is therefore important that staff involved understand the principles of paediatric special components, criteria for transfusion, how to prescribe and administer paediatric components, and the need for long-term follow-up when considering the consequences of transfusion.

This chapter briefly describes the transfusion management of the most important perinatal and paediatric disorders where specialized transfusion support is essential. The three sections (transfusion of the fetus, neonate and older child) discuss treatment of disorders including haemolytic disease of the fetus and newborn (HDFN), alloimmune and autoimmune thrombocytopenia, neonatal coagulopathy, transfusion support for children on paediatric intensive care and for those with haemoglobinopathies. While historical practice has been based mostly on expert opinion, there is an increasingly evidence-based approach in several areas. There is variation in neonatal component provision and transfusion practice between countries [2] and in general this chapter describes UK recommendations.

General issues

Adverse outcomes of paediatric transfusion

Reports to the UK national haemovigilance scheme, the Serious Hazards of Transfusion (SHOT) scheme, have suggested a disproportionate number of adverse outcomes of transfusion in paediatric patients compared to adults, particularly in infants and neonates [1]. A significant proportion of reports relate to transfusion errors such as transfusion of an incorrect blood component, including components lacking special requirements. For the neonatal and infant age groups, there have been relatively fewer reports of adverse reactions to transfusion than in older children, and it is likely that these are underreported, perhaps because they may have a more subtle presentation in these patients or are masked by intercurrent illness.

In the UK, a number of measures have been introduced to reduce the theoretical risk of transfusion transmission of variant CJD (vCJD) to all recipients, including universal leucocyte reduction of blood components, and there are increased measures for recipients born after 1 January 1996, such as providing imported FFP.

Practical Transfusion Medicine, Fourth Edition. Edited by Michael F. Murphy, Derwood H. Pamphilon and Nancy M. Heddle.
© 2013 John Wiley & Sons, Ltd. Published 2013 by John Wiley & Sons, Ltd.

Recognized hazards of transfusion in neonates

Transfusion of neonates has become safer, especially with the more widespread use of satellite packs. The most important recognized hazards of transfusion in neonates are:

- infection: bacterial or viral;
- hypocalcaemia (more common in neonates than in infants or children);
- volume overload;
- citrate toxicity;
- rebound hypoglycaemia (high glucose levels from blood additives);
- hyperkalemia (from large-volume transfusion);
- thrombocytopenia (after exchange transfusion);
- transfusion-associated graft-versus-host disease (TA-GvHD) (if nonirradiated blood components are given to those at risk; see below and Chapter 11).

There are theoretical concerns over potential toxicity of adenine and mannitol if given in large volumes to neonates [3], but a randomized trial showed apparent safety of these additives in neonatal cardiac surgery [4], and they are widely used for neonatal cardiac surgery in the UK with no evidence of adverse effects. Several retrospective studies have also reported an association between red blood transfusions and subsequent necrotizing enterocolitis (NEC) in neonates [5, 6], but proof of a causal association requires prospective studies.

Strategies to minimize transfusion risk in neonates

(a) Provision of special components for the fetal/neonatal age group (principles and UK practice):

- Reduction of infection risk:
  - cytomegalovirus (CMV)-safe: for UK, seronegative 'accredited' donors who have donated at least twice in the previous 2 years; for the United States, leucocyte-reduced blood may be considered as CMV-safe without in addition being tested as CMV seronegative; the precise efficacy of combining both leucocyte reduction and CMV-seronegativity to prevent transfusion transmission of CMV to neonates is not known, and there is a current observational study to try to define this in neonates <1500 g birth weight [7];
  - for UK, pathogen-inactivated FFP imported from a country with low risk of vCJD (also for all recipients born after 1 January 1996).
- Reduction of risk of morbidity from antibodies in donor plasma:
  - screen donors for high titre anti-A, anti-B and atypical antibodies;
  - for neonates who are not group O, do not use group O FFP and avoid group O platelets where possible.
- Reduction of risk of hyperkalaemia in large-volume transfusion (e.g. neonatal exchange):
  - use fresh blood (<5 days old).
- Reduction of risk of toxicity from additives in large-volume transfusion:
  - use citrate-phosphate-dextrose (CPD) for intrauterine transfusion (IUT) and neonatal exchange transfusions; saline-adenine-glucose-mannitol (SAG-M) for other large volume and top-up transfusions (in order to reduce the plasma content of the units and hence the theoretical risk of transfusion transmission of vCJD). Some countries resuspend red cells for neonatal exchange in plasma.
- Provision of haematocrit appropriate to clinical situation:
  - high (0.70–0.85) for IUT, to reduce volume overload; intermediate (0.5–0.6) for neonatal exchange transfusion; broader range (0.5–0.7) for neonatal top-up transfusion.
- Irradiation of cellular components to prevent TA-GvHD for at-risk patients (see below).

(b) The following strategies have been shown to reduce the need for red cell transfusion and/or donor exposure in neonates:

- development and implementation of transfusion guidelines;
- minimizing iatrogenic blood sampling;
- prevention and treatment of haematinic deficiencies (iron and folic acid);
- use of dedicated satellite packs ('paedipacks');
- judicious use of erythropoietin (see below);
- autologous cord blood transfusion through delayed clamping of the cord at delivery.

Prescription and administration of blood for neonates and children

There are frequent reports of overtransfusion of neonates and small children due to the prescription of blood components in 'units' rather than 'mL'. It is therefore recommended that transfusion prescriptions for these patients should be calculated in mL/kg and written up as a precise volume over a given time. Small-volume administration sets are available for transfusions to neonates in order to reduce the proportion of dead space in the giving set.

The fetus and neonate: crossmatching and general considerations

Management of the fetus and neonate in specific transfusion situations is discussed in detail below. The general principles for transfusion are summarized here:
• Prior to the first transfusion, samples should be obtained from the mother for ABO, RhD grouping and antibody screening and from the fetus/neonate for ABO, RhD and direct antiglobulin test (DAT) (plus an antibody screen if no maternal sample is available).
• In the fetus/neonate, the ABO group is determined on the cells only (as most infants do not produce anti-A and anti-B until 3–6 months of age).
• Red cells that are ABO compatible with maternal and neonatal plasma, RhD identical with neonate or negative should be used (note if exchange or 'top-up' transfusion is required for HDFN due to ABO incompatibility, group O red cells with low titre anti-A and -B or group O red cells suspended in AB plasma should be used).
• Group O blood is acceptable; units with high titre anti-A/anti-B must be excluded.
• If the mother's blood group is unknown, blood for the fetus/neonate should be crossmatched against the baby's plasma.
• If no atypical antibodies are present in the maternal (or infant) sample, and if the DAT of the infant is negative, crossmatching is not necessary for the first 4 months of postnatal life. It is preferable to use the maternal sample for the antibody screen: any significant antibodies may be at higher levels and therefore more easily detectable than in the infant plasma and it will also be easier to obtain sufficient sample.
• If the antibody screen or DAT is positive, full serological investigation and compatibility testing are necessary.

• Electronic crossmatch should only be used where it is controlled by an appropriate algorithm that takes into account maternal group and antibody screen and the baby's group and DAT. Red cells (and platelets if given) should be CMV safe and leucocyte reduced.
• Note that alloantibody formation is rare in the fetus and neonate and is usually associated with massive transfusion or with the use of fresh or whole blood.
• Gamma-irradiation of cellular blood components to reduce the risk of TA-GvHD is recommended for:
  – IUTs;
  – transfusions to neonates previously transfused *in utero*;
  – exchange transfusions as long as gamma-irradiation would not result in a delay in transfusion;
  – transfusions from a family member;
  – neonates with known or suspected inherited T-lymphocyte immune deficiencies (e.g. severe combined immunodeficiency).
These precautions are due to the immaturity of the fetal and neonatal immune system, which may lead to a reduced ability to reject transfused allogeneic lymphocytes, immune tolerance and the persistence of donor lymphocytes for up to 6–8 weeks after exchange transfusion.

Specific transfusion situations

Fetal transfusion

Fetal transfusions are a particularly specialized area of transfusion medicine, undertaken by fetal medicine specialists with the support of haematologists and transfusion medicine and laboratory staff. Intrauterine transfusions of red cells are given for the prevention and treatment of fetal anaemia, most commonly for HDFN and parvovirus infection (see Table 32.1 for causes of fetal anaemia). Intrauterine platelet transfusions may be given as part of the management of neonatal alloimmune thrombocytopenia (NAIT) (Chapter 5). Issues surrounding the investigation and management of suspected HDFN or NAIT are commonly encountered on neonatal units.

349

Table 32.1 Principal causes of fetal and neonatal anaemia.

Impaired red cell production
- Diamond–Blackfan anaemia
- *Congenital infection, e.g. parvovirus, CMV*
- Congenital Dyserythropoietic Anaemia
- Pearson's syndrome

Haemolytic anaemias
- *Alloimmune: haemolytic disease of the fetus and newborn (Rh, ABO, Kell, other)*
- Autoimmune, e.g. maternal autoimmune haemolysis
- Red cell membrane disorders, e.g. hereditary spherocytosis
- Red cell enzyme deficiencies, e.g. pyruvate kinase deficiency
- Some haemoglobinopathies, e.g. *α thalassaemia major,* HbH disease
- Infection, e.g. bacterial, syphilis, malaria, CMV, toxoplasma, Herpes simplex

Anaemia due to haemorrhage
- Occult haemorrhage before or around birth, e.g. *twin-to-twin,* fetomaternal
- Internal haemorrhage, e.g. intracranial, cephalhaematoma
- Iatrogenic: due to frequent blood sampling

Anaemia of prematurity
- Due to impaired red cell production, impaired erythropoietin production and reduced red cell lifespan
- Hb nadir usually 6.5–9 g/dL

Causes in italics commonly present in the fetus; other causes may present during fetal life but neonatal presentation is more common.

Haemolytic disease of the fetus and newborn

Red cell antibody testing in pregnancy

The three factors essential in the pathogenesis of HDFN are:
- maternal red cell alloantibodies that cross the placenta;
- fetal red blood cells that express antigens against which the antibodies are directed; and
- antibodies that are able to mediate red cell destruction.

Clinically relevant alloantibodies are almost always immunoglobulin G (IgG) and are reactive at 37°C. Women develop these antibodies as a result of previous transfusions, previous pregnancies or both. Identification of such antibodies is the main goal of antenatal screening.

The objectives of red cell antibody testing in pregnancy are to:
- identify red cell alloantibodies that are present at booking or develop during pregnancy;
- identify the pregnancy at risk of fetal or neonatal HDFN as a result of antibodies;
- identify the fetus requiring treatment *in utero* or in the neonatal period;
- identify RhD negative women who require anti-D prophylaxis (around 16% of women are RhD negative);
- ensure swift provision of compatible blood for obstetric emergencies (also see Chapter 26).

Red cell serology at the booking visit

At the booking visit, which should take place before the 16th week of pregnancy, all women should have their ABO and RhD group determined and should be screened for red cell alloantibodies. If red cell antibodies are detected at the booking visit and/or if there is a history of HDFN, the antibodies should be identified, quantified and monitored as outlined below. It is particularly important to monitor women with anti-D, anti-c and anti-K since these antibodies may be associated with severe HDFN affecting the fetus. Even if no red cell alloantibodies are detected at booking, all pregnant women should be retested at 28 weeks' gestation. Further testing of women without detectable antibodies is unnecessary since immunization later in pregnancy is unlikely to result in antibody levels sufficient to cause HDFN requiring treatment.

Partial D and weak D
D^u (weak D) individuals, rather than having 10 000–100 000 RhD proteins on the surface of each red cell, as is usually the case, have 50–5000 per red cell. This low antigen density may be difficult to detect but as they have minimal or no structural RhD abnormality they are regarded as D positive, do not form immune anti-D and therefore *do not* require prophylaxis with anti-D. Individuals who have significant structural abnormalities of the RhD antigen with part of the protein missing are described as having partial D status, e.g. D^{VI}. Partial D individuals can make anti-D against the epitopes of RhD that they lack if they are exposed to normal RhD antigens. Therefore partial D individuals *should* receive anti-D

prophylaxis and D negative red cell transfusions as if they were D negative. It is important that reagents for D grouping do not detect D^{VI} (so that these individuals group as D negative).

ABO antibodies

There is no need to test for ABO immune antibodies in antenatal samples as their presence is not predictive of HDFN and such antibodies very rarely cause significant haemolysis *in utero*.

Samples at delivery

In the case of babies born to women with clinically significant red cell alloantibodies (see below), a DAT should be carried out on cord blood. If it is positive, a red cell eluate may help identify the red cell antibody. Infants born to mothers with clinically significant antibodies should be monitored for 48–72 hours for the presence of haemolysis (see below for management of HDFN in the neonate).

A DAT should not be routinely performed on all D-positive infants of D-negative mothers as maternal prophylactic anti-D may result in a positive DAT in the baby. This antibody binding should not cause destruction of the baby's red cells, but the report of a positive DAT may result in unnecessary additional investigations and concern.

D-negative mothers with no previously detected anti-D should have prophylactic anti-D administered if the infant is D positive. A Kleihauer test should also be carried out on all such women to assess the requirement for additional anti-D (see below).

Clinically relevant red cell alloantibodies

The main antibodies implicated in HDFN are:
- Rh group – D, c, C, e, E, Ce and Cw;
- Kell group – K1, K2 and Kp^a;
- Duffy group – Fy^a;
- Kidd group – Jk^a.

Red cell alloantibodies *not* implicated in HDFN include anti-Le^a and anti-Le^b, anti-Lu^a, anti-P, anti-Xg^a and anti-Gerbish.

The antibodies most commonly implicated in severe to moderate HDFN are anti-D, anti-c and anti-K, and these are the three most likely to cause problems in the fetus as well as the neonate. Anti-K inhibits erythropoiesis as well as causing haemolysis.

Anti-D is the commonest cause of HDFN. This is because anti-D is highly immunogenic and a significant proportion of women are D negative (16%). Most anti-D antibodies are IgG1 or IgG1 plus IgG3. The presence of IgG3 alone, which has 100 times the destructive ability of IgG1, is uncommon and rarely associated with HDFN *in utero*, but can cause severe postnatal manifestations of HDN.

Anti-c is found most commonly in women with the R_1R_1 genotype (CDe/CDe), which occurs in 20% of pregnant women. Such women also have the propensity to make anti-E. HDFN due to anti-E is both less common and less severe. However, anti-E and anti-c in combination cause more severe HDFN than either antibody alone. Note that in such cases only the anti-E is detectable in eluates from cord blood red cells.

Anti-K1 is the most common red cell alloantibody outside the ABO and Rh system. K1 is the principal antigen of the Kell blood group system and is highly immunogenic; 5% of K1-negative individuals will produce anti-K1 if transfused with K1-positive blood. K1 has around twice the potency of c and E and 20 times the potency of Fy^a. Anti-K1 often causes severe HDFN; the haemolytic anaemia is compounded by suppression of erythropoiesis by anti-K1 inhibiting the growth of erythroid progenitor cells. Anti-K titres can be an unreliable predictor of the severity of HDFN. Therefore it is important to identify the fetuses at risk of HDFN by determining the fetal Kell genotype in all mothers with anti-K1 whose partners are heterozygous for K1 (since only 50% of such fetuses will be K1-positive). Moderate to severe HDFN may also be caused by anti-K2 (anticellano) and anti-Kp^a.

A number of other red cell alloantibodies have also been reported to cause HDFN of variable severity, e.g. anti-U. These initially present with a positive indirect antiglobulin test (IAT) in maternal serum; therefore all women with a positive IAT should have further investigation to identify any clinically relevant red cell alloantibodies.

Serological monitoring of pregnant women with anti-D, anti-c or anti-K

Women with these antibodies should be tested at monthly intervals to 28 weeks gestation and subsequently at fortnightly intervals. All samples should be checked in parallel with the previous sample. The women should be referred to a specialist fetal medicine unit if the antibody reaches a critical level and/or if it rises significantly. In addition, those women who have previously had a baby affected by HDFN should be referred before 20 weeks gestation for assessment irrespective of the antibody level.

For anti-D and anti-c, the antibodies can be quantified, and increases of 50% or more compared with the previous sample are significant irrespective of gestation. Anti-D levels of 4–15 IU/mL are associated with a moderate risk of HDFN, and should trigger referral to a specialist unit, and a level of >15 IU/mL indicates a high risk of hydrops fetalis. For anti-c, levels of 7.5–20 IU/mL are associated with a moderate risk of HDFN and a level of >20 IU/mL indicates a risk of severe HDFN. Paternal phenotyping provides further information on the risk to the fetus. Fetal RhD and c typing on maternal blood are reliable and should be performed where the father is heterozygous and there is a risk of HDFN either from previous history or the antibody levels.

For anti-K, the antibody titres may not accurately reflect the degree of fetal anaemia although samples should be titred for comparison during pregnancy. Amniocentesis is also not a good indicator of the severity of fetal anaemia since anaemia due to anti-K results from a combination of haemolysis and red cell hypoplasia. All women with anti-K should be referred to a specialist fetal medicine unit early in pregnancy unless the father is confirmed K negative, and fetal K typing should also be used if it is available.

Management of HDFN in the fetus

Fetal monitoring of 'at risk' pregnancies

The aims are to prevent hydrops developing *in utero* and to time delivery so that the baby has the best chance of survival. Fetal monitoring includes the following:
• Weekly Doppler ultrasonography of the fetal middle cerebral artery should be carried out to identify fetal anaemia; this is reliable up to 36 weeks gestation.
• Regular ultrasound scans should be carried out for fetal growth, hepatosplenomegaly and/or hydrops.
• Where expertise for fetal Doppler ultrasonography is unavailable, amniocentesis may be used to measure amniotic fluid bilirubin as an indirect measure of fetal haemolysis; the bilirubin is plotted on a graph of Liley

zones modified by Whitfield in order to predict the severity of HDFN and plan management.
• Fetal blood sampling should be carried out if severe HDFN before 24 weeks gestation is suspected, if there is a rapid rise in maternal antibody or if there has been a previous intrauterine death due to HDFN (fetal blood sampling carries a 1–3% fetal loss rate and may cause fetomaternal haemorrhage with further sensitization).
• IUT should be carried out if anaemia is severe and delivery is not possible due to extreme prematurity.

Intrauterine transfusion (IUT)

The aims of IUT are to:
• prevent or treat fetal hydrops before the fetus can be delivered;
• enable the pregnancy to advance to a gestational age that will ensure survival of the neonate (in practice, up to 36–37 weeks) with as few invasive procedures as possible.

These are achieved by starting the transfusion programme as late as safely possible but before hydrops develops and maximizing the intervals between transfusions by transfusing as large a volume of red cells as is considered safe. Transfusions may be intravascular, intraperitoneal or intracardiac. All transfusions are carried out with ultrasound guidance (Figure 32.1). During transfusion the point of the needle and fetal heart should be watched closely for signs of needle displacement, cardiac tamponade and bradycardia. The fetal loss rate associated with IUT is around 1–3% but is higher when the fetus is hydropic. IUT is generally indicated when the haematocrit falls to below 0.25 between 18 and 26 weeks gestation or to less than 0.3 after 26 weeks gestation. The aim of the transfusion is to raise the haematocrit to around 0.45 and repeat transfusion is often necessary after 2–3 weeks.

Intrauterine transfusion: component specification

• Plasma-reduced red cells with a haematocrit of 0.7–0.85.
• The red cells should be 5 days old or less, in CPD anticoagulant and sickle screen negative.
• The red cells should be group O (low titre haemolysin) or ABO identical with the fetus (if known), D negative and red cell antigen negative for the identified maternal antibody (in practice, if the mother has anti-c, R_1R_1 red cells are used). K-negative

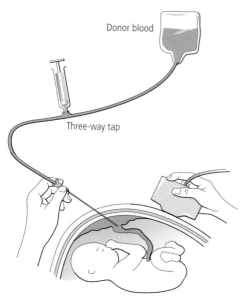

Fig 32.1 Intrauterine transfusion. Reproduced from Practical Transfusion Medicine 3rd Edition.

blood is recommended to reduce maternal alloimmunization risks.

• An IAT-crossmatch compatible with maternal serum and negative for the relevant antigen(s) determined by maternal antibody status should be carried out.

• Red cells for IUT should always be irradiated because of the risk of TA-GVHD.

• Red cells for IUT should be warmed to 37°C immediately prior to transfusion and transfused at a rate of 5–10 mL/minute.

Management of HDFN in the neonate

The severity of HDFN varies considerably from a hydropic infant with gross hepatosplenomegaly who needs immediate exchange transfusion to mild jaundice with or without anaemia.

The following tests should be carried out at delivery from all suspected cases:
• ABO and RhD group;
• DAT;
• serum unconjugated bilirubin;
• full blood count, reticulocyte count and blood film.

Affected babies should be monitored by checking their bilirubin and haemoglobin every 6 hours.

A rising bilirubin level may require treatment with exchange transfusion (see below) and/or phototherapy depending upon gestational age, postnatal age and birth weight (action charts are available for guidance; see Further reading, NICE, 2010). Phototherapy should be given from birth to all Rh-alloimmunized infants with haemolysis as the bilirubin can rise steeply after birth and this expectant approach will prevent the need for exchange transfusion in some infants. Phototherapy devices vary in efficacy and should have a minimum irradiance over the appropriate wavelengths [8]. Some studies have shown that administration of IVIG to neonates with HDFN reduces the need for exchange transfusion and it may be used for babies with HDFN where the bilirubin continues to rise significantly despite phototherapy [9].

'Late' anaemia presents at a few weeks of age in some babies with milder haemolytic disease who do not require exchange transfusion and in babies who have had earlier intrauterine transfusions; 'top-up' transfusion may be required. The blood film may show evidence of ongoing haemolysis and the anaemia is aggravated by the normal postnatal suppression of erythropoiesis.

Special features of HDFN due to ABO antibodies

• ABO haemolytic disease occurs only in offspring of women of blood group O and is confined to the 1% of such women that have high titre IgG antibodies.

• Haemolysis due to anti-A is more common (1 in 150 births) than anti-B.

• Hyperbilirubinaemia may be severe but anaemia is usually mild or absent.

• The blood film shows very large numbers of spherocytes with little or no increase in nucleated red cells.

• The DAT is usually, but not always, positive.

• It is not usually necessary to test for IgG antibodies in the plasma or on the red cells as the diagnosis can usually be easily made from the blood film appearances and positive DAT.

• Severe HDFN requiring exchange transfusion occurs in only 1 in 3000 births.

• If an exchange transfusion is required, this should be with group O red cells, with low titre anti-A and -B or with group O red cells suspended in AB plasma.

Principles of prevention of HDFN

Sensitization of D-negative pregnant women can be largely prevented by the combination of routine antenatal and postnatal anti-D prophylaxis. A dose of anti-D immunoglobulin of 125 IU (25 mg) given intramuscularly (IM) suppresses immunization by 1 mL of D-positive red cells (note that in the UK the dose of anti-D is given in IU whereas in other countries it is expressed in milligrams). While anti-D is extremely effective as prophylaxis, it cannot reverse immunization once it has occurred and has no effect on the development of non-D antibodies.

Antenatal anti-D prophylaxis

UK recommendations are for anti-D to be offered routinely to all nonsensitized D-negative pregnant women between 28 and 34 weeks of pregnancy as prophylaxis against sensitization by unrecognized small-volume fetomaternal haemorrhages. Variable prophylaxis regimens are used in the UK, either a dose of at least 500 IU (100 mg) at both 28 and 34 weeks or single dose of 1500 IU at 28–30 weeks.

Additional anti-D prophylaxis is given for potentially sensitizing events:
- amniocentesis, cordocentesis, chorionic villus sampling;
- other *in utero* therapeutic intervention/surgery;
- external cephalic version;
- fall/abdominal trauma;
- antepartum haemorrhage;
- ectopic pregnancy;
- intrauterine death (associated with chronic fetomaternal haemorrhage);
- miscarriage;
- therapeutic termination of pregnancy.

For potentially sensitizing events up to 12 weeks of pregnancy, anti-D (250 IU) is given for therapeutic termination of pregnancy but not for uncomplicated miscarriage or mild painless vaginal bleeds. Between 12 and 20 weeks, 250 IU anti-D is given following any potentially sensitizing events for nonsensitized mothers. For events after 20 weeks, in addition the volume of the fetomaternal haemorrhage (FMH) should be assessed (see below): for bleeds up to 4 mL at least 500 IU anti-D should be given, with higher doses for bleeds >4 mL. Anti-D should be given within 72 hours

of the sensitizing event. However, it may still be beneficial up to 10 days after the event.

Postnatal anti-D prophylaxis

Delivery of the baby is the most common time for fetal red cells to enter the maternal circulation and potentially cause sensitization. Post-delivery, the baby's blood group and D type should be checked, and if the baby is D positive an estimation of the volume of fetomaternal bleed should be performed on a maternal sample. If the baby is D positive, anti-D should be given within 72 hours of delivery. For an FMH of ≤4 mL, the anti-D dose is at least 500 IU in the UK (1000–1500 IU, 200–300 mg in the USA and some European countries) and following administration no further testing or follow-up is required. For larger FMHs, e.g. following traumatic births, Caesarean sections and manual removal of the placenta, higher doses are given depending on the volume of the bleed (see below).

Assessment of FMH

The acid elution (Kleihauer) test may be used for screening and initial quantification of an FMH. The principle of the Kleihauer test is that HbF-containing fetal red cells resist acid elution and therefore on staining appear dark pink in comparison to the unstained HbA-containing 'ghost' cells. By counting the numbers of pink-staining HbF-containing cells in several low power fields, having ascertained that the cells on the film are at a sufficient density, an initial estimate of the size of FMH can be made. Current UK guidelines [10] recommend that if <10 fetal cells are seen in 25 low power fields in the semi-quantitative Kleihauer test it can be assumed that the volume of FMH is <2 mL, but if there are ≥10 fetal cells accurate quantification is required. This may be performed by Kleihauer using higher power cell counting, but should also be confirmed by quantification of D-positive cells by flow cytometry. (Note that maternal hereditary persistence of fetal haemoglobin (HPFH) may cause a false positive Kleihauer to maternal HbF-containing red cells.)

Large fetomaternal bleeds

FMH ≥4 mL are considered to be 'significant' bleeds; 0.8% of women have an FMH of greater than 4 mL and 0.3% greater than 15 mL at delivery. If the bleed is ≥4 mL but less than the volume covered by the standard anti-D dose in use:

• a repeat test for fetal cells should be carried out on the mother 72 hours after the initial anti-D injection (if given IM, at 48 hours if intravenous) to confirm that the dose was sufficient;

• if fetal cells are still present and the baby is confirmed as D positive, repeat flow cytometry quantitation should be undertaken and further anti-D given to cover the remaining fetal cells; repeat testing for fetal cells should be performed at 72 hours with further anti-D and testing if necessary until no fetal cells are detected.

If the bleed is ≥4 mL and greater than the FMH volume that would be covered by the standard anti-D dose given, additional anti-D is required and there should be follow-up at 72 hours to check for clearance of fetal cells as above.

• The additional dose of anti-D required is 125 IU/mL for each additional mL of fetal red cells not already covered.

• For large bleeds, intravenous anti-D may be considered following specialist advice, and there is a different dose calculation.

Anti-D is not indicated in the following circumstances:

• patients who are already sensitized;
• those classified as weak D (e.g. D^u);
• if the infant is D negative;
• for women not capable of child-bearing (following transfusion of D-positive blood);
• for complete abortions <12 weeks gestation if there has been no surgical treatment.

It is possible that determination of fetal D type by molecular typing of free fetal DNA will be in widespread use for all pregnant D-negative women in the future to avoid giving unnecessary anti-D to women with a D-negative fetus.

Fetal platelet transfusion – neonatal alloimmune thrombocytopenia (NAIT)

NAIT is analogous to HDFN, with maternal alloantibodies to antigens on fetal platelets causing immune destruction both *in utero* and postnatally (for details see Chapter 5). Alloantibodies to HPA-1a, HPA-5b and HPA-3a account for almost all cases of

NAIT, the commonest being anti-HPA-1a (80–90% of cases). The main clinical problem in NAIT is intracranial haemorrhage, occurring in 10% of cases with long-term neurodevelopmental sequelae in 20% of survivors. The diagnosis of NAIT is made by demonstrating platelet alloantibodies in maternal plasma and incompatibility between parental platelet antigen genotypes (see Chapter 5).

Management of pregnancies at risk for NAIT (see also Chapter 5)

Prenatal management of NAIT remains controversial and all pregnancies should be monitored in a specialist fetal medicine centre with experience of NAIT.

• The principal options that have been used are an invasive approach using fetal transfusion with HPA-compatible platelets or a noninvasive approach relying on treatment of the mother with intravenous IgG and/or steroids. The latter approach is now recommended in most cases because of the risks associated with fetal blood sampling and transfusion.

• Platelets for intrauterine transfusion need to be HPA compatible with maternal antibody and hyperconcentrated to a platelet count of at least 2000×10^9/L. They must also be irradiated.

Management of neonate with suspected NAIT

• The platelet count must be monitored for at least 72 hours after birth as it may continue to fall during this time.

• Severely thrombocytopenic babies (platelets <30 × 10^9/L) with suspected or confirmed NAIT should be transfused with HPA-compatible platelets (HPA-1a/5b negative are available 'off the shelf' from transfusion centres in the UK).

• Babies with an intracranial haemorrhage in association with NAIT should have their platelet count maintained above 50×10^9/L with HPA-compatible platelets.

• If there is ongoing severe thrombocytopenia, intravenous IgG (total dose 2 g/kg over 2–5 days) may reduce the need for platelet transfusions until spontaneous recovery occurs 1–6 weeks after birth. However, it is only effective in about 75% of cases and the response is delayed for 24–48 hours.

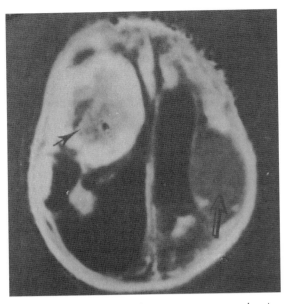

Fig 32.2 MRI studies: inversion recovery sequence showing subacute haematoma (black arrow) and chronic haematoma (open arrow). Adapted from de Vries LS, Connell J, Bydder GM *et al.* Recurrent intracranial haemorrhages *in utero* in an infant with alloimmune thrombocytopenia. Case report. *Br J Obstet Gynaecol* 1988; 95(3): 299–302.

• All babies with severe thrombocytopenia due to NAIT should have a cranial ultrasound to look for evidence of intracranial haemorrhage (Figure 32.2).

Neonatal transfusions

Red cells

Red cell transfusions to neonates may be:
• large volume, occurring once/twice:
  – exchange transfusion (80–200 mL/kg);
  – surgery, e.g. cardiac, extracorporeal membrane oxygenation (ECMO);
• small volume top-ups (most common, 10–20 mL/kg) occurring often through neonatal hospitalization.

Neonatal exchange transfusions

Exchange transfusion is used to treat severe anaemia at birth, particularly in the presence of heart failure and severe hyperbilirubinaemia. In the case of anaemia alone, a single volume (80–100 mL/kg) exchange is sufficient. For hyperbilirubinaemia, such as in HDFN,

the aim is to remove both antibody-coated red cells and excess bilirubin. Double-volume exchange (160–200 mL/kg) gives the best reduction in bilirubin (50%) and removes 90% of the infant's circulating RhD-positive cells. The pH of reconstituted whole blood or plasma-reduced red cells up to 5 days post-collection and storage used in exchange transfusion is around 7.0, which does not cause acidosis in the infant.

Exchange transfusion is a specialist procedure and should be undertaken only by experienced staff. The incidence of HDFN is declining partly due to the introduction of routine antenatal anti-D prophylaxis, so expertise in exchange transfusions is also reduced. Neonatal units should have access to written protocols. As neonatal red cells for exchange have a limited shelf life and the clinical situation can change rapidly, it is important that there is good liaison between laboratory staff, clinical haematologists and neonatologists to ensure timely provision of this specialized resource.

Indications for exchange transfusion

Hyperbilirubinaemia
Transfusions are indicated:
• when the serum bilirubin level indicates it is a necessity, at a threshold depending on the gestational and postnatal age of the baby (see the example of UK recommended treatment threshold graphs in Figure 32.3) and/or
• when there are clinical features and signs of acute bilirubin encephalopathy.

Anaemia
Evidence of anaemia is shown:
• when the cord haemoglobin is less than 8 g/dL.

Exchange transfusion in the neonate: component specification

• Plasma-reduced red cells with a haematocrit of 0.5–0.6 are recommended as packed cells may have a haematocrit up to 0.75 and cause a very high post-exchange haematocrit.
• The red cells should be less than 5 days old, collected into CPD anticoagulant, sickle screen negative, Kell negative. Some countries use reconstituted whole blood with red cells resuspended in plasma.
• The most recent British Committee for Standards in Haematology (BCSH) guidelines [11] state that

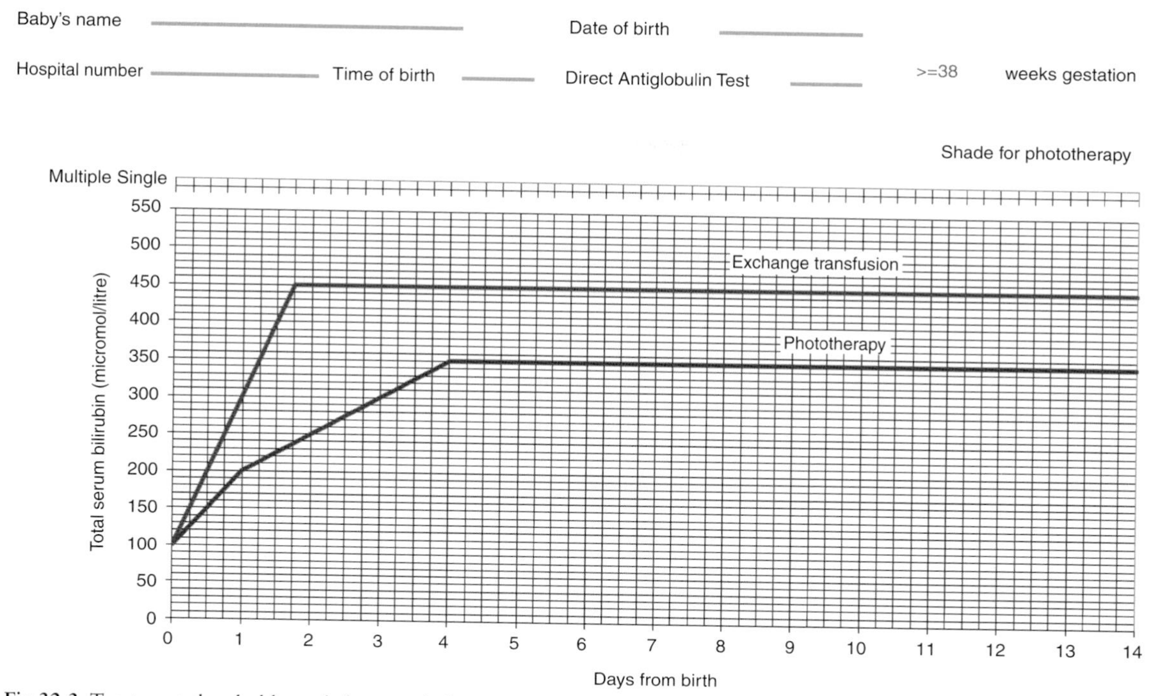

Baby's name _____   Date of birth _____

Hospital number _____   Time of birth _____   Direct Antiglobulin Test _____   >=38   weeks gestation

Shade for phototherapy

Fig 32.3 Treatment threshold graph for term babies with neonatal jaundice. *From:* National Institute for Health and Clinical Excellence (2010) *CG 98 Neonatal jaundice.* London: NICE. Available from www.nice.org.uk/guidance/CG98. Reproduced with permission.

red cells for neonatal exchange transfusion should be gamma-irradiated (and transfused within 24 hours of irradiation); gamma-irradiation is essential in the case of neonates who have previously received IUT and in all other cases is advisable unless to do so would lead to clinically relevant delay.

• Red cells for exchange should be warmed to 37°C immediately prior to transfusion.

Other large-volume neonatal transfusions

Large-volume transfusions, where the volume transfused approximates to the neonatal blood volume, are used for cardiac surgery and occasionally other surgery including for NEC. In the UK, the component provided for this situation has the same specification as for neonatal top-up transfusions and should be used within 5 days of donation (24 hours post-irradiation if required) in order to reduce the risk of hyperkalaemia in the recipient.

Neonatal resuscitation for severe anaemia post-delivery rarely requires a 'large-volume transfusion'

and many centres keep blood suitable for neonatal top-up transfusions on the labour ward for this indication.

Neonatal 'top-up' transfusions

Small-volume 'top-up' transfusions are commonly given to low birth weight preterm babies, with up to 80% of those weighing <1500 g at birth receiving at least one transfusion. These infants become anaemic in early life due to repeated iatrogenic losses, reduced red cell life span, low endogenous erythropoietin and a hyporegenerative bone marrow (see Table 32.2 for a summary of indications for transfusion). Strategies to limit transfusion including point-of-care testing have had limited success to date. Other attempts at delayed cord clamping and autologous placental transfusion have had a minor impact on allogeneic transfusion with potential risks [12].

Two recent randomized trials to investigate optimal transfusion triggers have had contradictory outcomes. These trials compared restrictive versus liberal

357

transfusion triggers for preterm infants (Iowa trial [13]; PINT trial [14]). Both had similar restrictive transfusion thresholds, but the Iowa liberal thresholds were higher than those for PINT. At short-term follow-up, the Iowa trial showed more frequent adverse neurological outcomes and incidence of apnoeas in the restrictive transfusion group, but that was not the case for the PINT trial. At 18–21 month follow-up in the PINT trial, there was a statistically significant cognitive delay for those in the restrictive group [15], supporting the suggestion that liberal transfusions may be neuroprotective. However, at an average 12-year follow-up of the Iowa group by MRI, the brain volumes of the liberally transfused but not the restrictive group were significantly smaller than controls, giving the opposite conclusion to PINT [16]. Overall, the use of restrictive thresholds only resulted in modest reductions in exposure to transfusion. A recent Cochrane review has concluded that it is prudent not to use triggers outside the restrictive and liberal thresholds in the studies described above until further trials are completed [17].

Guidelines for triggers for 'top-up' transfusion have been devised by committees in a number of countries, including the UK, Canada and the USA. Since there has been little objective evidence to guide practice, these guidelines are based on clinical experience and represent consensus views. Table 32.2 summarizes the indications for 'top-up' transfusions agreed by the BCSH neonatal and paediatric guidelines [18] and used in many UK neonatal intensive care units. These UK guidelines are in general closer to the restrictive than the liberal thresholds in the recent trials.

Table 32.2 Indications for neonatal 'top-up' transfusions. Adapted from British Committee for Standards in Haematology guidelines [18].

Clinical situation	Transfuse at
• Anaemia in the first 24 hours	Hb <12 g/dL
• Neonate receiving mechanical ventilation	Hb <12 g/dL
• Acute blood loss	10% blood volume lost
• Oxygen dependency (not ventilated)	Hb <8–10 g/dL
• Late anaemia, stable patient (off oxygen)	Hb 7 g/dL

Neonatal 'top-up' transfusions: component specification

• Small-volume 'top-up' transfusions can be given without further testing provided that there are no atypical maternal antibodies in maternal/infant serum and the infant's DAT is negative.
• Hct 0.5–0.7.
• CMV seronegative in the UK.
• The red cells should be ≤35 days old (in SAG-M).
• 'Paedipacks' (aliquotted donations from a single unit) should be used wherever possible for repeated transfusions to minimize donor exposure.
• The volume of a neonatal 'top-up' transfusion is usually 10–20 mL/kg.

Role of erythropoietin in reducing neonatal red cell transfusion

There have been numerous clinical trials of erythropoietin for the prevention or amelioration of neonatal anaemia, particularly anaemia of prematurity, since endogenous erythropoietin production is low in preterm babies for the first 6–8 weeks of life. These trials show that erythropoietin (250 units/kg/day 3 times per week for the first 6 weeks of life) can reduce red cell transfusions in well preterm babies but has a negligible effect on transfusion requirements of sick preterm babies, particularly those of less than 26 weeks gestation at birth. In practice, this means that erythropoietin has a limited role in neonates as it works best in those that need it least.

Therefore most neonatal units no longer use erythropoietin routinely. The situations in which erythropoietin can be useful are:
• in neonates whose parents refuse permission to use blood components;
• to prevent 'late anaemia' in babies with HDFN.

T antigen activation

Severe haemolytic transfusion reactions are occasionally seen in neonates or young children transfused with adult blood or fresh frozen plasma containing anti-T antibodies. This may be due to exposure or 'activation' of the T antigen on neonatal red cells, usually as a result of infection with clostridia, streptococci or pneumococci and/or in association with NEC. Up to 25% of infants with NEC have T antigen activation but so do many healthy neonates and haemolysis is extremely rare [19]. Therefore, although there remains some controversy, the majority of centres worldwide consider that no special provision for neonates with NEC is necessary and neither screen neonates for T activation nor donors for high titre anti-T.

Neonatal platelet transfusions

Neonatal thrombocytopenia

Severe thrombocytopenia (platelets $<50 \times 10^9$/L) occurs in ~2–5% of neonates on neonatal units. It is much more common in sick preterm infants, 30–40% of whom will develop thrombocytopenia in the first 4 weeks of life. Causes of neonatal thrombocytopenia are shown in Table 32.3. The most common cause presenting in the first few days of life is that associated with intrauterine growth restriction or maternal hypertension; however, the most important cause of severe thrombocytopenia (platelets $< 50 \times 10^9$/L) at birth is neonatal alloimmune thrombocytopenia (NAIT).

Table 32.3 Causes of neonatal thrombocytopenia.

Early onset (< 72 hours after birth)
Placental insufficiency (PET, IUGR, diabetes)
NAIT
Birth asphyxia
Perinatal infection (group B strep, *E. coli*, listeria)
Congenital infection (CMV, toxoplasmosis, rubella)
Maternal autoimmune (ITP, SLE)
Severe Rhesus HDFN
Thrombosis (renal vein, aortic)
Aneuploidy (trisomy – 21, 18, 13)
Congenital/inherited (TAR, Wiskott–Aldrich)
Late onset (>72 hours after birth)
Bacterial and fungal sepsis
Necrotizing enterocolitis
Congenital infection (CMV, toxoplasmosis, rubella)
Maternal autoimmune (ITP, SLE)
Congenital/inherited (TAR, Wiskott–Aldrich)

The most common causes are in bold type.
PET, pre-eclampsia; IUGR, intrauterine growth restriction; NAIT, neonatal alloimmune thrombocytopenia; strep, streptococcus; CMV, cytomegalovirus; ITP, idiopathic thrombocytopenic purpura; SLE, systemic lupus erythematosis; HDFN, haemolytic disease of the fetus and newborn; TAR, thrombocytopenia with absent radii.

Investigation of neonatal thrombocytopenia

In most cases the following tests will identify the diagnosis.
• Full blood count and film. The combination of erythroblastosis, high Hb, mild neutropenia without neutrophil left shift suggests that the cause is intrauterine growth restriction and/or maternal hypertension. However, neutrophil left shift and toxic granulation with more severe thrombocytopenia suggests that the cause is bacterial infection with or without DIC.
• Congenital infection screen. The most common congenital infection associated with neonatal thrombocytopenia is CMV.

Screening for NAIT should be carried out in any case of severe thrombocytopenia (platelets $<50 \times 10^9$/L) presenting in the first week of life unless there is very clear evidence of acute infection.

Neonatal thrombocytopenia due to maternal ITP

• Around 10% of infants of mothers with ITP or SLE develop neonatal thrombocytopenia secondary to transplacental passage of maternal platelet autoantibodies.
• Fetal platelet counts cannot be reliably predicted from maternal platelet counts nor from platelet serology.
• Thrombocytopenia is usually mild and intracranial haemorrhage occurs in less than 1% of at-risk babies.
• Platelet counts of babies born to mothers with ITP or SLE should be checked at birth and monitored daily for 2–3 days if below 200×10^9/L at birth.
• If the baby is well, treatment is unnecessary unless the platelet count falls below 20×10^9/L.
• Severe thrombocytopenia (platelets $<20 \times 10^9$/L): treatment with intravenous IgG (single dose 1 g/kg, repeated if necessary) is usually effective.
• Cranial ultrasound to look for intracranial haemorrhage should be performed in all neonates with severe thrombocytopenia.
• Platelet transfusion is reserved for life-threatening haemorrhage and should be given in conjunction with intravenous IgG.

Indications for platelet transfusion in neonates

Published guidelines for neonatal platelet transfusion acknowledge the lack of evidence on which to base

Table 32.4 Guidelines for platelet transfusion in neonatal thrombocytopenia.

- Platelet count $<30 \times 10^9$/L in otherwise well infants, including NAIT if no evidence of bleeding and no family history of intracranial haemorrhage
- Platelet count $<50 \times 10^9$/L in infants with:
  - clinical instability
  - concurrent coagulopathy
  - birth weight <1000 g and age <1 week
  - previous major bleeding (e.g. GMH-IVH)
  - current minor bleeding (e.g. petechiae)
  - planned surgery or exchange transfusion
  - platelet count falling and likely to fall below 30
  - NAIT if previous affected sibling with ICH
- Platelet count $<100 \times 10^9$/L in infants with: major bleeding

recommendations and aim for a safe approach. Suggested guidelines based on clinical experience are shown in Table 32.4. Some evidence suggests that prophylactic platelet transfusions are not required for healthy neonates until the platelet count falls to $20–30 \times 10^9$/L. However, a higher trigger level $(50 \times 10^9$/L) should be used for babies with the greatest risk of haemorrhage, especially extremely low birth weight neonates (<1000 g) in the first week of life.

A recent prospective observational study of outcomes of neonates with platelets below 60×10^9/L showed that although a third of these patients developed thrombocytopenia of $<20 \times 10^9$/L, only 9% developed major haemorrhage [20]. Those patients with major haemorrhage were mostly <28 weeks gestational age within the first 14 days of life. Prospective randomized trial data are required to inform future guidance for the most appropriate prophylactic platelet transfusion thresholds.

Neonatal platelet transfusion: component specification

- ABO and RhD identical or compatible.
- HPA compatible in infants with NAIT.
- CMV seronegative in UK.
- Apheresis, produced by standard techniques without further concentration.

- Irradiated if appropriate.
- Volume transfused usually 10–20 mL/kg.

Neonatal FFP and cryoprecipitate transfusion

There is much uncertainty around the appropriate use of FFP in neonates. A recent UK-wide survey of FFP transfusion practice showed that 42% of infant FFP transfusions were given as prophylaxis for abnormal coagulation in the absence of bleeding [21].

Definition of neonatal coagulopathy

Neonatal coagulopathy can be difficult to define. Plasma concentrations of different coagulation proteins mature at different rates and neonates have a different balance of procoagulant and anticoagulant proteins compared to older children. This results in different postnatal and gestational age-related coagulation ranges in the first months of life, particularly for the activated partial thromboplastin time (APTT), although overall neonatal haemostasis may be functionally as effective as in adults. There is a particular danger of misinterpreting neonatal results reported as the activated partial thromboplastin time ratio (APTR), calculated by dividing the neonatal APTT result by the midpoint of the local adult range, as these may appear inappropriately abnormal. Moreover, most laboratories rely on previously published neonatal ranges due to the difficulties in obtaining locally derived ranges in this age group. As the published ranges are likely to be using different analysers and reagents from the local laboratory, this needs to be taken into account when interpreting individual results.

Causes of haemorrhage in the newborn

In well infants the most common causes of bleeding are:
- vitamin K deficiency (haemorrhagic disease of the newborn);
- inherited disorders, particularly haemophilias;
- NAIT.

In sick infants the most common causes are:

• DIC – secondary to perinatal asphyxia, necrotizing enterocolitis or, less commonly, sepsis;
• liver disease.

Vitamin K deficiency bleeding (haemorrhagic disease of the newborn) (VKDB)

Vitamin K is necessary for posttranslational carboxylation of coagulation factors II, VII, IX and X and of the natural anticoagulants protein C and protein S. Levels of vitamin K and of all of these factors are physiologically low at birth. This physiological deficiency can be exacerbated by breast feeding, prematurity and liver disease, resulting in haemorrhagic disease of the newborn, often referred to as vitamin K deficiency bleeding (VKDB). Treatment of VKDB depends on the severity of bleeding. Mild cases should be given vitamin K (1 mg) intravenously or subcutaneously as this increases levels of active vitamin K deficiency coagulation factors within a few hours; where there is significant bleeding FFP may be given in addition to vitamin K.

There are three patterns of VKDB:
• Early VKDB presents in the first 24 hours of life, usually with severe haemorrhage. It is caused by severe vitamin K deficiency *in utero*, usually as a result of maternal medication that interferes with vitamin K, e.g. anticonvulsants.
• Classical VKDB presents at 2–7 days old in babies who have not received prophylactic vitamin K at birth. The risk is increased in breast-fed babies and in those with poor oral intake. The incidence in babies not receiving vitamin K supplementation is 0.25–1.7%.
• Late VKDB occurs 2 to 8 weeks after birth. It usually presents with sudden intracranial haemorrhage in an otherwise well, breast-fed term baby or in babies with liver disease.

Vitamin K prophylaxis

For prevention of neonatal vitamin K deficiency, both the American Academy of Pediatrics and the Department of Health in the UK recommend vitamin K supplementation at birth. Some studies have suggested a link between intramuscular vitamin K at birth and later childhood malignancies. Although other studies have not confirmed the link with malignancy, the controversy is unlikely to be resolved unequivocally in the short term. Current recommendations are that babies are given 1 mg vitamin K intramuscularly and if parents decline this they should be offered oral vitamin K, requiring multiple doses.

Indications for FFP and cryoprecipitate

Guidelines for the use of FFP, cryoprecipitate and albumin in neonates have been published by national committees in a number of countries. The guidelines aim to minimize their risks in the newborn both by the use of pathogen-inactivated products and by limiting their use for a small number of clinical indications. It is important to monitor the clinical and laboratory outcome of plasma transfusions.

The only indications for FFP in neonates recommended in the BCSH guidelines [18] and supported by evidence are: DIC, VKDB and inherited deficiencies of coagulation factors. Prophylactic FFP administered to preterm neonates at birth does not prevent intraventricular haemorrhage or improve outcome at 2 years of life. Similarly, FFP is not superior to other colloid or crystalloid solutions as a volume replacement solution in standard neonatal practice and there is no evidence to support its use to 'correct' the results of abnormal coagulation screens.

Neonatal FFP and cryoprecipitate: component specifications

• Current BCSH guidelines state that FFP for transfusion to neonates should preferably be of the same ABO group or group AB. Group O FFP should only be given to patients of group O.
• Plasma components may be standard or pathogen inactivated (although pathogen inactivated is not available in all countries). In the UK, single-donor FFP and cryoprecipiate for patients born after 1 January 1996 is imported from countries with low risk of vCJD. Plasma is inactivated by methylene blue with approximately 30% loss of activity of factors VIII, XI and fibrinogen as a result. Some hospitals in the UK use pooled solvent-detergent-treated imported FFP as an alternative (see Chapter 21 for further details).
• The FFP volume transfused is usually 10–20 mL/kg.

Neonatal neutropenia

Normal neutrophil levels vary with postnatal age, falling in healthy babies from around $5–10 \times 10^9$/L at birth to $2-6 \times 10^9$/L by the end of the first week of life. Neutropenia is therefore variably defined depending on postnatal age: less than 2.0×10^9/L at birth and less than 1.0×10^9/L from one week of age. The most common causes are neutropenia secondary to intrauterine growth restriction or maternal hypertension and neutropenia secondary to severe sepsis. The presence of neutrophil left shift and toxic granulation in a neutropenic neonate suggests acute bacterial infection.

Alloimmune neonatal neutropenia (see Chapter 5)

• This is analogous to HDFN: there is maternal sensitization to fetal neutrophil antigens during pregnancy.
• The most common implicated antibodies are anti-NA1 and anti-NA2.
• The estimated incidence of neonatal alloimmune neutropenia is 3% of live births but most cases are mild and asymptomatic and the diagnosis may be missed.
• Infants with severe neonatal alloimmune neutropenia develop severe cutaneous, respiratory or urinary tract infection.
• Treatment is with antibiotics and, if necessary, granulocyte colony-stimulating factor (rarely needed).

Granulocyte transfusions in neonates

There is no good evidence of the benefit of granulocyte transfusions for the treatment of neonatal infection. Both granulocyte colony-stimulating factor and granulocyte-macrophage colony-stimulating factor can be used to increase the neutrophil count in neutropenic neonates, but there is no clear evidence that this improves outcome.

Transfusion in older infants and children

General points

Although most children never require blood transfusion, there are several groups who are frequently transfused, including those on a paediatric intensive care unit (PICU) or undergoing cardiac surgery or ECMO, those with inherited transfusion-dependent disorders, such as thalassaemia major, and those undergoing intensive chemotherapy for haematological malignancies. For some of these patients, including those with thalassaemia major and sickle cell disease, bone marrow transplantation (BMT) or cord blood transplantation is a possible future treatment. Therefore all such children for whom BMT is a possible option should receive CMV-safe blood components. All children on regular transfusions should be vaccinated against hepatitis B as early as possible. Those on chronic transfusion therapy, particularly those with haemoglobinopathies, but also those with Congenital Dyserythropoietic Anaemia, aplastic anaemia and other bone marrow failure syndromes, should have an extended red cell phenotype (see below) performed prior to, or as soon as possible after, commencing regular transfusions. For chronically transfused paediatric patients, monitoring growth and development is an important outcome measure of efficacy.

Formula for calculating red cell transfusion volume in children

Several different formulas for calculating transfusion volume in children are in widespread use. Most formulas commonly used in the UK are based on the increase in Hb or haematocrit required and a 'transfusion factor'. The transfusion factor used varies from 3 to 5. There is a lack of evidence from prospective randomized trials to show which transfusion factor best predicts the rise in Hb/haematocrit and whether the same factor should be applied to all groups of children. Some recent retrospective studies suggest a transfusion factor of 5 better predicts the Hb/haematocrit in critically ill children but transfusion factors of 3 or 4 appear satisfactory for most children on long-term red cell transfusion. An example using a transfusion factor of 3 for packed red cell transfusion is shown here:

$$\text{Volume to transfuse (mL)} = \text{desired Hb (g/dL)} - \text{actual Hb (g/dL)} \times \text{weight (kg)} \times 3$$

A calculation for transfusion volume used in the USA is

$$\text{Volume of red cell (mL)} = \frac{\text{total blood volume (mL)} \times (\text{Hct desired} - \text{Hct observed})}{\text{Hct of donor unit}}$$

The normal rate of red cell transfusion is around 5 mL/kg/h.

Transfusion on paediatric intensive care unit (PICU)

There has been a recent randomized controlled trial of red cell transfusion in stable critically ill children on PICU (TRIPICU [22]), comparing a restrictive Hb trigger (7 g/dL) versus a liberal one (9.5 g/dL). There was no difference in the primary outcome (including mortality and new or progressive multiple organ dysfunction syndrome), suggesting that a restrictive transfusion strategy is reasonable for this group of patients.

Cardiac surgery and ECMO

Transfusion is frequently used in paediatric cardiac surgery including for priming of bypass circuits and treatment of postoperative bleeding and coagulopathy post-bypass. Transfusion practice in paediatric cardiac surgery is very variable, with major differences in the use of components across centres. There is a lack of recent large studies providing evidence for the age of blood to be used, anticoagulant and component support or for appropriate transfusion triggers in this situation, although the TRIPICU study [22] suggested that noncyanotic postoperative cardiac patients can be transfused at Hb of 7 g/dL without adverse outcome. ECMO is used post-bypass and for other situations of cardiopulmonary dysfunction/collapse. As with cardiac bypass, there is limited data to support specific blood component administration/transfusion triggers.

Paediatric massive transfusion

Trauma centres are increasingly setting up paediatric massive transfusion protocols in parallel with adult protocols, with fixed ratios of red cell to plasma transfusions, although there is little specific evidence for paediatric patients in this area.

Leukaemia, chemotherapy and BMT

Many aspects of the transfusion of children with leukaemia/cancer or undergoing haemopoietic stem cell transplantation (HSCT) are managed in a similar manner to adults. However, there are some that

Table 32.5 Indications for platelet transfusion in children with thrombocytopenia.

Platelet count $<10 \times 10^9$/L
Platelet count $<20 \times 10^9$/L and one or more of the following:
severe mucositis
DIC
anticoagulant therapy
platelets likely to fall $< 10 \times 10^9$/L before next evaluation
risk of bleeding due to a local tumour infiltration
Platelet count $20–40 \times 10^9$/L and one or more of the following:
DIC in association with induction therapy for leukaemia
extreme hyperleucocytosis
prior to lumbar puncture or central venous line insertion

DIC, disseminated intravascular coagulation.

deserve particular consideration in the paediatric situation.

Platelet transfusion in children undergoing chemotherapy or HSCT
- Indications for platelet transfusion in children are consensus based; those developed by the BCSH are shown in Table 32.5. In general, in noninfected, well children a platelet count of 10×10^9/L can be used as a transfusion trigger but higher thresholds are used for children who are sick and/or bleeding.
- The optimal platelet count for routine lumbar punctures for children on treatment for leukaemia is uncertain, but current recommendations are $20–40 \times 10^9$/L.
- Platelets should be ABO-compatible where possible because of the risk of haemolysis.
- Platelets should be RhD compatible and D negative girls *should* receive D negative platelets whenever possible, and if not should be administered anti-D.
- A transfusion of 10–20 mL/kg is given to children under 15 kg and an apheresis unit (maximum 300 mL) for children over 15 kg.

Granulocyte transfusion in children undergoing chemotherapy or HSCT
- There is no evidence to support the use of prophylactic granulocyte transfusions.
- Empirical data from some studies support their use where there is severe bacterial or fungal infection in

neutropenic children, including SCT, but they increase the risk of platelet refractoriness.

• Granulocytes for transfusion should be ABO, RhD and crossmatch compatible.

• Granulocytes for all recipients should always be irradiated and be CMV serologically negative.

HSCT donors

• Children who act as HSCT donors for their sibling(s) may require blood transfusion to cover blood lost during the procedure; however, this is avoided wherever possible. Allogeneic blood transfused to the donor during the bone marrow harvest should always be irradiated.

• Peripheral stem cell collections by apheresis are routinely performed in children in specialized centres.

Autologous donation of red cells is now no longer undertaken except in exceptional circumstances.

Transfusion support for children with haemoglobinopathies (also see Chapter 29)

Thalassaemia major

By definition all patients with thalassemia major are transfusion-dependent. Transfusion therapy is determined by the degree of anaemia and evidence of failure to thrive. Most children start transfusion when their haemoglobin drops below 6 g/dL.

Current BCSH [18] and Thalassaemia International Federation [23] guidelines recommend transfusion:

• to maintain an *average* Hb of 12 g/dl;
• to maintain a *pretransfusion* Hb of 9–10.5 g/dL;
• to prevent marrow hyperplasia, skeletal changes and organomegaly by inhibiting erythropoiesis;
• extended red cell phenotyping should be carried out before starting transfusions;
• transfusion requirements should be adjusted to accommodate growth;
• splenectomy may be considered if hypersplenism develops and causes a sustained increase in red cell requirements;
• iron chelation therapy should be considered after 10 transfusions and started once the ferritin is >1000 ng/mL (if possible starting after the age of 2 years because of desferrioxamine toxicity);
• since BMT and cord blood transplantation are the only cure, families should be offered HLA typing of siblings as possible bone marrow donors and/or cryopreservation of HLA-matched sibling cord blood.

Table 32.6 Indications for transfusion in sickle cell disease.

• 'Top-up'	splenic sequestration* hepatic sequestration* aplastic crises*
• Exchange transfusion	chest syndrome* stroke* mesenteric syndrome (abdominal crisis) multisystem organ failure
• Hypertransfusion	stroke (to prevent recurrence)* primary stroke prevention (raised TCD velocity)* renal failure (to prevent/delay deterioration) chronic sickle lung disease
• Surgery	selected patients pre-operatively (e.g. joint replacement)

*proven value
TCD – Transcranial Doppler

Sickle cell disease

Red cell transfusion in children with sickle cell disease should not be routine but reserved for specific indications (Table 32.6). Extended red cell phenotyping before the first transfusion is very important because up to 35% of patients otherwise develop red cell alloimmunization and may be very difficult to crossmatch. The majority of antibodies are in the Rh or Kell systems and may be transient and very difficult to detect, leading to a risk of delayed transfusion reactions.

Indications for 'top-up' transfusion in sickle cell disease Indications include splenic or hepatic sequestration and aplastic crisis. The aim is to raise the haemoglobin to the child's normal steady state (the haemoglobin should never be raised acutely to >10 g/dL since this is likely to cause an increase in blood viscosity).

Indications for exchange transfusion in sickle cell disease

• Acute chest syndrome
• Mesenteric (abdominal) syndrome
• Stroke
• Selected patients preoperatively
• Multiorgan failure

The aim is to reduce sickling and increase oxygen carriage without an increase in viscosity

Indications for hypertransfusion in sickle cell disease
• Prevent recurrence of stroke (i.e. secondary prevention of stroke)
• Prevent the development of stroke in children with sickle cell disease with Doppler evidence of cerebrovascular infarction/haemorrhage in the absence of clinical evidence of stroke (i.e. primary prevention of stroke)
• Delay or prevent deterioration in end organ failure (e.g. chronic sickle lung)
The aims are to maintain the percentage of HbS below 25% and the Hb between 10 and 14.5 g/dL.

Indications for preoperative transfusion in sickle cell disease
The BCSH guidelines are based on observational studies and one large randomized controlled study as there are few other available data. On the basis of these guidelines and recent information from the TAPS trial [24]:
• Top-up transfusion (Hb 8–10 g/dL) is as effective as exchange transfusion and may be safer.
• Although minor, low risk procedures (e.g. grommet insertion) and moderate risk surgery (e.g. tonsillectomy, laparoscopic cholecystectomy) may be undertaken without transfusion in some patients, the recent TAPS study [24] showed that patients with HbSS undergoing low and moderate risk surgery had an increased risk of adverse events without transfusion; the authors recommended on the basis of their results that preoperative transfusion to a haemoglobin of about 10 g/dL should be part of the standard management of patients with HbSS for low and moderate risk surgery.
• Exchange transfusion should be performed preoperatively for major procedures such as hip/knee replacement, organ transplantation, eye surgery and considered for major abdominal surgery.

Practical aspects of transfusion in sickle cell disease
• Extended red cell phenotyping (for Rh K, Fy, Jk, MNS and U) should be carried out; this should be done before the first transfusion and may be usefully arranged at an outpatient clinic follow-up during the first year of life.

• The R_0 blood group (cDe/cDe) is common in patients of African or Caribbean origin: all R_0 patients should receive C-negative, E-negative blood (i.e. rr or R_0).
• The use of sickle trait positive blood should be avoided by testing donor blood for HbS.
• During exchange transfusion in the acute situation, a total exchange of 1.5–2 times blood volume is required to achieve an HbS level of 20% or less; this may take 2–3 procedures if carried out manually. Automated exchange using a cell separator allows the exchange to be completed as a single procedure. The volume of packed cells (in mL) for each exchange is weight (kg) × 30.
• Normal saline (not FFP or albumin) should be used as volume replacement at the beginning of the exchange prior to starting venesection to avoid dropping the circulating blood volume.

Key points

1 Special components are available for fetal and paediatric transfusion to improve transfusion safety and optimize efficacy.
2 Transfusion management of HDFN in the fetus and neonate is complex and requires careful multidisciplinary input.
3 Neonatal red cell top-up transfusions have been the subject of recent trials but the outcomes are not clear-cut; current guidelines are in general closer to the restrictive than liberal thresholds in the trials.
4 Neonatal thrombocytopenia is common in neonatal units; there is a lack of evidence about appropriate triggers for prophylactic platelet transfusions and these are the subject of a current randomized trial.
5 Neonatal coagulopathy is difficult to define in practice and a significant proportion of FFP transfusions are given prophylactically to infants with presumed abnormal coagulation tests in the absence of bleeding.
6 There are specific recommendations for red cell transfusions for older children on PICU and for platelet transfusions for those undergoing chemotherapy.
7 Children with thalassaemia need careful transfusion management to allow normal growth and development and to minimize iron overload.

8 Transfusions for children with sickle cell disease may be given for acute complications or as part of a chronic hypertransfusion programme for primary or secondary prevention of stroke.

References

1 Stainsby D, Jones H, Wells AW et al. Adverse outcomes of blood transfusion in children: analysis of UK reports of the serious hazards of transfusion scheme 1996–2005. Br J Haematol 2008; 141: 73–79.

2 New HV, Stanworth SJ, Engelfriet CP et al. Neonatal transfusions. Vox Sanguinis 2009; 96: 62–85.

3 Luban NLC, Strauss RG & Hume HA. Commentary on the safety of red cells preserved in extended-storage media for neonatal transfusions. Transfusion 1991; 31: 229–235.

4 Mou SS, Giroir BP, Molitor-Kirsch EA et al. Fresh whole blood versus reconstituted blood for pump priming in heart surgery in infants. N Engl J Med. 2004; 351: 1635–1644.

5 Blau J, Calo JM, Dozor D et al. Transfusion-related acute gut injury: necrotizing enterocolitis in very low birth weight neonates after packed red blood cell transfusion. J Pediatr 2011; 158: 403–409.

6 Christensen RD. Association between red blood transfusions and necrotizing enterocolitis. J Pediatr 2011; 158: 349–350.

7 Josephson CD, Castillejo MI, Caliendo AM et al. Prevention of transfusion-transmitted cytomegalovirus in low-birth weight infants (≤1500 g) using cytomegalovirus-seronegative and leukoreduced transfusions. Transfus Med Rev 2011; 25: 125–132.

8 Bhutani VK; Committee on Fetus and Newborn, American Academy of Pediatrics. Phototherapy to prevent severe neonatal hyperbilirubinemia in the newborn infant 35 or more weeks of gestation. Pediatrics 2011; 128: e1046–1052.

9 American Academy of Pediatrics Subcommittee on Hyperbilirubinemia. Management of hyperbilirubinemia in the newborn infant 35 or more weeks of gestation. Pediatrics 2004; 114: 297–316.

10 British Committee for Standards in Haematology. Guidelines for the estimation of fetomaternal haemorrhage; 2009. Available at: http://www.bcshguidelines.com/documents/BCSH_FMH_bcsh_sept2009.pdf.

11 British Committee for Standards in Haematology. Guidelines on the use of irradiated blood components. Br J Haematol 2010; 152: 35–51.

12 Strauss RG & Widness JA. Autologous or allogeneic: cord blood red blood cells still are investigational. Transfus Med Rev 2012; 26: 91–92.

13 Bell EF, Strauss RG, Widness JA et al. Randomized trial of liberal versus restrictive guidelines for red blood cell transfusion in preterm infants. Pediatrics 2005; 115: 1685–1691.

14 Kirpalani H, Whyte RK, Andersen C et al. The Premature Infants in Need of Transfusion (PINT) study: a randomized, controlled trial of a restrictive (low) versus liberal (high) transfusion threshold for extremely low birth weight infants. J Pediatr 2006; 149: 301–307.

15 Whyte RK, Kirpalani H, Asztalos EV et al. Neurodevelopmental outcome of extremely low birth weight infants randomly assigned to restrictive or liberal hemoglobin thresholds for blood transfusion. Pediatrics 2009; 123: 207–213.

16 Nopoulos PC, Conrad AL, Bell EF et al. Long-term outcome of brain structure in premature infants: effects of liberal vs restricted red blood cell transfusions. Arch Pediatr Adolesc Med 2011; 165: 443–450.

17 Whyte R & Kirpalani H. Low versus high haemoglobin concentration threshold for blood transfusion for preventing morbidity and mortality in very low birth weight infants. Cochrane Database Syst Rev 2011; 11: CD000512.

18 British Committee for Standards in Haematology. Transfusion guideline for neonates and older children. Br J Haematol 2004; 124: 433–453.
 • 2005 amendment to the guidelines on transfusion for neonates and older children. Br J Haematol 2006; 136: 514–516.
 • 2007 amendment to the transfusion guidelines for neonates and older children (specification of imported FFP). Available at: http://www.bcshguidelines.com/documents/FFP_neonate_Amendment_1_17_Oct_2007.pdf.

19 Boralessa H, Modi N, Cockburn H, Malde R, Edwards M, Roberts I & Letsky E. RBC T activation and hemolysis in a neonatal intensive care population: implications for transfusion practice. Transfusion 2002; 42: 1428–1434.

20 Stanworth SJ, Clarke P, Watts T et al. Prospective, observational study of outcomes in neonates with severe thrombocytopenia. Pediatrics. 2009; 124: e826–834.

21 Stanworth SJ, Grant-Casey J, Lowe D et al. The use of fresh-frozen plasma in England: high levels of inappropriate use in adults and children. Transfusion 2011; 51: 62–70.

22 Lacroix J, Hebert PC, Hutchison JS et al. Transfusion strategies for patients in pediatric intensive care units. N Engl J Med 2007; 356: 1609–1619.

23 Cappellini M-D, Cohen A, Eleftheriou A et al. Guidelines for the clinical management of thalassaemia, 2nd edn revised; 2008. Available at: http://www.thalassaemia.org.cy/pdf/Guidelines_2nd_revised_edition_EN.pdf.

24 Howard, J, Malfroy, M, Llewelyn, C *et al.* Pre-operative transfusion reduces serious adverse events in patients with sickle cell disease (SCD): results from the Transfusion Alternatives Preoperatively in Sickle Cell Disease (TAPS) randomised controlled multicentre clinical trial. *Blood (ASH annual meeting abstracts)* 2011; 118: 9.

Further reading

Aher S & Ohlsson A. Late erythropoietin for preventing red blood cell transfusion in preterm and/or low birth weight infants. *Cochrane Database Syst Rev* 2006; 3: CD004868.

British Committee for Standards in Haematology. Guideline for blood grouping and antibody testing in pregnancy; 2006. Available at: http://www.bcshguidelines.com/documents/antibody_testing_pregnancy_bcsh_07062006.pdf.

British Committee for Standards in Haematology. Guideline on the administration of blood components; 2009. Available at: http://www.bcshguidelines.com/documents/Admin_blood_components_bcsh_05012010.pdf.

Egbor M, Knott P & Bhide, A. Red-cell and platelet allommunisation in pregnancy. *Best Pract Res Clin Obstet Gynaecol* 2012: 26; 119–132.

National Institute for Health and Clinical Excellence. *CG 98 Neonatal Jaundice.* London: NICE; 2010. Available at: www.nice.org.uk/guidance/CG98.

Patra K, Storfer-Isser A, Siner B, Moore J & Hack M. Adverse events associated with neonatal exchange transfusion in the 1990s. *J Pediatr* 2004; 144: 626–631.

Puckett RM & Offringa M. Prophylactic vitamin K for vitamin K deficiency bleeding in neonates. *Cochrane Database Syst Rev* 2000; 4: CD002776.

33 Recombinant proteins in diagnosis and therapy

Marion Scott

NHS Blood and Transplant, Bristol, UK

Introduction

Many potentially useful human proteins for therapeutic, diagnostic and research use are expressed in the body at very low concentrations and it is difficult, if not impossible, to isolate them by conventional biochemical methods. Other proteins, such as antibodies of a particular specificity, are difficult to purify from a complex mixture of very similar proteins. However, once the gene encoding a protein has been cloned and sequenced, it becomes possible to express the protein at high concentrations, using virally derived expression vectors that are designed to produce full-length proteins at high levels in various different *in vitro* culture 'host' cell systems. Some blood proteins, such as the coagulation factors to treat haemophilia, have been efficiently purified by fractionation of pooled human plasma, but have been shown to have the potential of transmitting diseases, such as HIV and HCV. The cloning and expression of these proteins has led to the availability of recombinant coagulation factors for the treatment of haemophilia, with reduced risk of infection. As the recombinant coagulation factors are grown *in vitro*, there is also the advantage of an unlimited supply of constant guaranteed product. Similar drivers have led researchers to try and develop recombinant replacements for specific immunoglobulins currently fractionated from high titre blood donations, such as anti-D. Some concern has been expressed about the safety of such recombinant products, as they may potentially contain viruses or other infectious agents arising from the host cells used to express the protein, or the culture medium components used to grow the host cells. Increasing awareness of the risks from pooled polyclonal blood components have been heightened by concerns about variant Creutzfeldt–Jakob disease (vCJD) in the UK. Are the potential risks from such biotechnology products any worse than the risks from blood components derived from pooled human plasma?

Apart from cloning and expressing such naturally occurring proteins, it is possible using recombinant DNA technology to produce modified forms of the proteins that do not occur naturally and that might have desired therapeutic effects or diagnostic advantages.

General methods for recombinant protein expression

The choice of the host cell system to use for recombinant protein expression relies on several factors. Bacterial expression systems, such as *Escherichia coli*, are the cheapest, simplest and most effective, but cannot be used for many types of human proteins that require eukaryotic posttranslational modifications for biological activity, e.g. glycosylation, since prokaryotes lack the enzymes that catalyse many of the posttranslational modifications found on eukaryotic proteins.

Practical Transfusion Medicine, Fourth Edition. Edited by Michael F. Murphy, Derwood H. Pamphilon and Nancy M. Heddle.
© 2013 John Wiley & Sons, Ltd. Published 2013 by John Wiley & Sons, Ltd.

Table 33.1 Production systems for recombinant mammalian proteins.

System	Cost	Production timescale	Scale-up capacity	Product quality	Glycosylation	Contamination risks
Bacteria	Low	Short	High	Low	None	Endotoxins
Yeast	Medium	Medium	High	Medium	Incorrect	Low risk
Plants	Low	Long	High	High	Some differences	Low risk, but environmental concerns
Insect cells	Medium	Medium	High	Medium	Incorrect	Low risk
Mammalian cells	High	Long	Low	Very high	Correct	Animal viruses
Transgenic animals	High	Very long	Low	Very high	Correct	Animal viruses

Proteins produced in prokaryotes may not be folded properly and/or can be insoluble, forming inclusion bodies. Genetically modified strains of yeast that have human glycosylation pathways have been produced for the efficient production of human glycoforms of recombinant proteins. Insect cells have also been used for recombinant protein expression, using baculoviral vectors. Transgenic animals have also been produced, with targeted production of recombinant proteins in milk. A comparison of different production systems for recombinant proteins is shown in Table 33.1.

For many types of human proteins, expression in a mammalian system is the best option, as this is the approach most likely to yield soluble, biologically active proteins, although it is considerably more expensive than expression in *E. coli*, yeast or insect cells. Cell lines commonly used are NS0 (mouse myeloma), CHO (Chinese hamster ovary) and COS-7 (African green monkey fibroblast).

A number of techniques have been developed for rapid, one-stage purification of recombinant proteins. Epitope tags are short amino acid sequences for which commercial monoclonal antibodies are available, and can be placed anywhere within the protein where it will not disrupt the protein's function. It is also common to create fusion proteins, i.e. to create a single open reading frame that encodes a well-characterized protein such as glutathione-S-transferase (GST) together with the sequence of the protein of interest. When the tag protein is produced, the protein of interest is produced as well, as one fusion protein. Fusion proteins are useful because they enable rapid purification by affinity chromatography, and the fused tag can be removed after purification using a specific protease.

Plasmids used for expression commonly contain a viral promoter sequence, an antibiotic resistance gene, a fusion tag sequence and a restriction endonuclease site for insertion of the coding sequence of interest (Figure 33.1). cDNA coding for the protein sequence of interest is normally derived by reverse transcriptase polymerase chain reaction (RT-PCR) from cells expressing the protein, using sequence specific primers to amplify the region required. This cDNA is then inserted into the expression vector and used to transfect a mammalian cell line. Growth in medium containing the antibiotic to which the vector codes resistance results in selection of transfected cells only. Production of the fusion protein can then be detected using antibodies to the fusion tag sequence, and the fusion protein purified and characterized. Some expression vectors do not insert into the host cell nuclear material and give rise to transient expression. Other vectors insert into the host cell DNA and give rise to stable expression.

Recombinant antibodies

Limitations of rodent monoclonal antibodies

Conventional monoclonal antibody technology uses immunization of mice or rats with antigen to yield hyperimmunized spleen cells, which are then fused with nonsecreting myeloma cell lines to yield hybridoma cell lines that can be grown *in vitro* to produce monoclonal antibodies [1]. Effectively the fusion process inserts the DNA from the spleen cells into the myeloma cells. Whilst many such conventional monoclonal antibodies were very successfully developed

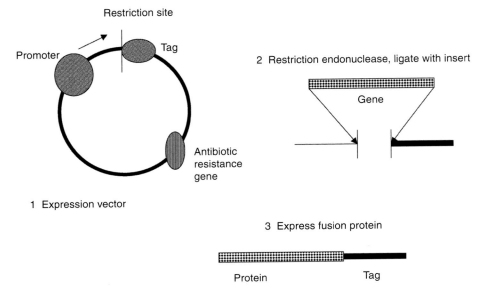

Restriction site

Promoter

Tag

2 Restriction endonuclease, ligate with insert

Gene

Antibiotic
resistance
gene

1 Expression vector

3 Express fusion protein

Protein   Tag

Fig 33.1 Production of recombinant fusion proteins.

into diagnostic reagents (such as the high avidity anti-A and anti-B now used routinely worldwide for blood grouping), it was not possible to produce antibodies of certain specificities in rodents, and attempts to use rodent monoclonal antibodies in man as therapeutics rapidly ran into problems, as the recipients developed a strong human antirodent response, which rapidly cleared the antibodies from the body.

Humanizing rodent monoclonals

The early promise of monoclonal antibodies as therapeutics was not realized and many became disillusioned with the concept of the 'magic bullet'. The success rate of rodent monoclonal antibodies that entered clinical trials was only 9% over the 20 years from 1980 to 2000. However, when the possibility of making recombinant antibodies became available in 1986, things rapidly changed. Using recombinant DNA technology, it was possible to replace the mouse constant domains of antibodies with corresponding human domains and express these chimeric recombinant immunoglobulin molecules in cell lines [2]. Further engineering work also allowed the replacement of the framework regions of the mouse variable domains with human framework regions, resulting in virtually fully humanized antibodies [3].

Human recombinant antibodies

Human circulating B cells can be selected from immune individuals and transformed into cell lines that can be grown in culture by transformation with Epstein–Barr virus (EBV). The cDNA coding for the antibodies can then be derived from these cells using RT-PCR, ligated into expression vectors and expressed in a suitable mammalian host cell line.

Alternatively phage display technology can be used (Figures 33.2 and 33.3). Bacteriophages that infect *E. coli* are modified such that they carry the cDNA encoding for antibody variable domains, whilst at the same time they express the antibody protein on their surface. This permits *in vitro* selection of antibodies of the required specificity and then expansion in *E. coli*. RT-PCR is used to amplify all of the heavy and light chain variable domains in a buffy coat sample. PCR is then used to assemble these randomly into VH and VL pairs, by inclusion of DNA encoding for a flexible linker chain between the heavy and light chain domains. A 'tag' sequence is also included to aid detection and purification. These linked heavy and light chain domains are known as single-chain Fv (scFv). The scFv constructs are then ligated into a phage display vector. The scFv domain is ligated into the vector next to regions that code for the PIII phage coat

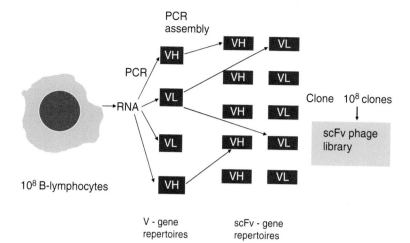

Fig 33.2 Generation of scFv phage libraries.

protein. The recombinant phage then expresses the scFv protein alongside their PIII coat protein at the tip of the phage. Phage libraries can be panned against antigens, and those phage selected that are displaying scFv that bind to the antigen. Selected phage are eluted from the antigen, expanded by culture in *E. coli* and then repanned against antigen. Selected human scFv can then removed from the phage vector and can be ligated to cloned human IgG constant domains

to express full-length human recombinant antibody molecules. One large advantage of this approach is that antibodies can be derived from phage display libraries made from nonimmunized individuals and that normally restricted antibodies (e.g. anti-self) can be derived [4].

Using these approaches, 30 recombinant antibodies are now successfully licensed for clinical use in a variety of applications with around 300 more in the pipeline, and they are now among the most commercially successful biotech drugs, with three in the top ten best selling drugs worldwide [5].

Human recombinant monoclonal anti-D

Despite the overall success in the production of rodent monoclonal antibodies to human ABO blood group antigens, no such monoclonal antibodies have been produced to the Rh antigens. Various different approaches have been developed to produce human monoclonal antibodies specific for RhD.

Early work used the immortalization of human B cells by infection with EBV. Improvements in the stability of human cell lines have been achieved by back-crossing human anti-D secreting EBV lines to a mouse–human heterohybridoma line or to a mouse myeloma line [6]. Use of these approaches has enabled the production of a large number of blood group-specific human anti-Rh monoclonal antibodies. The cDNA coding for these antibodies has then been expressed in suitable mammalian host cell lines to

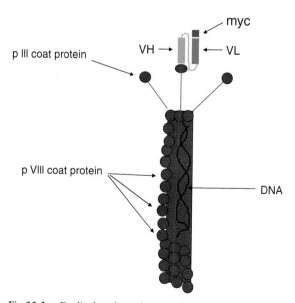

Fig 33.3 scFv displayed on phage surface.

produce recombinant anti-D suitable for therapeutic use (i.e. free from EBV).

Candidate monoclonal anti-Ds for immunoprophylaxis are selected, first, on their ability to bind to the RhD antigen via the Fv part of the molecule and, second, on their ability to interact with Fc receptors via the Fc part of the molecule to bring about immunomodulation. The exact mechanism of immunosuppression by anti-D is not known, but it is clear that it involves interaction of anti-D with Fc receptors. To be effective, prophylactic antibody must be capable of not only binding to the RhD antigen on the red cells via its Fv regions but also interacting with the effector cells of the immune system via its Fc region. Selection of recombinant monoclonal anti-D for therapeutic use therefore depends on not only the antigen specificity and avidity of the monoclonal antibody but also its functional activity in interacting with effector cells. To suppress immunization, IgG-coated RBC need to be rapidly cleared from the maternal circulation and localized in the spleen. It has been suggested that D antigen-specific B cells in the spleen are then deactivated by the simultaneous binding of the Fc region of the anti-D to $Fc\gamma RIIb$ together with binding of the B-cell receptor to the D antigen. Interactions of anti-D with $Fc\gamma RI$, $Fc\gamma RIIb$ and $Fc\gamma RIIIa$ may thus all be required for effective immunosuppression.

IgG monoclonal anti-D antibodies have been evaluated in various *in vitro* systems to test how effective the antibodies are at interacting with immune system effector cells. Each assay tests efficacy at binding to different Fc receptors. Rosette formation of sensitized cells with monocytes and phagocytes, adherence of sensitized cells to monocyte monolayers and chemiluminescent measurements of the oxidative burst caused when monocytes react with sensitized red cell are all *in vitro* measures of interaction with $Fc\gamma RI$. Antibody-dependent cellular cytotoxicity measurements by radiolabelled chromium release from natural killer cells measures interaction with $Fc\gamma RIIIa$. It is not clear at present how well performance in these various *in vitro* assays will predict *in vivo* efficacy.

Two monoclonal anti-D antibodies, BRAD-3 and BRAD-5, were selected for clinical study because of their high activity in *in vitro* functional assays, high avidity and specificity for the immunodominant epitope region of the RhD antigen and initial studies in D-negative male volunteers showed expected half-lives

and pharmacokinetics after injection. Further studies on the antibodies administered with ^{51}Cr-labelled D-positive red cells demonstrated accelerated red cell clearance in all subjects and provided preliminary evidence for protection from immunization [7]. One determinant of affinity for $Fc\gamma RIII$ is the glycosylation pattern of the immunoglobulin heavy chains, which may be determined by the nature of the host cell in which the antibody is expressed. A glycosylation pattern of low fucose content has been shown to confer enhanced ADCC activity. A human recombinant monoclonal anti-D selected to have such high affinity $Fc\gamma RIII$ binding activity has been shown to promote a similar clearance of antibody-coated RhD RBCs in healthy volunteers to polyclonal anti-RhD immunoglobulin [8]. Roledumab, a commercial product based on this antibody is currently in phase 2 clinical trials.

It is clear from the clinical trials to date that recombinant anti-D has the potential to replace polyclonal prophylactic anti-D. There is a case for universal antenatal prophylaxis if sufficient supplies of anti-D are available. How quickly recombinant anti-D becomes available will largely be determined by commercial investment and regulatory procedures.

Antiprion recombinant antibodies

A range of monoclonal antibodies to human recombinant prion proteins has been produced by immunizing prion knockout mice. Selected antibodies have been developed into a diagnostic test for bovine spongiform encephalopathy using homogenized bovine brain post mortem. Work is currently underway to try and increase the sensitivity of the assay to make it suitable for screening human blood for vCJD. It has been shown that these mouse monoclonal antibodies can prevent the spread of vCJD prion disease in a mouse model [9]. Currently efforts aim to engineer human chimeric and humanized versions of these mouse antibodies to progress this work into clinical trials for the potential treatment of vCJD.

Anti-HPA-1a recombinant antibodies

scFv specific for the human platelet antigen HPA-1a have been derived from a phage display library and ligated to scFv specific for the RhD antigen on red blood cells, and the novel bispecific recombinant antibody can be used in a mixed passive haemagglutination test for the HPA-1a antigen on platelets. The scFv has also been expressed as a full-length human IgG antibody by ligation to the constant domains of human IgG1, and this antibody had been used either fluorescently labelled or enzyme labelled in other diagnostic tests for the HPA-1a antigen on platelets.

'Null' recombinant antibodies

Using site directed mutagenesis, the Fc domains of human IgG antibodies have been mutated to have as little biological function as possible. Recombinant anti-D and anti-HPA-1a antibodies have been produced with this 'null' Fc region. *In vitro* studies have shown that these 'null' antibodies can effectively compete with clinically significant antibodies and prevent them, causing immune destruction of red cells and platelets, respectively. A clinical trial in male volunteers showed that the 'null' anti-D protected D-positive red cells from clearance by anti-D *in vivo* [10]. The aim is to see if the 'null' anti-HPA-1a antibody can be administered to HPA-1a-negative pregnant women who are carrying HPA-1a-positive fetuses and prevent neonatal alloimmune thrombocytopaenia by crossing the placenta and competing with maternal anti-HPA-1a that can cause destruction of fetal platelets (see also Chapter 5).

Recombinant phenotyping reagents

Many monoclonal human IgG antibodies have been produced that react with blood group antigens, but these must be used in enzyme or antiglobulin techniques that are not suited to hig throughput, automated blood grouping machines. By cloning the variable regions of these antibodies, it is possible to ligate them to the constant domains of human IgM antibodies and express hybrid recombinant molecules in myeloma cells. These antibodies are highly potent because they combine the high affinity of the affinity-matured IgG antibodies with the polymeric structure of IgM [11]. They are very potent direct agglutinins that can readily be used in automated blood grouping machines.

Recombinant antigens

Blood group antigens

Detection and identification of clinically significant blood group, platelet and granulocyte antibodies currently rely on the availability of high quality antibody screening and identification cells that cover all clinically significant antigens and carry them in combinations such that the specificity of antibodies can be deduced. The quality of these panels of cells is critical and their variability has been shown in UK National External Quality Assessment Scheme exercises to be the main cause of error in the detection and identification of antibodies. Quantitation of antibodies during pregnancy is carried out using titration or autoanalyser technology, both of which show high levels of variation, such that it is difficult to set levels at which clinical action is required.

Most of the relevant antigens have been sequenced and cloned. Some have been inserted in expression vectors and expressed in the membranes of *in vitro* cultured cells, e.g. expression of the Rh protein in K562 human erythroleukaemia cells. For some antigens it is possible to amplify just the extracellular domain of the protein that carries the antigen and express a soluble recombinant protein that carries antigenic activity. This has been demonstrated for the Kell, Lutheran, Duffy, MNSs and Cartwright red cell antigens, HPA-1a and HPA-1b platelet antigens and HNA-1 and HNA-2 granulocyte antigens [12].

The target of this work is to be able to produce microarrays of recombinant antigens that could then be used for high throughput antibody screening, identification, subclass determination and quantitation of antibodies in transfusion recipients and pregnant women.

Microbial antigens

In a similar way, recombinant microbial antigens have been produced to test blood donor plasma for the presence of antimicrobial antibodies, and thus exposure to transfusion transmitted diseases. Viral antigens and tests have been produced in this way, and more recently tests for parasites, such as those causing malaria (*Plasmodium falciparum* and *P. vivax*) and Chagas (*Trypanosoma cruzi*), have been produced and shown to have good specificity and sensitivity for screening blood donors [12].

373

Recombinant enzymes

It has long been known that it is possible to treat group A, B or AB red cells with glycosidase enzymes and convert them to group O, such that they would theoretically be a safe blood transfusion product for any ABO blood group recipient. However, the naturally occurring enzymes have poor kinetic properties and difficult-to-achieve pH optima, such that the process was not economically viable or able to pass rigorous quality assurance requirements for clinical use. New recombinant enzymes have now been produced from bacterial glycosidases with remarkably improved kinetic properties, such that the enzymes reproducibly cleave the A and B antigens with low enzyme protein consumption, short incubation times and at neutral pH [13]. Clinical trials evaluating the safety and efficacy of such recombinant enzyme-treated red cells are looking promising.

Recombinant coagulation factors

Recombinant coagulation factors have been successfully used for the treatment of haemophilia for several years. Recombinant protein technology has virtually eliminated transmissible disease risk from these products, such that the recombinant products are the products of choice for haemophiliacs. In the UK, most patients with severe haemophilia now receive recombinant factor VIII and factor IX. Recombinant factor VIIa was originally developed for the treatment of haemophilia patients who had developed inhibitory alloantibodies to factors VIII and IX, and is licensed for this application (see Chapter 37).

Recombinant haemoglobin is considered in Chapter 36 and *recombinant erythropoietin* in Chapters 28 and 34.

Conclusions

Recombinant protein technology has rapidly advanced over the last 25 years and we are now starting to see the routine use of recombinant proteins in transfusion medicine. Recombinant proteins will probably totally replace coagulation factors and specific immunoglobulins that are currently produced from fractionated pooled plasma. However, it is unlikely that recombinant products will replace intravenous immunoglobulin or albumin. Intravenous immunoglobulin works because of its broad specificity – it would be very difficult/impossible to mimic this successfully with a recombinant product. Albumin could be produced as a recombinant protein, but this is unlikely to be economically viable, compared to the ease of production from plasma. Only evidence of disease transmission by plasma-derived albumin could drive the production of recombinant albumin.

Further specific recombinant immunoglobulins are being produced that are not currently available as blood components – anti-HCV and anti-vCJD – and the efficacy of these needs to be investigated in clinical trials. Blood group antigens are now available as recombinant molecules, such that there may no longer be a need to use red cells, platelets and granulocytes for antibody screening, identification and quantitation.

Key points

1 Proteins expressed at low levels naturally can be cloned and expressed as recombinant proteins at high levels.
2 The sequence of recombinant proteins can be altered to give properties not found in naturally occurring proteins.
3 Human recombinant antibodies can be produced from nonimmune donors.
4 Murine monoclonal antibodies can be humanized for clinical use.
5 Recombinant antibodies with inactive Fc regions can be produced as blocking antibodies.
6 Recombinant antigens can be used for screening, identification and quantification of clinically significant antibodies.
7 Recombinant coagulation factors have largely replaced those derived from pooled plasma.

References

1 Kohler G & Milstein C. Continuous cultures of fused cells secreting antibody of predefined specificity. *Nature* 1975; 256: 495–497.

2 Morrison SL. Chimeric human antibody molecules: mouse antigen binding domains with human constant region domains. *Proc Natl Acad Sci USA* 1984; 81: 6851–6855.

3 Jones PT. Replacing the complementarity determining regions in a human antibody with those from a mouse. *Nature* 1986; 321: 522–525.

4 Marks JD, Hoogenboom HR, Bonnert TP *et al.* By-passing immunisation. Human antibodies from V-gene libraries displayed on phage. *J Molec Biol* 1991; 222: 581–592.

5 Reichert JM. Antibody-based therapeutics to watch in 2011. *mAbs* 2011; 3: 76–99.

6 Thompson KM, Melamed MD, Eagle K *et al.* Production of human monoclonal IgG and IgM antibodies with anti-D Rhesus specificity using heterohybridomas. *Immunology* 1986; 58: 157–160.

7 Kumpel BM, Goodrick MJ, Pamphilon DH *et al.* Human RhD monoclonal antibodies (BRAD-3 and BRAD-5) cause accelerated clearance of RhD red blood cells and suppression of RhD immunization in RhD– volunteers. *Blood* 1995; 86: 1701–1709.

8 Beliard R, Waegemans T, Notelet D *et al.* A human anti-D monoclonal antibody selected for enhanced FcgammaRIII engagement clears RhD+ autologous red cells in human volunteers as efficiently as polyclonal anti-D antibodies. *Br J Haematol* 2008; 141: 109–119.

9 White AR, Enever P, Tayebi M *et al.* Monoclonal antibodies inhibit prion replication and delay the development of prion disease. *Nature* 2003; 422: 80–83.

10 Armour KL, Parry-Jones DR, Beharry N *et al.* Intravascular survival of red cells coated with a mutated human anti-D antibody engineered to lack destructive activity. *Blood* 2006; 107: 2619–2626.

11 Gilmour JEM, Pittman S, Nesbitt R & Scott ML. Effect of the presence or absence of J chain on expression of recombinant anti-Kell immunoglobulin M. *Transfus Med* 2008; 18: 167–174.

12 Ridgwell K, Dixey J & Scott ML. Production of soluble recombinant proteins with Kell, Duffy and Lutheran blood group activity, and their use in screening human sera for Kell, Duffy and Lutheran antibodies. *Transfus Med* 2007; 5: 384–394.

13 Olsson ML & Clausen H. Modifying the red cell surface: towards an ABO-universal blood supply. *Br J Haematol* 2008; 140: 3–12.

Further reading

Abes R & Teillaud JL. Impact of glycosylation on effector functions of therapeutic IgG. *Pharmaceuticals* 2010; 3: 146–157.

Chang CD, Cheng KY, Jiang LX *et al.* Evaluation of a prototype *Trypanosoma cruzi* antibody assay with recombinant antigens on a fully automated chemiluminescence analyzer for blood donor screening. *Transfusion* 2006; 46: 1737–1744.

Corwin HL. The role of erythropoietin therapy in the care of the critically ill. *Transfus Med Rev* 2006; 20: 27–33.

Goodnough LT & Shander AS. Recombinant factor VIIa: safety and efficacy. *Curr Opin Hematol* 2007; 14: 504–509.

Kitchen AD, Lowe PH, Lalloo K & Chiodini PL. Evaluation of a malarial antibody assay for use in the screening of blood and tissue products for clinical use. *Vox Sanguinis* 2004; 87: 150–155.

Mondon P, Dubreuil O, Bouyadi K & Kharrat H. Human antibody libraries. *Front Biosci* 2008; 13: 1117–1129.

Rasmussen SK, Rasmussen LK, Weilgunny D & Tolstrup AB. Manufacture of recombinant polyclonal antibodies. *Biotechnol Lett* 2007; 29: 845–852.

Spencer KA, Osorio FA & Hiscox JA. Recombinant viral proteins for use in diagnostic ELISA to detect virus infection. *Vaccine* 2007; 25: 5653–5659.

Stanworth SJ, Birchall J, Doree CJ & Hyde C. Recombinant factor VIIa for the prevention and treatment of bleeding in patients without haemophilia. *Cochrane Database Syst Rev* 2007; CD005011.

Tsai CH, Fang TY, Ho NT & Ho C. Novel recombinant hemoglobin, rHb (beta N108Q), with low oxygen affinity, high co-operativity and stability against autooxidation. *Biochemistry* 2000; 39: 13719–13729.

Wilson J, Yao GL, Raftery J *et al.* A systematic review and economic evaluation of epoetin alpha, epoetin beta and darbepoetin alpha. *Health Technol Assess* 2007; 11: 1–202.

PART FIVE

Alternatives to Transfusion

34 Principles of patient blood management

Aryeh Shander[1] & Lawrence Tim Goodnough[2]

[1]Department of Anesthesiology, Critical Care and Hyperbaric Medicine, Englewood Hospital and Medical Center, Englewood, New Jersey, USA and Mount Sinai School of Medicine, New York, USA
[2]Departments of Pathology and Medicine, Stanford University, Stanford, California, USA

Introduction

The paradigm shift in transfusion medicine towards the restrictive use of allogeneic blood components and the avoidance of unnecessary transfusions has arisen for several reasons. Transfusion can be a life-saving therapy when indicated and appropriately administered. On the other hand, unnecessary transfusions result in potential risks without clear benefits. Although some of the better-known risks and complications of allogeneic transfusions (discussed in detail later in this chapter) have been mitigated through advances in blood screening, processing and banking (notwithstanding the occasional newly emerging infectious risks such as prions), other mainly noninfectious risks remain. Moreover, several studies have demonstrated that clinical outcomes of patients who receive allogeneic blood components are often worse (or not any better) compared with their nontransfused peers. It remains subject to debate whether worse outcomes are due to the transfusions or the underlying conditions leading to transfusion (e.g. anaemia and comorbidities).

The changing landscape of balance between supply and demand for donated banked blood is another important factor. Increasing life expectancy in the developed nations is a triumph for health care systems, but has the consequence of increasing the number of transfusion recipients (e.g. elderly patients with chronic comorbidities) relative to potential donors (e.g. healthy young adults). It is reasonable to assume that the prospect of the potential demand for allogeneic blood outpacing its potential supply is a matter of 'when' not 'if' [1]. Additionally, the ongoing scrutiny on the reported harmful effects of *ex vivo* storage of banked blood (i.e. the storage lesion) is likely to redefine the acceptable shelf life of banked blood, exerting further pressure on inventory management and supply. Finally, the perplexing direct and indirect costs associated with allogeneic blood transfusions (incurred by the donors, recipients, health care centres and the society as a whole) are being increasingly acknowledged.

Despite all this, thousands of patients continue to receive transfusions every day and many are inappropriately transfused [2], as indicated by the vastly variable transfusion rates across clinicians and hospitals not explainable by patients' characteristics or procedures alone [3]. All these and other factors call for more judicious use of allogeneic blood components and employing effective alternative modalities as well as a shift from a 'product-centred' to 'patient-centred' transfusion practice as advocated by Patient Blood Management (PBM) [4].

What is patient blood management?

The concept of PBM is relatively new, but it can be viewed as logical evolution of strategies proposed and

Practical Transfusion Medicine, Fourth Edition. Edited by Michael F. Murphy, Derwood H. Pamphilon and Nancy M. Heddle.
© 2013 John Wiley & Sons, Ltd. Published 2013 by John Wiley & Sons, Ltd.

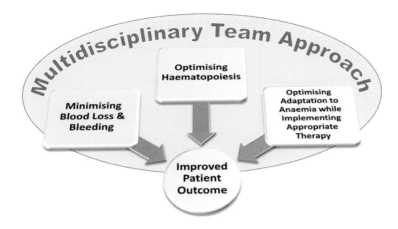

Fig 34.1 Pillars of patient blood management, addressing the common risk factors of transfusion in a coordinated, multidisciplinary effort to improve patient outcomes.

utilized initially to care for patients who were not willing (or able) to receive transfusions (i.e. 'blood-less' medicine and surgery), followed by wider application of these strategies for a broader spectrum of patients with the goal of restricting or eliminating the use of allogeneic blood components (i.e. blood conservation). PBM is defined as 'the timely application of evidence-based medical and surgical concepts designed to maintain haemoglobin concentration (Hb), optimise haemostasis and minimise blood loss in an effort to improve patient outcome'.[1] What makes PBM distinct is its emphasis on improving the clinical outcomes of the patients through the use of preventive measures. The term PBM begins with 'patient' and the word 'transfusion' is missing from the definition, implying that the patients and their health outcomes are given priority over other processes, including reducing blood utilization, although the latter is most often also achieved during implementing PBM.

Although PBM strategies are often envisioned during care of elective surgical patients, they can be adjusted and applied during the care of all patients who may be candidates for transfusion at some stages of their medical treatment. For instance, patients undergoing nonelective surgeries, trauma patients, patients undergoing chemoradiotherapy and patients suffering from nonsurgical bleeding can all be treated using PBM strategies and benefit from them. PBM

strategies include a combination of medications and devices as well as medical and/or surgical techniques applied via an interdisciplinary team approach. To be most effective, the interdisciplinary approach relies on a plan of care tailored to the specific needs and conditions of the patients. The treating physician must assume a proactive role in PBM, anticipating the complications and adjusting the treatment plan as necessary.

Given the link between allogeneic transfusion and unfavourable outcomes, identification and management of the risk factors of predisposing patients to being transfused is a centrepiece of PBM. It has been shown that the majority of transfusions in elective, urgent and emergent surgical patients can be attributed to the presence of anaemia, amount of blood loss and the failure to implement evidence-based recommendations to make transfusion decisions [5]. Accordingly, PBM relies on three main strategies, known as 'pillars of PBM' to manage these risks (Figure 34.1) [6]:
– optimizing haemopoiesis;
– minimizing blood loss and bleeding;
– harnessing and optimizing physiological adaptation to anaemia while implementing appropriate therapy.

Several therapeutic options and approaches are available under each strategy, and given the rapid pace of advancements in medical research, readers should refer to current references for the most updated information on each modality. Combined use of these strategies is expected to reduce the risk of patients being exposed to allogeneic blood transfusions. However, close attention must be paid to the independent

[1] From the Society for the Advancement of Blood Management (SABM) at: http://www.sabm.org/public/.

impact of each approach on the clinical outcomes of the patients. The case of aprotinin represents a cautionary example: although the antifibrinolytic agent was found to be highly effective in reducing surgical blood loss and transfusions, its independent association with increased risk of death and other serious complications resulted in its withdrawal from the market [7]. More recently, aprotinin has re-emerged in Canada to prevent life-threatening bleeding in patients undergoing cardiac bypass surgery, in the light of some issues raised on the interpretation of data that had previously resulted in its withdrawal. All in all, this example can clearly demonstrate the dynamic and ever-changing nature of PBM modalities and the need for their continuous study and assessment. It is rarely adequate to merely focus on the transfusion-sparing effect of modalities, and meaningful clinical endpoints should also be included in the studies – a concept that is fundamental to PBM.

Optimizing haemopoiesis

The importance of preventive measures in PBM can be best viewed in its first pillar. Anaemia is a leading risk factor of allogeneic red cell transfusion, a valuable warning sign of serious underlying diseases and an independent predictor of morbidity and mortality. The negative impact of anaemia has even been reported in mildly anaemic patients. Based on recent reports and depending on studied populations, preoperative anaemia can be present in as many as 75% of patients undergoing elective surgeries. Similarly high frequencies have been reported in critically ill patients and those admitted with ischemic or chronic heart disease – all patients who are likely to be more susceptible to the detrimental effect of anaemia and who are commonly transfused. Hence, proper screening for and management of anaemia provides an excellent opportunity to improve the clinical outcomes of these patients. Recent guidelines developed by a multidisciplinary panel for the Network for Advancement of Transfusion Alternatives (NATA) call for determination of Hb as early as 28 days before any scheduled orthopaedic surgeries to allow adequate time for diagnosis and treatment, with the ultimate goal of diagnosing the underlying cause of anaemia and normalizing the Hb by the day of surgery (see Goodnough *et al.* [8]). Such an approach is reasonable for all patients scheduled for any high-blood-loss procedures, not only orthopaedic surgeries. There is often no justification to subject an anaemic patient to increased risk of transfusion by proceeding with an elective procedure; proper management of anaemia and rescheduling the procedure is the more sensible approach.

The proposed algorithm (Figure 34.2) for evaluation of anaemia includes assessment of the iron status followed by renal function, other nutritional deficiencies and the presence of other chronic diseases. The management strategies should be adjusted based on the underlying cause and may include iron therapy (oral or intravenous, IV), folic acid/vitamin B_{12} supplements, erythropoiesis stimulating agents (ESAs) and referral to specialists for further investigation. ESAs are particularly effective in promoting erythropoiesis and increasing Hb in a relatively short period of time in various surgical and nonsurgical patient populations, producing an equivalent of 1 unit of RBC per week of treatment [9]. However, the associated risk of thrombotic and other serious complications reported for these agents requires that their use be closely monitored and adjusted according to individual patient's needs. Particularly, studies indicate that the associated risks increasingly outweigh the benefits of the ESA therapy as Hb approaches the normal range in patients with chronic kidney disease or cancer. Studies have showed that IV iron is capable of enhancing the therapeutic effect of ESAs, reducing their needed dose, in addition to being an effective haematinic agent on its own (with or without iron pre-existing iron deficiency). Hence, IV iron has been proposed as a relatively safe and effective complement and even an alternative to ESA therapy to improve Hb and patient outcomes while reducing allogeneic blood transfusions. IV iron is often superior to oral iron supplements, given its faster and more effective action, better tolerability and the possibility to provide a total dose in a single infusion using some iron formulations. Serious complications are rare and less frequent in newer IV iron preparations. Other agents such as androgens may also be considered to stimulate haemopoiesis. Despite promising initial results from phase I trials, emergence of neutralizing antibodies hindered the clinical studies on recombinant thrombopoietin as a therapy to increase platelet counts. Newer thrombopoiesis stimulating agents (TSAs) have been developed and are undergoing clinical trials; more data are needed to assess whether these can

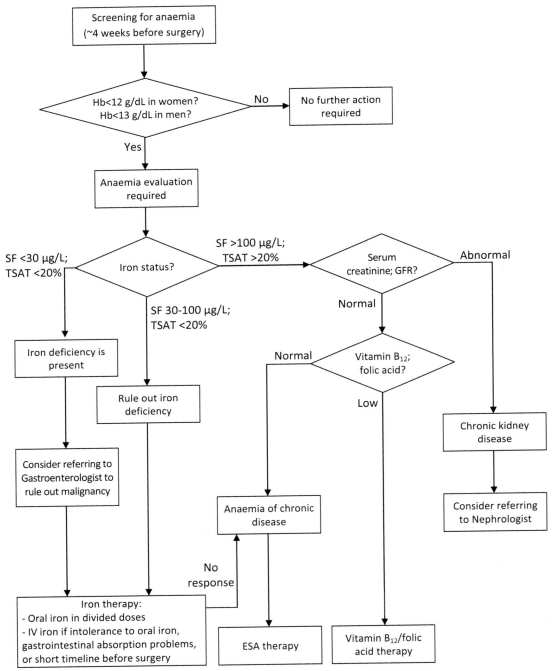

Fig 34.2 Algorithm for detection, evaluation and management of anaemia in patients scheduled for elective surgeries (modified from Goodnough *et al.* [8]). ESA, erythropoiesis stimulating agent; GFR, glomerular filtration rate; Hb, haemoglobin; SF, serum ferritin; TSAT, transferrin saturation.

provide additional tools to optimize haemopoiesis as a potential PBM strategy.

Attention towards anaemia and haemopoiesis should not be limited to the preoperative period. Anaemia is a common finding in the postoperative period, critically ill patients and patients undergoing various medical treatments such as chemoradiotherapy. In all these and other cases, careful screening and management of anaemia will reduce the risk of transfusion while ensuring that the patients are spared from the detrimental impact of anaemia on their clinical outcomes.

Minimizing blood loss

A key perspective in PBM is that the patient's own blood should be viewed as a unique and valuable resource that must be protected against unwarranted loss. Patients can lose blood due to various pathologies (e.g. gastrointestinal bleeding) as well as iatrogenic causes (e.g. excessive phlebotomy for laboratory testing). Surgical bleeding is an obvious source, but other more cryptic sources of blood loss should also be considered. During hospital stay, patients are often subjected to frequent diagnostic blood draws, which can quickly amount to clinically significant blood loss (possibly exceeding 500 mL). In a recent multicentre study (see Salisbury *et al.* [10]), 20% of nonanaemic patients admitted with acute myocardial infarction developed anaemia during their stay and the risk of developing anaemia increased by 18% (15% after multivariate adjustment) for every 50 mL of blood drawn. Mean total phlebotomy volume varied significantly among the studied hospitals [10]. Use of paediatric-sized tubes to collect the blood sample and avoiding 'standing' orders with no or little potential to affect treatment are ways to reduce this source of blood loss.

Detailed history taking and physical examination with attention to potential bleeding disorders is of the utmost importance. The presence of bleeding disorders in the past medical history or family history should be considered as red flags and further investigated. Current medications should be scrutinized for agents that could cause anaemia or interfere with coagulation. Oral anticoagulant therapy and the associated prolonged international normalized ratio (INR) are commonly encountered in patients scheduled for surgery. If not properly managed, these patients may be faced with an increased risk of surgical blood loss (if coagulopathy is significant) or an increased risk of receiving unnecessary and avoidable plasma transfusions – both undesirable outcomes. It should be noted that the often-assumed association between mildly prolonged INR and increased risk of bleeding is not supported by clinical studies. Moreover, allogeneic plasma units may not contain sufficient levels of various coagulation factors, rendering them essentially incapable of correcting mildly prolonged INR. When stable, these patients can be more appropriately managed by discontinuing or adjusting the dose of the anticoagulant and rescheduling the elective procedure. The same approach can be used for patients on antiplatelet therapy ahead of elective high blood-loss procedures. In all cases, potential risks and benefits of anticoagulants in the few days leading to the surgery should be carefully considered [11].

Control of surgical blood loss is another important approach in PBM. Surgical planning and rehearsal, use of less or minimally invasive approaches, use of tourniquets and optimized patient placing and positioning to reduce local blood flow to the site of surgery, avoidance of unnecessary hypothermia, appropriate use of other fluids to maintain normovolaemia, meticulous haemostasis and use of electrocautery and other haemostatic surgical tools instead of traditional scalpels are among the options to reduce surgical blood loss and improve patient outcomes. A growing list of haemostatic agents are available for use in surgical wounds. Topical dressings, sealants and adhesives can reduce bleeding through mechanical blockage and/or active promotion of clot formation or inhibition of fibrinolysis. Among systemic haemostatic agents, lysine analogues (tranexamic acid (TXA) and ε-aminocaproic acid (EACA)) – small molecules with antifibrinolytic activity via inhibiting the conversion of plasminogen to plasmin – have been shown to be relatively safe and highly effective in reducing blood loss and transfusion [7] and in improving patient outcomes. More evidence is needed to support systemic administration of clotting factors such as recombinant activated factor VII (rFVIIa), factor XIII and fibrinogen as safe and effective PBM strategies [12]. Some of these and other pharmacological agents are discussed in more details in Chapter 37.

Autotransfusion techniques are the other available approaches to reduce blood loss or mitigate its effect

Table 34.1 Comparison of key features of most common autotransfusion techniques for use in patient blood management

Key features	Autotransfusion techniques		
	PAD	ANH	CS
Timing of blood collection	Weeks leading to surgery	On the surgery day before incision	During and after surgery
Only applicable to elective procedures	Yes	No	No
Location where blood collection occurs	Out of the operating room in the hospital or outpatient clinic	In the operating room	In the operating room, postanaesthesia care unit, or postoperative recovery room
Source of collected blood	Phlebotomy	Phlebotomy	Shed blood in the field or drains
Specific replacement of collected blood	None; haematinics may be needed to avoid anaemia	Colloids or crystalloids (volume replacement)	None
Potential to optimize haemopoiesis	Yes, particularly if haematinics are used	No	No
Type of infused blood	Stored whole blood	Fresh whole blood	Variable; usually washed or filtered and resuspended RBCs
Risk of contamination with unwanted materials	Unlikely	Unlikely	Possible but clinical significance undetermined
Possibility of storage lesion	Yes	Minimal	Minimal
Possibility of transfusion errors	Yes	Unlikely	Unlikely
Possibility of wastage of blood	Yes	Yes	No (collected blood would have otherwise been lost)
Preparation and logistics	Inconvenient to the patient as multiple hospital visits are required	Minimal	Acquisition and maintenance of the CS machine
Other notable risks and disadvantages	Possibility of rendering patient anaemic and increasing the risk of transfusion by the day of surgery	Potential risks of haemodilution if too aggressive; other risks specific to the used colloids and crystalloids (type and volume)	None other than the quality of the collected blood and the potential for the presence of unwanted cells or materials

ANH, acute normovolaemic hemodilution; CS, red blood cell salvage; PAD, preoperative autologous transfusion.

without use of allogeneic blood. Table 34.1 provides a head-to-head comparison of the key features and characteristics of the three more common autotransfusion techniques (also see Chapter 35). Preoperative autologous donation (PAD) is occasionally considered as an alternative to allogeneic blood transfusion in patients undergoing elective surgery. In this procedure, patients donate about a unit of their blood per week during the weeks leading to the surgery to be stored and reinfused back to them if required during the surgery or immediate postoperative period. PAD use has been declining due to several limitations including significant costs and inconvenience to the patients, risk of becoming anaemic due to the required aggressive phlebotomies and the associated increased risk of needing allogeneic blood in the perioperative period, the need for ESA and iron, folate and vitamin B_{12} supplementation to compensate for the blood draws, potential risk of clerical error, potential harmful effects of storage and the relatively high possibility that many units of PAD blood are not eventually used and are discarded, further shadowing the cost effectiveness of this procedure [13].

Acute normovolaemic haemodilution (ANH) is a simple, low cost autotransfusion technique, especially effective in surgeries with high expected blood loss. In this procedure, a precalculated volume of patient's blood is removed and replaced by crystalloid or colloid solutions before or after the induction of anaesthesia to achieve a predetermined target haematocrit while maintaining the patient normovolaemic. During surgery, patients bleed 'diluted' blood and therefore the lost blood contains fewer cells and factors, effectively reducing the actual amount of blood loss. Collected blood is kept in the operating room and is transfused to patients at wound closure, or whenever blood transfusion is indicated. ANH does not involve any extensive preoperative arrangements and it can be done in both elective and urgent procedures. Moreover, since ANH blood is stored at the patient's bedside, there is no storage and processing cost and risk of clerical errors or harmful effects of storage. Despite theoretical benefits, studies have shown conflicting results on the efficacy of ANH in reducing allogeneic transfusions [14]. Nonetheless, ANH appears to be effective, particularly in procedures characterized by significant blood loss. Platelet-rich plasmapheresis (PRP) is an autotransfusion technique resembling ANH that involves removing a part of the patient's platelets from the circulation ahead of the surgery. The autologous platelets can be reinfused to the patient at the end of surgery to optimize haemostasis [15].

Cell salvage involves recovery of the patient's shed blood from the surgical field, sponges and drains. The procedure can be done during or after the surgery. This blood is then washed, filtered and reinfused back to the patient. Cell salvage has the clear advantage that it relies on a resource that is otherwise wasted and lost. Several studies have supported the efficacy of cell salvage in reducing blood loss and transfusions [16]. However, given the nature of the procedure and the collected blood, controversy exists on the potential link between cell salvage and loss of coagulation factors (because of washing), haemolysis

and increased risk of introducing unwanted materials and contaminations (e.g. bacteria, debris, amniotic fluid or tumour cells) into the blood circulation. Use of leucocyte reduction filters in cell salvage devices appears to be an effective measure to remove the unwanted materials, and available evidence supports the use of cell salvage in most patients undergoing procedures with significant blood loss [17]. Autologous transfusion techniques are discussed in more detail in Chapter 35.

Throughout the care, particularly during the postoperative period, patients should be closely monitored for abnormal bleeding. Postoperative bleeding in excess of what is normally expected should be immediately investigated and controlled, and the patient should be readily transferred back to the operating room for re-exploration if bleeding persists.

Harnessing and optimizing physiological adaptation to anaemia while implementing appropriate therapy

The first pillar of PBM calls for 'anaemia vigilance' among clinicians to actively look for anaemia and manage it in patients. What is meant by the third pillar here is that when an anaemic patient is undergoing proper management and waiting for the treatments (e.g. haematinics) to exert their effects, additional faster-acting appropriate management strategies (other than transfusions) should also be pursued to reduce the immediate negative impact of anaemia, and allogeneic blood transfusions must be used properly and appropriately only when clear indications exist and potential benefits are expected to outweigh the risks (i.e. evidence-based transfusion practice).

As anaemia develops, the body responds by a number of physiological adaptations that may occur anywhere from the cellular and subcellular level to the whole system level. Examples include increased ventilation and Hb oxygen saturation, increased cardiac output, reduced systemic vascular resistance, active control of local blood flow, increased tissue oxygen extraction and cellular metabolic adaptations, all with the goal of maintaining the balance between oxygen supply and demand. Interventions can be done to support and optimize these physiological adaptations to anaemia. Examples include supplemental

385

oxygen therapy, maintaining adequate perfusion and normovolaemia, and avoiding tachycardia and other conditions associated with increased unnecessary demand.

As untreated anaemia becomes more severe, adaptive mechanisms begin to fail and the oxygen delivery and supply becomes inadequate to meet the demand at some point depending on the individual tissue and organ. When this occurs, the risk of tissue hypoxia and ischaemia quickly increases and, if left untreated, the patient condition and clinical outcomes deteriorate. When a patient is moving in this direction and is likely to experience tissue hypoxia and ischaemia, measures must be employed to improve the oxygen delivery capacity of the blood quickly and this is when allogeneic blood transfusions are indicated and necessary. Similarly, it may be required to raise a patient's platelet count or increase coagulation factors quickly. Timely and appropriate transfusion of blood components is the other important aspect of the third pillar of PBM.

Numerous studies, including controlled trials, have shown that 'restrictive' transfusion strategies (usually based on Hb levels of 7–8 g/dL as triggers) are safe and effective in the management of patients who are commonly considered for transfusion, and often achieve better outcomes. Although the term 'restrictive' may imply that the patients are deprived of a beneficial treatment, it is used in this context in contrast to traditional 'liberal' transfusion triggers (namely the outdated and discredited Hb/haematocrit 10/30 rule), which are now widely believed to be excessive and harmful to the patients. Transfusion guidelines for various patient populations are available, and they all emphasize that blood and blood components should be transfused when 'clear' physiological need exists, rather than blindly based on arbitrary Hb or haematocrit 'triggers'. The goal should be treating the patient, rather than attaining a certain Hb level [18, 19]. Nonetheless and despite certain limitations, Hb or haematocrit levels remain the most commonly used criteria for making transfusion decisions. Most current guidelines agree that transfusions are usually indicated in patients with Hb levels below 6 g/dL, and they are almost never indicated in patients with Hb levels above 10 g/dL; Hb levels between these two ends constitute a grey zone in which the benefits of transfusion are unclear, with factors such as advanced age and comorbidities (e.g. heart disease) often considered in making the decision [19]. Yet, the

lowest permissible Hb level varies among individual patients, depending on their physiopathological status and rate and trend of blood loss. Therefore, signs of inadequate oxygen delivery and ischaemia (e.g. relative hypotension or tachycardia, new ischaemic ST-segment changes, increased oxygen extraction rate and decreased oxygen consumption) in the context of anaemia and normovolaemia and the absence of other probable causes are usually indications for transfusion regardless of Hb [20].

Conclusions

A feedback cycle exists between anaemia, allogeneic blood transfusions and unfavourable patient outcomes. In addition to anaemia increasing the risk of transfusions, anaemia and transfusion are both independent risk factors for adverse outcomes. New or aggravated pre-existing comorbidities can in turn exacerbate anaemia (e.g. via inflammation) and/or increase the risk of a patient being transfused (e.g. a new or worsened ischaemic heart disease resulting in the patient being more liberally transfused in fear of ischaemia). PBM provides strategies to break these vicious cycles and improve patient outcomes [5].

Figure 34.3 depicts the schematic effects of PBM strategies on a hypothetical patient's Hb, the Hb threshold at which oxygen demand overtakes the supply (the so-called critical Hb) and the likelihood of receiving allogeneic blood transfusions, compared with a hypothetical patient treated according to more 'conventional' strategies. Individual strategies used in PBM show various levels of effectiveness in reducing transfusions and improving patient outcomes as supported by numerous studies. However, PBM is more effective when appropriate strategies are implemented in combination and as part of multimodality, multidisciplinary programmes. Data on effectiveness of implementation of PBM strategies in concert to achieve its goal are beginning to emerge, but more data are needed to establish and quantify better the impact of PBM on patient outcomes [21]. PBM strategies are rapidly evolving to reflect the latest findings in the field. Newer technologies such as point-of-care coagulation testing and continuous Hb monitoring are promising tools to assess better the patients' needs and adjust their management, but more clinical evidence is needed to support their widespread use. Advances in

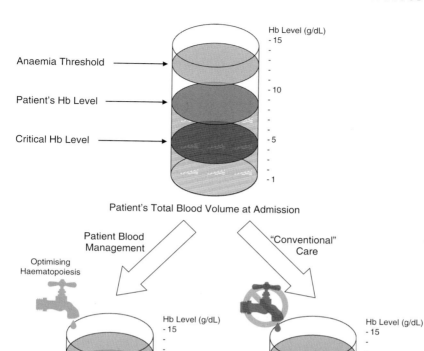

Fig 34.3 Schematic comparison of patient blood management (PBM) versus more 'conventional' care and the impact on allogeneic blood transfusions. A hypothetical patient is admitted with pre-existing anaemia. Proper management according to PBM strategies would result in increased haemoglobin concentration (Hb; represented by the upper tap), reduced blood loss (represented by the lower tap), potentially lower critical Hb level and more judicious use of blood components, altogether reducing allogeneic blood transfusions and improving patient outcomes. Conversely, undetected and unmanaged anaemia, uncontrolled blood loss and liberal transfusion strategies would result in the patient receiving (potentially unnecessary and harmful) allogeneic blood transfusions without remarkable benefits.

our understanding of the circulation system in physiological and pathological conditions, oxygen demand of organs, tolerance of anaemia and adaptive measures and coagulation, as well as more refined surgical techniques and more specific pharmacologic agents, have revolutionized our approach to transfusion. The trend is only expected to escalate in the years to come, with many more blood management modalities expected to become available. With all these exciting developments in mind, one should not forget that, in all cases, improving the patients' clinical outcomes is the first and foremost goal of PBM.

387

Key points

1 A vicious cycle often exists between anaemia, allogeneic blood transfusions and unfavourable patient outcomes, with anaemia and transfusion being independent risk factors of worse outcomes.

2 Many patients are inappropriately transfused, as indicated by the vastly variable transfusion rates not explainable by patients' characteristics or procedures alone.

3 There is urgent need for adopting more judicious use of allogeneic blood and a shift from a 'product-centred' to 'patient-centred' transfusion practice.

4 Patient blood management (PBM) is 'the timely application of evidence-based medical and surgical concepts designed to maintain Hb, optimise haemostasis and minimise blood loss in an effort to improve patient outcome'.

5 What makes PBM distinct is its emphasis on improving the clinical outcomes of the patients through the use of preventive measures.

6 PBM strategies can be adjusted and applied during the care of all patients who may be candidates for transfusion at some stages of their treatment.

7 PBM achieves its goals through relying on three main strategies: optimizing haemopoiesis, minimizing bleeding and harnessing and optimizing physiological adaptation to anaemia while implementing appropriate therapy.

8 PBM is more effective when appropriate strategies are implemented in combination and as part of multimodality, multidisciplinary programmes.

References

1 Drackley A, Newbold KB, Paez A & Heddle N. Forecasting Ontario's blood supply and demand. *Transfusion* 2011; 52(2): 366–74.

2 Shander A, Fink A, Javidroozi M, Erhard J, Farmer SL, Corwin H *et al.* Appropriateness of allogeneic red blood cell transfusion: The International Consensus Conference on Transfusion Outcomes. *Transfus Med Rev* 2011; 25(3): 232–246.

3 Bennett-Guerrero E, Zhao Y, O'Brien SM, Ferguson Jr TB, Peterson ED, Gammie JS *et al.* Variation in use of blood transfusion in coronary artery bypass graft surgery. *J Am Med Assoc* 2010; 304(14): 1568–1575.

4 Goodnough LT & Shander A. Patient blood management. *Anesthesiology* 2012; 116(6): 1367–1376.

5 Gombotz H, Rehak PH, Shander A & Hofmann A. Blood use in elective surgery: the Austrian benchmark study. *Transfusion* 2007; 47(8): 1468–1480.

6 Thomson A, Farmer S, Hofmann A, Isbister J & Shander A. Patient blood management – a new paradigm for transfusion medicine? *ISBT Sci Ser* 2009; 4: 423–435.

7 Henry DA, Carless PA, Moxey AJ, O'Connell D, Stokes BJ, Fergusson DA *et al.* Anti-fibrinolytic use for minimising perioperative allogeneic blood transfusion. *Cochrane Database Syst Rev* 2011; (3): CD001886.

8 Goodnough LT, Maniatis A, Earnshaw P, Benoni G, Beris P, Bisbe E *et al.* Detection, evaluation, and management of preoperative anaemia in the elective orthopaedic surgical patient: NATA guidelines. *Br J Anaesth* 2011, January; 106(1): 13–22.

9 Bohlius J, Tonia T & Schwarzer G. Twist and shout: one decade of meta-analyses of erythropoiesis-stimulating agents in cancer patients. *Acta Haematol* 2011; 125(1–2): 55–67.

10 Salisbury AC, Reid KJ, Alexander KP, Masoudi FA, Lai SM, Chan PS *et al.* Diagnostic blood loss from phlebotomy and hospital-acquired anemia during acute myocardial infarction. *Arch Int Med* 2011; 171(18): 1646–1653.

11 Jacob M, Smedira N, Blackstone E, Williams S & Cho L. Effect of timing of chronic preoperative aspirin discontinuation on morbidity and mortality in coronary artery bypass surgery. *Circulation* 2011; 123(6): 577–583.

12 Lin Y, Stanworth S, Birchall J, Doree C & Hyde C. Use of recombinant factor VIIa for the prevention and treatment of bleeding in patients without hemophilia: a systematic review and meta-analysis. *CMAJ* 2011; 183(1): E9–19.

13 Goodnough LT. Autologous blood donation. *Anesthesiol Clin North America* 2005; 23(2): 263–270, vi.

14 Segal JB, Blasco-Colmenares E, Norris EJ & Guallar E. Preoperative acute normovolemic hemodilution: a meta-analysis. *Transfusion* 2004; 44(5): 632–644.

15 Carless PA, Rubens FD, Anthony DM, O'Connell D & Henry DA. Platelet-rich-plasmapheresis for minimising peri-operative allogeneic blood transfusion. *Cochrane Database Syst Rev* 2011; (3): CD004172.

16 Carless PA, Henry DA, Moxey AJ, O'Connell D, Brown T & Fergusson DA. Cell salvage for minimising perioperative allogeneic blood transfusion. *Cochrane Database Syst Rev* 2010; (4): CD001888.

17 Esper SA & Waters JH. Intra-operative cell salvage: a fresh look at the indications and contraindications. *Blood Transfus* 2011; 9(2):139–147.

18 Napolitano LM, Kurek S, Luchette FA, Corwin HL, Barie PS, Tisherman SA *et al.* Clinical practice guideline: red

blood cell transfusion in adult trauma and critical care. *Crit Care Med* 2009; 37(12): 3124–3157.

19 Practice guidelines for perioperative blood transfusion and adjuvant therapies: an updated report by the American Society of Anesthesiologists Task Force on Perioperative Blood Transfusion and Adjuvant Therapies. *Anesthesiology* 2006; 105(1): 198–208.

20 Madjdpour C & Spahn DR. Allogeneic red blood cell transfusion: physiology of oxygen transport. *Best Pract Res Clin Anaesthesiol* 2007; 21(2): 163–171.

21 Spahn DR. Anemia and patient blood management in hip and knee surgery: a systematic review of the literature. *Anesthesiology* 2010; 113(2): 482–495.

Further reading

Achneck HE, Sileshi B, Jamiolkowski RM, Albala DM, Shapiro ML & Lawson JH. A comprehensive review of topical hemostatic agents: efficacy and recommendations for use. *Ann Surg* 2010, February; 251(2):217–228.

Carless PA, Henry DA, Carson JL, Hebert PP, McClelland B & Ker K. Transfusion thresholds and other strategies for guiding allogeneic red blood cell transfusion. *Cochrane Database Syst Rev* 2010; (10): CD002042.

Goodnough LT & Shander A. Blood management. *Arch Pathol Lab Med* 2007, May; 131(5): 695–701.

Isbister JP, Shander A, Spahn DR, Erhard J, Farmer SL & Hofmann A. Adverse blood transfusion outcomes: establishing causation. *Transfus Med Rev* 2011, April; 25(2):89–101.

Munoz M, Garcia-Erce JA, Villar I & Thomas D. Blood conservation strategies in major orthopaedic surgery: efficacy, safety and European regulations. *Vox Sanguinis* 2009, January; 96(1):1–13.

Shander A, Javidroozi M, Ozawa S & Hare GM. What is really dangerous – anaemia or transfusion? *Br J Anaesth* 2011; 107(S1): i41–i59.

Shander A, Moskowitz DM & Javidroozi M. Blood conservation in practice: an overview. *Br J Hosp Med (Lond)* 2009, January; 70(1): 16–21.

Shander A, Spence RK & Auerbach M. Can intravenous iron therapy meet the unmet needs created by the new restrictions on erythropoietic stimulating agents? *Transfusion* 2010, March; 50(3): 719–732.

Society of Thoracic Surgeons Blood Conservation Guideline Task Force; Ferraris VA, Brown JR, Despotis GJ, Hammon JW, Reece TB et al. 2011 update to the Society of Thoracic Surgeons and the Society of Cardiovascular Anesthesiologists blood conservation clinical practice guidelines. *Ann Thorac Surg* 2011, March; 91(3): 944–982.

35 Autologous transfusion

Dafydd Thomas[1], Biddy Ridler[2] & John Thompson[2]

[1]Morriston Hospital, Swansea, Wales, UK
[2]Peninsula College of Medicine and Dentistry, Royal Devon and Exeter Hospitals, Exeter, UK

Autologous (patient's own) blood transfusion has come full circle. The salvage and reinfusion of blood lost during an amputation was first reported by Dr John Duncan in 1885. The development of blood storage, banking and understanding of serology then led to safe and effective transfusion support for medicine, surgery and obstetrics using donor blood. However, the increased cost of blood components, decreasing numbers of blood donors, increased demand, inappropriate use and successive threats of bacterial, viral and prion infection changed our emphasis at the end of the last century [1–3]. Perhaps the major driver was a medicolegal one, with a new benchmark, namely 'The public is entitled to expect that the blood they receive will be 100% safe [4]. The knowledge of the medical profession is not relevant in determining the legitimate expectation of the public and nor is the fact that the defect could not have been avoided in relevant circumstance. Once the risk is known about the product is defective even if the risk could not be identified in the particular product' (Lord Justice Burton, 2001).

As a result of haemovigilance several successful measures were introduced to improve blood safety and the various techniques for the provision of autologous blood have been refined, studied scientifically and audited.

The 'Appropriate Use of Blood' subcommittee was established by NHS Blood and Transplant in England to discuss and investigate strategies for blood conservation. It came to the conclusion that an integrated programme would be more successful than piecemeal implementation and that autologous blood transfusion should be part of a total quality management approach based on four strands (Table 35.1):

• preoperative identification of patients at increased risk of bleeding and optimization before surgery (e.g. correction of anaemia);
• perioperative blood salvage (collection of blood that would otherwise be lost in the surgical field or in postoperative drains);
• blood sparing methods such as drugs and surgical technique; and
• a strict postoperative transfusion protocol.

Reasons to consider autologous transfusion

Clinical transfusion practice should reduce the risks involved in blood transfusion. Strict blood donor exclusion criteria together with extensive testing of blood to decrease the risk of transfusion-transmitted infection has reassured clinicians and maintained demand for donor blood. Blood conservation strategies should minimize the use of donor blood by withholding transfusion until strictly clinically necessary and employing techniques such as autologous transfusion. In some situations, autologous transfusion is definitely indicated, such as in patients with rare blood groups or complex red cell antibodies for whom it

Practical Transfusion Medicine, Fourth Edition. Edited by Michael F. Murphy, Derwood H. Pamphilon and Nancy M. Heddle.
© 2013 John Wiley & Sons, Ltd. Published 2013 by John Wiley & Sons, Ltd.

Table 35.1 An approach to blood conservation and the reduction of risk associated with blood transfusion in patients having elective surgery.

- Check the blood count well in advance of surgery and correct any treatable anaemia
- Ask about antiplatelet or anticoagulant drugs the patient is taking and consider if any should be stopped
- Abide by the maximum/blood ordering schedule that should be available in your organization
- Check antibody status and blood group so group-specific blood can be used in an emergency
- Consider whether the patient has a hereditary or acquired bleeding tendency and investigate/treat as appropriate
- During surgery consider technical methods to reduce bleeding
- Postoperatively, consider whether blood transfusion is clinically indicated (transfusion trigger) and, if it is, consider how many units are required to achieve the desired Hb (transfusion target)
- If operation would normally require blood transfusion, consider the option of autologous blood transfusion

Such as:

Technique	Situations in which it might be considered
Intraoperative cell salvage	Any patient with estimated blood loss >0.5 L; especially suitable for massive blood loss
Postoperative cell salvage	Patients with postoperative drain loss from a clean site

is difficult to source compatible blood. Autologous transfusion should also be used instead of, or to supplement the use of, donor blood, in situations where it has been shown to be effective and safe. It has been suggested that more than 20% of surgical demand can be met by autologous transfusion [5] and other blood conservation methods such as preoperative anaemia optimization [6]. Certain procedures can be undertaken with virtually no donor blood support (see Chapter 34), conserving supplies for areas of medicine where there are few alternatives, such as haematological oncology and the increased use in upper gastrointestinal haemorrhage.

Blood conservation strategies

Since the third edition of *Practical Transfusion Medicine*, there has been considerable research, audit and re-evaluation of blood sparing strategies, with the result that several are no longer used in clinical practice.

Pre-deposit autologous donation

This technique was much vaunted as a means of donating and reserving one's own blood prior to elective surgery [7]. Several observational (but very few randomized) studies were published. The problems were as follows:

- Patients were chronically anaemic at the time of surgery, with little reserve for bleeding and so they were subsequently transfused more frequently.
- Anaemia increases the bleeding time and therefore surgical blood loss.
- The practical difficulties were significant both for the patient and the participating hospital.
- Cancelled operations meant that blood could go out of date.
- Prospective randomized trials showed comparatively modest savings in donor blood transfusion.
- Careful blood transfusion protocols in the control groups seriously reduced overall transfusion and surgical teams began to introduce other more effective techniques to reduce blood loss, because they knew they were being observed.
- There was a lower threshold for transfusing the pre-deposited blood (because it was there), but there was still the potential for clerical or other errors.

Pre-deposit may be useful in certain special situations, such as in paediatric surgery, where there is a great incentive to avoid transfusion-associated infection. In such cases, it can be assisted by stimulating the patient's bone marrow with recombinant erythropoietin and iron (usually parenterally) to increase haemoglobin (Hb) concentration. Directed pre-deposit from relatives was abandoned for ethical reasons as it would place relatives under pressure to reveal lifestyle choices that they might want to keep private.

Acute normovolaemic haemodilution

Acute normovolaemic haemodilution (ANH) seemed to have great promise but is seldom practised outside specialist surgical areas. Blood is withdrawn at the beginning of surgery and replaced with a balance of colloid (usually complexed starch) and clear fluid to maintain normovolaemia. The patient consequently bleeds dilute blood during the procedure, so decreasing red cell loss. After surgical blood loss ceases, the fresh autologous blood is returned. The problems are as follows:
• There is no level 1 scientific evidence (from a properly powered randomized controlled trial) to show that ANH actually reduces donor blood exposure.
• ANH takes on average 20 minutes to perform and theatre time is precious.
• Haemodilution may increase bleeding by reducing the haematocrit and diluting clotting factors.
• Haemodilution may precipitate cardiac ischaemia and even myocardial infarction.

Most studies of ANH were not randomized or used ANH in conjunction with other methods, so it was difficult to ascribe benefit to one or the other. In addition, although theoretical formulas could be used to determine exactly how much blood could be withdrawn, in clinical practice most authors reported comparatively modest volumes of ANH. There may be circumstances where high volume ANH could be employed in fit patients at low risk of myocardial ischaemia, particularly paediatric spinal surgery. Pilot studies have been successful and randomized trials in niche areas are awaited.

Other techniques that have been abandoned

• Routine preoperative coagulation tests (unless there is a positive personal or family history of bleeding).
• Transfusion if Hb >10 g/dL (accepted as unnecessary).
• Aprotinin (withdrawn by the manufacturer because of renal failure and decreased survival).
• Ultrafiltration to remove excess water after cardiac bypass.
• Leucocyte filters in bypass circuits (may activate white cells).

• Platelet-rich plasmapheresis (no benefit).
• Unwashed mediastinal blood (may lead to coagulopathy).
• DDAVP (unless there is an established platelet defect such as uraemia or von Willebrand's disease).
• Bovine thrombin-derived haemostatic sealants in cardiac surgery (can provoke antibody response and allergy), although the new generation selected male donor products are less likely to cause these problems.

Effective methods for blood conservation

The following techniques are accepted and should be part of a hospital's blood conservation strategy:
• Total quality management – continuous audit and improvement of the process of blood transfusion in the perioperative setting (see Chapters 27 and 34).
• Intraoperative cell salvage (ICS).
• Postoperative cell salvage (PCS) from wound drains.
• *Appropriate* transfusion and acceptance of the very low risk of viral and other risks.
• Transfusion if Hb < 7 g/dL postoperatively.
• Stopping drugs associated with increased bleeding such as aspirin (unless a high cardiac risk) or clopidogrel (unless a drug eluting coronary stent was inserted in the last 6 months).
• Blood component therapy if active oozing and supported by abnormal tests and thromboelastography.
• Near patient Hb testing.
• Limited sampling in intensive care (reduced volume tubes, near patient testing).

Before surgery: optimizing Hb and haemostasis

This process involves preassessing a patient in advance of surgery and taking steps to reduce the requirements for transfusion. 'Preparing Patients for Surgery' clinics can also identify medical or social reasons that may have led to an operation being cancelled and therefore increase a hospital's efficiency.

If a patient is anaemic, it is important to investigate the underlying cause. For example, iron deficiency may be due to a gastrointestinal malignancy. If a patient with iron deficiency anaemia is started on iron, the Hb can be expected to rise by about 1 g/dL per week. It is therefore important to check the blood count sufficiently far in advance of surgery to allow time for treatment to be given if required. Patients presenting for surgery with a normal Hb will require transfusion at a later stage or may even avoid blood transfusion altogether. A personal 'goal' is useful for the patient and their general practitioner; e.g. Hb >12 g/dL prior to elective hip replacement.

Newer formulations of intravenous iron have fewer adverse reactions than were associated with these preparations in the past. Intravenous iron is almost immediately available for red cell production. Research is being undertaken to determine whether administration of intravenous iron as late as the pre-operative day can improve red cell production in response to surgical anaemia and thus decrease the use of donor blood.

It is important to consider patient factors that might cause excessive blood loss during surgery and that can be corrected in advance. Patients on aspirin or clopidogrel for secondary prevention can stop it 5–7 days before surgery (except if the patient is at high risk of suffering a myocardial infarction or has a drug-eluting coronary stent). Patients in atrial fibrillation on warfarin can discontinue the drug a few days before surgery. The newer oral anticogulants such as dagibatran and rivaroxaban are likely to rise in popularity over the next few years. For dagibatran, which has a half-life of 12–17 h, the thrombin clotting time, ecarin clotting time and TT determined by Hemo-clot(R) thrombin inhibitor assay are sensitive tests to qualitatively evaluate the anticoagulant effects. The activated partial thromboplastin time (aPTT) can provide a useful qualitative assessment of anticoagulant activity but is less sensitive. The factor Xa inhibitor rivaroxaban has a shorter (7–11 h) half-life, so simple withdrawal should suffice, except for emergency surgery, when prothrombin concentrates can be used to reverse the anticoagulant effect.

If it is imperative to continue anticoagulation, such as in cases of mechanical heart valve replacement, the patient may be given intravenous heparin to cover the surgical period. It is important to take a bleeding history when the patient is seen prior to surgery. Screening tests and specific treatment may be required (see Chapter 25). Bleeding diatheses must be considered in patients with renal or liver disease. Agents such as desmopressin (DDAVP) or tranexamic acid may enhance surgical haemostasis [8] (see Chapter 37).

During surgery: reduction in blood loss

Blood loss in many operations has fallen significantly with advancing surgical and anaesthetic techniques. Use of harmonic scalpels, laparoscopy and careful surgical technique has had a huge impact on blood usage. The maintenance of normothermia ensures optimum coagulation and has also been shown to decrease blood loss.

There are several techniques specific to cardiac surgery that have been the subject of good-quality clinical trials. Protamine sulfate has an anticoagulant effect when used in excess, so reduced doses are now given following bypass surgery. The dose can be titrated using the activated clotting time, or more simply a 50% dose given. In vascular surgery, heparin is no longer reversed. Heparin-bonded bypass circuits can be used to reduce the dose of systemic heparin required. Shed mediastinal blood can be reinfused if washed (see below).

During/after surgery: when to transfuse

No blood transfusion is without risks, but equally the administration of blood may be life saving. In making the decision to transfuse, the balance of risks must be considered for each individual. Factors influencing the decision to transfuse include the Hb, the patient's life expectancy, i.e. age/prognosis (many of the adverse effects of transfusion-transmitted infection or immune modulation are delayed) and, above all, clinical judgement about the patient's ability to tolerate anaemia, including the presence of other factors such as cardiac or respiratory disease and sepsis.

Transfusion triggers

Data from patients who refuse blood on religious grounds or who live in parts of the world where blood is scarce or dangerous have helped our understanding of the effects of anaemia. In otherwise healthy patients the following transfusion triggers for stable anaemia might be considered:

- <4 g/dL: transfuse unless fit, asymptomatic and Hb rising;
- 4–7 g/dL: transfusion usually necessary;

CHAPTER 35

- 7–10 g/dL: transfusion not usually necessary; and
- >10 g/dL: transfusion rarely required [6, 9].

A randomized trial of patients in intensive care showed that less severely ill patients (Acute Physiology and Chronic Health Evaluation II score <20) and patients under 55 years actually had a survival advantage if the Hb was maintained between 7 and 9 g/dL rather than between 10 and 12 g/dL. For patients with clinically significant cardiac disease the mortality was similar in both groups [10].

For otherwise fit patients with a previously normal Hb who are actively bleeding, the following guidelines are appropriate:
- Blood loss <15% blood volume: give fluids; no need to transfuse.
- Blood loss 15–30% blood volume: consider transfusion.
- Blood loss 30–40% blood volume: transfusion usually necessary.
- Blood loss >40% blood volume: transfusion indicated.

Note that blood volume is about 70 mL/kg in adults, so that 20% of blood volume is approximately 1 L. For patients with a short life expectancy or those with chronic anaemia and impaired red cell production, the main trigger for transfusion should be the patient's *symptoms*.

Transfusion targets

In addition to considering when to transfuse, a target Hb should be established for each clinical scenario using the best data available (see above and Chapter 27). It is also important to consider how many units to give. In other words, the *dose* of blood should depend on the estimated blood volume based on the patient's weight.

When a patient is actively bleeding, replacement of red cells should be guided by an estimate of blood loss. A guide to how many units are required to achieve the target is shown in Table 35.2. Single-unit transfusions have previously been discouraged. However, Table 35.2 shows that it might be reasonable to give one unit to a small elderly woman who is symptomatic with an Hb of 7 g/dL to bring it up to just under 9 g/dL. The transfusion of blood just because it has been made available for the patient should be avoided. If blood is not used, it can be returned to the blood bank and

Table 35.2 Guide to number of units required to achieve the 'target' haemoglobin (Hb).

Amount of Hb in 1 unit of red cells
Example: volume bled 450 mL × average Hb 13 g/dL = 58 g/unit

	Weight (kg)		
	43	57	71
Blood volume (70 mL/kg in adults)	3 L	4 L	5 L
Increase in Hb after one unit transfusion (g/dL)	1.9	1.6	1.2

used for another patient. Near patient testing with a device such as the Haemocue is an *essential* component of modern theatre practice for incremental transfusion management. This is also gradually becoming standard for ward practice.

Techniques for providing autologous blood

ICS now seems to offer the most cost-effective method of autologous transfusion. Future issues in blood supply and demand combined with the discovery of other bloodborne diseases may change this view and result in a re-examination of PAD and ANH. Autologous blood must be clearly labelled and be distinct from donor blood. An example of an autologous blood label is shown in Figure 35.1; autologous units are more easily identified if their labels are printed a different colour to those used for allogeneic blood.

Cell salvage

Principle
During surgical operations when blood loss is expected, blood can be collected, processed and then returned to the patient. This can be done either intraoperatively or postoperatively depending on the type of operation. This process can be cost effective even when small volumes of blood (i.e. more than 500 mL) are collected. The amount salvaged not only decreases the use of allogeneic blood but in many instances completely removes the need for allogeneic blood transfusion, i.e. 'bloodless surgery'.

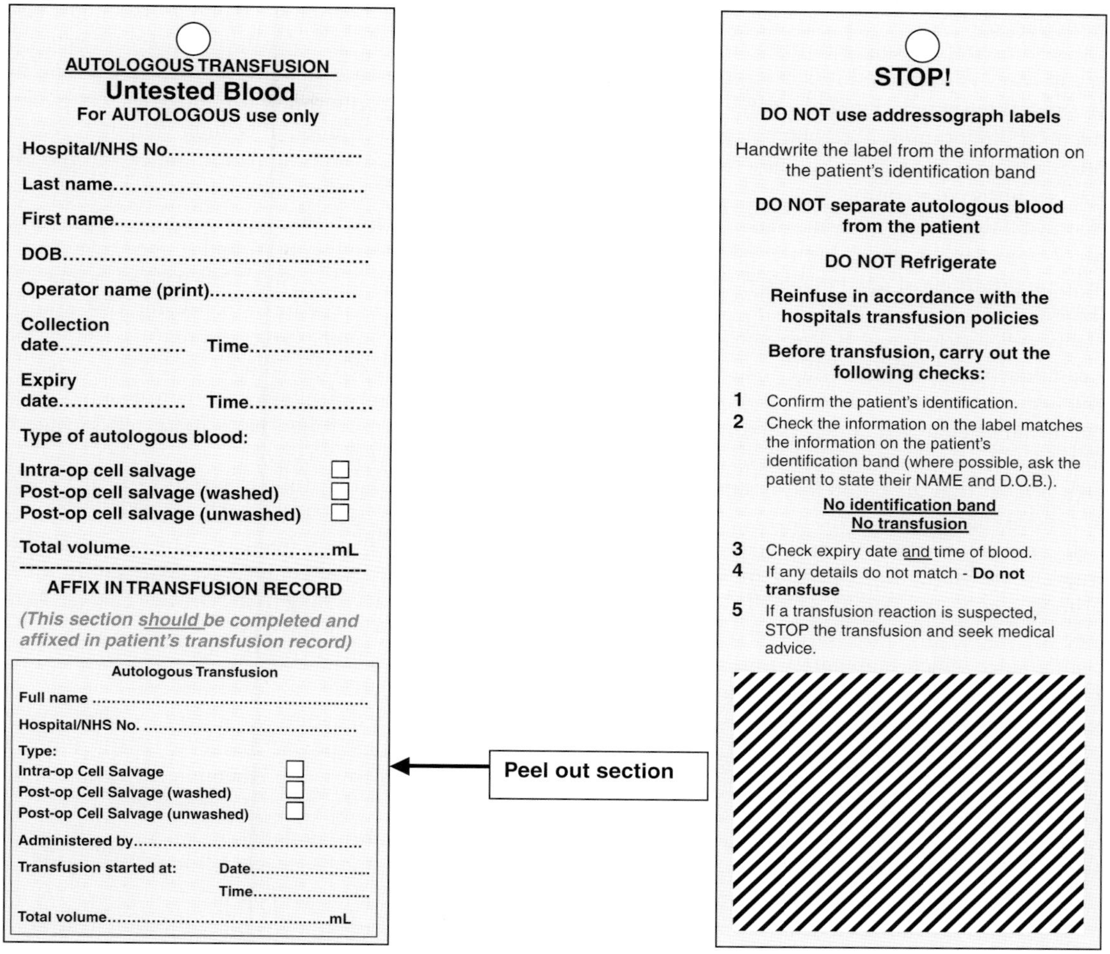
AUTOLOGOUS TRANSFUSION
Untested Blood
For AUTOLOGOUS use only
Hospital/NHS No.................................
Last name...
First name..
DOB..
Operator name (print)...........................
Collection
date..................... Time.......................
Expiry
date..................... Time.......................
Type of autologous blood:
Intra-op cell salvage ☐
Post-op cell salvage (washed) ☐
Post-op cell salvage (unwashed) ☐
Total volume.................................mL
AFFIX IN TRANSFUSION RECORD
(This section should be completed and affixed in patient's transfusion record)
Autologous Transfusion
Full name ....
Hospital/NHS No. ....
Type:
Intra-op Cell Salvage ☐
Post-op Cell Salvage (washed) ☐
Post-op Cell Salvage (unwashed) ☐
Administered by..
Transfusion started at: Date..........................
Time..........................
Total volume..mL

Peel out section

STOP!
DO NOT use addressograph labels
Handwrite the label from the information on the patient's identification band
DO NOT separate autologous blood from the patient
DO NOT Refrigerate
Reinfuse in accordance with the hospitals transfusion policies
Before transfusion, carry out the following checks:
1 Confirm the patient's identification.
2 Check the information on the label matches the information on the patient's identification band (where possible, ask the patient to state their NAME and D.O.B.).
No identification band
No transfusion
3 Check expiry date and time of blood.
4 If any details do not match - **Do not transfuse**
5 If a transfusion reaction is suspected, STOP the transfusion and seek medical advice.

Fig 35.1 Autologous labels (provided by the UK Cell Salvage Action Group).

Intraoperative cell salvage

Intraoperative cell salvage (ICS) involves the collection and reinfusion of red cells lost during surgery [11]. This may be performed as follows:

- Single-unit reinfusion devices (only used in fully anticoagulated patients). These are simple and cheap for low volume losses.
- Continuous reinfusion of unprocessed blood using a dialysis technique. This may be used in conjunction with cardiac bypass but is not of proven benefit and may be associated with risk of haemolysis and high dose heparin reinfusion leading to coagulopathy.
- Reinfusion of processed blood (discussed below).

There are a number of machines available that wash red cells by centrifugation and resuspend them in saline (examples are shown in Plates 35.1 to 35.4 in the plate section). Blood is aspirated from the wound site and mixed with heparin or citrate anticoagulant via dual-lumen suction before it enters the reservoir of the machine. The cycle can be either run automatically or controlled manually. In general, about 75% of red cells can be recovered for reinfusion back into the patient. The machines can deliver the equivalent of 10 units of blood per hour. Swabs laden with blood can be wrung out into a bowl of normal saline and then suctioned into the device for processing to further increase yield.

Advantages of ICS
- There is a considerable reduction in donor blood usage in cases where blood loss is large (>1 L). Suitable operations might include open heart surgery, cystectomy and ruptured ectopic pregnancy, aortic aneurysm repair and spinal surgery (especially paediatric scoliosis correction).
- It is available to *all* patients having appropriate surgery regardless of medical fitness.
- In some situations of uncontrolled blood loss it may be life saving.
- Unlike other techniques, ICS can be used selectively in cases where the actual, rather than the predicted, blood loss is high.
- Blood can be collected in the reservoir and the decision to use the machine and harness can be deferred until it is clear that the blood loss is sufficient to warrant processing.
- Cell salvage is generally accepted by Jehovah's Witnesses, provided the collected blood remains in continuity with the patient. Finally, and perhaps most importantly, the processed red cells stay by the patient's side, which eliminates almost entirely the risk of receiving the wrong blood. Identification error remains one of the biggest risks of blood transfusion.

Disadvantages/risks of ICS
Adverse events to autologous blood transfusion are now reported to the Serious Hazard of Transfusion (SHOT) scheme in the UK. In 2010 there were 15 reported events including clerical error and hypotension during reinfusion through ultrafiltration under pressure. With regard to specific concerns:
- The reinfusion of haemolysed salvaged blood is unlikely, providing the wash process is undertaken correctly. Currently available machines operate on an automatic washing process. A sensor monitors the effluent from the wash cycle, which continues until the liquid being discarded is completely clear, suggesting removal of all free Hb, fragmented red cells and other contaminants. Quality control samples should be assayed and logged for all individual machines.
- There have been no deaths associated with air embolism, due to improved design and greater awareness of such problems. Air embolism was only reported with very early machines, but collected blood should not be used with pressurized reinfusion devices.

- It does not recover all the blood lost so donor blood may be required in massive haemorrhage. Platelets and coagulation factors are removed by the washing process so supplementation with allogeneic coagulation factors may be required after high volume ICS (> six cycles depending on coagulation indices) in the same way as it may be required after massive blood transfusion (see Chapter 26).
- It requires a capital outlay and trained operators, so ICS can be used only in hospitals with sufficient numbers of suitable procedures to become cost effective. As the cost of donor blood continues to rise with the introduction of safety measures such as universal leucocyte reduction of blood and increasingly sensitive and expensive microbiology testing, cell salvage has become more cost effective.

It is important to follow agreed standard operating procedures, to document all stages of the process and maintain an audit database. Operators should be properly trained and competency assessed. In the UK this should be according to the UK Cell Salvage Action Group (UKCSAG) guidelines.

Indications for ICS
The primary indication is surgery, where expected blood loss is likely to be in excess of 500 mL. Even when blood loss is unpredictable, the collection of operative blood loss may be worthwhile. Providing this blood is anticoagulated, it can be processed and reinfused as red cells suspended in saline if sufficient volumes are collected. The processing kits are separately packaged so only the collection reservoir is wasted if small volumes are salvaged following a decision not to proceed to processing. ICS is cost-neutral providing one unit of packed red cells is reinfused. Even if a small volume of ICS blood is retransfused, raising the patient's Hb level to exceed the agreed transfusion trigger will obviate the need for donor blood.

Relative contraindications
There are a number of situations where the use of cell salvage has been discouraged. In the presence of massive haemorrhage, however, ICS may avoid hypovolaemic shock.
- Malignant cells. Although leucocyte filters may remove the majority of cancer cells, and small numbers may not be clinically significant compared with the numbers that enter the circulation during surgery,

some would advocate the use of gamma-irradiation in this setting, but this is logistically difficult to arrange. Several studies have reported large numbers of patients receiving cell salvage during cancer surgery, particularly in urology. To date there have been no reports of lung metastasis or decreased survival. The technique should be discussed on an individual basis with patients, with special arrangements for consent. The National Institute for Health and Clinical Excellence (NICE) has now approved ICS in urological malignancy in the UK, and all recipients of ICS in cancer surgery should be involved in audit or clinical trials.

• Infection. Although the balance of risk depends on the clinical urgency for salvaged blood, antibiotics may be added to the anticoagulant solution and given parenterally to the patient to treat bacteraemia. Several trials have confirmed the value of ICS in trauma where the quality of life gain for younger fitter patients is very high.

• Amniotic fluid in the operative field, which may cause embolism/disseminated intravascular coagulation. Studies show that circulating amniotic fluid is common during normal and Caesarean delivery. It is removed during the normal wash cycle and adverse events are rare. ICS can be life saving in complicated pregnancy such as placenta accreta. Filtering of the salvaged blood removes lamellar bodies and fetal squames and may enhance patient safety. NICE now approves ICS in obstetric practice.

• Sickle cell disease. Cells may sickle in the machine due to low oxygen tension and therefore red cell yield would be low. This is a theoretical reason to avoid using ICS in the presence of sickle cell disease.

• Where topical clotting agents such as fibrin glue have been used or iodine has been used to wash out the abdomen. In practice, these contaminants promote thrombin generation or haemolyse red cells. Even if these agents are collected they are washed out during the centrifugal process, but it is recommended to temporarily cease suction, irrigate the surgical area with at least 1 L of IV grade normal saline and then recommence processing.

• There have been reports of hypotension associated with the reinfusion of ICS blood in obstetric practice, when negatively charged leucocyte depletion filters have been used. This may occur if the blood is infused under pressure. To date there are no clear data but it is important to avoid pressure reinfusion. This may limit the speed of reinfusion in cases of massive haemorrhage.

Postoperative cell salvage

Postoperative cell salvage (PCS) involves the collection of blood from surgical drains followed by reinfusion with or without processing. The blood recovered is dilute, partially haemolysed and defibrinogenated and contains high levels of cytokines unless washed. There is a clear advantage in terms of enhanced recovery following knee replacement and it may be that cellular activation and enhanced nitric oxide levels during nonwashed PCS are a positive contributory factor in boosting immunity [1]. Randomized trials comparing washed and nonwashed PCS with allogeneic blood are awaited. If the collected wound drainage blood is simply reinfused, some centres limit the quantity reinfused. Others recommend that all blood is washed and resuspended in saline. This can be done either with the apheresis machines used in the main theatre suite or with the newer and more compact processing machines that wash collected blood by the patient's bedside.

The current state of the art in postoperative drainage centres on audits to look at the precise volumes reinfused and its cost effectiveness as a blood sparing technique.

Key points

1 Autologous transfusion should be considered as part of a total quality management strategy for minimizing the risk associated with transfusion for all patients having surgery.

2 Planning and appropriate treatment in advance of or during surgery can reduce transfusion requirements.

3 An audit of ICS and PCS activity can give useful local data and inform clinicians about indicated surgical cases.

4 Before transfusing a patient always consider the strict clinical indications and how many allogeneic units are required.

5 ICS and PCS are the most effective methods of autologous transfusion.

6 The reinfused red cells are capable of carrying oxygen immediately to the tissues.

References

1 Gharehbaghian A, Haque KM, Truman C *et al*. Effect of autologous salvaged blood on postoperative natural killer cell precursor frequency. *Lancet* 2004; 363:1025–1030.

2 Goodnough LT, Brecher ME, Kanter MH & AuBuchon JP. Transfusion medicine. Part 1. *N Engl J Med* 1999; 340: 438–447.

3 Goodnough LT, Brecher ME, Kanter MH & AuBuchon JP. Transfusion medicine. Part 2. *N Engl J Med* 1999; 340: 525–533.

4 Calman KC. Cancer: science and society and the communication of risk. *Br Med J* 1996; 313: 799–802.

5 Consensus Statement. Autologous transfusion: 3 years on. What is new? What has happened? *Transfus Med* 1999; 9: 285–286.

6 American Society of Anesthesiologists Task Force on Perioperative Blood Transfusion and Adjuvant Therapies. Practice guidelines for perioperative blood transfusion and adjuvant therapies: an updated report by the American Society of Anesthesiologists Task Force on Perioperative Blood Transfusion and Adjuvant Therapies. *Anesthesiology* 2006; 105: 198–208.

7 British Committee for Standards in Haematology. Guidelines for policies on alternatives to allogeneic blood transfusion 1. Predeposit autologous blood donation and transfusion. *Transfus Med* 2007; 17: 354–365.

8 CRASH-2 Trial Collaborators. Effects of tranexamic acid on death, vascular occlusive events, and blood transfusion in trauma patients with significant haemorrhage (CRASH-2): a randomised, placebo-controlled trial. *Lancet* 2010; 376(9734): 23–32.

9 Carless PA, Henry DA, Carson JL, Hebert PP, McClelland B & Ker K. Transfusion thresholds and other strategies for guiding allogeneic red blood cell transfusion. *Cochrane Database Syst Rev* 2010; CD002042.

10 Hebert PC, Wells G, Blachman MA *et al*. A multicentre, randomized, controlled clinical trial of transfusion requirements in critical care. Transfusion Requirements in Critical Care Investigators, Canadian Critical Care Trials Group. *N Engl J Med* 1999; 340: 409–417.

11 Ashworth A & Klein A. Cell salvage as part of a blood conservation strategy in anaesthesia. *Br J Anaesth* 2010; 105: 401–416.

Further reading

Maniatis A, Van der Linden P & Hardy J-F (eds). *Alternatives to Blood Transfusion Medicine*, 2nd edn. Oxford: Wiley Blackwell; 2011.

Shander A, Javidroozi M, Ozawa S & Hare GMT. What is really dangerous: anaemia or transfusion? *Br J Anaesth* 2011; 107 (Suppl. 1): i41–i59.

Speiss BD, Spence RK & Shander A (eds). *Perioperative Transfusion Medicine*, 2nd edn. Philadelphia, PA: Lippincott Williams & Wilkins; 2006.

Thomas D, Thompson J & Ridler B (eds). *A Manual for Blood Conservation*. Shrewsbury: tfm Publishing Ltd; 2005.

36 Blood substitutes

David J. Roberts[1] & Chris V. Prowse[2]

[1]University of Oxford, NHS Blood and Transplant and Department of Haematology, John Radcliffe Hospital, Oxford, UK

[2]Edinburgh University, Edinburgh, Scotland, UK

Collecting and fractionating human blood for medical use is an expensive and time-consuming process. Large donor panels must be recruited and tested to maintain a constant supply of safe, phenotyped cellular and protein fractions of whole blood. Collection and processing of blood are complex procedures. Moreover blood transfusion carries risks and has significant, and in some cases unavoidable, side effects [1]. There are obvious attractions to the potential replacement of transfusion of cellular components with alternative products that do not have the same dependence on a readily available blood donor population, can be treated to reduce infectious and noninfectious risks, do not require crossmatching and that have a less-restrictive shelf life than the current red cell and platelet components provided by transfusion services [2]. Such products would be of particular interest in battlefield and emergency situations and the armed services have been a major funder of research in this field [3] (Table 36.1).

Despite this and research programmes that stretch back to the earlier half of the last century there are, as yet, no licensed products in this field, other than one haemoglobin solution in South Africa. Hopes of making artificial blood substitutes have also been dampened by a persuasive systematic review of red cell haemoglobin substitutes that has revealed that aggregated data from many small trials show a high morbidity and mortality from thrombotic events including myocardial infarction [4]. At the same time our understanding of stem cell biology and haematopoietic development has made the growth of red blood cells, platelets and neutrophils *in vitro* a real possibility. An alternative approach of 'virtual blood substitutes' to achieve the desired effect without transfusion is described below.

In broad terms there are three categories of blood substitute under development:
• products that are still based on the use of donor-derived blood cells (human or animal);
• synthetic products that achieve the same endpoint by mirroring the function of the natural product or by novel mechanisms;
• 'virtual' blood substitutes (see Table 36.2), using growth factors to stimulate endogenous haemopoiesis or drugs to secure haemostasis.

The outstanding 'virtual' blood substitutes are the haemopoietic growth factors that can stimulate production of red cells and platelets and mobilize white cells and stem cells. Increasing the effectiveness of circulating platelets with 1-deamino-8-D-arginine vasopressin (DDAVP) or the use of recombinant factor VIIa, inhibiting fibrinolysis by tranexamic acid or ε-aminocaproic acid, or securing haemostasis by the use of fibrin sealant are well-established methods of reducing bleeding and through avoiding red cell and/or platelet transfusion are classic 'virtual' blood substitutes [5–7]. The pivotal CRASH-2 trial showed that tranexamic acid reduced mortality in major trauma when given up to three hours after injury [8]. This

Practical Transfusion Medicine, Fourth Edition. Edited by Michael F. Murphy, Derwood H. Pamphilon and Nancy M. Heddle.
© 2013 John Wiley & Sons, Ltd. Published 2013 by John Wiley & Sons, Ltd.

Table 36.1 Potential 'real' blood substitutes.

Red blood cells	Crosslinked haemoglobin tetramers
	Recombinant haemoglobin tetramers
	Polymerized haemoglobin
	Conjugated haemoglobins
	Encapsulated haemoglobin
	Perfluorocarbons
	In vitro expansion of red blood cells
Platelets	Freeze-dried platelets
	Infusible platelet membranes
	Fibrinogen-coated microspheres
	Peptide-coated red cells
	Glycoprotein receptor carrying liposomes
	Megakaryocytes
	In vitro expansion of megakaryocytes
White blood cells	*In vitro* generation of antiviral and antitumour cytotoxic lymphocytes
	In vitro generation of dendritic cells
Stem cells	*In vitro* expansion of stem cells

landmark study has stimulated renewed interest in this therapy and recent studies have suggested tranexamic acid may be effective in reducing blood loss in orthopaedic surgery and reducing mortality in battlefield trauma. Further major trials of tranexamic acid are planned in obstetric and upper gastrointestinal haemorrhage.

Table 36.2 Virtual blood substitutes.

Red blood cells	Erythropoietin
Leucocytes	Antibiotics, antiviral and antifungal agents
	Active immunization
	G-CSF and GM-CSF
Platelets	TPO
	PEGylated recombinant human megakaryocyte growth and development factor (MGDF)
	Interleukin 11
	TPO mimetics – microbial peptides
Haemostatic &	Aprotinin
Pharmacological	DDAVP
Agents	episilon-aminocaproic acid and tranexamic acid
	Recombinant coagulation factor VIIa
	Fibrin sealants

This chapter discusses the 'real' red cell and platelet substitutes in development. The virtual blood substitutes are covered in Chapters 25, 35 and 37. Understanding the potential role of blood substitutes and the practical and theoretical obstacles to their introduction into clinical practice provides illuminating lessons about the physiology of blood and modern biotechnology.

Red cell substitutes

Modified haemoglobin-based blood substitutes

Red blood cells have a number of functions beyond oxygen and carbon dioxide transport, including:
• modulation of oxygen delivery under conditions of low pH and/or high pCO$_2$ (the Bohr effect);
• encapsulation of haemoglobin to prolong circulating half-life;
• modulation of vascular tone via effects on nitric oxide (NO) concentrations;
• reduction of methaemoglobin.

These functions depend on a complex and elegant interplay between the haemoglobin molecule, the red cell enzymes, the internal milieu and the red cell membrane [8]. Perhaps, not surprisingly, the higher order functions of the red cell have proved difficult to mimic in artificial components.

Early attempts to transfuse purified unmodified haemoglobin did show that the oxygen-carrying capacity could be restored. However, transfusion of unmodified haemoglobin causes a number of problems [9]. The main side effects can be summarized as follows:
• Isolated tetramers are unstable and dissociate to globin dimers and monomers. As the tetramers dissociate, the allosteric cooperativity and the modulation of oxygen affinity by bound 2,3-diphosphogylcerate (2,3-DPG) are lost, giving a reduced oxygen carrying capacity. The P_{50} (the partial pressure of O_2 at which haemoglobin is half-saturated with oxygen) is reduced from 26 to less than 10 mmHg (Figure 36.1a).
• Globin chains, and to some extent tetramers, are filtered by the kidneys and precipitate in the renal tubules, causing renal dysfunction.
• Isolated tetramers transit the vascular endothelium and scavenge NO, so reducing NO availability in

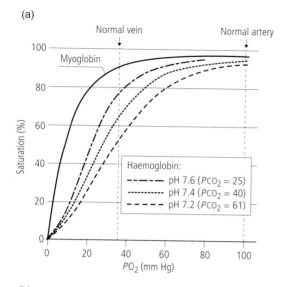

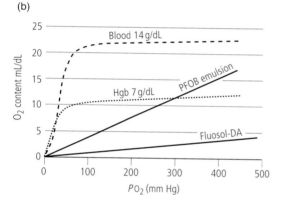

Fig 36.1 (a) Oxygen affinity of haemoglobin tetramers and monomers. Oxygen-dissociation curve of myoglobin or dissociated haemoglobin monomers compared with that of haemoglobin at two pH values. PO_2, partial pressure of oxygen. (b) Oxygen affinity of PFCs. Comparison of oxygen-carrying capacity of whole blood and fluorocarbons. Whole blood with a haemoglobin content of 14 g/dL possesses an arterial O_2 content of 20 mL/dL at a PO_2 of 100 mmHg. By contrast, fluorocarbon emulsions carry less O_2 at a given partial pressure of oxygen. A 90% PFOB emulsion can carry 10 mL of O_2 at a PO_2 of 300 mmHg. Perfluorodecalin (*Fluosol-DA 20*), which used early emulsification technology to achieve a 20% fluorocarbon emulsion, can only carry 2–3 mL of O_2/dL at PO_2 of 300 mmHg.

the extravascular compartment causes vasoconstriction and oesophageal spasm.

Reduction of NO has dramatic effects on the vascular physiology and can result in not only vasoconstriction but also inflammation and platelet activation. Several modifications have been made to free haemoglobin tetramers to overcome these problems. Currently, Several second-generation red cell substitutes, including intramolecularly crosslinked haemoglobin, conjugated haemoglobin and polymerized haemoglobin, have been the subject of clinical trials and the third generation of substitutes of artificial red blood cells is under development and at the stage of animal trials (for summary see Table 36.3). It is also now clear that haemoglobin-based blood substitutes do not reduce transfusion requirements but merely defer it as they are cleared quickly. The strategy for the possible use of these therapies is now focused on improving oxygen delivery in specific situations. In the USA, the FDA have stated that they will only consider licensing red cell substitutes for three indications:
• regional perfusion, e.g. percutaneous transcoronary angioplasty, enhancing radiation therapy of tumours;
• acute haemorrhaghic shock;
• for use in the perioperative period.

Intramolecularly crosslinked haemoglobin

Diaspirin crosslinked haemoglobin

The crosslinking of haemoglobin tetramers with bis-(3,5-dibromosalicyl) fumarate yields diaspirin crosslinked haemoglobins with a high P_{50} for good oxygen delivery, e.g. *Hemassist*. However, haemoglobin tetramers still cause significant smooth muscle spasm, leading to oesophageal spasm and increases in blood pressure. The product has now been withdrawn due to an excess death rate in a clinical trial in trauma patients.

Recombinant haemoglobin

Large-scale production of recombinant haemoglobin in *Escherichia coli* and yeast has been established by Somatogen, who were purchased by Baxter in 1998. Using recombinant DNA technology the alpha

Table 36.3 Red cell substitutes under trial or development.

	Product/company	Current status
Intramolecularly crosslinked haemoglobin		
Diaspirin crosslinked haemoglobin	*Hemassist*, Baxter Healthcare (USA)	Failed phase III trials
Recombinant haemoglobin	*Optro/rHb2.0*, Somatogen Inc. with Baxter (USA)	Shelved
Polynitroxylated haemoglobin tetramers	*Hemozyme*, SynZyme(USA)	Shelved
Sebacoyl-linked haemoglobin tetramers	*OxyVita* IPBL Pharmaceuticals	Shelved
Polymerized haemoglobin		
Glutaraldehyde crosslinked haemoglobin	*Polyheme*, Northfield (USA)	Shelved
Glutaraldehyde crosslinked bovine haemoglobin*	*Hemopure*, Biopure (USA)	Shelved
O-raffinose crosslinked haemoglobin	*Hemolink*, Hemosol (Canada)	Failed phase III trials
Conjugated haemoglobin		
Polyoxyethylene: haemoglobin	*PHP*, Apex Bioscience (USA)	In phase III trials
Polyethylene glycol: bovine haemoglobin	Enzon (USA)	In phase Ib/II trials
Polyethylene glycol: human haemoglobin	*Hemospan*, Sangart (USA)	Shelved
Bovine Hb polymer containing SOD and catalase	*PolyHb-SOD-CAT*, McGill University	Pre-clinical
Covalent complex bovine haemoglobin with GSSG, adenosine and ATP	*Hemotech*, HemoBiotech Inc.	Pre-clinical
Encapsulated haemoglobin Perfluorocarbons		
Liposome-encapsulated haemoglobin	Terumo (Japan), US Navy	Pre-clinical
Perfluorocarbons		
Synthetic fluorocarbron/emulsifer	*Perftoran*	Licensed in Russia and Mexico
	Oxygent, Alliance (USA)	Phase III trials planned
	Oxycyte	Side effects concern in phase I trials

*Licensed in South Africa for anaemia therapy.

globin chains were fused to yield an undissociable 'tetramer'. It was also possible to engineer haemoglobin molecules to reduce NO affinity. Baxter has announced withdrawal from this development.

Polymerized haemoglobin

Haemoglobin may be crosslinked by bifunctional chemicals to form polymers or haemoglobin molecules can be directly linked to a high molecular weight nonprotein carrier. In either form renal filtration and smooth muscle dysfunction may be reduced. The oxygen-carrying capacity, reduced by the loss of 2,3-DPG binding, may be restored by other modifications. Three forms of crosslinked polymerized haemoglobin were produced for clinical trials.

Glutaraldehyde crosslinked haemoglobin

Human haemoglobin has been crosslinked with glutaraldehyde and pyridoxal phosphate added to the 2,3-DPG pocket to increase P_{50} (*Polyheme*,

Northfield, Inc.). The second polymerized product is a glutaraldehyde crosslinked bovine haemoglobin (*Hemopure*, Biopure). This product is licensed in South Africa and a similar product is already licensed for canine use.

O-raffinose crosslinked haemoglobin

The third form of polymerized haemoglobin is one with oxidized O-raffinose crosslinking, which produces a haemoglobin polymer with a high P_{50}. However, the product contains biologically significant amounts of crosslinked haemoglobin tetramers, which can and do cause smooth muscle spasm in the gastrointestinal tract.

Conjugated haemoglobin

Polymeric haemoglobin may also be made by crosslinking haemoglobin, not to itself but to high molecular weight polyoxyethylene (*PHP*, Apex Bioscience) or to polyethylene glycol (*PEG-Hb*, Enzon Inc.; *Hemospan*, Sangart Inc.) These methods increase the half-life of the preparations and reduce NO-mediated vasoactivity. The Apex Bioscience and Enzon products have been at trial in sepsis and to improve solid tumour radiation therapy. *Hemospan* is unusual in having a deliberately low P_{50} to prevent the release of oxygen until the haemoglobin reaches the capillaries, and phase I trials have shown it lacks the vasoactivity of most other preparations and can result in smooth muscle spasm.

The use of these haemoglobin-based blood substitutes was reviewed by Nathanson and colleagues following an FDA-sponsored workshop to consider the reasons behind the slow development of these products [4, 9]. The group reviewed the clinical effectiveness of *Hemassist*, *Hemopure*, *Hemolink*, *PolyHeme* and *Hemospan*. It proved very difficult to assemble the data from many small trials, which in some cases had never been made public, but they were able to use data presented to the FDA and from press releases. The meta-analysis reached many startling conclusions. First, these haemoglobin-based blood substitutes were associated with an increased mortality (relative risk 1.3) and myocardial infarction (relative risk 2.7). Second, and perhaps more disturbingly, the trials that could have reached this conclusion were completed in 2000 but no mechanism existed to ensure such

clinically significant data on morbidity and mortality from a medicinal product reached the public domain. It was evident that several subsequent trials had been granted ethical permission without the full data on the dangers of the products available to the review boards. Development of these products has now ceased [10].

Second-generation haemoglobin-based blood substitutes

Development has continued on other modifications to haemoglobin that may make it useful and safe as a blood substitute. Flexible cross-linkers may generates well-defined octamers or bis-tetramers that show cooperative oxygen binding and remain within the circulation [11]. Within the red cell, haemoglobin may also enhance the production of NO by reduction of nitrite. It appear that bis-tetramers and haemoglobin linked to polyethylene glycol (PEGylated-Hb) retain nitrite reductase activity and so enhance NO bioavailability and vasodilation [12]. These results are promising but the clinical effectiveness and safety of these products remains to be established.

Artificial red blood cells – encapsulated haemoglobins

The third generation of haemoglobin-based red cell substitutes include artificial red blood cells. The modern formulations have used phospholipid vesicles (0.2 μm in diameter) with sialic acid analogues added to the membranes to reduce the clearance by the reticuloendothelial system. Further improvements to microencapsulated haemoglobin under investigation are:

• inclusion of catalase and superoxide dismutase to reduce oxygen radical and methaemoglobin formation and

• use of biodegradable polylactides and polyglycolides in artificial membranes or nanoparticles to increase haemoglobin concentration to 15 g/dL in small nanometre diameter vesicles.

These second- and third-generation haemoglobin substitutes are at the early stage of animal trials. It seems feasible that further development may produce artificial erythrocytes or haemoglobin polymers that may mimic some of the complex, higher order functions of 'real' red cells.

Clinical use of haemoglobin-based red cell substitutes

The problems that have been revealed regarding not only the lack of effectiveness but also the increased morbidity and mortality of haemoglobin-based blood substitutes has diminished but not extinguished enthusiasm for their development and clinical use. It seems certain that any product entering clinical trials will be subject to much greater scrutiny and evaluation of known side effects in well-designed animal trials before entering human Phase I trials [13]. It looks very difficult to achieve sustained increased delivery in total oxygen in clinical use or reduction in use of allogeneic blood cells. It is of interest to remember that a recent systematic review has demonstrated that reducing trigger levels can by itself reduce allogeneic transfusion by up to 40% [14]. Nevertheless, there is much interest in using these blood substitutes to improve local oxygen delivery in critically ischaemic areas by manipulating the molecular size and oxygen affinity of haemoglobin-based therapies [15].

Red blood cells grown *in vitro*

All red cells are ultimately derived from self-renewing stem cells that reside in the periosteal niche in the bone marrow. These stem cells can also circulate and both bone marrow and peripheral blood-derived stem cells can be isolated and used for haematopoietic stem cell transplants. Isolated stem cells can be induced to differentiate into early and late erythroblasts and finally enucleated reticulocytes using defined ambient oxygen concentrations, cytokine mixtures with or without stromal or supporting cells [16, 17]. These models have been used to understand the normal and pathological development of red cells. However, the expansion of erythroid cells has been sufficiently refined to grow enough red cells *in vitro* for transfusion into humans [17]. The derived red cells appear to have a normal structure and function although the type of haemoglobin chains that are present depends on the source of the stem cells and the degree of switching from the fetal to adult pattern of haemoglobin gene expression. Red cells derived *in vitro* would all be young red cells or reticulocytes while red cells from a donor are comprised of red blood cells with an age distribution from reticulocytes to cells that are near the end of their lifespan. Therefore, red cells grown *in vitro* may have a long lifespan and so enhanced survival in the recipient compared to red cells collected from a donor.

There are now other possible sources of stem cells. Embryonic stem cells can be isolated and maintained in culture. They can be induced to develop into all cell linages including red blood cells. The number of embryonic stem cells lines is limited but now it is possible to form induced pluripotent stem cells (iPSCs) from fibroblasts or other apparently terminally differentiated cells by 'reprogramming' these mature cells by the expression of just a few transcription factors [18]. The ultimate potential of iPS cells to make mature erythroid cells with normal phenotypes is not yet clear but these methods would have the enormous advantage of generating self-renewing stem cells from donors with defined red cell, white or platelet antigen phenotypes for specific applications in diagnostic or therapeutic uses, e.g. as rare blood groups or as exact matches for recipients with multiple alloantibodies. While the red cell work is the furthest advanced, it is also possible to develop platelets and neutrophils *in vitro* from stem cells from cord or adult blood or from embryonic or induced pluripotent stem cells.

There are many technical problems to be overcome if red cells, neutrophil or platelets derived *in vitro* are to become a reality. Maintaining the cultures will require industrial scale methods and artificial supports to allow the large volume of cells to develop in culture. Nevertheless, these applications, which could not have been seriously contemplated only a few years ago, are now at advanced stages of development in many laboratories and over the next few years we can expect to see human trials of these products.

Perfluorocarbons

Principle

Liquid perfluorocarbons (PFC) are synthetic hydrocarbons in which most of the hydrogen atoms have been substituted by fluorine atoms. The low intermolecular attractions result in a high capacity to dissolve gases such that the oxygen content of a PFC is up to 20 times that of water [19].

These chemicals have inherent limitations including a short intravascular half-life ($\sim$12 h), insolublity in water requiring emulsification with surfactants and limited oxygen-carrying capacity–the amount of oxygen carried is directly proportional to the inspired oxygen concentration (see Figure 36.1b). This requires patients to breathe oxygen-rich air, limiting their use to operating rooms and intensive care settings.

First-generation fluorocarbons

Fluosol-DA 20, an emulsion of 20% perfluorodecalin, is the only oxygen-carrying volume expander licensed in the USA. It was initially hoped it would gain widespread use but trials showed no efficacy in patients who refused blood transfusions. The only indication for which it has been approved is percutaneous transluminal coronary angioplasty, although some trials showed no benefit in combination with tissue plasminogen activator (tPA) over tPA alone. The inherent limitations of this perfluorocarbon are compounded by the side effects, which include:

- marked uptake by the reticuloendothelial system;
- disruption of pulmonary surfactant leading to ventilation/perfusion defects in the lungs; and
- complement activation resulting in anaphylaxis.

Fluosol has been approved to date by the US Food and Drug Administration and licensed for use in nine countries, not for the use of reducing the amount of allogeneic blood units transfused but for use during cardiac angioplasty. However, the storage and rewarming of this emulsion proved problematic and production has ceased.

Perftoran is an improved first-generation perfluorocarbon. The emulsified product consists of particles of approximately 1 μm diameter, apparently allowing them to evade clearance by macrophages and so have a longer half-life and fewer side effects. It is, however, only produced in Russia and has been licensed for use there and in Mexico.

Oxygent

This second-generation perfluorocarbon, based on perfluoro-octylbromide (PFOB), has been trialled by Alliance Pharmaceutical Company and contains egg yolk phospholipids as emulsifier. This composition confers several advantages over previous products including:

- greater oxygen-carrying capacity (see Figure 36.1b);
- reduced or absent complement activation;

- reduced interference with pulmonary surfactants; and
- improved stability and shelf life.

The small size of PFCs has suggested that they may improve oxygenation in ischaemic or infarcted tissues or increase oxygenation in tumours and so increase sensitization to radiotherapy or chemotherapy. Trials have been performed in a number of perioperative settings, most notably in cardiac surgery, in conjunction with acute normovolaemic haemodilution (ANH). Such trials have shown a delay in the time to reach the trigger levels for allogeneic transfusion, but a large pivotal trial was recently suspended due to concerns about the excess rate of stroke. This has now been ascribed to overenthusiastic ANH rather than the use of the PFC. Side effects of flushing and flu-like symptoms and delayed fever, headaches and nausea, as a result of macrophage activation, and a transient thrombocytopenia occur in some patients and may limit clinical applications.

It is currently approved for Phase II trials in the USA and Phase II trials in Europe. Some results are promising but a recent trial in cardiac surgery showed an excess of stoke compared to controls, suggesting that systemic side effects have not been eliminated. Further trials will be watched carefully.

Third-generation perfluorocarbons

Third-generation PFCs are under development. *Oxycyte* is based on F-*tert*-butylcyclohexane and is being studied as an 'oxygen therapeutic'. The aim of these products is not to replace allogeneic blood components but to supplement their use or effectiveness in specific situations. A Phase I safety study in traumatic brain injury has been completed and Phase II studies are underway in Switzerland and Israel.

Platelet substitutes

Platelet concentrates are widely used in the management of thrombocytopenia and abnormal platelet function. These products have allowed the development of chemotherapy regimens that cause prolonged absence of platelet production and have made extracorporeal bypass a safe, routine procedure. However, both the supply and use of fresh platelets pose particular problems due to storage being limited to

5 days due to gradual loss efficacy and the risk of bacterial contamination. Supply also requires the maintenance of large, well-characterized donor panels and specialized centres for apheresis procurement. Repeated platelet transfusions are frequently accompanied by the development of antiplatelet antibodies, usually directed against major histocompatibility complex (MHC) class I antigens or against other platelet surface antigens.

Artificial platelet substitutes hold the promise of avoiding these logistic, technical and medical problems and so achieving cheaper, safer and more readily available therapy for thrombocytopenia. However, as for red cells, replacement of the natural product has not been straightforward. Attempts to replace platelets can again be divided into 'real' and 'virtual' platelet substitutes. Virtual platelet substitutes range from improved clinical guidelines and their implementation (Chapters 23 and 34), through drugs that may reduce blood loss (Chapter 37) to compounds that stimulate platelet production. Although not strictly speaking a platelet substitute, the development of pathogen reduction technologies for platelets may eliminate bacteria, viruses and leucocytes from this product, so reducing transfusion-transmitted infection, febrile nonhaemolytic transfusion reactions and transfusion-associated graft-versus-host disease.

Substitutes for platelets have not yet been licensed but several products are under development (Table 36.1). The most promising are summarized below.

Platelet membrane preparations

In the search for an alternative to fresh platelet concentrates, freeze-dried platelets were initially shown to be superior to frozen and thawed platelets in tests of haemostasis *in vitro*. Freeze-dried platelets were subsequently shown to be as effective as stored platelets *in vitro* and to provide haemostasis in thrombocytopenic animals. Clinical evaluation is planned. Compared to platelet concentrates, freeze-dried platelets have the apparent advantages of reduced viral and bacterial load as a result of paraformaldehyde treatment. However, they have some disadvantages:
• must be made from fresh platelets and
• may still stimulate an alloimmune response.

Infusible platelet membranes are derived from stored platelets as membrane fragments that seem to promote haemostasis without causing thrombosis in animals [20]. They are the only platelet substitute to have undergone clinical trial, where they were shown in a small number of patients to be effective in individuals refractory to standard platelet transfusion studies. The advantages of infusible plasma membranes over platelet concentrates include:
• reduced viral and bacterial load;
• reduced expression of HLA class I antigens; and
• may be made from outdated platelets.

However, these membrane preparations are clearly recognized by the innate immune system and rapidly cleared by splenic macrophages. The short circulating half-life of these agents poses a substantial obstacle to their clinical use.

Synthetic platelets

Beyond the manipulation of platelet membranes the search for a useful substitute for platelet concentrates has led to a totally synthetic approach (Figure 36.2). Microspheres of human albumin coated with human fibrinogen (*Synthocytes*, *Thrombospheres*) reduce bleeding time and acute blood loss in thrombocytopenic animals. They have no immediate toxicity in rodents or primates. Fibrinogen-coated microspheres would have the advantages of:
• sterility;
• production independent of platelet concentrates; and
• absence of HLA class I and platelet surface alloantigens.

Interestingly, these microspheres appear to promote the formation of a platelet plug by interacting with residual normal platelets. It seems likely that both lyophilized platelet and infusible plasma membranes may also function in a similar manner. Liposomes with inserted platelet receptors are also under investigation as a platelet alternative.

The efficacy of lyophilized platelets, infusible platelet membranes and fibrinogen-coated microspheres in the prophylaxis of bleeding in severely thrombocytopenic patients will require careful evaluation and there has been little progress in this field over the last decade. More immediate applications for these platelet substitutes may be in improving haemostasis where the platelet count is moderately reduced and as alternative or adjuvant therapy where patients have

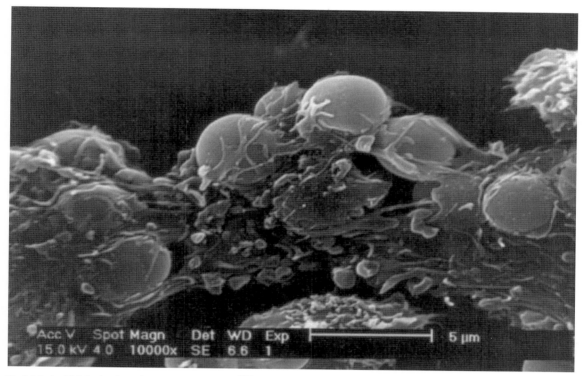

Fig 36.2 Artificial platelet substitutes–*Synthocytes*™. Electron micrograph showing the interaction of *Synthocytes*™ and normal platelets on a collagen surface.

become refractory to platelet transfusions through alloimmunization.

Summary

Real red blood and platelet substitutes have yet to reach the clinic. Simple substitutes lack the more complex and important function of whole cells. The development of first and second generation of haemoglobin-based blood substitutes has been halted after a pivotal systematic review showed that they were associated with excess mortality and an increased risk of myocardial infraction compared with controls. There are a number of other haemoglobin substitutes in development that are being designed to have no vasoactive effects and that may increase NO delivery locally. Incorporation of haemoglobin in polymers or nanoparticles may also yield a safe and effective product. The perfluorocarbons have also been beset by serious side effects, but second- and third-generation products are in early clinical trials.

Progress with platelet substitutes has also been slow. Synthetic microspheres that provide platelet-like activity may be free of viral contamination and polymorphic molecules, but would seem unlikely to be as effective as fresh platelets with the possible exception of treating haemorrhage, e.g. in patients with immune platelet refractoriness with no compatible donors.

Therefore, while nontoxic substitutes with reasonable biological activity are likely to be available, it is far from clear whether they will replace cells derived from donors for the majority of clinical uses. The new understanding of stem cell biology and differentiation has revealed the possibility of growing red blood cells and platelets *in vitro*. The conclusion drawn five years ago still seems valid, namely, at the risk of making speculative assessments, it seems more likely that real blood substitutes will find small niche applications and the virtual blood substitutes and improved prescribing will reduce the use of donor-derived products.

Key points

1 A series of modified haemoglobin-based blood substitutes have been developed to try to avoid dependence on donors, any infectious risk and unwanted immune responses.
2 Red blood cells have a number of functions beyond oxygen and carbon dioxide transport including NO generation and control of vascular responses that have proved difficult to mimic with blood substitutes. Existing haemoglobin-based blood substitutes have proven to be unsafe, causing myocardial infarction and increasing mortality.
3 Newer crosslinked and polymerized haemoglobin-based blood substitutes may have a better vascular response profile but are in an early phase of clinical development.
4 Platelet substitutes have been developed but have not been shown to be clinically effective.
5 It may be possible to grow red blood cells, platelets and neutrophils *in vitro* from stem cells for therapeutic use.
6 It is likely that blood substitutes in development will only have niche applications for the foreseeable future.

References

1 Shander A, Javidroozi M, Ozawa S & Hare GM. What is really dangerous: anaemia or transfusion? *Br J Anaesth* 2011; 107 (Suppl. 1): i41–59.
2 Jacobs T and Fischer J. When a long shot is worth a shot. *Nature Biotechnol* 2005; 23: 805.
3 Auker CR & McCarron RM. US Navy experience with research on, and development of, hemoglobin-based oxygen carriers. *J Trauma* 2011; 70 (5 Suppl.): S40–S41.
4 Natanson C, Kern SJ, Lurie P, Banks SM & Wolfe SM. Cell-free hemoglobin-based blood substitutes and risk of myocardial infarction and death: a meta-analysis. *J Am Med Assoc* 2008; 299: 2304–2312.
5 Dhillon S. Fibrin sealant (evicel® [quixil®/crosseal™]): a review of its use as supportive treatment for haemostasis in surgery. *Drugs* 2011; 71: 1893–1915.
6 Morrison JJ, Dubose JJ, Rasmussen TE & Midwinter MJ. Military Application of Tranexamic Acid in Trauma Emergency Resuscitation (MATTERs) Study. *Arch Surg* 2012; 147: 113–119.
7 Safo MK, Ahmed MH, Ghatge MS & Boyiri T. Hemoglobin–ligand binding: understanding Hb function and allostery on atomic level. *Biochim Biophys Acta* 2011; 1814: 797–809.
8 CRASH-2 trial collaborators; Shakur H, Roberts I, Bautista R, Caballero J, Coats T, Dewan Y, El-Sayed H, Gogichaishvili T, Gupta S, Herrera J, Hunt B, Iribhogbe P, Izurieta M, Khamis H, Komolafe E, Marrero MA, Mejía-Mantilla J, Miranda J, Morales C, Olaomi O, Olldashi F, Perel P, Peto R, Ramana PV, Ravi RR & Yutthakasemsunt S. Effects of tranexamic acid on death, vascular occlusive events, and blood transfusion in trauma patients with significant haemorrhage (CRASH-2): a randomised, placebo-controlled trial. *Lancet* 2010;376: 23–32.
9 Estep T, Bucci E, Farmer M, Greenburg G, Harrington J, Kim HW, Klein H, Mitchell P, Nemo G, Olsen K, Palmer A, Valeri CR & Winslow R. Basic science focus on blood substitutes: a summary of the NHLBI Division of Blood Diseases and Resources Working Group Workshop 2006. *Transfusion* 2008; 48: 776–782.
10 Jaspen B. FDA shoots down Northfield Labs blood substitute. *Chicago Tribune* 2009, April; 36.
11 Harris DR & Palmer AF. Modern cross-linking strategies for synthesizing acellular hemoglobin-based oxygen carriers. *Biotechnol Prog* 2008; 24: 1215–1225.
12 Lui FE & Kluger R. Enhancing nitrite reductase activity of modified hemoglobin: bis-tetramers and their PEGylated derivatives. *Biochemistry* 2009; 48: 11912–11919.
13 Fergusson DA & McIntyre L. The future of clinical trials evaluating blood substitutes. *J Am Med Assoc* 2008; 299: 2324–2326.
14 Carson JL, Carless PA & Hebert PC. Transfusion thresholds and other strategies for guiding allogeneic red blood cell transfusion. *Cochrane Database Syst Rev* 2012; 4: CD002042.
15 Kluger R. Red cell substitutes from hemoglobin – do we start all over again? *Curr Opin Chem Biol* 2010; 14: 538–543.
16 Migliaccio AR, Whitsett C & Migliaccio G. Erythroid cells *in vitro*: from developmental biology to blood transfusion products. *Curr Opin Hematol* 2009; 16: 259–268.
17 Giarratana MC, Rouard H, Dumont A, Kiger L, Safeukui I, Le Pennec PY, François S, Trugnan G, Peyrard T, Marie T, Jolly S, Hebert N, Mazurier C, Mario N, Harmand L, Lapillonne H, Devaux JY & Douay L. Proof of principle for transfusion of *in vitro*-generated red blood cells. *Blood* 2011; 118: 5071–5079.

18 Okita K & Yamanaka S. Induced pluripotent stem cells: opportunities and challenges. *Phil Trans R Soc Lond B Biol Sci* 2011; 366: 2198–2207.

19 Lane TA. Perflurochemical-based artifical oxygen carrying red cell substitutes. *Transfus Sci* 1995; 16: 19–31.

20 Chao FC, Kim BK, Houranieh AM *et al*. Infusible platelet membrane (IPM) is a potential substitute for platelets in transfusion: correction of prolonged bleeding time in thrombocytopenic rabbits. *Thromb Haemost* 1993; 69: 750.

Further reading

Baudin-Creuza V, Chauvierre C, Domingues E, Kiger L, Leclerc L, Vasseur C, Celier C & Marden MC. Octamers and nanoparticles as hemoglobin based blood substitutes. *Biochim Biophys Acta Prot Proteom* 2008; 1784: 1448–1453.

Blajchman MA. Substitutes and alternatives to platelet transfusions in thrombocytopenic patients. *J Thromb Haemost* 2003; 1: 1637–1641.

Blood substitute. Wikipedia. http://en.wikipedia.org/wiki/Blood_substitute. Accessed 10 June 2012.

Estep T, Bucci E, Farmer M, Greenburg G, Harrington J, Kim HW, Klein H, Mitchell P, Nemo G, Olsen K *et al*. Basic science focus on blood substitutes: a summary of the NHLBI Division of Blood Diseases and Resources Working Group Workshop, March 1, 2006. *Transfusion* 2008; 48: 776–782.

Gladwin MT, Grubina R & Doyle MP. The new chemical biology of nitrite reactions with hemoglobin: R-state catalysis, oxidative denitrosylation, and nitrite reductase/anhydrase. *Acc Chem Res* 2009; 42: 157–167.

Ker K, Kiriya J, Perel P, Edwards P, Shakur H & Roberts I. Avoidable mortality from giving tranexamic acid to bleeding trauma patients: an estimation based on WHO mortality data, a systematic literature review and data from the CRASH-2 trial. *BMC Emerg Med* 2012; 12: 3.

37

Pharmacological agents and recombinant activated factor VIIa

Beverley J. Hunt[1] & Simon J. Stanworth[2]

[1]Kings College, London, UK and Departments of Haematology, Pathology and Rheumatology, Guy's and St Thomas' NHS Foundation Trust, London, UK
[2]NHS Blood and Transplant, John Radcliffe Hospital, Oxford, UK

Introduction

There continues to be interest in the use of pharmacological agents to reduce bleeding, in light of the concerns about blood safety and new data on the efficacy and safety of tranexamic acid. Pharmacological agents are used in two ways: either to prevent excessive bleeding or to treat established bleeding. The agents used can be broadly classified into four groups: antifibrinolytics, topical sealants, desmopressin and the recombinant prohaemostatic factors such as recombinant activated factor VIIa (rFVIIa).

Antifibrinolytics

These include the lysine analogues, tranexamic acid (TA) and epsilon-amino caproic acid (EACA), which are competitive inhibitors of plasminogen binding to fibrin and endothelial receptors, and aprotinin, a (related) serine protease inhibitor that inhibits a number of haemostatic enzymes but principally has a powerful direct antiplasmin effect. *In vitro* TA has approximately ten times the antifibrinolytic activity of EACA and is therefore assumed to be a more potent antihaemorrhagic agent. A Cochrane systematic review has shown that TA and other lysine analogues are efficacious in reducing bleeding and blood usage perioperatively, but the publication of the Clinical Randomization of an Antifibrinolytic in Significant

Haemorrhage 2 (CRASH-2) trial has pushed TA to the fore, as an efficacious, safe and cost-effective tool in reducing mortality in bleeding trauma patients.

Tranexamic acid in traumatic bleeding

The CRASH-2 study was a randomized controlled trial (RCT) of TA versus placebo in the management of bleeding after trauma recruited 20 000 patients worldwide [1]. The primary outcome was death in hospital within four weeks of injury. All-cause mortality was reduced significantly with tranexamic acid (1463 (14.5%) tranexamic acid group versus 1613 (16.0%) placebo group; relative risk, 0.91; 95% CI, 0.85–0.97; $p = 0.0035$). The risk of death due to bleeding was significantly reduced by 9% (489 (4.9%) versus 574 (5.7%); relative risk, 0.85; 95% CI, 0.76–0.96; $p = 0.0077$). Not only was the drug shown to be efficacious in reducing death but it was also shown to be safe as there were no adverse events and, importantly for a drug that affects haemostasis, there were no increased thrombotic events; indeed there was a trend to a lower rate of arterial events in those receiving TA. Further analysis of the data showed that benefit was greatest the earlier that TA was given after injury and that there was a possibility of negative benefit given after 3–6 hours from injury [2]. This has resulted in a worldwide change in the practical management of massive bleeding; for example, there is a National Health Service England programme of implementation to ensure

Practical Transfusion Medicine, Fourth Edition. Edited by Michael F. Murphy, Derwood H. Pamphilon and Nancy M. Heddle.
© 2013 John Wiley & Sons, Ltd. Published 2013 by John Wiley & Sons, Ltd.

that TA is given by paramedics and ambulance staff on site prior to hospital injury.

The cost effectiveness of using TA in trauma has been calculated in three countries [3]: Tanzania as an example of a low-income country, India as a middle-income country and the UK as a high-income country. The cost of giving TA to 1000 patients was $17 483 in Tanzania, $19 550 in India and $30 830 in the UK. The estimated incremental cost per life year gained of administering TA is $48, $66 and $64 in Tanzania, India and the UK respectively, making it highly cost effective. The WHO has recently classed it as an essential drug.

Interestingly CRASH-2 showed no reduction in the use of blood components in those treated with TA. A recently published study of the use of TA in a military study has suggested that this is due to the higher survival rate with TA: living patients will require further blood components. Indeed, in the military study the group receiving TA had a 24% survival rate and required more blood than the control group.

Perioperative use of the lysine analogues

A Cochrane systematic review [4] analysed data from over 211 RCTs of the perioperative use of antifibrinolytics in over 20 000 participants. It suggested that TA and EACA were nonstatistically slightly less efficacious in reducing the need for transfusion and the need for re-operation than aprotinin (as expected from their lower K_i against plasmin) (Table 37.1).

A continuous infusion is given perioperatively. The dose of TA that has been used is variable, 2.5–100 mg/kg over 20 minutes preoperatively followed by 0.25–4 mg/kg/h delivered over 1–12 hours and 1 mg/kg for 10 hours. Antifibrinolytics can also be given to treat established fibrinolysis: the recommended dose for TA is up to 1–2 g by slow IV infusion.

Obstetric haemorrhage

The CRASH-2 clinical trialists have now embarked on an RCT of TA in obstetric haemorrhage, aiming to randomize 14 000 women over 5 years to tranexamic acid of 1 gm followed by another 1 gm for continued bleeding versus placebo [5].

Aprotinin

The original and licensed regimen of aprotinin for use in high risk cardiac surgery [6, 7] was for 2M Kallikrein inhibitory units (KIU) to the patient, 2M KIU to the cardiopulmonary (CPB) circuit and 50 000 KIU per hour during CPB. This reduced postoperative drainage loss by 81% and total haemoglobin loss by 89%. Since aprotinin is a bovine protein and thus can provoke an immunological reaction, a test dose is required. Aprotinin can also be used in established fibrinolytic bleeding; 500 000 KIU intravenous (IV) is a good antiplasmin dose.

Aprotinin was shown to reduce perioperative bleeding in over 80 randomized controlled studies. Indeed, it has been used as an example by Sir Iain Chalmers as an example of the need for systematic reviews [8]; how was it ethical to randomize patients to placebo in the later trials when so much data was already showing that it reduced blood loss significantly? In fact, worse was to come. The error of using a reduction in blood loss as a surrogate marker of reduction in premature mortality was shown. For several large open studies of the use of antifibrinolytics in cardiac surgery it was suggested that although it reduced bleeding, it was associated with increased risk of death and renal dysfunction compared with other antifibrinolytics [9]. The later BART study, an RCT comparing aprotinin versus EACA versus TA was halted by the data monitoring committee due to concerns about the death rate in patients receiving aprotinin [10]. A total of

Table 37.1 The summary statistics from a Cochrane systematic review of antifibrinolytic use for minimizing perioperative allogeneic blood transfusion. Reproduced from Guerriero et al. [4].

Agent	Risk reduction in the use of red cell transfusion (85% CI)	Risk reduction in the need for re-operation for bleeding (95% CI)
Aprotinin	34%, i.e. RR = 0.66 (0.61–0.71)	0.48 (0.35–0.68)
Tranexamic acid	0.61 (0.54–0.69)	0.67 (0.41–1.09)
EACA	0.75 (0.58–0.96)	0.35 (0.11–1.17)

CI, confidence interval; EACA, epsilon aminocaproic acid.

74 patients (9.5%) in the aprotinin group had massive bleeding, as compared with 93 (12.1%) in the TA group and 94 (12.1%) in the EACA group (relative risk in the aprotinin group for both comparisons, 0.79; 95% confidence interval (CI), 0.59–1.05). At 30 days the rate of death from any cause was 6.0% in the aprotinin group, as compared to 3.9% in the TA group (relative risk, 1.55; 95% CI, 0.99–2.42) and 4.0 in the EACA group (relative risk, 1.52; 95% CI, 0.98–2.36). The relative risk of death in the aprotinin group as compared with that in both groups receiving lysine analogues was 1.53 (95% CI, 1.06–2.22). There was voluntary suspension of marketing aprotinin. Subsequently the use of aprotinin has declined and TA has largely replaced it.

Mechanism of action of antifibrinolytics

TA and EACA are synthetic lysine analogues that bind to the lysine binding sites on fibrinogen and other plasminogen receptors present on white cells and endothelium that would normally bind plasminogen, i.e. a competitive inhibitor.

Aprotinin is a basic serine protease inhibitor extracted from bovine lung. In high doses (150–200 KIU), it inhibits kallikrein; the licensed regimen achieves blood levels of about 200 KIU/mL [11, 12]. However, even in lower concentrations, aprotinin is a powerful inhibitor of plasmin, which appears to be the main mechanism for its effect on bleeding; its molar potency *in vitro* is 100 and 1000 times that of tranexamic acid (TA) and epsilon amino caproic acid (EACA).

Antifibrinolytics may also have a minor effect in preserving platelet membrane receptors, possibly by inhibiting plasmin-mediated degradation.

Monitoring the antikallikrein effect of aprotinin

Aprotinin by inhibiting kallikrein prolongs *in vitro* tests of the intrinsic system including the activated clotting time (ACT), which is used to monitor heparin during cardiopulmonary bypass. Kallikrein normally operates a positive feedback on the generation of factor XII. In order to allow for adequate levels of heparin, the ACT should be run greater than the normal level of 500 seconds, ideally at 750 seconds to compensate and allow for 'normal' heparin levels. The activator in the ACT has traditionally been celite,

but kaolin has been used instead in some ACT tubes, for it is less affected by aprotinin and thus ACTs can be monitored in the normal way.

Desmopressin

Desmopressin acetate (DDAVP) is a synthetic vasopressin analogue that is relatively devoid of vasoconstrictor activity. It increases the plasma concentrations and activity of von Willebrand factor (vWF) two- to fivefold by inducing the release of vWF from Weibel Palade bodies in the endothelium. It also stimulates the release of tissue plasminogen activator from the endothelium and promotes platelet activation. DDAVP shortens the bleeding time in patients with von Willebrand's disease, platelet function defects and uraemia and so is used for these indications.

Despite the success of early trials, a Cochrane systematic review of all 18 RCTs where DDAVP was given to reduce the use of allogeneic red cells concluded that there was no benefit from DDAVP in minimizing perioperative allogeneic red cell transfusion [13]. Side effects include flushing and an antidiuretic effect.

Topical sealants

Topical sealants can be used to stop oozing from small, sometimes inaccessible, blood vessels during surgery when conventional surgical techniques are not feasible. A number of sealants are licensed and used in surgery and trauma including:
- liver and spleen lacerations;
- dental extraction in patients with bleeding disorders;
- gastric ulcers;
- vascular grafts;
- sealing of dural leaks; and
- as an alternative to sutures.

Fibrin sealants mimic the final part of the coagulation cascade in that a source of thrombin is added to fibrinogen concentrates in the presence of calcium and a clot forms. They can be administered by a 'gun', which produces mixing of the reagents. Some sealants have two additional ingredients: factor XIII and aprotinin to stabilize the clot.

The initial source of thrombin was of bovine origin, which led to the development of a postoperative bleeding due to the formation of antibodies to bovine thrombin, which cross-react against human factor V, leading to acquired factor V deficiency [14].

Although they are derived from blood components, fibrin sealants have a lower risk of transmitting infection than donor blood. A Cochrane systematic review of their efficacy found a total of seven trials, including 388 patients, that showed a reduction of exposure to red cell transfusion by a relative 54%, but the trials were of poor methodological quality and larger more rigorous trials are needed [15].

Other topical sealants are available such as FloSeal, which is a thrombin-gelatin haemostatic matrix; Tachosil, a horse collagen sponge with human fibrinogen and thrombin; HemoStase, a purified plant polysaccharide; and CT3 surgical sealant, which is a novel absorbable polyethylene gyycol/collagen biopolymer sealant. There are inadequate data on reducing morbidity, mortality, length of stay and post-operative complication rate to know whether their use is efficacious and cost effective.

Recombinant activated factor VIIa

Recombinant activated factor VII (rFVIIa) was developed as a treatment for bleeding episodes in haemophiliac patients with inhibitors to factor VIII or IX. It is approved in Europe for this indication and for the management of:
• haemophilia A or B with inhibitors;
• acquired haemopilia;
• congenital FVII deficiency; and
• Glanzmann's thrombasthenia with refractoriness to platelet transfusion with antibodies to GPIIb/IIIa and/or HLA antigens.

However, rFVIIa has also been used widely as an 'off label' treatment in patients with platelet dysfunction, thrombocytopenia and massive transfusion after major surgery or trauma in patients without a pre-existing coagulopathy. Initially the body of evidence for these indications was disappointingly mainly from case reports and case series, but now data exists from 25 RCTs (see below).

Mechanism of action of pharmacological doses of rFVIIa

About 1% of circulating factor VII is in the activated form and the amount of rFVIIa required for bypass is larger than this. Certainly in haemophilia patients the doses required are much higher than those that generate a plasma concentration adequate for its binding to tissue factor. Disagreement revolves around the issue of whether rFVIIa has an effect independent of tissue factor. It has been demonstrated *in vitro* that rFVIIa is able to weakly bind activated platelets and cause activation of FX. The explanation of rFVIIa needing to bind to platelets may explain why rFVIIa is located only at the site of bleeding. Others hold the view that VIIa binds to tissue factor in the normal way. Whatever the mechanism, coagulation occurs locally at the site of bleeding without disseminated activation.

Hereditary clotting factor deficiencies

Haemophilia with an inhibitor or acquired haemophilia
Like the endogenous protein, rFVIIa has a short half-life, approximately 2.7 hours in adults, but the half-life in children and in bleeding haemophiliacs is shorter. The dosing interval in treating haemophiliac bleeding episodes is 2 hourly, lengthened up to 4 hourly later in the course of treatment. A loading bolus followed by a continuous infusion of rFVIIa is also used. Even though the recommended dosage is 90 µg/kg, it is clear that the optimal dose and dosing intervals of rFVIIa have not been established with certainty; higher doses up to 300 µg/kg have proved to be more clinically efficacious in some patients.

Whilst the prothrombin time (PT) and activated partial thromboplastin time (APTT) are shortened after treatment with pharmacological doses of rFVIIa, these are indirect correlates of its action. The measurement of FVII clotting activity (FVIIa:C) in the treatment of haemophilia-related bleeding has led to a recommendation of a minimum level of 6–10 IU/mL and peak levels of greater than 30–50 IU/mL when giving IV boluses. These levels appear to be associated with clinical improvement in haemostasis. The use of thromboelastography and thrombin generation has also been explored in trying to find an *in vitro* measure that correlates with clinical response.

Inherited factor VII deficiency
Bleeding episodes in patients with inherited factor VII deficiency have responded to lower doses of rFVIIa than required in haemophiliacs with inhibitors: doses ranging from 15 to 20 µg/kg every 2–3 hours until

cessation of bleeding are recommended. Patients with factor VII deficiency are the only known patients to develop antifactor VIIa antibodies after treatment.

Other congenital bleeding disorders

There are anecdotal reports of the successful use of rFVIIa in bleeding in von Willebrand's disease. Some consider rFVIIa to be the agent of choice in patients with factor XI deficiency, with similar low doses as used in those with factor VII deficiency.

Inherited platelet defects

Patients with rare, congenital platelet defects have had successful treatment of bleeding episodes and undergone surgery safely with rFVIIa treatment. These include disorders such as Glanzmann thrombasthenia (abnormalities of the platelet fibrinogen receptor glycoprotein IIb/IIIa) and Bernard Soulier syndrome (lack of the glycoprotein Ib platelet receptor).

Platelet dysfunction occurs in uraemia and with aspirin, clopidogrel and glycoprotein (GP) IIb/IIIa inhibitors in acute coronary syndromes. rFVIIa has been reported to control bleeding anecdotally in these situations.

Off-licence use in patient groups other than haemophilia

Many bleeding patients without haemophilia have now been treated, off-licence, with rFVIIa [16, 17]. The patients' settings are very diverse, including surgery (especially cardiac), gastrointestinal bleeding, liver dysfunction, intracranial haemorrhage and trauma, for example. Patients with liver dysfunction often have disproportionately low factor VII levels compared to the other vitamin K-dependent factors. rFVIIa normalizes the PT in liver disease with a single dose of 5–80 μg/kg, the dose depending on the patient. In trauma, following early reports of the use of rVIIa, there was an avalanche of reports of rFVIIa being used in uncontrolled bleeding after surgery and trauma. Much of these early patterns of use were driven by case reports and small case series, open to real problems of publication bias and confounding.

Randomized controlled trial evidence

Data from 25 RCTs enrolling around 3500 patients have now evaluated the use of rFVIIa as both prophylaxis to prevent bleeding (14 trials) or therapeutically to treat major bleeding (11 trials), in patients without haemophilia. This literature provides a more robust means of assessing the effectiveness and safety of rVIIA. When combined in meta-analysis [18], the trials showed modest reductions in total blood loss or red cell transfusion requirements (equivalent to less than one unit of red cell transfusion). However, the reductions were likely to be overestimated due to the limitations of the data. For other endpoints, including clinically relevant outcomes, there were no consistent indications of benefit and almost all of the findings in support of and against the effectiveness of rFVIIa could be due to chance (the exception was thromboembolic events, see below). Other limitations applied in many trials, e.g. uncertainty about the protocols for use of blood components.

A first randomized placebo-controlled trial of rFVIIa in blunt and penetrating trauma after patients had been transfused eight units of red cells suggested trends to requiring less red cells in those with penetrating injuries, without differences in thromboembolic events, but the findings were not replicated in a larger trial [19]. One issue for the trauma trials is the data, which show that rFVIIa is less effective in those who are acidotic or in severe shock. As for trauma, in the studies of patients with intracranial bleeding, although there were promising results in earlier therapeutic studies, the findings were not replicated in subsequent larger trials.

In both prophylactic and therapeutic groups of trials, there was an overall trend to increased thromboembolic events [18]. The forest plots for total arterial thromboembolic events are shown in Figure 37.1 and reach statistical significance. Thromboembolic disease is multifactorial and for many of the patients in the clinical settings of the included studies, a higher risk of thrombosis might be expected, for example, related to immobilization and stroke. Underestimation of the rates of thromboembolic events from the RCTs compared to current hospital practice is also likely, as a history of thrombosis or vaso-occlusive disease was a common criterion for exclusion in most of the included studies. Levi et al. published the rate of thrombotic events in all published RCTs of rVIIa and company data [20]. They also showed no increased rate of venous thromboembolism but significantly higher rates of arterial events; e.g. 2.9% of those who had rVIIa had coronary thrombosis compared with

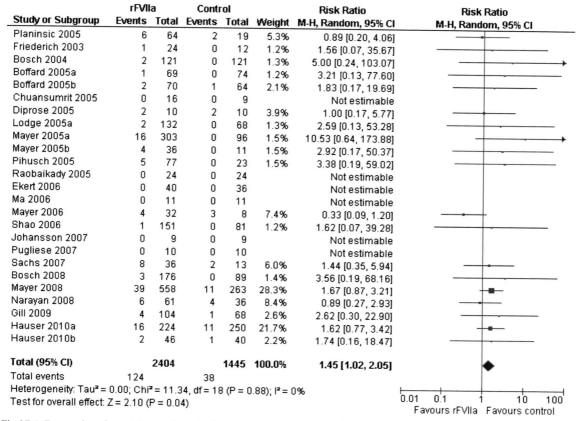

Study or Subgroup	rFVIIa Events	Total	Control Events	Total	Weight	Risk Ratio M-H, Random, 95% CI
Planinsic 2005	6	64	2	19	5.3%	0.89 [0.20, 4.06]
Friederich 2003	1	24	0	12	1.2%	1.56 [0.07, 35.67]
Bosch 2004	2	121	0	121	1.3%	5.00 [0.24, 103.07]
Boffard 2005a	1	69	0	74	1.2%	3.21 [0.13, 77.60]
Boffard 2005b	2	70	1	64	2.1%	1.83 [0.17, 19.69]
Chuansumrit 2005	0	16	0	9		Not estimable
Diprose 2005	2	10	2	10	3.9%	1.00 [0.17, 5.77]
Lodge 2005a	2	132	0	68	1.3%	2.59 [0.13, 53.28]
Mayer 2005a	16	303	0	96	1.5%	10.53 [0.64, 173.88]
Mayer 2005b	4	36	0	11	1.5%	2.92 [0.17, 50.37]
Pihusch 2005	5	77	0	23	1.5%	3.38 [0.19, 59.02]
Raobaikady 2005	0	24	0	24		Not estimable
Ekert 2006	0	40	0	36		Not estimable
Ma 2006	0	11	0	11		Not estimable
Mayer 2006	4	32	3	8	7.4%	0.33 [0.09, 1.20]
Shao 2006	1	151	0	81	1.2%	1.62 [0.07, 39.28]
Johansson 2007	0	9	0	9		Not estimable
Pugliese 2007	0	10	0	10		Not estimable
Sachs 2007	8	36	2	13	6.0%	1.44 [0.35, 5.94]
Bosch 2008	3	176	0	89	1.4%	3.56 [0.19, 68.16]
Mayer 2008	39	558	11	263	28.3%	1.67 [0.87, 3.21]
Narayan 2008	6	61	4	36	8.4%	0.89 [0.27, 2.93]
Gill 2009	4	104	1	68	2.6%	2.62 [0.30, 22.90]
Hauser 2010a	16	224	11	250	21.7%	1.62 [0.77, 3.42]
Hauser 2010b	2	46	1	40	2.2%	1.74 [0.16, 18.47]
Total (95% CI)		**2404**		**1445**	**100.0%**	**1.45 [1.02, 2.05]**
Total events	124		38			

Heterogeneity: Tau² = 0.00; Chi² = 11.34, df = 18 (P = 0.88); I² = 0%
Test for overall effect: Z = 2.10 (P = 0.04)

Fig 37.1 Forest plot of arterial thromboembolic events in randomized trials of rVIIA. Reproduced from Simpson *et al.* [18].

1.1% of controls. Rates of arterial events were particularly high in those over 65 years (9% versus 3.6%, $p = 0.003$) and the rates were especially high in those over 75 years (10.8% versus 4.1%, $p = 0.02$). Concerns about the thrombotic risk, especially increased rate of arterial events associated with the off-licence use of rVIIa led to a Black Box warning from the FDA in the USA early in 2010.

Safety considerations

The mechanism of rFVIIa in initiating haemostasis led to concerns that widespread coagulation could be precipitated, particularly if tissue factor were expressed in atherosclerotic vessels; in which case, administration of rFVIIa could cause acute thrombosis. However, more than 7 000 000 doses of rFVIIa have been given to haemophiliacs with a 1% incidence of serious adverse events including myocardial infarction, stroke and venous thromboembolism. Moreover, a recently published meta-analysis of seven RCTs using rFVIIa in surgical procedures showed no increased risk of thromboembolism or mortality rates.

Conclusions

Pharmacological agents are now considered part of the management of major bleeding after trauma or surgery, but key questions pertaining to their safety and efficacy remain unanswered for many. Practically, TA and EACA have been shown to be efficacious and safe and should be used in preference to aprotinin.

The extent of rVIIa's efficacy, dosage and frequency of use remains unclear. Its use is limited by its high rate of arterial thrombosis, especially in those over 65, and its cost and lack of licence for many indications. It would seem prudent for each hospital to draw guidelines on the use of rFVIIa for 'rescue therapy' whereby it is used only when 'best practice' management of blood component therapy has failed.

Key points

1 Antifibrinolytics have been shown to reduce the use of allogeneic red cells during surgery. At the current time, TA and EACA are recommended over aprotinin in view of concerns about the safety of the latter.
2 TA reduces mortality in bleeding trauma patients and should be given as early as possible after injury to maximize its effect.
3 Topical sealants, although widely used, need more research to assess their full risk–benefit analysis.
4 Desmopressin has not been shown to be beneficial in reducing bleeding in surgical patients.
5 The efficacy of rFVIIa in off-licence 'rescue therapy' in bleeding patients is uncertain and is associated with an increased rate of arterial thrombosis, especially in the elderly. It might be considered as part of a local protocol after 'best practice' use of blood component therapy has failed.

References

1 Henry DA, Carless PA, Moxley AJ et al. Anti-fibrinolytic use for minimising perioperative allogeneic blood transfusion. Cochrane Database Syst Rev 2007; CD001886.
2 CRASH-2 trial collaborators; Shakur H, Roberts I, Bautista R, Caballero J, Coats T, Dewan Y, El-Sayed H, Gogichaishvili T, Gupta S, Herrera J, Hunt B, Iribhogbe P, Izurieta M, Khamis H, Komolafe E, Marrero MA, Mejía-Mantilla J, Miranda J, Morales C, Olaomi O, Olldashi F, Perel P, Peto R, Ramana PV, Ravi RR & Yutthakasemsunt S. Effects of tranexamic acid on death, vascular occlusive events, and blood transfusion in trauma patients with significant haemorrhage (CRASH-2): a randomised, placebo-controlled trial. Lancet 2010, 3 July; 376(9734): 23–32. Epub 14 June 2010.
3 CRASH-2 collaborators; Roberts I, Shakur H, Afolabi A, Brohi K, Coats T, Dewan Y, Gando S, Guyatt G, Hunt BJ, Morales C, Perel P, Prieto-Merino D & Woolley T. The importance of early treatment with tranexamic acid in bleeding trauma patients: an exploratory analysis of the CRASH-2 randomised controlled trial. Lancet 2011, 26 March; 377(9771): 1096–1101, e1–2.
4 Guerriero C, Cairns J, Perel P, Shakur H & Roberts I. CRASH 2 trial collaborators. Cost-effectiveness analysis of administering tranexamic acid to bleeding trauma patients using evidence from the CRASH-2 trial. PLoS One 2011, 3 May; 6(5): e18987.
5 Shakur H, Elbourne D, Gülmezoglu M, Alfirevic Z, Ronsmans C, Allen E & Roberts I. The WOMAN Trial (World Maternal Antifibrinolytic Trial): tranexamic acid for the treatment of postpartum haemorrhage: an international randomised, double blind placebo controlled trial. Trials 2010, 16 April; 11: 40.
6 Royston D, Bidstrup BP, Taylor KM & Sapsford RN. Effect of aprotinin on need for blood transfusion after repeat open-heart surgery. Lancet 1987; 2: 1289–1291.
7 Karkouti K, Beattie WS, Dattilo KM et al. A propensity score case–control comparison of aprotinin and tranexamic acid in high transfusion – risk cardiac surgery. Transfusion 2006; 46: 327–338.
8 Chalmers I. The scandalous failure of scientists to cumulate scientifically. Abstract to paper presented at The Ninth World Congress on Health Information and Libraries, 20–23 September 2005, Salvador, Brazil. Available at: http://www.icml9.org/program/activity.php?lang=en&id=36 (cited 5 October 2005).
9 Mangano DT, Tudor IC & Dietzel C, for Multicentre Study of Perioperative Ischemia Group and Ischemia Research and Education Foundation. The risk associated with aprotinin in cardiac surgery. N Engl J Med 2006; 354: 353–365.
10 Fergusson DA, Hebert PC, Mazer CD et al. A comparison of aprotinin and lysine analogues in high-risk cardiac surgery. N Engl J Med 2008; 358: 2319–2331.
11 Segal H & Hunt BJ. Aprotinin: pharmacological reduction of perioperative bleeding. Lancet 2000; 355: 1289–1290.
12 Hunt BJ, Segal H & Yacoub M. Aprotinin and heparin monitoring during cardiopulmonary bypass. Circulation 1992; 86: 410–412.
13 Carless PA, Henry DA, Moxet AJ et al. Desmopressin for minimising perioperative allogeneic blood transfusion. Cochrane Database Syst Rev 2004;CD001884.
14 Banninger H, Hardegger T, Tobler A et al. Fibrin glue in surgery: frequent developments of inhibitors of bovine thrombin and human factor V. Br J Haematol 1993; 85: 528–532.
15 Carless PA, Henry DA & Anthony DM. Fibrin sealant use for minimising peri-operative allogeneic blood transfusion. Cochrane Database Syst Rev 2003; CD004171.
16 Martinowirz U, Kenet G, Lubetski A, Luboshitz J & Segal E. Recombinant activated factor VII for adjunctive hemorrhage control in trauma. J Trauma 2001; 51: 431–438.

17 Shao YF, Yang JM, Chau GY *et al.* Safety and haemostatic effect of recombinant activated factor VII in cirrhotic patients undergoing partial hepatectomy: a multicentre, randomized, double blind, placebo-controlled trial. *Am J Surg* 2006; 191: 245–249.

18 Simpson E, Lin Y, Stanworth S, Birchall J, Doree C & Hyde C. Recombinant factor VIIa for the prevention and treatment of bleeding in patients without haemophilia. *Cochrane Database of Syst Rev* 2011; 2: CD005011. DOI: 10.1002/14651858.CD005011.pub3.

19 Boffard KD, Bruno Riou B, Brian Warren B *et al.* Recombinant factor VIIa as adjunctive therapy for bleeding control in severely injured trauma patients: two parallel randomized, placebo-controlled, double-blind clinical trials. *J Trauma* 2005; 59: 8–15.

20 Levi M, Levy JH, Andersen HF & Truloff D. Safety of recombinant activated factor VII in randomized clinical trials. *N Engl J Med* 2010, 4 November; 363(19): 1791–800. Erratum in *N Engl J Med* 2011 17 November; 365(20): 1944.

Further reading

Freemantle N & Irs A. Observational evidence for determining drug safety. *Br Med J* 2008; 336: 627–628.

Dzik WH, Blajchman MA, Fergusson D, Hameed M, Henry B, Kirkpatrick AW, Korogyi T, Logsetty S, Skeate RC, Stanworth S, Macadams C & Muirhead B. Clinical review: Canadian National Advisory Committee on Blood and Blood Products – Massive Transfusion Consensus Conference 2011: report of the panel. *Crit Care* 2011, December 8; 15(6): 242.

Roberts HR, Monroe DM & White GC. The use of recombinant factor VIIa in the treatment of bleeding disorders. *Blood* 2004; 104: 3858–3864.

Rossaint R, Bouillon B, Cerny V, Coats TJ, Duranteau J, Fernandez-Mondejar E, Hunt BJ, Komadina R, Nardi G, Neugebauer E *et al.* Management of bleeding following major trauma: an updated European guideline. *Crit Care* 2010; 14: R52.

PART SIX

Cellular and Tissue Therapy and Organ Transplantation

38 Regulation and accreditation in cellular therapy

Derwood H. Pamphilon[1] *& Zbigniew M. Szczepiorkowski*[2]

[1]Retired from NHS Blood and Transplant, Bristol, UK
[2]Transfusion Medicine Service, Cellular Therapy Center, Dartmouth-Hitchcock Medical Center and Geisel School of Medicine at Dartmouth, Hanover, New Hampshire, USA

Introduction

In recent years there have been considerable advances in cellular therapies. The most widely used type of cellular therapy has been haemopoietic stem cell transplantation (HSCT) from its inception in 1968. In many cases patients with haematological and nonhaematological diseases are cured after HSCT. There have also been advances in the immunotherapy of cancer and viral infections and in the use of cellular therapy for tissue regeneration and repair.

A number of different agencies and professional bodies are involved in the regulation and accreditation of cellular therapy both in the USA and Europe. The regulations and standards depend on the source of the cell to be transplanted, the way it is used and the nature of any manipulations carried out. As a result of this the last decade has seen a seemingly bewildering growth in regulatory and accreditation requirements and these have put pressure on both clinical and laboratory services.

The drivers for these are:
- traceability of products from donor to recipient;
- microbiological safety;
- enhanced product quality.

There are multiple organizations involved in the process of accreditation and standard setting of haemopoietic stem cell transplant programmes.

Figure 38.1 illustrates the timeline of this involvement by different organizations.

Haemopoietic stem cell transplant activity

The numbers of transplants has increased considerably in recent years so that between 50 and 70 000 are performed each year. The majority are autografts and related (usually sibling) donor procedures, although World Marrow Donor Association (WMDA) data show that the number of transplants using unrelated donor stem cells increased from 3237 in 1997 to 10 981 in 2008 [1]. The overall number of unrelated donors available on international registries reported to the WMDA in its 10th Annual Report increased from 4.8 to 14.6 million during that time period. In the last 10–15 years there has been a switch to the use of peripheral blood progenitor cells (PBPC), which are now regarded as the source of choice in 98% of autografts and 74% of allografts in Europe as well as a great increase in the use of cord blood (CB) units so that, in patients under the age of 16, they now account for 30% of transplants and its use is increasing in adults as well.

In 1990, 4200 HSCTs were reported to the European Blood and Marrow Transplant Group (EBMT), a number that had risen by 2008 to 26 810

Practical Transfusion Medicine, Fourth Edition. Edited by Michael F. Murphy, Derwood H. Pamphilon and Nancy M. Heddle.
© 2013 John Wiley & Sons, Ltd. Published 2013 by John Wiley & Sons, Ltd.

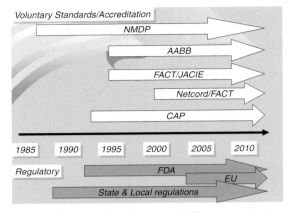

Fig 38.1 Timeline of involvement of different organizations in the field of cellular therapy.
AABB (formerly the American Association of Blood Banks); CAP, College of American Pathologists; FACT, Foundation for the Accreditation of Cellular Therapy; EU, European Union; FDA, US Food and Drug Administration; JACIE, Joint Accreditation Committee (ISCT and EBMT); NMDP, National Marrow Donor Program.

(Figure 38.2). Autologous transplants comprised 65% of these and 35% were allografts; 46% of first-time allografts are now from identical siblings and 49% from unrelated HSCT has increased in all diseases

reported to the EBMT and CIBMTR with the exception of chronic myeloid leukaemia (CML), where the advent of the tyrosine kinase inhibitor imatinib has reduced numbers (see Chapter 41).

The structure of SCT programmes

Figure 38.3 shows the journey of an allogeneic stem cell product from a registry or sibling donor or CB unit where a blood sample is typed in the histocompatibility and immunogenetics (H&I) laboratory to determine the HLA type, via the marrow, peripheral blood or CB collection facility and the cell processing laboratory to the clinical transplant unit. The various accreditation and regulatory bodies involved and their area of involvement are shown.

European Union Directives and Legislation

Documents published in Europe in 1978 and 1994 stressed the need for international standardization of tissue and cell collection practices and the harmonization of legislation relating to the collection and transplantation of substances of human origin. It was

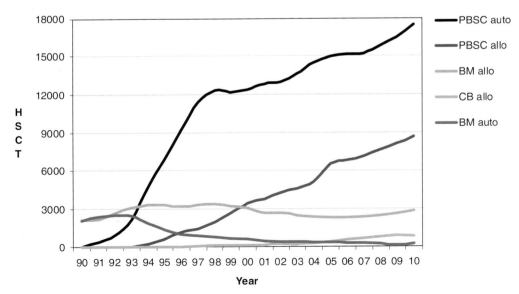

Fig 38.2 Trends in allogeneic and autologous BM and PB HSCT 1990–2010 (data from Helen Baldomero, EBMT).

422

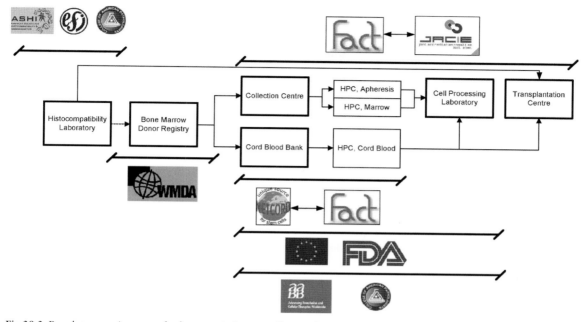

Fig 38.3 Regulatory environment for haemopoietic stem cell transplantation.
Note that this figure does not reflect all potential regulatory reporting requirements for transplantation centres.

recommended that there should be functional definitions of tissue banks and that such banks should be:
• nonprofit making;
• licensed by national health authorities;
• the cells collected should be tested for infectious disease markers (IDMs);
• appropriate records should be kept;
• there should be consent for removal or collection of cells and tissues.

In 2004 the European Union (EU) Directive on Tissues and Cells was published as Directive 2004/23/EC [2]. In 2006 two technical annexes supplying more detailed information were published as Commission Directives 2006/17/EC (donation, procurement and testing) and 2006/86/EC (coding, processing, preservation, storage and distribution) [3, 4]. The Directives are legally binding with a requirement that they are transposed into European law.

In 2005 Competent Authorities (CA) were appointed or established in the UK and other European Member States and these subsequently became responsible for the licensing of facilities storing tissues or cells. In the UK the Human Tissue (Quality and Safety for Human Application) Regulations,

which translate the EU Directive into UK law, were published in 2006 and in 2007; all three directives were fully implemented. Other EU countries have also made similar arrangements. The Directive states that it 'lays down standards of quality and safety for human tissues and cells intended for human applications, in order to ensure a high level of protection of human health' and that it was established to 'help to reassure the public that human tissues and cells that are procured in another Member State, nonetheless carry the same guarantees as those in their own country'. Of relevance to HPC transplantation and immunotherapy, the following cells and tissues are included within the scope of the Directive:
• haemopoietic stem cells from peripheral blood, bone marrow and CB;
• donor leucocytes and other cellular therapies;
• adult and embryonic stem cells.

The various sections of the Directive describe:
(i) the requirements for the person in charge of a cellular therapy or tissue facility (the responsible person or designated individual);
(ii) the arrangements for the facility itself and its staffing;

(iii) the role of the CA and the need for 2-yearly inspections;

(iv) the requirements for consent;

(v) traceablilty with retention of key records for a period of 30 years;

(vi) the reporting of adverse events and reactions to the CA;

(vii) conditions to be met when stem cells are imported or exported.

The Human Tissue Act (HT Act) 2004

This key piece of legislation serves as a good example of how national legislation for cell and tissue collection and processing operates [5, 6]. It was introduced in the UK in 2006, repealing and replacing the HT Act of 1961 as well as the Anatomy Act (1989) and Human Organ Transplants Act (1989). It established the Human Tissue Authority (HTA) as the CA for the UK. Its aim is to regulate the collection, storage, use and disposal of human bodies, body parts, organs and tissues.

The HT Act ensured that consent became the fundamental principle underpinning the lawful storage and use of organs and tissues. In addition, the Act also applies to the removal of transplantable material from the deceased. Consent is required when tissue is removed from the living or deceased for the purposes of:

• anatomical examination;
• determining the cause of death;
• obtaining scientific or medical information about a person relevant to another;
• public display;
• research in connection with disorders or functioning of the human body (unless the material is made anonymous and for specific, ethically approved research);
• transplantation.

The HT Act is supported by two governmental regulations (Statutory Instruments 2006 no. 1659 (37) and 2006 no. 1260 (38)), directions issued by the HTA to help explain and interpret the Act and also a number of Codes of Practice, of which three are particularly relevant to cell and tissue therapies [7]. These are:

(i) consent;

(ii) removal, collection, retention and disposal of organs and tissues;

(iii) donation of allogeneic bone marrow and peripheral blood stem cells for transplantation.

Obtaining legally valid consent is extremely important and the HTA states that it is a positive act, that it is voluntary and may be withdrawn at any time. Appropriate information should be provided and the person giving consent must have the capacity to do so. Children may consent if they are competent to do so. Consent prior to death is sufficient for organ and tissue donation and relatives have no legal right to overrule such consent.

The United States Food and Drug Administration (FDA)

The Food and Drug Administration (FDA) of the Department of Health and Human Services of the USA has been involved in the area of cellular therapy since early 1990s [8]. Through a series of public meetings and notices in the Federal Register the FDA recognized the need for regulatory oversight in the area of cell, gene and tissue therapies and products. Initial guidance documents were issued in 1993, 1996, 1997 and 1998 based on the Public Health Service Act, Section 361 (42 USC 264).

FDA Good Tissue Practice (GTP) Regulations for human cells, tissues and tissue-based products (HCT/Ps) require institutions shipping HPC, Cord Blood; HPC, Apheresis; and TC, Apheresis, but not HPC, Marrow, to be registered with FDA as manufacturers. There are specific requirements for donors who may be eligible/ineligible based on a suitability determination and defined in final guidance documents (see below). An annual update is required.

The regulatory approach implemented by the FDA based on the 1997 proposal for regulation included cellular therapy products (named HCT/P – human cells, tissues and tissue-based products) with gene therapy and tissues rather than with blood components. This different approach had significant implications for the field by defining minimal requirements for establishments involved in manufacturing of HCT/P. The FDA also introduced a concept of risk assessment which includes: (1) the relationship between the donor and the recipient (i.e. autologous, allogeneic related, allogeneic unrelated); (2) the amount of processing and manipulation (nonmanipulated, minimally manipulated and more than minimally manipulated); and (3) the purpose for which the tissues are used (homologous and nonhomologous use, where homologous use is defined as repair, replacement or supplementation of a recipient's cells or tissues with an HCT/P that performs the same basic functions in the recipients as in the donor).

The last of the aspects of risk assessment has been debated by the cellular therapy community as one that assigns potentially a different level of regulatory scrutiny based on the intended use despite equivalent risk in the first two areas, such as donor and the level of manipulation.

For very practical reasons it is common among cellular therapy practitioners in the USA to discuss products as '351' and '361' products. This nomenclature relates to two different sections of the Public Health Service Act. The 361 products are covered in 21 Code of Federal Regulations (CFR) 1271 A, B, C, D, E, F (i.e. Good Tissue Practice), while the 351 products are covered in multiple regulations including 21 CFR 1271 C, D; 21 CFR 207.20 (f); 21 CFR 210–211; 21 CFR 807.20 (d); 21 CFR 820.1 (a); 21 CFR 312 (investigational new drug regulations (IND)) and others. The 361 products are defined in 21 CFR 1271.10 as (1) minimally manipulated; (2) intended for homologous use; (3) do not involve combination with a drug or a device, except for a sterilizing, preserving or storage agent, if the agent does not raise new clinical safety concerns; and (4) does not have a systemic effect and is not dependent upon the metabolic activity of living cells for its primary function, or has a systemic effect and is for autologous use, or for allogeneic use in a first-degree and second-degree blood relative, or for reproductive use. All products that do not fulfil these requirements are considered 351 products.

Based on the assignment of 351 and 361 products there are different requirements for biological product deviation reporting.

It is important to note that there are tissues excluded from 21 CFR 1271 that include vascularized organs; whole blood and blood components; human milk and minimally manipulated bone marrow. Thus, HPC, Marrow (minimally manipulated), is regulated by different set of regulations, which are under the authority of the Health Resources and Services Administration (HRSA).

For a thorough discussion of FDA regulatory activities and current guidance documents the reader is referred to the agency website http://www.fda .gov/cber/gene.htm and http://www.fda.gov/cber/tiss.htm.

The ultimate goal of the FDA regulatory structure is to bring cellular therapy products to the licensed status. In October 2009, the FDA issued the guidance document regarding the biological licence application for HPC, Cord Blood. The regulations required that after October 2011 all CB units would be either licensed by the CB banks or issued based on the IND [9] (see the guidance document for more information). These requirements led to a significant effort by the CB banks to submit a biological licence application (BLA) to the FDA for approval. There are several CB banks that submitted BLAs and are in different stages of licence issuance. At the time of writing (November 2012) only three products, Hemacord (New York Blood Center); HPC Cord Blood (University of Colorado Medical School) and Duracord (Duke University School of Medicine) have been licensed.

The CB units that are not licensed are issued under IND protocol (e.g. NMDP is a holder of one of the INDs).

Nongovernmental (voluntary) accreditation

Many programmes elect to be accredited by one of the voluntary accrediting organizations in addition to observing governmental regulations. There are multiple reasons for voluntary accreditation ranging from recognition by healthcare insurance providers for reimbursement purposes through improved quality of care to fulfilling requirements by some of the local governmental regulations (e.g. Commonwealth of Massachusetts requires FACT accreditation from all Transplantation Centres).

All accrediting organizations require adherence to local and governmental laws and regulations in addition to individual standards established by each of them. Each voluntary organization has a slightly different approach to the accreditation process, but generally an applicant facility needs to meet or exceed standards promulgated by the accrediting organization. The published standards, which are typically updated in defined time intervals, describe a minimum level of expectations. Table 38.1 summarizes major differences (and similarities) between different accrediting organizations.

Table 38.1 Overview of voluntary accreditation/registry organizations.

	FACT	JACIE	Netcord/ FACT	AABB	CAP	NMDP	WMDA
Membership	No	No	No	No	No	Yes	Yes
Accreditation	Yes	Yes	Yes	Yes	Yes	No	Yes
Scope							
Registries	na	na	na	na	na	na	++
Recruitment	na	na	na	na	na	++	+
Donor	+	+	++	+	+	++	++
Collection	++	++	++	++	++	++	+
Processing	++	++	++	++	++	++	na
Transplantation	++	++	na	na	na	++	na
Products							
HPC, Apheresis	Yes	Yes	No	Yes	Yes	Yes	Yes
HPC, Marrow	Yes	Yes	No	Yes	Yes	Yes	Yes
HPC, Cord Blood	No	No	Yes	Yes	Yes	Yes	Yes
TC, Lymphocytes	Yes	Yes	No	Yes	Yes	Yes	No
Other CTCs	No/Yes**	No/Yes**	No	Yes	No	No	No
Standards structure	Checklist	Checklist	Checklist	ISO based	Checklist	Checklist	Checklist
Current edition/version*	5th	5th	4th	5th	2011/7	21st	2011
Accredited facilities (non-US/US)							
Registries	na	na	na	na	na	na	20
Cord blood banks	na	na	22/9†	38/28†	Unknown	5/21	Unknown***
Collection/processing/ transplant	17/170†	112	na	HPC 4/90† Somatic cells 3/3†	Unknown	34/148 tc† 6/42 dc† 16/79 cc† 15/84 ac†	na

FACT, Foundation for the Accreditation of Cellular Therapy; JACIE, Joint Accreditation Committee (ISCT and EBMT); aaBB, formerly American Association for Blood Banks; CAP, College of American Pathologists; NMDP, National Marrow Donor Program; WMDA, World Marrow Donor Association; CTC, Cellular Therapy Products; tc, transplant centre; dc, donor centre; cc, collection centre; ac, apheresis centre; na, not applicable.
*As of 1 January 2012.
**Processing facility can be accredited for other cellular therapy products.
***Presently Netcord–FACT accredited cord blood banks can obtain WDMA accreditation (per WDMA website).
†Figures shown as non-US/US.

Standards are prepared by a group of experts within the organization, typically called 'Standards Committee', which establish minimum expectations for the facilities willing to participate in the accrediting programme. The draft standards are presented for public comments, which then may or may not be incorporated into the final standards. Some organizations, notably CAP, do not present the standards (in this particular case checklist questions) for comments.

Once the final version of the standards is approved a tool is created, which is used during the inspection process.

The accreditation process generally consists of three phases: phase I – the application step, when the applicant facility submits necessary documentation to the accrediting body and certifies that it is compliant with the standards; phase II – the confirmation step, when the accrediting body using on-site inspection confirms that the applicant facility truly follows the standards; and phase III – the recognition step, when a certificate of accreditation is being issued based on the documentation submitted and the results of on-site inspection and, if necessary, satisfying responses to identified shortcomings in the applicant facility. The accreditation certificate has an expiration date and stipulates that if there are any significant changes in the programme structure and/or performance these will be promptly reported to the accrediting body. Each of the accrediting organizations may have additional requirements.

(i) FACT and JACIE

In 1994 the Foundation for Accreditation of Cell Therapy (FACT) in the USA initiated a voluntary inspection and accreditation scheme for cell therapy facilities. Five years later its European counterpart, the Joint Accreditation Committee of the ISCT (International Society for Cell Therapy) and EBMT (JACIE), was founded. FACT–JACIE is a voluntary system that accredits clinical transplant programmes as well as the cell collection, processing and banking elements that are covered by current EU legislation [10]. Whilst FACT–JACIE accreditation is not compulsory, there are pressures for the clinical, collection and laboratory parts of HSCT programmes to comply with their requirements in some countries. These include purchasing agreements with healthcare funders. The primary aim of FACT and JACIE is to improve the quality of HSCT in North America, Europe and elsewhere by providing a means whereby transplant centres, HPC collection facilities and processing facilities can demonstrate high quality practice. This is achieved through external inspection of facilities to ensure compliance with the FACT–JACIE standards. A further aim is to ensure consistency between the standards and other national and international standards, including the EU Tissues and Cells Directive (Directive 2004/23/EC) and the related Commission Directives 2006/17/EC and 2006/86/EC (see above).

FACT–JACIE accreditation is voluntary, but provides a means whereby transplant facilities can demonstrate that they are working within a quality system that covers all aspects of the transplantation process and that they can show compliance with the requirements of insurance companies or national

and/or international regulatory authorities. Accreditation of HPC transplant facilities is through on-line submission of documentation and Centres may apply for accreditation as complete programmes comprising a clinical programme, collection facility and processing laboratory or, for example, as a single collection or processing facility that may serve a number of clinical programmes.

The FACT–JACIE standards

The 5th edition of the standards was published in 2012 and covers all aspects of clinical transplant programmes, bone marrow and peripheral blood stem cell collection facilities, as well as processing laboratories. The standards also apply to the use of therapeutic cells (TC) derived from the peripheral blood or bone marrow, including donor lymphocytes and mesenchymal stem cells. The standards cover the clinical use of HPC(CB) by clinical programmes but not the collection or banking of CB, which is covered by the related Netcord–FACT standards and inspected and accredited by FACT–Netcord (see below). The standards are available on the FACT and JACIE websites and are structured as shown in Table 38.2, and contain essential principles that apply throughout:
- Establishment and maintenance of a Quality Management Programme (QMP).
- Requirement for documentation of policies, procedures, actions, requests, which extends to all aspects of transplant activity. For example, the initial diagnosis of a patient must be documented in the clinical notes using source material or reports. A request from the clinical unit to the laboratory for issue of cells must be made in writing. A potential donor must not only be properly evaluated for eligibility but the programme must have clear written criteria for what constitutes an eligible donor and must clearly document whether the donor meets these criteria.
- Personnel must not only be appropriately qualified, they must be trained in the procedures they regularly perform and their competency to perform the task after training must be assessed and documented.
- Validation of all equipment and procedures. Validation is a term used to describe the activity required to prove that any procedure, process, equipment, material, activity or system actually leads to the expected results. For example, a new apheresis machine must be shown to produce the expected results in terms of cell yields.

427

Table 38.2 Structure of the 5th edition of the FACT–JACIE standards.

Clinical (B)	Collection (C+Cm)	Processing (D)
General	General	General
Clinical Unit	Collection Facility	Processing Facility
Personnel	Personnel	Personnel
Quality Management	Quality Management	Quality Management
Policies and Procedures	Policies and Procedures	Policies and Procedures
Donor Selection, Evaluation, and Management	Donor Evaluation and Management	Process Controls
Therapy Administration	Coding and Labeling	Coding and Labeling
Clinical Research	Process Controls	Distribution
Data Management	Cellular Therapy Product Storage	Storage
	Cellular Therapy Product Transportation and Shipping	Transportation, Shipping, and Receipt
Records	Records	Disposal
	Direct Distribution to Clinical Program	Records

Also important is the requirement for close cooperation and interaction between the different parts of the programme, especially important where a clinical programme may use an offsite collection and/or processing facility.

Quality management (QM)

An active quality management programme (QMP) is essential to the FACT–JACIE standards. A QMP is a mechanism to ensure that procedures are being carried out by all staff members in line with agreed standards. In a transplant programme, this ensures that the clinical, collection and laboratory units are all working together to achieve good communication, effective common work practices and increased guarantees for patients. It is a means of rapidly identifying errors or accidents and resolving them so that the possibility of repetition is minimized. It assists in training and clearly identifies the roles and responsibilities of all staff. Once the required level of quality has been achieved, the remaining challenge is to maintain this standard of practice. With a working quality management system in place and adequate resources, the fundamental elements necessary to sustain the programme are continued staff commitment and vigilance. The culture and systems for quality management are well established in laboratories but are relatively new in clinical units and many programmes have experienced difficulty setting up a QMP to cover the clinical programme and collection facility. It is recommended that HSCT programmes have dedicated quality managers.

Experience of centres implementing FACT and JACIE

It was anticipated that implementation of the FACT–JACIE standards would pose some difficulties for applicant centres, particularly in relation to establishing a quality management system (QMS). It was also anticipated that there would be resource implications in terms of staff time because of the amount of detailed documentation that is required to demonstrate compliance with the standards. To assess this in Europe a survey was designed to assess the difficulties experienced by centres in preparing for JACIE accreditation and the results showed that the most difficult part of preparation was implementing the quality management (QM) system, adverse event reporting system and other documentation. Lack of a culture of QM was cited as an important problem. The extra resources most frequently required were a quality manager and a data manager. Only 19% of centres needed to improve their physical facilities. There is clearly an important need for training of clinical staff (doctors and nurses) in QM. It is also important for centres to have a designated quality manager who has appropriate experience in QMS.

Improvements clearly depend on the level of existing services, so that failure to demonstrate improvement in, for example, facilities or data management may reflect good pre-existing resources. In other areas, e.g. adverse event reporting, the systems for monitoring performance were only set up as part of implementing JACIE, so it is difficult to monitor improvements without an established baseline for comparison. Indeed, implementation of JACIE may have the paradoxical effect of seeming to increase adverse events because these were not previously adequately reported. All centres felt that accreditation was worth the effort invested. In addition, with the implementation of the EU Directive on Safety of Tissues and Cells (2004/23/EC) it is likely that collection and processing facilities will increasingly view compliance with JACIE standards as important in providing evidence that they are complying with the requirements of the Directive.

A detailed analysis of transplant outcome in 107 000 European patients transplanted between 1999 and 2007 showed that acquisition of JACIE accreditation was associated with improvement in overall patient survival [11].

(ii) Netcord–FACT

In the same way that FACT–JACIE cooperate to produce a globally agreed set of standards and a guidance manual for accreditation of HSCT programmes, FACT collaborates with Netcord, which is an international organization for CB banking [12]. Their combined, international standards, first issued in 2000, are the gold standard for CB banks worldwide. The most recent standards (4th edition) were published in 2010. They comprise five sections that cover CB bank quality management, operations, donor management and collection, processing, donor selection and release. It should be noted that clinical transplantation is dealt with in the FACT–JACIE standards. The next edition is expected in 2013.

(iii) AABB

Established in 1947, AABB is an international, not-for-profit association dedicated to the advancement of science and the practice of transfusion medicine and related biological therapies. AABB membership consists of approximately 1800 institutions and over 8000 individuals, including physicians, scientists, administrators, medical technologists, nurses, researchers, blood donor recruiters and public relations personnel. Members are located in all 50 states and 80 foreign countries. In 1958, the *Standards for a Blood Transfusion Service* was published, and an independent accreditation programme was established. The AABB approach to the field of cellular therapies has aimed to balance flexibility in an outcome-based approach with the need for rigorous evidence-based standards. The standards are written using an ISO-based template. The ten chapter headings are based on the AABB Quality System Essentials (QSEs), published in 1997 as AABB Association Bulletin 97-4. The 10 QSEs correlate directly with ISO. The AABB Standards for Cellular Therapy Services (5th edition published in 2011) [13], which are revised and updated every 18 months, cover all cellular therapy product and cell sources including autologous, allogeneic and cadaveric donors. AABB also coordinates the production of a cell therapy product Circular of Information (COI) [14].

Under a QM system approach, each chapter progresses from general policies to specific procedures. The chapters are:
- Organization
- Resources
- Equipment
- Agreements
- Process Control
- Documents and Records
- Deviations and Nonconforming Products or Services
- Internal and External Assessments
- Process Improvement
- Safety and Facilities

The chapters open with broad statements (a part of the template for all AABB standards, which are amended, if necessary, to fit a particular field), which are followed by more specific standards and, finally, end with reference standards, which are most prescriptive. The reference standards are generally presented as tables or lists of activities/requirements.

The AABB accreditation is valid for 2 years and each accredited institution is assessed every 24 months. Recently, the AABB, following other accrediting organizations, introduced unannounced assessments.

These occur on any day within 90 days of the accreditation expiration date.

(iv) College of American Pathologists

The College of American Pathologists (CAP) (www .cap.org) is a medical society serving nearly 16 000 physician members and the laboratory community throughout the world [15]. It is the world's largest association composed exclusively of pathologists and is widely considered the leader in laboratory quality assurance. The nearly 16 000 pathologist members of the CAP represent board-certified pathologists and pathologists in training worldwide. More than 6000 laboratories are accredited by the CAP and approximately 23 000 laboratories are enrolled in the College's proficiency testing programmes. There are two proficiency tests currently offered for the cellular therapy products, SCP (Stem Cell Test) and CBT (Cord Blood Test).

The CAP primarily accredits laboratories in clinical and anatomical pathology, but the accreditation process also includes other entities such as cellular therapy laboratories, HLA laboratories and reproductive laboratories.

The accreditation process, called the Laboratory Accreditation Program, is based on fulfilling the CAP checklist (self-assessment and on-site inspection), which consists of three major parts: the discipline specific checklist(s), the laboratory general checklist and the all common checklist. Each checklist component consists of subject header, declarative statement and evidence of compliance. These elements are designed to help both the inspectee and inspector in fulfilling the intent of the requirement. Furthermore, the inspectors are trained to use the ROAD (Read, Observe, Ask, Discover) inspection technique.

The questions on tissue banking were added to the transfusion medicine checklist in 1993. There were five questions covering the following: (1) documentation defining the authority, responsibility and accountability of the programme; (2) records documenting the type of processing and infectious disease testing for each tissue stored; (3) procedures defining storage conditions of the different tissues handled and retention of records; (4) records showing proper storage conditions; and (5) records allowing for identification of the donor and recipient for each tissue handled. In 2004 the CAP expanded the tissues section of the checklist and significantly expanded the haemopoietic progenitor cells section of the checklist. In general, the CAP checklists undergo frequent review by the CAP's scientific resource committees and the Commission on Laboratory Accreditation. New editions are released once a year.

The Reproductive Laboratory Accreditation checklist was created in 1993 and contains requirements for gametes and embryos. The September 2007 edition was revised to address or clarify requirements to prepare CAP-accredited laboratories better for their FDA inspections.

The CAP inspection is performed every other year and the inspection team consists of professionals from a CAP accredited facility that is led by a team leader who is an appropriately qualified Fellow of the College. The inspections generally last two days. The accredited facilities are also required to perform self-evaluation in the year when there is no on-site inspection. Any identified shortcomings need to be documented and addressed.

(v) The World Marrow Donor Association

The WMDA is an international organization that publishes standards to which HSCT donor registries wishing to achieve accreditation for their activities must adhere [16]. These standards are available on the WMDA website (www.worldmarrow.org) and include benchmark standards with which all registries must comply in order to be accredited for the first time, the rest being optional. For subsequent accreditation, the registry must comply with all of the standards. Important areas described by the standards include general organization of the donor registry, donor recruitment, assessment, counselling, histocompatibility and immunogenetic characterization of donors, other testing including an infectious disease marker, IT requirements, donor searches, collection and transport of cells. At the present time accreditation is given after a detailed review of documentation submitted by the registry by independent reviewers but site visits are not done, although a pilot scheme to introduce them is under way. Accreditation is valid for 5 years.

(vi) Histocompatibility Accreditation [17, 18]

The American Society for Histocompatibility and Immunogenetics (ASHI) and its European counterpart – the European Federation of Immunogenetics (EFI) – accredit H&I laboratories after reviewing documentation and conducting a site visit. The College of American Pathologists also accredits histocompatibility laboratories. The accreditation by CAP fulfils requirements of the National Marrow Donor Program 21st edition of standards (October 2011), but at the time of writing has not been accepted by the FACT–JACIE standards. This creates an unfortunate situation where the transplant programmes cannot utilize CAP accredited histocompatibility laboratories for HLA testing.

Conclusions: How do HSCT programmes respond to the challenge?

The requirements of regulatory and accreditation bodies place huge demands on transplant programmes. In some cases they may need to construct new and improved facilities for HSC collection, processing and storage. A key feature is the need to develop robust quality management programmes as described above, which will include detailed policies and procedures to cover all their activities. Initial staff training and ensuring ongoing competency are crucial. HSCT programmes should remember that deficiencies commonly found at inspection involve the QMP, policies and procedures, donor assessment and testing and the labelling of cell therapy products. The interaction between the different component parts of programmes should work seamlessly and where, for example, cell processing or laboratory testing is performed outside the programme by external agencies, then service level agreements will need to be in place. Most units that achieve compliance with regulatory and accreditation standards feel that the exercise has been worthwhile and that the quality of the services that they offer has been improved.

Key points

1 There have been considerable advances in cellular therapy in the last 20 years and newer developments include the use of cell therapy products for regenerative medicine and immunotherapy.
2 The accreditation and regulatory environment has become increasingly complex and its aim is to enhance product quality and safety.
3 The development of robust quality systems is central to achieving compliance with these new requirements.
4 Some regulations are mandatory, e.g. the EU Directive and FDA requirements, whilst others, such as FACT–JACIE or AABB accreditation, are voluntary.
5 Increased resource is required to successfully implement the changes needed to achieve compliance.

References

1 World Marrow Donor Association Annual Report. Available at: http://www.worldmarrow.org/.
2 Directive 2004/23/EC of the European Parliament and Council on setting standards of quality and safety for the donation, procurement, testing, processing, preservation, storage and distribution of human tissues and cells. Available at: www.transfusionguidelines.org.uk.
3 Commission Directive 2006/17/EC implementing Directive 2004/23/EC of the European Parliament and Council as regards certain technical requirements for the donation, procurement and testing of human tissues and cells. Available at: www.transfusionguidelines.org.uk.
4 Commission Directive 2006/86/EC implementing Directive 2004/23/EC of the European Parliament and Council as regards traceability requirements, notification of severe adverse reactions and events and certain technical requirements for the coding, processing, preservation, storage and distribution of human tissues and cells. Available at: www.transfusionguidelines.org.uk.
5 The Human Tissue Act 2004 (except Scotland), ISBN 0 10 543004 8. Available at: www.hta.gov.uk.
6 The Human Tissue Act 2006 (Scotland), ISBN 0-10-590094-X. Available at: www.show.scot.nhs.uk.
7 Human Tissue Authority (HTA): Codes of Practice for Consent (Code 1), for Donation of Organs, Tissues and Cells (Code 2), for Removal, Storage and Disposal of Human Organs and Tissues (Code 5), for Donation of Allogeneic Bone Marrow and Peripheral Blood Stem Cells for Transplantation (Code 6) and for Import and Export of Human Bodies, Body Parts and Tissue (Code 8). Available at: http://www.hta.gov.uk.
8 FDA documents. Available at: www.fda.gov/cber/tiss.htm and www.fda.gov/cber/gene.htm.
9 Guidance for Industry Minimally Manipulated, Unrelated Allogeneic Placental/Umbilical CB Intended for Hematopoietic Reconstitution for Specified Indications; October 2009. Available at: http://www.fda.gov/cber/guidelines.htm.

10 Standards for Haematopoietic Progenitor Cell Collection, Processing and Transplantation, fifth edn, from the Foundation for the Accreditation of Cell Therapy (FACT) and the Joint Accreditation Committee of ISCT–Europe and EBMT (JACIE); 2012. Available at: www.jacie.org.

11 NETCORD–FACT International Standards for CB Collection, Processing, Testing, Banking, Selection and Release, 4th edn; 2010. Available from www.factwebsite.org.

12 AABB Standards for Cellular Therapy Services, 5th edition; 2011. Available from: www.aabb.org.

13 Circular of Information for the Use of Cellular Therapy Products, version 2009. Available from: www.aabb.org and www.factwebsite.org.

14 CAP Checklist. Available at www.cap.org under Accreditation and Laboratory Improvement.

15 World Marrow Donor Association (WMDA) Standards, March 2011. Available at www.worldmarrow.org.

16 Standards for Histocompatibility Testing: the American Society for Histocompatibility and Immunogenetics (ASHI) standards; 2011. Available at http://www.ashi-hla.org/images/uploads/2011ASHIStandards_Guidance.pdf.

17 Standards for Histocompatibility Testing: the European Federation for Immunogenetics (EFI) standards; 2010. Available at www.efiweb.org.

18 Hurley CK. (1999) Histocompatibility Testing Guidelines for Haematopoietic Stem Cell Transplantation using Volunteer Donors: Report from the World Marrow Donor Association. Quality Assurance and Donor Registries Working Groups of the World Marrow Donor Association. *Bone Marrow Transplantation* 1999; 24(2): 119–121.

Further reading

Cornish JM. JACIE accreditation in paediatric haemopoietic SCT. *Bone Marrow Transplant* 2008, October; 42 (Suppl. 2): S82–86. Review.

Gratwohl A, Brand R, Niederwieser D, Baldomero H, Chabannon C, Cornelissen J, de Witte T, Ljungman P, McDonald F, McGrath E, Passweg J, Peters C, Rocha V, Slaper-Cortenbach I, Sureda A, Tichelli A & Apperley J. Introduction of a quality management system and outcome after hematopoietic stem-cell transplantation. *J Clin Oncol* 2011, 20 May; 29(15): 1980–1986. Epub 11 April 2011.

Hurley CK, Foeken L, Horowitz M, Lindberg B, McGregor M & Sacchi N; WMDA Accreditation and Regulatory Committees. Standards, regulations and accreditation for registries involved in the worldwide exchange of hematopoietic stem cell donors and products. *Bone Marrow Transplant* 2010, May; 45(5): 819–824. Epub 22 February 2010.

Pamphilon D, Apperley JF, Samson D, Slaper-Cortenbach I & McGrath E. JACIE accreditation in 2008: demonstrating excellence in stem cell transplantation. *Hematol Oncol Stem Cell Ther* 2009; 2(2): 311–319.

Wall DA. Regulatory issues in cord blood banking and transplantation. *Best Pract Res Clin Haematol* 2010, June; 23(2): 171–177. Review. PMID: 20837328 [PubMed – indexed for MEDLINE].

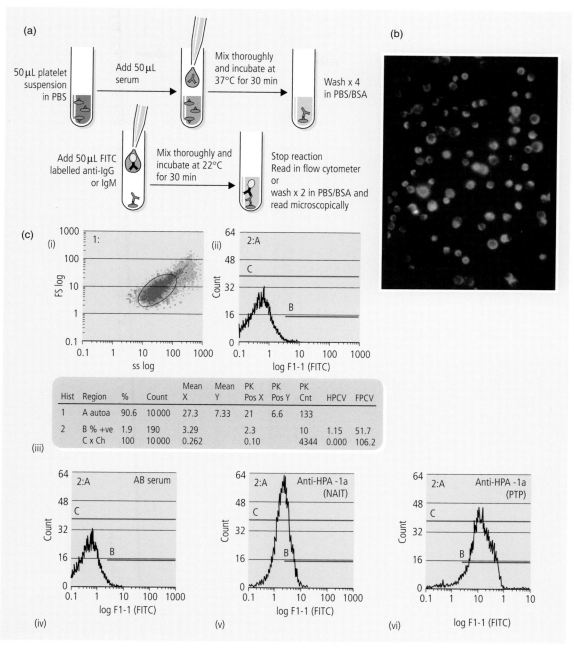

Plate 5.1 Indirect platelet immunofluorescence test. (a) Outline of assay. (b) Results of microscopic analysis of PIFT showing a strongly positive reaction. (c) Results of flow cytometric analysis of PIFT. (i) The platelet population is identified from forward/side scatter characteristics and the population is gated for analysis. (ii) and (iii) Results may be analysed in terms of mean (or median) channel fluorescence (region 'C') or the percentage of the population that is fluorescent (region 'B'). Figures (iv) to (vi) show plots of fluorescence intensity versus number of events for (iv) a negative sample, (v) a sample containing weak anti-HPA-1a and (vi) a potent anti-HPA-1a.

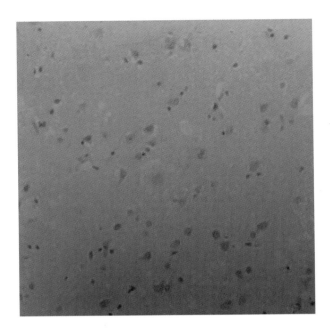

Plate 15.1 Section through the brain of a patient with CJD demonstrating spongiform degeneration of neuronal tissue and a florid amyloid plaque (centre). Reproduced with the permission of Professor James Ironside.

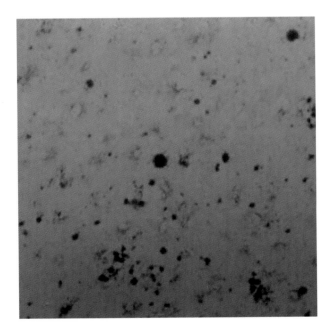

Plate 15.2 Section through the brain of a patient with variant CJD with immunohistochemical staining for PrP demonstrating abnormal accumulation of PrPSc throughout the brain. Reproduced with the permission of Professor James Ironside.

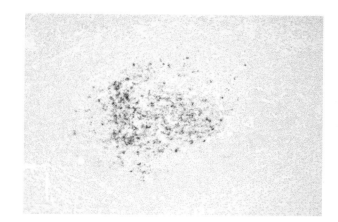

Plate 15.3 Section through the lymphoid tissue of a patient with variant CJD with immunohistochemical staining for PrP demonstrating abnormal accumulation of PrPSc in follicular dendritic cells. Reproduced with the permission of Professor James Ironside.

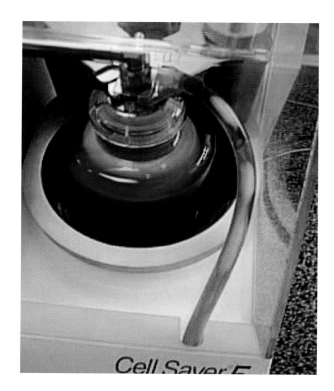

Plate 35.1 Centrifuge bowl within an apheresis machine showing the dense red cell layer towards the outside of the bowl and separation from the buffy coat and plasma layers.

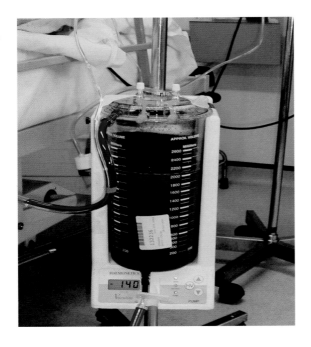

Plate 35.2 Collection reservoir, which may be used either operatively or postoperatively to collect the spilt blood or wound drainage.

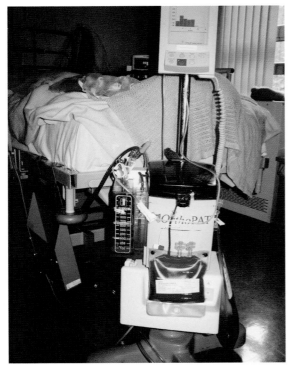

Plate 35.3 Equipment is now available that can wash salvaged blood in the ward environment.

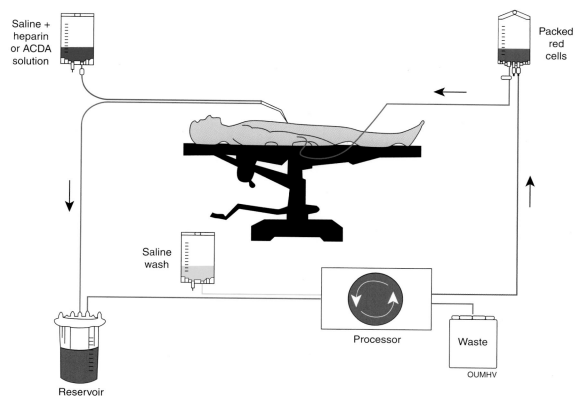

Saline +
heparin
or ACDA
solution

Packed
red
cells

Saline
wash

Processor

Waste

OUMHV

Reservoir

Plate 35.4 Diagram of complete cell saver setup (provided by the UK Cell Salvage Action Group).

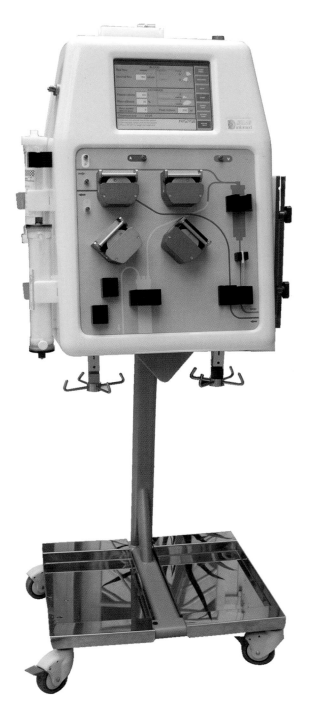

Plate 39.1 Infomed HF440, an example of a multitherapy filtration device.

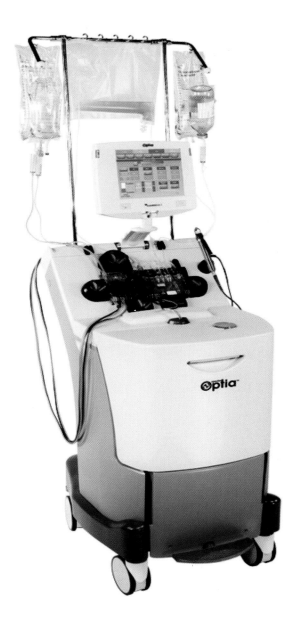

Plate 39.2 Spectra Optia (TerumoBCT), an example of a continuous flow apheresis device.

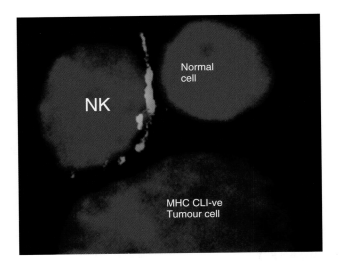

Plate 43.1 Capping of KIR molecules on NK cell. Anti-KIR antibody (green) shows colocalization of KIR and MHC class I molecules at the synapse between the NK and autologous normal cell. In contrast, the MHC-negative tumour cell fails to initiate capping of the KIR molecules.

39

Stem cell collection and therapeutic apheresis

Khaled El-Ghariani[1] & *Zbigniew M. Szczepiorkowski*[2]

[1]NHS Blood and Transplant and Sheffield Teaching Hospitals NHS Trust and University of Sheffield, Sheffield, UK

[2]Transfusion Medicine Service, Cellular Therapy Center, Dartmouth-Hitchcock Medical Centre and Geisel School of Medicine at Dartmouth, Hanover, New Hampshire, USA

The word *apheresis* is derived from the Greek meaning 'a withdrawal'. Therapeutic apheresis is the process of using apheresis technology to manipulate patient's circulatory contents through removal or exchange, to achieve a therapeutic goal. The rationale for this is that it will remove or reduce a substance or substances implicated in the pathology of the disease being treated. Plasma exchange is the process of exchanging part of the patient's plasma with suitable replacement fluid. Different cellular components can be removed with high precision. Red cells can be exchanged, circulating stem cells and lymphocytes can be collected for transplantation and the excess white cells or platelets that are present in myeloproliferative disorders can be removed. Molecules such as low density lipoproteins and immunoglobulins can be specifically removed through the use of adsorption columns. A decision to offer these treatments to patients should be based on factors such as temporary benefits of apheresis, potential adverse effects and the availability and efficacy of other treatment modalities.

Cell separators

Efficient cell separators are currently available. These machines are equipped with sophisticated software and safety alarm systems to detect air and changes in access or inflow pressure. Apheresis technology is based on either filtration or centrifugal systems. Filtration systems use permeable membranes to separate blood into its cellular and noncellular components by subjecting it to sieving through a membrane with suitably sized pores. An example of a filtration system is the Infomed HF440 (Plate 39.1 in the plate section). Centrifugal systems use G forces to separate blood into different components. Centrifugation of blood within apheresis machines results in sedimentation of its components into distinct layers. Based on increasing density, these layers are plasma, platelets, monocytes, lymphocytes and haemopoietic progenitor cells (HPCs), granulocytes and red cells.

Apheresis machines use either continuous- or intermittent-flow technology. In the continuous-flow machines, blood is continuously pumped into a spinning disposable harness where separation takes place and components are either diverted to a collection bag or returned to the patient as required. These machines often require two points of access to the circulation, one for withdrawal and another for return blood to the subject. Examples of continuous-flow systems are Spectra Optia (TerumoBCT) (Plate 39.2 in the plate section), Amicus (Fenwal) and Com.Tec (Fresenius Kabi). Intermittent-flow machines collect blood into a bowl during the draw cycle and then centrifuge it down to separate plasma and cellular components. Different components are diverted to the collection bag or returned to the patient along with replacement fluid during the return cycle. This process requires a

Practical Transfusion Medicine, Fourth Edition. Edited by Michael F. Murphy, Derwood H. Pamphilon and Nancy M. Heddle.
© 2013 John Wiley & Sons, Ltd. Published 2013 by John Wiley & Sons, Ltd.

single point of access to the circulation. An example of a presently marketed intermittent-flow system is the UVAR XTS (Therakos). Apheresis systems are primed with normal saline to displace air from the harness and also to ensure isovolumia, an important prerequisite for patients with haemodynamic instability or sickle cell disease. In children and small adults, the extracorporeal volume may be relatively high and the system will need to be primed by a mixture of packed red blood cells and normal saline or albumin [1]. Cell separators must be qualified and maintained according to the manufacturer's recommendations and must be operated by trained personnel.

Patient assessment and treatment planning

A physician experienced in the use of cell separators should undertake clinical assessment, to weigh the patient's current health status and expected benefit against potential risks and inconveniences. Plasma exchange often provides relief of the patient's symptoms for variable lengths of time and it is usually only part of the patient's treatment plan. Informed consent must be obtained from all competent patients and from authorized family members when the patient is not able to be consented. Laboratory evaluations before the first procedure should be tailored to the patient's clinical status; these may include a full blood count, coagulation screen and biochemistry. These tests are repeated thereafter as required. Apheresis treatment plans will include the type of vascular access, volume to be exchanged, type of replacement fluid, frequency of procedures and monitoring of response to therapy. Adequate vascular access is crucial. Peripheral veins, usually located in the antecubital fossa, should be evaluated by apheresis staff early in planning and should be used wherever possible, especially for patients requiring a limited number of procedures. Central venous catheterization, though, is associated with an increased risk of complications related to apheresis procedures and is required for patients who have inadequate peripheral veins or who require frequent procedures. A rigid double-lumen catheter should be used. Trained staff must undertake central vein cannulation and postinsertion catheter care [2]. Maximum effort should be exerted to avoid failure of vascular access during the procedure; such failure is associated with disappointment to both patients and staff.

Haemopoietic progenitor cell (HPC) mobilization

Currently, haemopoietic cell transplantation in adults is more commonly undertaken using mobilized peripheral blood (PB) rather than bone marrow as a source of stem cells (see also Chapter 36). This is because HPC, Apheresis [HPC(A)] engrafts faster than marrow and can be harvested without the need for hospital admission or general anaesthesia [3]. In the steady state, HPCs circulate in the peripheral blood, albeit in very low numbers, of less than 0.1% of the total white blood cell count. To ensure adequate graft, mobilization of such cells from the marrow into the peripheral circulation is necessary. Granulocyte colony-stimulating factor (G-CSF) is used to mobilize healthy donors, whereas mobilization of autologous cells can be achieved by growth factors, mainly G-CSF and/or the administration of chemotherapy such as cyclophosphamide or disease-specific combination chemotherapy. Granulocyte-macrophage colony-stimulating factor (GM-CSF) is less effective and more toxic than G-CSF to be used routinely for most donors. The mechanism of HPC mobilization started to unravel revealing involvement of a number of different molecules. One of them is CXCR4 expressed by HPCs among other cells. The ligand of this receptor is stromal-derived factor 1 (SDF-1; CXCL12), which is produced by marrow stromal cells. The association of CXCR4 with its ligand mediates stem cell homing, trafficking and retention. Proteolytic enzymes, such as elastase, cathepsin G and matrix metalloproteinase-g, released from neutrophils following administration of chemotherapy and/or G-CSF, are thought to degrade molecules such as CXCR4 and SDF-1, which are important for anchoring stem cells to marrow stroma and induce mobilization. Also, G-CSF may have an inhibitory effect on expression of CXCR4 mRNA and the reduced expression of CXCR4 receptors enhance mobilization.

Most healthy donors are mobilized by G-CSF at a dose of 10 μg/kg/day. Progenitor cells usually peak after the fourth injection when harvesting starts and the procedure may be repeated until the target number of stem cells is achieved. Donor age, steady-state CD34 levels and the dose of G-CSF may impact on the CD34+ cell mobilization. G-CSF used in healthy donors has proven to be both effective and reasonably safe [4]. The most common symptoms are bone pain, headaches, fatigue and nausea. Reduction in arterial oxygenation has also been noted. Rare but serious effects of G-CSF have been reported. Splenic enlargement is very common and there are a few case reports of splenic rupture, either spontaneously or precipitated by minor trauma or viral infection. Donors are encouraged to report any pain or discomfort that they may experience over the splenic region. G-CSF has a procoagulant effect and may increase the risk of myocardial infarction or ischaemic strokes in susceptible individuals. The effects of G-CSF on genomic stability and possible long-term leukaemogenesis remain unclear; however, this concern justifies long-term follow-up of G-CSF-stimulated donors. Pegylation of G-CSF is a process in which a polyethylene glycol (PEG) moiety is conjugated to a G-CSF molecule. This increases its molecular mass, reduces its renal excretion and prolongs its half-life in excess of 30 hours. Data are accumulating to support the use of one or two injections of pegylated G-CSF to mobilize autologous stem cells [5]. Two branded forms of G-CSF (Granocyte and Neupogen) have been available since the early 1990s. Extensive data are available concerning their safety. Recently G-CSF biosimilar agents have become available. These are alternative biological versions of G-CSF with significantly lower cost. The long-term safety of biosimilars is not yet known and therefore their use in mobilizing allogeneic donors is not recommended [6].

The response of individuals to mobilization regimens is variable and some donors fail to mobilize enough HPCs into circulation, to allow collection of an adequate graft. Such poor mobilization is more common in autologous than allogeneic donors. Stem cell damage due to old age, previous exposure to chemotherapy and radiotherapy, or disease involvement of bone marrow is associated with poor mobilization in autologous donors. Stem cell toxic agents such as melphalan and carmustine and other commonly used chemotherapy agents such as fludarabine and lenalidomide are specifically known to impair mobilization. The percentage of donors who mobilize poorly varies widely between published studies. This is most likely due to inconsistency in the definition of poor mobilization and the differences in the donor groups studied. Patterns of donors' responses to mobilization treatment are likely to continue to change in

the future, depending on changes in types of diseases treated, the patients' age profiles and comorbidities. Also, the effects of new cancer treatments need to be defined. A few reports suggested that therapies such as rituximab and bortezomib may not adversely affect mobilization. The mechanism of poor mobilization in healthy donors is unclear. However, experiments in mice have suggested a genetic control of the vigour and timing of mobilization. Individuals who prove to be hard to mobilize may respond favourably to mobilization at a later date or by using different mobilization treatment. If clinically indicated, it is worth undertaking further mobilization attempts in such individuals. Table 39.1 lists the options available to manage poor mobilization.

Plerixafor (Mozobil) is a CXCR4 antagonist that blocks this receptor reversibly and inhibits its interaction with SDF-1. This leads to HPC release into the circulation. Plerixafor synergizes with G-CSF and is usually administered the night before the planned first day of collection, at 240 μg/m^2 subcutaneous injection. The introduction of plerixafor has provided

Table 39.1 Management options for poor mobilization.

1 Patients should be considered for stem cell mobilization and harvesting, if required, early in the course of their illness and before stem cell toxic agents are used in their treatment.

2 Leucocytapheresis is repeated daily for several days and a larger blood volume is processed to maximize yield. Leucocytapheresis may be started at a lower CD34+ cells count (e.g. 5–10 × 10^6/μL) in patients who are likely to be hard to mobilize.

3 Salvage plerixafor is introduced the day before the planned first day of apheresis if the CD34+ cell count and total leucocyte count predict mobilization failure.

4 Mobilization is repeated at a later date to allow marrow recovery using higher dose G-CSF ± chemotherapy ± plerixafor. Cells obtained from two mobilization attempts are likely to be adequate.

5 New agents such as stem cell factor (ancestim) could be used, ideally within the context of a clinical trial to evaluate this approach [21].

6 Marginally low numbers of stem cells are accepted for transplantation.

7 Bone marrow is harvested instead. However, bone marrow from poor mobilizers may not be of good enough quality and delayed engraftment may follow.

clinical practice with a safe and effective new mobilizing agent [7, 8]. Although current use of plerixafor is limited by increased drug cost, its judicious use in an appropriately selected patient population has been proven to be cost effective [9] and the drug has been approved by the US Food and Drug Administration (FDA) and the European Medicine Evaluation Agency (EMEA) for autologous HPC donations for patients with myeloma and non-Hodgkin's lymphoma. Because most patients are good mobilizers, the universal use of plerixafor is not justified. Plerixafor could be used in patients who have previously failed mobilization with a success rate of up to 70% [10]. However, use of plerixafor during the first mobilization of selected high risk patients could be more helpful by eliminating the need for a second mobilization, reducing the number of apheresis sessions required and avoiding delays in transplantation. This could be achieved by adopting a 'just-in-time' policy where patients' total leucocyte (white blood count) and blood CD34+ cell counts are monitored. Those with high leucocyte count (e.g. $>10 \times 10^9$/L) and low CD34+ cell count (e.g. $<15 \times 10^6$/µl) would be identified as potential mobilization failure and given plerixafor during their first mobilization attempt [11].

PB HPC collection (leucocytapheresis)

Leucocytapheresis, following chemotherapy and G-CSF mobilization, could commence when leucocyte counts are rising ($\geq 1 \times 10^9$/L). However, currently, most centres use surface expression of CD34 on PB cells, measured by flow cytometry, to predict the optimal time to start HPC collection, to predict the success of collection and to enumerate HPC in the collected product [12]. CD34 is a heavily glycosylated phosphoglycoprotein expressed on progenitor cells of all lineages within the lymphohaemopoietic system, but not on mature cells. Endothelial progenitors, marrow stromal cells and osteoclasts also express CD34. Approximately, 1.5% of aspirated normal marrow mononuclear cells, less than 0.1% of nonmobilized PB and approximately 0.5% of cord blood cells are CD34+. The function of CD34 molecules remains elusive; however, analysis of its structure indicates that these molecules may have a role in cellular signal transduction and/or cell adhesion. CD34 is a surrogate marker for stem cells. Purified autologous CD34+ cells mediate haemopoietic engraftment whereas CD34– cells do not engraft. There is a clear correlation between the number of CD34+ cells infused and the rate of subsequent recovery of both neutrophils and platelets posttransplant [13]. Compared with marrow harvests, G-CSF mobilized grafts contain three- to fourfold higher CD34+ cells and about a 10- to 20-fold increase in CD3+ T cells. An optimal number of infused HPC(A) required for transplantation is not fully defined. However, to ensure timely engraftment and graft survival, there is a consensus to infuse at least 2.0×10^6/kg recipient body weight of CD34+ cells for autologous transplant and 4×10^6/kg of recipient body weight for allogeneic transplant [13]. A higher allogeneic cell number is required with increased HLA disparity between donor and recipient. In addition, a higher number of cells should be collected if tandem transplant or graft manipulation is contemplated. The maximum number of cells to be infused is not defined. However, in the autologous setting, the inconvenience and cost of harvesting of much higher cell numbers are not justified by improvement of clinical outcome. In some studies, infusion of very high numbers of allogeneic cells was found to be associated with a higher risk of extensive chronic graft-versus-host disease (GVHD) [13].

Administration of G-CSF just before leucocytapheresis should be avoided. G-CSF injections are usually followed by temporary reduction of circulating stem cells lasting for about 4 hours. The optimal harvesting time is between 4 and 12 hours after subcutaneous injection of G-CSF. Serial measurement of PB CD34+ cell count in autologous donors is usually obtained as soon as their total leucocyte approaches 1×10^9/L. Collection, started at a level of 20 CD34+ cells/µl, gives the best yield. However, collection may also start at 10/µL or even 5/µL in donors who may not mobilize so well. Healthy donors usually follow a more predicted course and their peak mobilization is usually reached at day 5, after four G-CSF injections. Some donors require further injections either because of delayed mobilization or because not enough cells were collected at the first collection.

Collection of HPC(A) is a technically challenging procedure and different machines collect cells with different efficiency and selectivity. Machine efficiency is measured by the percentage of CD34+ cells that can be collected at a specific peripheral CD34+ cell count. The collected yield can be enhanced by the machine's ability to process more volumes of donor blood within a reasonable period of time and without inconvenience to the donor. Selective machines manage to target HPC(A) with less contamination by other unwanted blood cells. This reduces platelets and red cell contamination of the harvest, which is important in two respects: first, such contamination affects stem cell cryopreservation and may increase infusion complications and, second, collection of other cells such as platelets may lead to thrombocytopenia in the donor.

Apheresis units should observe good manufacturing practice and qualify new machines against published data, as well as against existing equipment, to ensure that new technologies are safe and convenient to the donors, as well as able to meet required product specifications [14]. This is particularly important in cases where the unit deals with special donor groups such as children, or heavily pretreated autologous patients, who tend to mobilize poorly.

There are other important operational features of apheresis machines that should be taken into consideration. The volume of the end product should be optimized to minimize the amount of dimethylsulfoxide (DMSO) yet maximize viability of HPCs during transport and storage. Smaller volumes are easy to cryopreserve, require a smaller storage space and are associated with less DMSO infusion toxicity. However, it is equally important that the contamination of the final product with granulocytes is minimized, as they were shown to be the primary cause of infusion-related adverse reactions. Machines that have smaller extracorporeal volumes are less likely to cause transient anaemia and hypovolaemia in small subjects and children and so avert the need to prime with blood. Machines that are using a single point of access (i.e. single needle) to circulation are usually associated with an ability to process a smaller volume of blood and so give a lower yield of CD34+ cells.

Several machines, such as COBE Spectra, COBE Spectra Optia, Amicus (Fenwal) and Com.Tec (Fresenius Kabi), are able to collect stem cells with different efficiencies and selectivity. COBE Spectra is a commonly used apheresis machine. A new development of this technology, Spectra Optia is found to be at least equally efficient but also less sensitive to changes in blood flow due to less than optimal venous access. This machine, similarly to already marketed for this use Amicus and Com.Tec, is automated and has small end harvest and extracorporeal volumes [14].

A total of 2–3 patient blood volumes are usually processed by the apheresis machine at each leucocytapheresis procedure. Large-volume leucocytapheresis (processing of 3–6 blood volumes over a longer period of time or by increasing the blood flow into the apheresis machine) has been tried and shown to collect significantly higher CD34+ yields. This may reduce the number of leucocytapheresis procedures required and also limit exposure to G-CSF [15]. Although this practice is associated with donor inconvenience, citrate toxicity and platelet loss, it has been used successfully and extensively – particularly for allogeneic donors.

Plasma exchange

Plasma exchange is an effective treatment for many conditions, mainly immune in nature. Exchanging patient's plasma is associated with removal of a pathological substance or substances; an example is immunoglobulin in situations of hyperviscosity or autoimmune disorders such as myasthenia gravis. The removed plasma is most commonly replaced with human albumin solution (HAS) of 4.5%. (In the USA, it is called human serum albumin and is usually 5%). Up to one-third of the exchange volume can be replaced by normal saline if the patient's starting albumin level is normal; otherwise hypotension and/or peripheral oedema may follow. HAS is used because it provides the necessary oncotic pressure with fewer allergic reactions and an impressive safety record with regard to infection transmission. In other clinical scenarios, the exchange process is required not only to remove factors implicated in the disease pathogenesis but also to replace necessary plasma constituents. In thrombotic thrombocytopenic purpura (TTP), for example, plasma exchange removes autoantibodies to the von Willebrand factor-cleaving protease, an important enzyme otherwise known as ADAMTS13, and the associated ultralarge von Willebrand factor multimers. Plasma exchange is also required to replace the missing ADAMTS13; hence fresh frozen plasma (FFP) is used as a replacement fluid for TTP. Solvent detergent plasma is the recommended replacement fluid for TTP in the UK, while in the USA this product is not currently available. Clotting factors may also require replacement during the course of plasma exchange. A therapeutic dose of FFP (10–15 ml/kg) may be included as the last replacement fluid

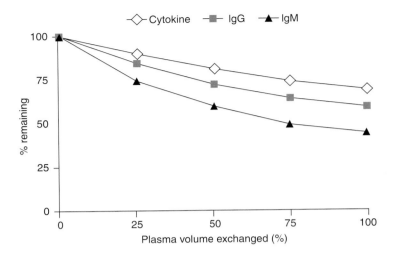

Fig 39.1 Kinetics of plasma exchange. Reproduced with permission from El-Ghariani and Unsworth [16].

to be infused in cases where repeated exchange with albumin has depleted clotting factors in patients at a high risk of bleeding.

Plasma exchange treatment plans include determination of the amount of plasma to be exchanged in relation to the patient's estimated plasma volume and how to space the procedures to ensure efficiency. An exchange of 1.0–1.5 of the patient's plasma volume will exchange 63–78% of their plasma and is therapeutically effective in most situations. Larger volume exchange is associated with inconvenience, use of larger amounts of replacement fluid and brings little extra benefit (Figure 39.1) [16]. The frequency and total number of exchanges depend on the disease being treated and on the patient's response. Hyperviscosity, TTP and Goodpasture's syndrome require daily exchanges; others may respond to a course, e.g. five exchanges over 7–10 days.

Response to treatment varies between patients. Criteria to monitor response to treatment should be agreed early in the treatment plan to avoid under-treatment, overtreatment or the continuation of ineffective treatment. TTP is monitored by measuring the platelet count and other parameters of haemolysis whilst Guillain–Barré syndrome and myasthenia gravis are assessed by clinical neurological improvement. Evidence is accumulating regarding the effectiveness, or otherwise, of different apheresis procedures to treat various disease processes (Table 39.2). The American Society for Apheresis (ASFA) publishes a guideline document every 3 years with assignment of

Table 39.2 Disorders for which apheresis is accepted as first-line therapy, either as a stand-alone treatment or in conjunction with other modes of treatment (ASFA Category I indications®). Adapted from the American Society for Apheresis guidelines, 5th edition and Szczepiorkowski ZM *et al. J Clin Apheresis* 2010, 25: 83–177 [17].

Plasma exchange
  Thrombotic thrombocytopenic purpura
  Hyperviscosity in monoclonal gammopathies
  Cryoglobulinemia
  Antiglomerular basement membrane disease
    (Goodpasture's syndrome)
  Myasthenia gravis
  Paraproteinemic polyneuropathies (IgG/IgA)
  Guillain–Barré syndrome
  Chronic inflammatory demyelinating
    polyradiculoneuropathy
Red cell exchange
  Life- and organ-threatening sickle cell crisis
Photopheresis
  Erythrodermic cutaneous T-cell lymphoma
  Heart transplant rejection prophylaxis
Selective lipid removal (usually by adsorption column) for
    homozygote familial hypercholesterolemia
Leucocytapheresis for hyperleucocytosis causing leucostasis

ASFA Category (I to IV) and Recommendation Grade for different diseases [17].

Although large randomized trials support the use of plasma exchange in the treatment of Guillain–Barré syndrome, intravenous immunoglobulin (IVIG)

is equally effective. Given the ease of administration, IVIG is usually a first-choice therapy. However, either of the two treatment modalities can be used if the other fails. Chronic inflammatory demyelinating polyneuropathy also responds to both plasma exchange and IVIG and the former can be used for maintenance treatment. In myasthenia gravis, plasma exchange has a clear therapeutic effect; however, the disease control is temporary and may be followed by a rebound. Plasma exchange is used to treat emergencies such as respiratory failure or swallowing difficulties and to prepare patients for thymectomy. Plasma exchange must be accompanied by an appropriate immunosuppressive regime if it is to be of long-term benefit in myasthenia gravis.

Paraproteinaemia causing clinically evident and progressive hyperviscosity syndrome is a medical emergency requiring urgent plasma exchange to lower the concentration of the responsible paraprotein. IgM, the largest immunoglobulin and mostly intravascular, is most likely to cause hyperviscosity. IgA and IgG3 tend to aggregate and, after IgM, are more likely than other isotypes or subclasses to be associated with hyperviscosity. One to three treatments will usually alleviate symptoms long enough for chemotherapy to take effect. These patients are often severely anaemic. They should not be transfused until the viscosity has been lowered as a rise in haematocrit can precipitate a serious worsening of their symptoms. Plasma exchange can also be life saving in cryoglobulinaemia associated with a fulminant clinical picture. Replacement fluids should always be warmed. At the same time, the cause of the cryoglobulinaemia must be determined and definitive chemotherapy instituted if appropriate. Plasma exchange plays a limited role in the treatment of autoimmune cytopenia; however, it is the treatment of choice for TTP and should be started as soon as the diagnosis is strongly suspected. Daily plasma exchange is needed for at least 2 days after the platelet count has returned to normal (i.e. over 150×10^9/L) and lactate dehydrogenase (LDH) is within the normal range. Plasma infusion can also be used to treat TTP if plasma exchange is not immediately available.

Plasma exchange is required as an adjuvant therapy in antiglomerular basement membrane disease (Goodpasture's syndrome). In the presence of pulmonary haemorrhage, it is important not to overload the patient with replacement fluids as this may provoke further bleeding. Plasma exchange may be used in certain cases of pauci-immune rapidly progressive glomerulonephritis and systemic vasculitis. Such cases need to be discussed with a specialist. Plasma exchange has no proven role in the management of systemic lupus erythematosus nephritis (SLE) or uncomplicated rheumatoid arthritis.

Red cell exchange

Red cell exchange involves the removal of a patient's red cells and concomitant infusion of allogeneic donor cells. This procedure, evolved as a manual procedure, can be performed by apheresis machines and is most commonly used to treat sickle cell disease and some parasitic infections such as malaria or babesiosis. A major advantage of this automated procedure is the isovolaemic nature of the exchange, which is important in preventing further complications occurring. A single red cell volume exchange removes approximately 60% of the red cells originally present in the patient's circulation. The patient's haematocrit, the fraction of the patient's red cells to be left in circulation after the exchange, the desirable final haematocrit and the haematocrit of the replacement fluid can be entered into the apheresis device's software, which then calculates the volume of red cells to be removed and estimates the volume of red cells to be used as replacement.

Exchange using normal red cells as a replacement fluid is beneficial in the treatment and prevention of certain sickle cell crises. Exchange should aim at raising the haemoglobin A to 70–80% to avoid further vasoclusive crises and treat the ongoing one. However, the final haematocrit following exchange should not exceed 30%. Hyperviscosity, associated with a higher haematocrit, is associated with a reduction in oxygen delivery. Neurological events after partial exchange, usually for priapism, have been observed and thought to be due to high end haemoglobin levels, a situation also known as ASPEN syndrome (an eponym for association of sickle cell disease, priapism, exchange transfusion and neurological events coined by Siegel et al. in 1993 [18]). Red cell exchange may not shorten an uncomplicated painful sickle cell crisis but may be considered in severe and frequent debilitating crises. A patient who survives an acute ischaemic stroke could be maintained on a regular exchange programme to prevent recurrence. For acute chest syndrome, life- or organ-threatening complications, red cell exchange can provide rapid reduction of sickle haemoglobin and is less likely to cause iron accumulation. Red cell exchange in sickle cell disease is associated with concerns such as increased requirement of allogeneic blood, which is associated with the risk of red cell alloimmunization.

Red cell exchange is an adjuvant therapy that should be considered for severely ill patients with malaria if parasitaemia is more than 10% or if the patient has severe malaria manifested by altered mental status, nonvolume overload pulmonary oedema or renal complications. Treatment is discontinued after achieving ≤5% residual parasitaemia. Absolute erythrocytosis causing hyperviscosity, thromboembolism or bleeding should be treated by tackling its primary cause and possibly by phlebotomy to maintain a normal haematocrit. However, erythrocytapheresis is also used to treat certain patients with polycythaemia, where removed red cells are replaced with albumin or saline to maintain isovolemia. This procedure is particularly useful in patients with polycythaemia vera, complicated by acute thromboembolism, severe microvascular complications or bleeding, especially if the patient is haemodynamically unstable.

Extracorporeal photochemotherapy (photopheresis)

Extracorporeal photochemotherapy (ECP) is a process in which the patient's mononuclear cells (MNC) are collected and exposed to ultraviolet A light (UVA) in the presence of photoactivating agents such as 8-methoxypsoralen (8-MOP). This process brings about immunomodulation, which can be therapeutically beneficial to patients with advanced cutaneous T-cell lymphoma (CTCL), GVHD and cardiac transplant rejection [19]. The mechanism of action of ECP is not fully understood; however, ECP induces lymphocyte apoptosis, which leads to changes in cytokine secretion patterns, more tolerant antigen presenting cells (APCs), induction of Treg cells and suppression of CD8+ effector cells. Interestingly, ECP does not lead to an increased incidence of opportunistic infection, a feature that is particularly useful in patients with extensive skin lesions. ECP can be best achieved by collecting MNC using a specialized cell separator such as the THERAKOS™ CELLEX™ system (most commonly used in the UK and USA). This machine delivers a calculated UVA radiation dose into the MNC suspension pretreated with 8-MOP, before returning the cells to the patient's circulation. Heparin and, less commonly, ACD-A are used as anticoagulants. Alternatively, ECP can be completed using a combination of a cell separator to collect leucocytes, 8-MOP is added to the apheresis product and the suspension is then exposed to UVA using an irradiation source (UV light box), such as the UV-matic irradiator and then re-infused. This practice is commonly used in Europe, but strict adherence to good manufacturing practice (GMP) regulations for re-infused products is required. ECP is contraindicated in the presence of psoralen hypersensitivity.

There is some evidence for the use of ECP in erythrodermic CTCL and steroid-refractory GVHD, but randomized controlled studies are needed. There is good evidence supporting the use of ECP in preventing cardiac rejection following transplantation. Randomized controlled trials have also shown a therapeutic benefit in type 1 diabetes mellitus, but the inconvenience associated with the procedure outweighs the clinical benefit. Patients with advanced CTCL (stage III/IV) typically receive ECP on two consecutive days once per month. For the management of chronic GVHD, an accelerated regime has been used to gain rapid control of the disease with two consecutive treatments administered initially every 2 weeks. In the USA often a higher frequency of two procedures per week for 12 weeks is used. ECP is a treatment option for patients with steroid refractory acute GVHD [20].

Complications of therapeutic apheresis

Complications occur in up to 10% of procedures; most are mild but, rarely, serious complications including deaths have been reported. Given the advances in technology, machine-related problems are unusual. Failure of the machine that will prevent red cell return can result in red cell loss of up to 200 ml of blood in newer instruments while up to 350 ml in older instruments. Central catheter-related complications, such as pneumothorax, internal bleeding, thrombosis and infections, are more common and can be serious. Allergic reactions to replacement fluids are uncommon but can be significant. These include anaphylactic reactions, hypotension and urticarial rashes.

Reactions to HAS are now rare as the preparations contain lower amounts of significant contaminants than previously, especially of vasoactive kinins. HAS essentially carries no risk of infection and it does not increase the citrate return. Dilution of coagulation factors can occur following repeated plasma exchanges and may require the addition of FFP to the replacement fluid. FFP poses the risk of bloodborne infection (although virally inactivated products are now available), allergic reactions and also contributes to the citrate load as it contains approximately 14% citrate anticoagulant by volume. Side effects of the citrate anticoagulant, almost universally used, are particularly common. These result from hypocalcaemia and include paraesthesiae (digital and perioral), abdominal cramps and, rarely, cardiac dysrhythmias and seizures. Citrate toxicity usually responds to simple measures such as slowing the rate of return and providing extra calcium orally. Intravenous calcium may be required. Patients with renal failure who are receiving large amounts of citrate during plasma exchange may develop a profound metabolic alkalosis. Patients receiving repeated treatments over a long period of time can lose significant quantities of calcium. Complications during therapeutic apheresis may arise from underlying pathology or comorbidity. It is important that the clinical status is assessed prior to exchange. Where risks are increased, but benefit is likely, a suitable location for the procedure such as a high dependency unit may be required.

Key points

1 A physician experienced in the use of cell separators should assess the patient's need to have a therapeutic apheresis procedure taking into consideration potential risks and inconvenience.
2 Adequate vascular access is crucial. Central venous catheterization needs to be undertaken by trained staff to minimize risks to patients.
3 G-CSF with or without chemotherapy is currently the gold standard for HPC mobilization.
4 Donors who prove to be hard to mobilize may respond favourably to the addition of plerixafor to the G-CSF mobilization protocol.
5 Human albumin solution (4.5%) is the most commonly used replacement fluid for plasma exchange.

Occasionally, plasma, possibly solvent detergent product, is needed.
6 Photopheresis induces immunomodulation without immunosuppression and is indicated for certain stages of cutaneous T-cell lymphoma, GVHD and solid organ transplant rejection.

References

1 Kim HC. Therapeutic apheresis in pediatric patients. In: BC Mcleod, ZM Szczepiorkowski, R Weinstein *et al.* (eds), *Apheresis Priniciples and Practice*, 3rd edn. Bethesda, MD: AABB Press; 2010.
2 Guidance on the use of ultrasound locating devices for placing central venous catheters, National Institute for Clinical Excellence, September 2002, ISBN: 1-84257-213-X. Available at: http://www.nice.org.uk.
3 To LB, Roberts MM, Haylock DN *et al.* Comparison of haematological recovery times and supportive care requirements of autologous recovery phase peripheral blood stem cell transplants, autologous bone marrow transplants and allogeneic bone marrow transplants. *Bone Marrow Transplantation* 1992; 9(4): 277–284.
4 Pulsipher MA, Chitphakdithai P, Miller JP *et al.* Adverse events among 2408 unrelated donors of peripheral blood stem cells: results of a prospective trial from the National Marrow Donor Program. *Blood* 2009; 113: 3604–3611.
5 Tricot G, Barlogie B & Zangari M. Mobilization of peripheral blood stem cells in myeloma with either pegfilgrastim or filgrastim following chemotherapy. *Haematologica* 2008; 93: 1739–1742.
6 Shaw BE, Confer DL, Hwang WY *et al.* Concerns about the use of biosimilar granulocyte colony-stimulating factors for the mobilization of stem cells in normal donors: position of the World Marrow Donor Association. *Haematologica* 2011; 96(7): 942–947.
7 Di Persio JF, Micallef IN, Stiff PJ *et al.* Phase III prospective randomized double-blind placebo-controlled trial of plerixafor plus granulocyte colony-stimulating factor compared with placebo plus granulocyte colony-stimulating factor for autologous stem-cell mobilization and transplantation for patients with non-Hodgkin's lymphoma. *J Clin Oncol* 2009; 27(28): 4767–4773.
8 Di Persio JF, Stadtmauer EA, Nademanee A *et al.* Plerixafor and G-CSF versus placebo and G-CSF to mobilize hematopoietic stem cells for autologous stem cell transplantation in patients with multiple myeloma, *Blood* 2009; 113(23): 5720–5726.
9 Costa LJ, Alexander ET & Hogan KR. Development and validation of a decision-making algorithm to guide the use of plerixafor for autologous hematopoietic stem cell

mobilization. *Bone Marrow Transplantation* 2010; 46: 64–69.

10 Durate RF, Shaw BE, Marin P *et al.* Plerixafor plus granulocyte CSF can mobilize hematopoietic stem cells from multiple myeloma and lymphoma patients failing previous mobilization attempts: EU compassionate use data. *Bone Marrow Transplantation* 2011; 46: 52–58.

11 Li J, Hamilton E, Vaughn L *et al.* Effective and cost analysis of 'just-in-time' salvage plerixafor administration in autologous transplant patients with poor stem cell mobilization kinetics. *Transfusion* 2011; 51: 2175–2182.

12 Gutensohn K, Magens MM, Kuehnl P *et al.* Increasing the economic efficacy of peripheral blood progenitor cell collections by monitoring peripheral blood CD34+ concentrations. *Transfusion* 2010; 50(3): 656–662.

13 Heimfeld S. HLA-identical stem cell transplantation: is there an optimal CD34 cell dose? *Bone Marrow Transplantation* 2003; 31: 839–845.

14 Reinhardt P, Brauninger S, Bialleck H *et al.* Automatic interface-control apheresis collection of stem/progenitor cells: results from an autologous donor validation trial of a novel stem cell apheresis device. *Transfusion* 2011, 51(6): 1321–1330.

15 Abrahamsen JF, Stamnesfet S & Liseth K. Large-volume leukopheresis yields more viable CD34+ cells and colony-forming units than normal-volume leukopheresis, especially in patients who mobilize low numbers of CD34+ cells. *Transfusion* 2005; 45: 248–253.

16 El-Ghariani K & Unsworth DJ. Therapeutic apheresis – plasmapheresis. *Clin Med* 2006; (4): 343–347.

17 Szczepiorkowski ZM, Winters JL, Bandarenko N *et al.* Guideline on the use of therapeutic apheresis in clinical practice – evidence-based approach from the Apheresis Applications Committee of the American Society for Apheresis. *J Clin Apheresis* 2010; 25: 83–177.

18 Siegel JF, Rich MA & Brock WA. Association of sickle cell disease, priapism, exchange transfusion and neurological events: ASPEN syndrome. *J Urology* 1993; 150(5 Pt 1): 1480–1482.

19 McKenna KE, Whittaker S, Rhodes LE *et al.* Evidence-based practice of photopheresis 1987–2001: a report of a workshop of the British Photodermatology Group and the UK Skin Lymphoma Group. *Br J Dermatol* 2006; 154: 7–20.

20 Perfetti P, Carlier P, Strada P *et al.* Extracorporal photopheresis for the treatment of steroid refractory acute GVHD. *Bone Marrow Transplantation* 2008, 42: 609–617.

21 Lapierre V, Rossi J-F, Azar N *et al.* Ancestim (r-metHu SCF) plus filgrastim and/or chemotherapy for mobilization of blood progenitors in 513 poorly mobilizing cancer patients: the French compassionate experience. *Bone Marrow Transplantation* 2011, 46: 936–942.

Further reading

Bensinger W, DiPersio JF & McCarty JM. Improving stem cell mobilization strategies: future directions. *Bone Marrow Transplantation* 2009, 43: 181–195.

Cashen AF, Lazarus HM & Devine SM. Mobilizing stem cells from normal donors: is it possible to improve upon G-CSF? *Bone Marrow Transplant* 2007; 39: 577–588.

George JN. How I treat patients with thrombotic thrombocytopenic purpura. *Blood* 2010, 116: 4060–4069.

Gertz MA. Current status of stem cell mobilization. *Br J Haematol* 2010; 150: 647–662.

Scarisbrick J. Extracorporeal photopheresis: what is it and when should it be used? *Clin Expl Dermatol* 2009; 34: 757–760.

Scarisbrick JJ, Taylor P, Holtick U *et al.* UK consensus statement on the use of extracorporeal photopheresis for treatment of cutaneous T-cell lymphoma and chronic graft-versus-host disease. *Br J Dermatol* 2008; 158(4): 659–678.

Siddiq S, Pamphilon D, Brunskill S *et al.* Bone marrow harvest versus peripheral stem cell collection for haemopoietic stem cell donation in healthy donors. *Cochrane Database Syst Rev* 2009, Issue 1: CD006406. DOI: 10.1002/14651858. CD006406.pub2.

To LB, Leversque J-P & Herbert KE. How I treat patients who mobilize hematopoietic stem cells poorly. *Blood* 2011; 118: 4530–4540.

40 Haemopoietic stem cell processing and storage

Ronan Foley & Pamela O'Hoski

Department of Pathology and Molecular Medicine, McMaster University,
Hamilton, Ontario, Canada

Background

Historically obtained from the posterior pelvis of a donor under general anaesthesia, haemopoietic progenitor cells (HPCs) can now be obtained from peripheral blood as well as from the umbilical cord and placenta post-delivery. Recognition that haemopoietic growth factors (i.e. G-CSF) administered either alone or following chemotherapy results in significant mobilization of a blend of cell populations (including HPCs) into the peripheral blood has had a profound impact on stem cell collection both for autologous transplantation and for healthy stem cell donors. Identification of HPCs correlates with expression of the CD34+ antigen. Other markers such as the absence of CD38 or the presence of CD133, Flk2/Flt3 as well as aldehyde dehydrogenase activity may be more specific but remain investigational. Functional evaluation of colony-forming units (CFUs) of myeloid, erythroid, megakaryocytic and long-term culture initiating cells may be useful functional assays that can complement immunophenotypic analysis.

Terminology to describe HPC and other cell-based human products derived from a bone marrow harvest (HPC, Marrow), from mobilized apheresis peripheral blood (HPC, Apheresis), from umbilical cord (HPC, Cord Blood) or from steady-state apheresis for donor lymphocyte infusion (DLI) (Therapeutic Cells, T cells) (Table 40.1) have been suggested by the International Society for Blood Transfusion (ISBT 128

nomenclature). Each source exhibits different biological properties and graft compositions. If one compares a bone marrow graft (approximately 700–1500 ml) to mobilized blood progenitor cells (100–400 ml) collected by leucapheresis distinct differences are noted. A mobilized peripheral blood component typically contains a greater number of CD34+ progenitors but also a greater number of T-lymphocytes, which has raised concern for a greater incidence of chronic GVHD in patients undergoing allogeneic BMT [1]. Conversely, when a nonmyeloablative transplant is performed a higher dose of CD34+ cells may be of greater importance to ensure engraftment and stable chimerism, thus favouring an HPC, Apheresis product. A unit of cord blood (HPC, Cord Blood) may have less progenitor cells, but compensates with a higher proliferative potential and a lower risk of GVHD [2].

Transplant procedures

Autologous SCT

Expanding clinical indications support the use of autologous SCT in a variety of clinical settings, including multiple myeloma (single or tandem) and relapsed non-Hodgkin and Hodgkin lymphoma (B and T diffuse large cell, mantle cell lymphoma, Burkitts and follicular lymphoma). Autologous SCT is also a therapeutic option for patients with gonadal or

Practical Transfusion Medicine, Fourth Edition. Edited by Michael F. Murphy, Derwood H. Pamphilon and Nancy M. Heddle.
© 2013 John Wiley & Sons, Ltd. Published 2013 by John Wiley & Sons, Ltd.

443

Table 40.1 Human haemopoietic progenitor cells (HPCs).

Name	Donor	Options	Storage
HPC, Marrow Collect 10–15 mL/kg recipient weight with maximum 20 mL/kg donor weight Dose $2-4 \times 10^8$/kg recipient weight	Matched related donor	Standard intraoperative marrow harvest adults or children	Usually infused following collection
	Matched unrelated donor	Steady state versus donor treated with mobilization agent such as Filgrastim (investigational)	Cryopreservation post buffy coat concentration
	Autologous (rare)		
HPC, Apheresis Process 12–25 litres of donor blood	Autologous patient (common)	Apheresis product collected following a stem cell mobilization agent (G-CSF, pegylated G-CSF, glycosolated G-CSF, GM-CSF, SCF, AMD-3100) +/– Chemotherapy	Auto SCT – cryopreserved
	Matched related donor	Mobilize with 5–10 µg/kg G-CSF	AlloSCT – infused following collection or cryopreserved
	Matched unrelated donor	Mobilize with 5–10 µg/kg G-CSF	
	Haploidentical donor	Mobilize with 16 µg/kg G-CSF	CD34+ selection, T-cell depletion and cryopreservation
TC, Apheresis or TC-T Cells Donor lymphocyte infusion	Matched related donor	Same donor as original HPC product but not mobilized – steady state Dose = CD3+/lymphocyte/kg recipient weight	First dose following collection
	Matched unrelated donor		Graduated doses cryopreserved
HPC – Cord	Cord blood approximately 100 mL	Consenting parent(s) >3.0×10^7/kg recipient weight *In utero* *Ex utero*	Red cell depleted then all cryopreserved

retroperitoneal germ cell tumors refractory to cisplatin-based chemotherapy. At present autologous progenitor cells are almost exclusively obtained by leucapheresis. Use of HPC, Apheresis reduces the time to engraftment with shorter hospitalization, less transfusional support and the use of antimicrobials [3].

Allogeneic SCT

Allogeneic SCT involves replacement of a diseased bone marrow with haemopoietic elements from a healthy donor. It is now known that engraftment of both HPCs as well as donor immune T-lymphocytes are essential for long-term haemopoiesis and disease control. Donor lymphocytes contribute to both graft-versus-leukaemia (GVL) as well as graft-versus-host disease (GVHD). Shifting the balance of therapeutic efficacy solely from stem cell replacement to maintenance of a transplanted donor immune system has led to reduced intensity nonmyeloablative or 'mini' allogeneic transplants.

Allogeneic donors may be from a related sibling or obtained from a bone marrow registry. Matches are based on the human leucocyte antigen (HLA) system comprised of genes on chromosome 6 that encode cell-surface antigen presenting proteins linked to our immune system. The major histocompatibility complex (MHC) is made up of two basic classes involved in antigen presentation and subsequent immune activation. MHC class I includes HLA-A, HLA-B and HLA-C, whereas MHC class II includes HLA-DR, HLA-DQ and HLA DP. The proteins encoded by HLA define self and directly instruct the immune system to recognize self-versus-nonself. HLA typing previously employed simple serological testing (antibody-based) to provide low resolution typing. Although useful in the related setting, there have been concerns regarding sole use of low resolution typing use in unrelated donors. Many HLA laboratories now perform high resolution (HR) molecular typing to ensure that a potential unrelated donor/recipient pair is as highly matched as possible.

If an unrelated match cannot be found remaining options include related haploidentical transplantation or allogeneic transplant using stored cord blood. Haploidentical SCT involves a related donor/parent who has only a partial HLA match. Due to significant HLA barriers large-volume CD34+ product must be rigorously purified (T-depleted). This may result in lasting immune deficiency with a high risk of fulminant infection (viral, CMV, EBV) or relapse.

Donor lymphocyte infusions (DLI)

The cell products infused for DLI collected from the original HPC donor in an unstimulated state are called Therapeutic Cells-Apheresis and Therapeutic Cells-T Cells. DLI may be used to help convert mixed donor chimerism to full donor chimerism after allogeneic HPC transplant or as pre-emptive therapy for treatment of an early relapse by providing a direct GVL effect.

HPC products

Bone marrow

Use of bone marrow (HPC, Marrow) has decreased in recent years as other sources of progenitor cells have become available but in certain circumstances, like transplanting paediatric patients or patients with aplastic anaemia, a role for bone marrow still exists. Collecting bone marrow involves placing the donor under general anaesthesia and then aspirating 10–15 ml/kg recipient weight (maximum 20 ml/kg donor weight) from the posterior iliac crests and placing the product in a collection bag containing ACD/heparin anticoagulant. Collected product is passed through 500 and 200 μm filters to remove bone and other debris prior to infusion or further processing. The target nucleated cell dose (automated counter) is 2–4×10^8 /kg recipient weight. Use of marrow CD34+ enumeration suggests a CD34+ cell dose $>3.0 \times 10^6$/kg correlates with improved recovery and 5-year survival while $<1.2 \times 10^6$/kg correlates with inferior recovery [4, 5].

Peripheral blood

Mobilization of CD34+ progenitor cells into blood with collection by leucapheresis (HPC, Apheresis) is the method of choice for patients undergoing autologous SCT. This procedure is based on obtaining sufficient CD34+ progenitor cells (defined as a minimum of 2.0×10^6 CD34+ cells/recipient weight and an optimal of 5.0×10^6 CD34+ cells/recipient weight). Ideally the mobilization strategy employed should result in an optimal product with predictable engraftment performance, minimal side effects, a reasonable DMSO volume and diminished risk of contamination with tumor cells. Lower doses of infused CD34+ cells can result in delayed or failed platelet engraftment, Case-by-case decisions are made to proceed with auto SCT when less than 2.0×10^6/kg CD34+ cells based on the clinical situation and stability of the underlying disease. For patients undergoing auto SCT two strategies can be employed: either growth factor(s) alone or growth factors that follow administration of chemotherapy. Use of growth factor(s) alone results in a more predictable schedule, less neutropenia-associated infections and reduced cost, but is associated with a higher chance of mobilization failure. A combined chemotherapy/growth factor approach is associated with greater toxicity and less predictability. The benefits of using chemotherapy include disease control during the procedure and theoretical benefit of reduced tumor cell contamination.

As an alternative to undergoing a marrow harvest, an allogeneic donor may be asked to provide mobilized peripheral blood progenitors collected by leucapheresis. Administration of G-CSF alone is the currently accepted strategy for mobilization of normal healthy donors. Use of HPC, Apheresis as opposed to HPC, Marrow appears to improve the time to haemopoietic recovery and offers a greater GVL effect [6], but carries a potentially higher risk of chronic extensive GVHD. Retrospective studies suggest children and adolescents with acute leukaemia or aplastic anaemia have inferior outcomes when an HPC, Apheresis graft is used [7].

Umbilical cord blood

Characteristics of banked cord products include highly functional HPCs, less CMV contamination and a lower risk of GVHD. It is generally accepted that the kinetics of haemopoietic recovery are significantly slower when using HPC, Cord Blood. This may relate to fewer and less mature HPCs. A minimum target of approximately 3.0×10^7 nucleated cells per recipient weight per unit of cord blood is required. A higher dose may be considered depending on HLA disparity. Measurement of CD34+ cells/recipient kg weight may be more informative. The mean collection volume for a cord sample is approximately 100 ml (50–200 ml) including anticoagulant [8]. Several techniques for cord blood collection may be performed either prior to or following delivery of the placenta. Closed system collection techniques have improved rates of bacterial contamination. Cells can be stored in a smaller volume by immediately removing plasma and red blood cells. Characterization of the cord unit includes: volume, weight, total nucleated count, CD34+ cell count, colony-forming analysis, ABO/Rh and HLA typing, full panel transmissible disease testing and haemoglobin electrophoresis [9]. Cord units should be processed quickly and immediately stored at 4°C with cryopreservation to occur as soon as possible. Once properly stored, it is currently not known how long HPC, Cord Blood components remain viable. *In vitro* analysis has suggested reasonable viability to as long as 15 years, perhaps longer [10]. In an effort to hasten time to reconstitution in larger adult recipients, double UCB are now being considered [11]. The strategy appears to improve significantly the time to engraftment. When evaluated 100 days posttransplant, typically only one cord unit, often the unit with a higher CD34+ count, seems to dominate reconstitution.

Donor lymphocytes

The collected product is known as TC, Apheresis and if the entire product is infused immediately it retains this name. In some instances there is concern that administration of a large single dose of donor T cells may precipitate fatal GVHD rather than the desired GVL. Graduated doses of donor T cells are often administered over time. Lymphocyte content is calculated using automated or manual differential as well as flow cytometry (CD3+). The laboratory will aliquot doses (defined by institution or protocol) based on $CD3+ \times 10^6/$ kg of recipient weight, often giving the first dose fresh but cryopreserving other doses.

HPC product assessment and specialized procedures

CD34 enumeration

Flow cytometry on a fresh HPC product provides CD34+ enumeration in a timely manner (1 hour). Given the importance of accurate CD34+ enumeration the procedure should follow a standardized and validated methodology (i.e. 'The ISHAGE guidelines for CD34+ cell determination by flow cytometry') [12]. A CD34+ enumeration kit includes CD45-FITC/CD34-PE, isotype control PE, stem cell microbeads (known concentration/μL), lysing solution (ammonium chloride) and a viability dye 7-amino actinomycin D (7-AAD). HPC samples stored at 18–20°C should be processed within a few hours and samples kept overnight should be stored at 2–6°C. Total viable CD34, apoptotic and necrotic cells can be measured with calculations based on product volume.

CD34+ enumeration from peripheral blood on the morning of collection may be instructive and predictive. An absolute CD34+ cell number expressed per microlitre appears to be the most useful variable. In a recent analysis we assessed 258 donors undergoing autologous SCT. Greater than 20 CD34+/μL correlated with a successful collection ('good mobilizers'), as opposed to donors with <10/μL ('poor mobilizers') (Table 40.2). Newer mobilization agents such as CXCR-4 binding inhibitors (AMD3100) and stem cell factor (hu-SCF) may be administered to auto SCT patients identified as high risk for mobilization failure.

Table 40.2 Predictive value of peripheral blood (PB) pre-CD34+ enumeration.

PB CD34+/μL	Positive predictive value (%)	Sensitivity (%)	Specificity (%)
≥10	86.4	100	60.2
≥15	91.8	97.2	78.1
≥20	93.6	95.1	83.5
≥30	96.6	90.7	91.7
≥40	98.8	86.9	97.3

Analysis of 258 patients undergoing auto SCT for multiple myeloma and non-Hodgkin lymphoma. On the morning of collection a peripheral blood sample was analysed by flow cytometry. The absolute CD34+/μL value predicted the ability to successfully collect a target of 2.0×10^6 CD34+/kg in a large-volume apheresis collection.

Viability assays

Trypan blue (TB) is a simple exclusion dye test indicating cell viability, which can be routinely performed in any laboratory. Cells that fail to exclude dye are considered nonviable and are readily identified. Use of fluorescent stains with dark-field microscopy may reduce background staining. 7-Aminoactinomycin (7-AAD) is a fluorescent chemical with affinity for GC-rich DNA. Nonviable cells lack membrane integrity and will take up 7-AAD, which can be measured by flow cytometry. If performing viability for cryopreserved HPC product it is important to keep in mind that small aliquots will have different cooling properties that may diminish viability. Thus viability results from a cryovial are simply an estimate of viability for an actual product contained in a bag.

In vitro HPC assays

Functional analysis of HPCs can be performed using cells grown in semi-solid methylcellulose (MC) to identify colony-forming units (CFU). Resultant CFU-erythroid, CFU-granulocyte, CFU-mixed (CFU-GEMM) and CFU-megakaryocyte colonies help to characterize the short-term multipotency of a given HPC product. These assays are time consuming (2 weeks) and do not provide real-time information for products that are administered shortly after collection. Facilities managing HPC, Cord products that are stored frozen over long periods may offer colony assay results along with CD34 content in order to characterize the available unit better. These assays do have utility in the evaluation of long-term storage and for validation of newer cryopreservation strategies. Longer cultures (2 months) on stromal cell layers followed by MC culture assess long-term culture initiating cells (LTC-IC) and may provide functional evidence for pluripotent HPCs.

Sterility testing

Sterility testing suitable to detect clinically significant bacteria and fungal contamination of an HPC product must be performed at a minimum postprocessing. It is our preference to collect cultures when the product arrives in the laboratory and after each step of processing. Most centres accomplish this by collection of aerobic and anaerobic blood cultures from the product. In some cases paediatric bottles can be used to minimize the volume of sample removed from the product. Cultures should be performed: (i) at the end of HPC product collection and the end of processing for cryopreservation and (ii) after each step of any reprocessing (washing cells, manipulation on cell processor, post CD34+ selection). Cultures may also be obtained from each bag at the time of re-infusion. If an investigative cell-based product is administered additional analysis for sterility, mycoplasma, endotoxin, identity, adventitial virus, purity and potency are required.

ABO incompatibility

HLA-matched HPC SCT can proceed even if the blood groups of donor and recipient do not match. There are two types of ABO mismatch, each with its own interventions, which may need to occur before the transplant product can be infused [13]. ABO major mismatch results when the recipient's plasma contains a potent ABO antibody directed against donor's red cells. HPC, Apheresis products have a haematocrit of 5–10%, whereas the red cell content of HPC, Marrow haematocrit is much higher, ranging from 25 to 30%. Significant intravascular lysis of red cells will cause a haemolytic transfusion reaction if the product is infused without an intervention to decrease the level of the ABO antibody. Recipient's with ABO antibody titre against donor's red cells greater than 1:16 should be prepared by performing several apheresis procedures to replace plasma with 5% albumin. The titre of antibody can be further reduced by infusing plasma containing soluble ABO substance that matches the problem antibody. These measures are generally sufficient to allow safe infusion of HPC, Apheresis, but significant residual antibody after other interventions may require processing of HPC, Marrow to remove most of the red cell content. Red cell depletion of marrow is most commonly performed using a blood processor such as the Cobe 2991 with or without the addition of a sedimenting agent like hydroxethyl starch (HES). Red cell content at completion of processing should be as low as possible while minimizing loss of progenitor cells.

An ABO minor mismatch results when the donor's plasma contains a potent antibody directed against recipient's red cells. The need for intervention is less common in this setting as the ratio of antibody to red cell antigen is much lower, but it is wise to assess the level of donor antibody against the intended recipient's red cells. The presence of an antibody with a titre above 1:256 may necessitate group O red cell exchange of the recipient if the product is HPC, Apheresis. HPC, Marrow should undergo plasma depletion to remove at least 80% of antibody either through manual centrifugation or in semi-closed mode using a Cobe 2991 or similar blood processor.

CD34+ enrichment

CD34+ enrichment of HPC products is performed for a variety of reasons: haploidentical transplant, reduction of potential tumour burden in autologous HPC products and providing a T-cell depleted product to a recipient at high risk of GVHD. Both HPC, Apheresis and HPC, Marrow can be CD34 enriched but the marrow product must first be processed to a buffy coat concentrate to reduce volume and red cell content. Commercially available monoclonal antibody-based CD34+ enrichment devices have proven highly effective. The CliniMacs™ instrument from Miltenyi Biotec produces an extremely pure product (average 98% T-cell depletion) while recovering 65–75% of initial CD34+ content. Briefly, the HPC product is labelled with antibody to CD34 antigen, which is attached to an iron dextran particle; then the product is run through a column that sits between the poles of a powerful electromagnet. Labelled cells are retained

in the column until all the product is processed; then the magnet recedes and the CD34-enriched product is eluted into clinical grade PBS buffer containing 0.5% human serum albumin. The final product can be infused fresh or cryopreserved for use in the future.

Ex vivo expansion

Given the limitations of inadequate numbers of HPCs in some products (HPC, Cord Blood, poor mobilizers) the ability to *ex vivo* expand stem and progenitor cells has significant clinical potential. Numerous strategies to date have included cultures in combinations of cytokines including Flt-3 ligand, SCF, IL-3, IL-6, IL-11, G-CSF, GM-CSF and TPO grown with or without bone marrow stromal cells. In these studies it is important to determine if expansion is occurring in committed progenitor cells (short-term haemopoietic reconstitution) as opposed to early progenitor cell expansion (long-term reconstitution). Despite numerous efforts, attempts at clinical expansion have been limited to date and remain investigational. The ability to expand committed progenitors in an effort to improve short-term neutrophil and platelet recovery may be more feasible [14]. The ability to expand early progenitors has significant implications for investigational trials employing gene therapy.

T-cell depletion

Despite the use of potent immunosuppressive agents (i.e. Methotrexate, Cyclosporine) GVHD remains a common (up to 50%) complication for patients undergoing allogeneic SCT. GVHD is primarily mediated by T-lymphocytes, which can be successfully removed from the graft prior to administration. T-cell depletion can clearly reduce GVHD, but also may hinder engraftment, increase the incidence of leukaemic relapse and the risk of infections including posttransplant lymphoproliferative disorders. *Ex vivo* procedures include physical separation by density gradient (counterflow centrifugal elutriation), depletion with lectins, cytotoxic drugs and the use of anti-T-cell antibodies (examples are CD2, CD3, CD5, CD8, CD25 and CD52) alone or in combination (complement, conjugated to toxin). Despite an ability to significantly eliminate T cells to as low as $<1 \times 10^5$ CD3+ cells/kg recipient weight and attenuate acute GVHD, no differences in chronic GVHD, transplant-related mortality and disease-free survival have been proven to date [15].

Storage of HPC products

In many instances the HPC product is stored for short periods of time (hours) in an unmanipulated liquid state. Reported temperatures suitable for short-term storage range from 4 to 37°C (see Table 40.3). Ambient temperature is often preferred for short-term storage of HPC, Marrow [16] but 'ambient' should be a specific temperature range, e.g. 18 to 22°C. HPC collected by apheresis can be held at room temperature for 1–2 hours if further processing is to occur imminently, but are most commonly stored at 4°C when longer storage is required. A lower temperature may minimize damage by nonspecific cytokine release from granulocytes and mononuclear cells. There is a progressive loss of progenitor cells during nonfrozen storage with the rate of loss influenced by cell concentration, quantity and type of other cells contained in the product, the storage bag and the storage temperature [17]. What is most important is that the definition of ideal conditions for storage be validated at the stem cell facility. Validation should include temperature, cell concentration (if the product is to be held overnight before processing the leucocyte count should be diluted with donor plasma to below a concentration below 2×10^8/mL), additives in the product, addition of extra plasma to dilute cell counts, viability and, if the technology is available, progenitor assays.

The length of time the product can be stored should also be established by in-house viability measurements at the end of intended storage and an expiry date and time set for each type of product handled. All equipment used for storage must also be validated to maintain the established temperature range. Storage requirements should include designating a location dedicated only for HPC products and a separate, clearly labelled location for any product that must be quarantined. A mechanism for monitoring and documenting temperature that includes local and remote alarms must be in place. If the product is stored at 'ambient temperature', the temperature of the location of storage must be documented. There should be a posted contingency plan that deals with temperature or mechanical failure of the designated storage equipment.

Cryopreservation

The majority of allogeneic products are not cryopreserved; however, centres that perform large numbers of allogeneic transplants may cryopreserve collected product to allow increased flexibility in the timing of the transplant related to the donor collection. In other cases donor availability or a change in the recipient's condition may dictate that the collected product be cryopreserved. Virtually all products to be used for autologous SCT are cryopreserved in order to allow time to administer multiday conditioning regimens and ensure infusion of progenitor cells occurs once toxic chemotherapy drugs have been cleared from the circulation.

HPC products to be cryopreserved must be transported to the processing laboratory in a designated transport cooler that has been validated for transport time and temperature. On arrival the receiving staff document minimum/maximum and actual temperatures of transport and the product visual inspection for colour, leakage and correct labelling.

All materials to be used in the cryopreservation process should have lot number and expiration date recorded. Visual inspection of all equipment and reagents must also be performed and recorded. The product will be manipulated in a biohazard safety cabinet so appropriate cleaning, disinfection and checks of a magnehelic gauge to ensure proper airflow are done in advance so that all is ready when the product arrives. HPC, Marrow and HPC, Cord products require processing to reduce mature red cell content and volume reduction before cryopreservation processing can occur. In most instances the haematocrit of HPC, A is between 5 and 10%, which does not represent enough mature red cell contamination to cause a problem so these products can be cryopreserved without removal of mature red cells. Plasma collected from the donor (apheresis) or retained from red cell depletion (referred to as concurrent plasma) should always accompany the product to the processing laboratory in case there is a need to dilute the product.

Sterility testing must be performed on the product on arrival and after the addition of the cryoprotectant

449

Table 40.3 Stem cell laboratory processing procedures.

Procedure	Methods	Indication
Red cell depletion of HPC, Marrow	Semi-automated – Cobe 2991 cell processor with or without HES Manual centifugation	Major ABO/other antigens Cryopreservation of HPC, Cord Blood
Plasma depletion of HPC, Marrow	Semi-automated – Cobe 2991 cell processor Manual centrifugation	Minor ABO mismatch
Buffy coat concentration	Centrifugation Semi-automated – Cobe 2991 cell processor	Volume reduction Cryopreservation of HPC -Marrow
Sterility	Bacterial fungal detection Investigational products (mycoplasma, adventitial virus, endotoxin)	HPC products precryopreservation and post – thaw Cryoprotectant solutions
Viability	Dye exclusion (TB), fluorescence microscopy 7-AAD – flow cytometry	Products to be used after more than 2 years of storage
CD34/CD3 enumeration	Flow cytometry (i.e. ISHAGE)	HPC, Apheresis HPC, Marrow HPC-C (optional) TC, Apheresis
Functional HPC assays	CFU assays, LTC-IC	Viability post long-term storage Viability postinvestigative procedure (purging) Validation of new procedure to document HPC loss Assess stored cryopreserved product post 'warming event'
CD34 enrichment	Immunomagnetic bead-based separation	Related haploidentical SCT 'purge' technique Selected cases (GVHD prophlaxis) Clinical trial
T-cell depletion	Antibody-based +/− toxin Elutriation	Investigational Selected cases Clinical trial
Cryopreservation	DMSO, HES/DMSO controlled-rate freezing or freeze in −80°C Liquid nitrogen storage below −150°C	Option for all HPC products

solution. It is also wise to collect a sterility sample from the prepared cryoprotectant solution to ensure reagents used are sterile. Once sterility samples are collected, samples are drawn for a nucleated cell count and CD34 assessment. Processing cannot begin until at least the nucleated cell count is known as products with a nucleated cell count higher than 4.5×10^8/mL require dilution by adding a calculated amount of concurrent donor plasma.

Techniques for cryopreservation are designed to interfere with mechanisms that cause cell damage or death during the freezing process [18]. HPC need to be protected from dehydration and ice crystal formation within the cell. Most often the cryoprotectant used to accomplish this protection is dimethyl sulfoxide (DMSO). Dimethyl sulfoxide is a 'penetrating cryoprotectant' that acts in two separate ways. First, when cooling is relatively slow ice crystals tend to form in the extra cellular space. Ice formation concentrates extracellular solutes resulting in increased osmolality. DMSO moderates the increasing concentration by slowing water absorption by the ice crystals. Second, rapid diffusion of DMSO through the cell membrane allows the intracellular concentration of DMSO to be equal to the extracellular concentration, which facilitates water to move from within to outside the cell without excessive osmotic stress and before ice crystal formation can occur.

At rapid rates of cooling intracellular ice can form even when cryoprotectant is used. The cooling rate should minimize ice formation potential and complement the cryoprotectant's adjustment of the solution's rate of cooling. The concentration of DMSO required in the solution is determined by the 'colligative effect'. Colligative refers to the properties of a solution (i.e. rate of freezing) being dependent on the number of particles (solute) and not the composition of the particles. The optimum concentration of DMSO to achieve good penetration of cells and moderation of the freezing point of the extracellular water is 10% volume in volume. Reduced concentrations of DMSO (5%) can be used if DMSO is combined with a macromolecular cryoprotectant like HES [19]. This macromolecule does not penetrate the cells but protects by forming a viscous noncrystalline glassy shell that retards the movement of water, preventing progressive dehydration. Cryoprotection can be accomplished by using macromolecules alone. Addition of DMSO to the solution raises the temperature at which the glassy shell forms. This facilitates intracellular dehydration necessary to avoid ice crystal formation while extracellular solute concentration is stopped by the glassy formation. The 'combined' cryoprotectant seems to afford better cell recoveries than the use of macromolecule alone. This type of cryoprotectant solution is a complex blend of salts, sugars, DMSO and plasma proteins and requires careful attention to the recipe and process when being prepared. Plasma proteins also have cryoprotectant properties and the addition of serum proteins to a cryoprotectant solution appears to improve HPC survival. The range of protein concentration and the source of protein used in cryoprotectant solutions are variable, with some groups preferring donor plasma as their source while others use 5% human serum albumin.

Processing of products to remove mature red cells should be performed prior to cryopreservation for HPC, Marrow and HPC, Cord Blood, where infusion of large quantities of free haemoglobin from lysed red cells may cause renal toxicity. Large quantities of red cells can also cause clumping of the product during processing. The concentration of mature red cells in HPC, Apheresis is not usually high enough to cause problems during processing or at infusion. Bone marrow product must be processed before cryopreservation, not only to remove red blood cells but also to eliminate fat and the majority of plasma volume. Processing: (i) allows cryopreservation of a buffy coat suspended at a desirable cell concentration, (ii) minimizes the volume of cryoprotectant that is used and later infused to the recipient and (iii) reduces the amount of freezer storage space required. Processing of the bone marrow product to achieve these ends can be performed manually using caution to use centrifuge speeds that keep the 'g' between 800 and 1000 to minimize progenitor cell damage. Alternatively, the product can be processed in a semi-automatic manner using a Cobe 2991 cell processor.

High cell concentrations in a product to be cryopreserved can result in poor recovery of progenitor cells. Very high cell concentrations can lead to post-thaw clumping of cells possibly due to leucocyte agglutination. High cell concentrations may lead to increased neutrophil death precryopreservation, with consequent release of cytokines that may damage the progenitor cells. HPC products with very low cell concentrations can also result in poor post-thaw viability; these products should be volume reduced to increase cell concentration. Most laboratories freeze HPCs at concentrations between 1.0 and 5.0×10^8/mL but successful cryopreservation outcomes have been reported using concentrations as high as 8×10^8/mL and as low as 1×10^6/mL.

Cryopreserved HPCs have been stored at temperatures as warm as $-80\,^\circ$C but there is risk of cell damage caused by recrystallization as water migrates from small to large crystals. Most centres avoid this risk by storing at or below $-120\,^\circ$C in mechanical freezers or in the vapour or liquid phase of nitrogen. Products and temperature monitoring devices should be placed well below the rim of liquid nitrogen freezers to minimize the increase of temperature caused by opening the lid. Product exposed to frequent temperature change is at risk of progressive damage to stored cells. This gradient effect can be minimized by using aluminium storage canisters and frameworks inside

451

freezers to allow better heat conductivity and moderation of temperature loss throughout the freezer. Storage of products immersed in liquid nitrogen provides a constant temperature of −196°C and insulation against temperature fluctuations. Measures must be taken to eliminate droplet or other contamination within the freezer as virus and bacteria can survive in liquid nitrogen and crosscontamination of products is a risk. Products immersed in liquid nitrogen should include some type of an overwrap on each bag before placing in the aluminium canister.

The duration of cryopreserved storage may be indefinite if temperatures are consistently maintained below −150°C. As previously noted, cord blood cells maintain functionality for 15 years or greater; a current report of autologous recipients receiving second transplants with product cryopreserved for up to 7 years describes engraftment kinetics identical to those seen at use for the first half of the product stored for only 1–2 months [20].

Thawing of cryopreserved haemopoietic progenitor cells

Thawing can occur at the patient bedside or in the laboratory depending on institutional policy. Recipient identification is verified and the product is retrieved from storage. Units should be transported to the thaw location in a liquid nitrogen dry shipper with continuous temperature monitoring. The temperature should be maintained below −120°C until immediately before the thaw.

In most instances thawing is performed in a 37°C waterbath. The water source can be freshly drawn tap or sterile water. If a waterbath maintained by thermostat is used there should be careful cleaning and disinfection between uses. Alternately, fresh water is placed into a sterile basin, using a new basin for each recipient. The monitored temperature range should remain between 35 and 39°C. If the cells are thawed too slowly there is risk of injury from ice recrystallization; if the temperature is too high there is loss of viability or clumping of protein material within the bag. To begin, the protective canister is opened and labels are confirmed by two technologists. If the cryopreserved product has been overwrapped at cryopreservation it can be placed into the prepared 37°C waterbath; otherwise the unit should be placed in a plastic bag prior to immersion to avoid water droplet contamination into exposed ports. The unit is gently massaged over 5 minutes to ensure all parts are liquid and there is no residual slush. Some centres collect a culture sample from each thawed bag immediately prior to infusion to document postprocessing sterility.

Toxicity of the cryoprotectant directly to HPCs has been described so exposure of thawed cells to DMSO should be limited both precryopreservation and at thaw. Cryoprotectant can cause toxicity to the recipient but if the dose of DMSO is carefully controlled it is not necessary to remove it prior to infusion. The DMSO dose should be limited to less than 1 gm/kg of recipient weight in a 24-hour period. If the total amount of DMSO exceeds this limit, infusion should occur over two days. In situations where DMSO is to be removed, serial dilutions of protein-based solution to avoid osmotic shock to cells can be employed. At completion cells are resuspended in a 5% protein-based solution.

Quality assurance

A quality programme defines the policies and environment necessary to attain acceptable outcomes and meet safety standards consistently. The components include SOPs that address all activities, standardized and controlled labelling, documentation/record keeping that ensures traceability, personnel qualifications and training, building, facilities and equipment validation, environmental monitoring, regular auditing and error and accident system/management. Regulatory authorities worldwide have placed major emphasis on the establishment of an effective quality programme along with strict compliance to best practices in clinical, collection and laboratory settings. At the processing laboratory the quality programme is the means by which good manufacturing practices are instituted and followed throughout product manufacturing and manipulation. Lot-to-lot variation is minimized and the safety, purity and potency of the product are guaranteed.

Key points

1 Clinical indications for both autologous and allogeneic stem cell transplants are increasing.

2 HPCs can be obtained from three sources: bone marrow, peripheral blood and umbilical cord blood. Characteristics of these products differ in terms of HPCs and other mature cells.

3 Validated methods for cryopreservation are a key requirement to ensure optimal graft performance following administration to a transplant recipient.

4 Quality assurance testing of products at multiple stages of processing is essential for safety, purity, identity, potency and stability.

5 Accurate nucleated cell counting, CD34+ enumeration, viability(/clonogenic) assays and sterility analysis before and after cryopreservation are essential.

6 An established quality assurance programme and formal accreditation are critical to establish high level standards in the field of HPC transplantation.

References

1 Stem Cell Trialists' Collaborative Group. Allogeneic peripheral blood stem-cell compared with bone marrow transplantation in the management of hematologic malignancies: an individual patient data meta-analysis of nine randomized trials. *J Clin Oncol* 2005; 23: 5074–5087.

2 Wagner JE, Barker JN, Defor TE *et al.* Transplantation of unrelated donor umbilical cord blood in 102 patients with malignant and nonmalignant diseases: influence of CD34 cell dose and HLA disparity on treatment-related mortality and survival. *Blood* 2002; 100: 1611–1618.

3 Vellenga E, van Agthoven M, Coockewit AJ *et al.* Autologous peripheral blood stem cell transplantation in patients with relapsed lymphoma results in accelerated haemopoietic reconstitution, improved quality of life and cost reduction compared with bone marrow transplantation: the Hovon 22 study. *Br J Haematol* 2001; 114: 319–326.

4 Bittencourt H, Rocha V, Chevret S *et al.* Association of CD34 cell dose with haemopoietic recovery, infections, and other outcomes after HLA-identical sibling bone marrow transplantation. *Blood* 2002; 99: 2726–2733.

5 Zubair AC, Zahrieh D, Daley H *et al.* Engraftment of autologous and allogeneic marrow HPCs after myeloablative therapy. *Transfusion* 2004; 44: 253–261.

6 Couban S, Simpson DR, Barnett MJ *et al.* A randomized multicenter comparison of bone marrow and peripheral blood in recipients of matched sibling allogeneic transplants for myeloid malignancies. *Blood* 2002; 100: 1525–1531.

7 Schrezenmeier H, Passweg JR, Marsh JC *et al.* Worse outcome and more chronic GVHD with peripheral blood progenitor cells than bone marrow in HLA-matched sibling donor transplants for young patients with severe acquired aplastic anemia. *Blood* 2007; 110: 1397–1400.

8 Reed W, Smith R, Dekovic F *et al.* Comprehensive banking of sibling donor cord blood for children with malignant and nonmalignant disease. *Blood* 2003; 101: 351.

9 Eichler H, Meckies J, Schmut N, *et al.* Aspects of donation and processing of stem cell transplants from umbilical cord blood. *Z Geburtshilfe Neonatol* 2001; 205: 218.

10 Broxmeyer HE, Srour EF, Hangoc G *et al.* High-efficiency recovery of functional haemopoietic progenitor cells from human cord blood cryopreserved for 15 years. *Proc Natl Acad Sci USA* 2003; 100: 645.

11 Wall DA, Chan KW. Selection of cord unit(s) for transplantation. *Bone Marrow Transplant* 2008; 42: 1.

12 Sutherland DR, Anderson L, Keeney M, Nayar R & Chin-Yee I. The ISHAGE guidelines for CD34 + determination by flow cytometry. International Society of Hematotherapy and Graft Engineering. *J Hematother* 1996; 5: 213–226.

13 Rowley SD, Donato ML *et al.* Red blood cell-incompatible allogeneic haemopoietic progenitor cell transplantation. *Bone Marrow Transplantation* 2011; 46: 1167–1185.

14 Paquette RL, Dergham ST, Karpf E *et al.* Ex vivo expanded unselected peripheral blood: progenitor cells reduce post transplantation neutropenia, thrombocytopenia, and anemia in patients with breast cancer. *Blood* 2000; 96: 2385.

15 Hale G, Zhang MJ, Bunjes D *et al.* Improving the outcome of bone marrow transplantation by using CD52 monoclonal antibodies to prevent graft-versus-host disease and graft rejection. *Blood* 1998; 92: 4581.

16 Antonenas V, Garvin F *et al.* Fresh PBSC harvest, but not bone marrow show temperature related loss of CD34 viability during storage and transport *Cytotherapy* 2006; 8: 158–165.

17 Peltengell R, Wall PJ *et al.* Viability of haemopoietic progenitors from whole blood, bone marrow and leucapheresis product. Effects of storage media, temperature and time. *Bone Marrow Transplantation* 1994, November; 14(5): 703–709.

18 Bakken AM Cryopreserving human stem cells. *Curr Stem Cell Res Ther* 2006, January; (1): 47–54.

19 Rowley SD, Feng Z *et al.* A randomized phase III trial of autologous blood stem cell transplantation comparing cryopreservation using dimethylsulfoxide versus dimethylsulfoxide with hydroxyethyl starch. *Bone Marrow Transplantation*, 2003; 31: 1043–1051.

20 Cameron G *et al.* Cryopreserved mobilised autologous blood progenitors stored for more than two years successfully support blood count recovery after high dose chemotherapy. *Cytotherapy* 2011, August; 13(7): 856–863.

Further reading

Martin-Henao GA, Torrico C, Azqueta C *et al.* Cryopreservation of HPC from apheresis at high cell concentrations does not impair the hematological recovery after transplantation. *Transfusion* 2005; 15: 1917–1924.

Thomas ED, Appelbaum FR, Blume KG, Forman SJ & Negrin RS *Haemopoietic Cell Transplantation*, 4th edn. Wiley-Blackwell; 2009.

41

Haemopoietic stem cell transplantation

I. Grant McQuaker[1] *& Ian M. Franklin*[2]

[1]BMT Unit, Beatson West of Scotland Cancer Centre, Glasgow, Scotland, UK
[2]Irish Blood Transfusion Service, National Blood Centre, Dublin, Republic of Ireland

Introduction

Although the treatment of haematological malignancies has improved significantly in the past 30 years, many patients have diseases that remain incurable with conventional therapeutic approaches. Bone marrow cells are exquisitely sensitive to chemotherapy and radiotherapy, and the recognition that radiation could kill bone marrow function permanently while other organs recovered or were largely unaffected suggested that bone marrow transplantation (BMT) might be feasible [1]. Initially the pretransplant chemoradiotherapy *conditioning* of the patient was thought to provide 'space' for the incoming cells to engraft, as well as killing any residual cancer cells. The transplant itself was perceived only as a haemopoietic 'rescue'. Subsequently, it was recognized that the person's own (autologous) bone marrow cells could be used for the same purpose. However, it became apparent that allogeneic transplants (between different individuals) produce an immune mediated graft-versus-leukaemia (GVL) effect, because patients with chronic graft-versus-host disease (GVHD) had improved disease-free survival [2]. Allogeneic BMT is therefore a combination of the chemotherapy and/or radiotherapy with an immune mediated effect against the leukaemia or other malignancy. Later, it was shown that some patients with chronic myeloid leukaemia, who had relapsed after an allogeneic HSCT, could return to full molecular remission after infusions of immune competent lymphocytes from the original donor [3].

This provided more direct proof of a GVL effect. Allogeneic BMT is now seen as more of an immunotherapy, in which the transplant itself is a major component in keeping the disease under control. This is why allogeneic BMT has a much lower recurrence rate, but also a higher incidence of posttransplant infections and immune-associated complications than an autologous transplant. Reduced intensity conditioning (RIC) transplants have been developed to harness the immunological benefits of allogeneic transplants, while avoiding much of the toxicity [4]. The RIC is insufficient to eradicate bone marrow cells but immune tolerance is induced to ensure engraftment of the incoming donor transplant. Although these RIC transplants are sometimes known as 'mini-transplants', they are still arduous procedures requiring great commitment from the patient.

Principles of haemopoietic stem cell transplants (HSCT)

The original bone marrow derived transplants are now more likely to be performed using peripheral blood stem cells (PBSCs) or even cord blood. The term haemopoietic stem cell is now more appropriate. HSCT is used:
• to enable intensification of chemotherapy and radiotherapy so that toxicity to the bone marrow is no longer an important factor in determining outcome and/or

Practical Transfusion Medicine, Fourth Edition. Edited by Michael F. Murphy, Derwood H. Pamphilon and Nancy M. Heddle.
© 2013 John Wiley & Sons, Ltd. Published 2013 by John Wiley & Sons, Ltd.

• to ensure complete engraftment of the donor marrow through immunosuppression of the host (patient), thus permitting tolerance to develop;
• to promote a GVL (or other tumour) effect.

Sources of stem cells

• *Allogeneic stem cells*. These come from another individual, traditionally a matched sibling. There is an increasing use of alternative donors, mainly unrelated adults from donor registries but also cord blood derived cells [5] (see Table 41.1). There is currently increasing interest in using haploidentical family donors. Unrelated transplants use volunteer donors from national and international registries. The toxicity and results of these procedures is improving steadily. HLA compatibility testing using molecular typing and sequencing of patient and recipient genes has resulted in much improved transplant outcomes. The use of umbilical cord blood, from unrelated donor cord blood banks, is increasing worldwide. It is still, in the main, for individuals with low body weight (<50 kg) because of the small number of stem cells in a cord sample. Using two cord donations may lead to more rapid engraftment and much reduced failed engraftment (10%). Additionally, a double cord transplant is associated with a reduced relapse rate and means that cord blood transplants for adults are now a realistic option [6]. The advantage of cord blood is that it is obtained from an immune naive source, so that HLA and other mismatches are tolerated with less GVHD than would be expected if an adult donor were used.
• *Syngeneic cells*. These come from an identical twin and have similar attributes to autologous stem cells.
• *Autologous*. These come from the patient.

The donor

Donors must always be treated with respect and not as a means to an end. In particular, the patient must not be used as a conduit to transmit information to a potential sibling donor. Ideally, a physician separate from the transplant team should take responsibility for donor care. Both the Human Tissues Authority (HTA) and the Joint Accreditation Committee of EBMT and the International Society for Cytotherapy

(ISC)-Europe (JACIE) have recommendations regarding donor care, and where the donor is a child an independent assessor is essential. Doctors involved in advising donors, whether family or unrelated, must be aware of current guidance and legislation in this area [7].

Often, especially if the donor is a sibling, there is only one available. However, if there is a choice of donor a range of factors must be considered before selecting the best donor, including the degree of HLA matching between the donor and recipient, the gender and age of the donor, CMV status and blood group. Young male donors are preferred. Multiparous female donors can increase the risk of GVHD, and usually have a lower body weight [8].

Collecting haemopoietic stem cells

Bone marrow cells may be obtained either directly by aspiration or from the peripheral blood (peripheral blood stem cells, PBSCs). Bone marrow harvesting involves bone marrow aspiration from both posterior iliac crests (under general anaesthesia). A minimum of 2×10^8/kg nucleated cells provides reliable engraftment posttransplant. PBSC mobilization is increasingly used instead of marrow harvesting, although some donors may be unfit for one method or the other or express a preference, which should be respected. In healthy donors this is achieved using the growth factor G-CSF, in patients undergoing autologous procedures, following chemotherapy and growth factor. It is likely that PBSC allografts produce more chronic, but not acute, GVHD than bone marrow transplants in siblings. This may be associated with less relapse in patients at high risk of recurrent disease – advanced-phase CML, for example – and so will still be favoured [9]. Comparative data in unrelated donor transplants also suggest that the use of PBSC is associated with more chronic GVHD but no difference in long-term survival [10].

Indications for haemopoietic stem cell transplants

Stem cell therapy is generally used when conventional dose treatment has failed or is expected to have a high likelihood of failure. The failure of primary therapy

Table 41.1 Comparison of sources of stem cells.

	Sibling	Family haploidentical donor	Unrelated adult volunteer	Umbilical cord blood
Availability	~1:3 have a sibling donor match	Almost every patient will have a donor (sibling/ parent/child)	>20 million donors worldwide; about 70% chance of finding a matched donor for those of Western European origin	~500 000 banked worldwide; 99% chance of finding a 4/6 HLA A,B,DR match
Matching requirements	Increasingly molecular matching with 9/10 allele match acceptable	5/10	Molecular matching with 9/10 allele match acceptable	Most data describes 4/6 matching by serology for Class 1 and molecular for Class 2 (DR)
Speed of availability	3–4 weeks, can be quicker	As per sibling	3–4 months, can be quicker but difficult	Potentially available in days from identifying the preferred cord blood(s)
Engraftment	PBSC ~14 days; BM ~21 days	As for sibling though higher risk of rejection	As for sibling	~20–30 days; platelets may be slower in adult size recipients
Acute GVHD (Grade II–IV)	25–50% (highest with multiparous female donors)	20–40%, though may be severe	30–70%	30–70%
Chronic GVHD	30–40% for BM; 40–70% for PBSC (highest with multiparous female donors)	10–20%	40–50% for BM; 50–70% for PBSC	20–50%
Second donations/ DLI availability	Availability dependent on donor	Yes, but high risk of GVHD	Availability dependent on donor	Unavailable
Risk to the donor	Small	Small	Small	None
Pretransplant testing complete (HLA and virology)	Once donor identified, takes a week or so	As per sibling	Once donor identified and requested, may take several weeks	At time of cryopreservation and unit available for issue

when a disease recurs is a clear endpoint. A perception that failure is likely is more subjective, although some objective evidence may be present. Examples would be chromosome abnormalities known to be associated with poor outcomes, such as the Philadelphia chromosome or 4,11 translocations in acute lymphoblastic leukaemia (ALL), and chromosome 7 deletions in acute myeloid leukaemia (AML). A slow initial response to treatment may suggest that relapse will be likely, as might a high tumour load (bulky disease or a high leucocyte count). Prognostic scoring systems are now available for a number of conditions

Table 41.2 Classification of indications for blood and marrow transplants.

Degree of consensus	Allogeneic HSCT	Autologous HSCT
Very high level of agreement	Poor risk AML CR1 AML other than CR1 Adults <35 years with ALL CR1 ALL other than CR1 CML CP1 if poorly responsive to TKI CML other than CP1 Poor risk myelodysplasia Very severe aplastic anaemia in children and young adults	Multiple myeloma first response Relapsed Hodgkin disease Relapsed aggressive non-Hodgkin lymphoma (NHL)
Some variation in practice between BMT units/nations	Multiple myeloma Chronic lymphocytic leukaemia Low grade NHL ALL patients >35 years CR1 Myelofibrosis	AML CR1 AML other than CR1
Little consensus as to evidence in support of indications. Clinical trials highly appropriate in these indications	Hodgkin's disease	CML other than CP1 Myelodysplasia Chronic lymphocytic leukaemia

All transplant procedures are arduous, even though mortality has fallen over the past years. In addition, the use of allogeneic donors causes major problems with immune reconstitution such that few patients over 60 years would be considered for such transplants. With improved tissue matching, the difference between sibling and unrelated transplants is less apparent. Reduced intensity conditioned transplants have increased these age thresholds. For autografting some groups have extended the limit to 75 years and the authors have experience of up to 69 years. Fitness of the patient and the likelihood of benefit are the most important considerations.
CR, complete remission (CR1, first complete remission); CP, chronic phase of CML.

and can be used to select patients who may benefit from transplantation.

The indications for HSCT have changed over time and will continue to do so [11]. Current indications for HSCT in 2012 are shown in Table 41.2.

Complications of transplantation

Patients who are being considered for any form of HSCT must be given full information about the procedure prior to giving consent. Although results are improving, all HSCT procedures carry major risks of mortality, morbidity and long-term complications. Some of these risks will be lifelong. Careful assessment of potential transplant candidates is mandatory [12].

Regimen-related toxicity

This refers to the immediate toxic effects of the radiotherapy or chemotherapy used for the transplant. Even the reduced intensity conditioning (RIC) protocols are sufficient to cause toxicity. Organs at risk of damage include the gut, with severe mucositis a major problem. Less commonly, liver, heart, lungs and kidneys may suffer transient or even permanent damage. Careful pretransplant assessment of each patient is essential. Damage to these tissues by the conditioning may be more likely to elicit an immune response from the donor cells, adding to the toxicity of the procedure. The use of RIC transplants does reduce this toxicity and enables some patients to receive transplants who might be unfit for full chemotherapy and radiotherapy conditioning. In addition, there are now validated pretransplant comorbidity scoring systems, which can estimate the risk transplant related mortality for individual patients and aid in decision making [13].

Rejection

Rejection is an immune-mediated event in which the pretransplant conditioning and immunosuppression are insufficient to prevent residual recipient immune cells eradicating donor cells. It only occurs in allogeneic transplants, although graft failure due to inadequate numbers of stem cells in the transplant and/or pre-existing damage to the marrow microenvironment can occur in autografts. HLA incompatibility between the patient and donor, and prior sensitization of the patient to HLA or other marrow cell antigens are risk factors for rejection. HLA sensitization should be prevented by using leucocyte-reduced blood components from presentation onwards [14].

GVHD

GVHD is caused by immune-competent T-lymphocytes in the donor recognizing recipient antigens in the patient as foreign, a process that begins with tissue damage caused by the conditioning therapy [15]. This is followed by antigen recognition, clonal T-cell expansion and then cytokine release, which increases and perpetuates the response. Despite prophylactic immunosuppression, more than half of patients receiving allogeneic transplants will develop acute GVHD in the first 100 days posttransplant. Acute GVHD is characterized by involvement of the skin, liver and gut.
• Skin: from an erythematous sunburn-like rash to a blistering, exfoliative erythroderma.
• Liver: typically the bile ducts are attacked and an obstructive jaundice-type picture develops. Milder forms may lead to elevated transaminases and cause considerable difficulties with diagnosis.
• Gastrointestinal tract: classically profuse watery diarrhoea develops, bloody in the most severe cases. Upper gastrointestinal upset is not uncommon, with nausea and sickness.

Relapse

Despite the intensive preparation for transplant a significant proportion of patients will suffer recurrent disease posttransplant. Patients at special risk are those not in remission at the time of transplant or patients with more advanced disease, i.e. has already relapsed once after chemotherapy. An absence of a GVL effect, as in autologous HSCT, or when no GVHD is seen, also increase relapse risk [2].

Infectious complications

The immune system of the transplant recipient must be suppressed to allow the graft to be accepted and antitumour therapy such as total body irradiation (TBI) ensures that the patient has minimal immune function at the time of the transplant. Even the RIC transplants have this risk, because they utilize intensive immunosuppression in order to ensure that the transplant is not rejected. The agents used (fludarabine and anti-T cell or panlymphoid monoclonal antibodies) induce prolonged and profound immune deficiency. Haemopoietic recovery takes at least 2–3 weeks, but recovery of neutrophils is only part of the reconstitution of the immune system that must occur for full recovery. BMT-related immune problems may be divided conveniently into three phases as follows. Immune deficiency is compounded at any point after BMT by the presence of active GVHD.

Immediate post-BMT phase
This phase is characterized by neutropenia as well as lymphopenia and hypogammaglobulinaemia. During this period the patient is managed with:
• protective isolation; filtered air to reduce fungal contamination is especially important;
• prophylactic antifungal, antiviral and antibacterial therapy is routine;
• pre-emptive use of therapeutic antimicrobials; broad-spectrum antibacterial agents at the first sign of fever, followed by antifungal treatment in the absence of prompt resolution;
• intravenous immunoglobulin may be used in some patient groups; and
• prophylactic neutrophil infusions are not used routinely; trials are needed urgently but are very difficult to design and deliver.

Early postengraftment period
The patient will now have some marrow function and, if GVHD is absent or controlled, may be able to leave

hospital. Although patients having autologous transplants rarely have major problems after this time, vigilance is necessary. Allogeneic HSCT recipients remain at risk of:

- bacterial infections related to central lines;
- fungal infection;
- cytomegalovirus (CMV). Most units will monitor for emerging CMV using a polymerase chain reaction (PCR)-based test, and treat positive results before there is evidence of disease. Such pre-emptive strategies are very effective and CMV is becoming a much less important cause of mortality after allogeneic SCT [16]. Such monitoring is also applied to other viruses such as adenovirus and EBV, which are becoming more important considerations as current SCT techniques produce more profound pre- and posttransplant immunosuppression;
- other viruses, especially respiratory virus and other herpes viruses such as herpes zoster (HZV);
- toxoplasmosis and pneumocystis.

Later problems

Patients who have active GVHD requiring immunosuppressive therapy will continue to have impaired immunity to pathogens, and most patients who have received unrelated donor transplants will have detectable abnormalities of the immune system. However, by three years posttransplant almost all patients not taking immunosuppressive drugs will have virtually normal immunity.

- (Re-)vaccination has a role to play but those patients still on immunosuppression will not respond optimally.
- Continued prophylaxis and vigilance are required.
- Hyposplenic cover. Patients who have had allogeneic transplants are hyposplenic and must receive vaccine against organisms such as *Pneumococcus*, *Meningococcus* and *Haemophilus influenzae B* (HIB), as well as receiving lifelong chemoprophylaxis, e.g. with amoxicillin.

Late effects

It might be thought that having endured a life-threatening primary disease followed by the immediate risks of HSCT outlined above, that survivors might be entitled to a respite from further problems. Unfortunately, a litany of potential problems can and do occur, including the following:

- cataracts (total body irradiation only);
- endocrine problems such as:
  - hypothyroidism;
  - growth retardation in children (especially TBI +/− steroids);
  - infertility;
- sexual dysfunction;
- second malignancies, which remains a risk even 20 years after the transplant;
- transfusion-transmitted viruses, e.g. hepatitis C;
- iron overload and liver dysfunction from red cell transfusions.

These problems mean that HSCT recipients require lifelong follow-up at a centre familiar with the range of late complications and with a sufficiently large practice to ensure that emerging problems are identified promptly. There are published recommendations for the follow-up of these patients [17].

BMT outcome

A discussion of the results of BMT for the wide range of indications now accepted is beyond the scope of this chapter. Current results from the International Bone Marrow Transplant Registry (IBMTR) are available on their web site and should be referred to so that only the most up to date information is used. Historically matched sibling donor transplantation is favoured over matched unrelated donor transplantation, which is favoured over transplantation with significant mismatches (cord and haploidentical transplants). However, there is no doubt that the differences in outcome are becoming less marked.

CML

Historically, CML has been one of the major and most widely accepted indications for allogeneic HSCT and excellent results were achieved, especially in young patients transplanted early after diagnosis. Since the advent of tyrosine kinase inhibitors (TKI), such as Imatinib, disease control is excellent in the majority of patients and so HSCT is no longer considered to be standard first-line treatment if a good response to TKI is achieved. Patients with more advanced stage CML or those who fail to respond or lose a response to TKI are considered for allogeneic SCT.

Acute leukaemia

For acute leukaemia, the precise details of each case are needed before a recommendation can be made. These include chromosome analysis and phenotype. For example, very few patients with Philadelphia chromosome-positive ALL will be cured without an allogeneic transplant.

Results for all patient groups at 3 years for leukaemia-free survival (LFS) in acute leukaemia in adults are on the order of:

• 50–60% in first complete remission (CR1): relapse risk 25%;
• 35–40% for second or subsequent complete remission: relapse risk 46%;
• 20–25% for patients transplanted not in remission: relapse risk 68%.

Registry data are of great importance but cannot replace the careful assessment of individual patients in the light of their specific prognostic factors. These may serve to improve or worsen the risks for a particular case, e.g. coexistent disease, toxic effects of prior chemotherapy, previous invasive fungal infection. Also, registries report only mature data, usually with a minimum of 3 years follow-up. The value of more recent developments requires the scrutiny of primary research publications and reports to specialist meetings.

Post-BMT chimerism and molecular monitoring

It has been possible to monitor leukaemic clones using sensitive molecular techniques for nearly 20 years now. More recently, molecular techniques have been applied to routine monitoring of donor and recipient chimerism posttransplant. RIC transplants often exhibit a period of mixed chimerism early posttransplant, when the presence of both residual host and donor haemopoiesis is detectable. Capillary

electrophoresis detection systems allow accurate quantitation of the relative contributions of host and donor to haemopoiesis, by detecting short tandem repeats (STR). Mixed chimerism is believed to be associated with a higher risk of graft rejection or relapse and optimal graft versus leukaemia responses are dependent upon full donor chimerism [18]. Donor lymphocyte infusions (DLI) of graded numbers of T-lymphocytes can be used to switch patients from mixed to full donor chimerism.

By using DLI early in relapse of CML after allogeneic HSCT and giving a specific dose of cells, it is possible to separate GVL from a GVHD response, although the particular subset of T cells that will generate GVL without the risk of GVHD has not been identified. DLI has been tried in numerous diseases with varying success.

Cytotoxic T-cell therapy

It has been known for some time that DLI targeted against Epstein–Barr virus (EBV) can be used to treat lymphoproliferative disorder (LPD) in children who have received an unrelated donor HSCT. In these cases intensive immunosuppression is given to ensure that the graft was not rejected and this led to increased reactivation of EBV, which triggered the LPD. By isolating T cells and exposing them to EBV *in vitro* it is possible to generate clonal cytotoxic T cells that recognize EBV antigens and kill the LPD cells. In the main this treatment has been highly effective in both the prophylactic and therapeutic management of EBV LPD [19].

Although it is possible to generate sufficient antitumour effect to induce remissions in LPD, the one disease that has been treated effectively with immunotherapy is a virus-associated malignancy. In the past few years more progress has been made in developing strategies for using cytotoxic T cells against viruses in the HSCT setting, particularly CMV, than for antitumour indications. Viruses possess foreign antigens not possessed by the human patient and the relative lack of progress in antitumour immunotherapy, beyond basic DLI approaches, suggests that identifying and exploiting tumour antigens remains elusive (see also Chapter 43).

461

Regulatory aspects of haemopoietic stem cell transplantation

An awareness of current regulations regarding HSCT is essential for medical, nursing and scientific staff responsible for the various parts of the service.

In the European Union (EU), competent authorities regulate tissue banks, which includes processing and storage of HSC. In the UK, for example, the Human Tissue Authority (HTA) is the competent authority to ensure that the EU Directive on Tissues and Cells is implemented, and has legal powers. A professional organization, JACIE, inspects and sets standards for the clinical and laboratory HSCT process. Although not having legal force, JACIE compliance is seen as essential to an active HSCT programme.

Conclusion

At present there are still no clearly developed indications or proven strategies for cellular immunotherapy other than for generating GVL against CML using DLI and for the prevention and treatment of EBV LPD. The exploitation of increasing knowledge of the immune system has not been easy. The most likely application appears to be in a more refined approach to the use of DLI posttransplant and the application of RIC transplants to more nonmalignant diseases where immune modulation may have a role.

Meanwhile, what is the long-term future for HSCT generally? These transplants can save life in many patients with incurable leukaemia and lymphomas. Patients who survive the first three years are likely to enjoy long-term survival, although life expectancy does not return to normal. RIC transplants extend the benefits to more patients who might have been unfit to undergo the rigours of a myeloablative procedure. Whether the use of RIC transplants in a wider range of malignant diseases is effective will become apparent in the next few years. Autologous transplants seem set to decline further in importance as improved chemotherapy, immunotherapy (Rituximab) and improved allogeneic HSCT reduces the number of patients for which they are applicable. Additional approaches are still needed to deal with those patients whose primary disease is poorly responsive to current chemoradiotherapy.

Key points

1 The increasing use of cord blood transplants generally, and particularly for adult/larger patients >50 kg.
2 The declining role for autologous transplants due to improvements in conventional treatment (for myeloma and lymphoma) or a greater emphasis on allogeneic stem cell transplantation (for adult acute leukaemia).
3 The importance of treating donors of stem cells as individuals and not as a means to an end.
4 The stem cell transplantation field is becoming increasingly regulated in Europe by both professional and statutory bodies.
5 That although reduced intensity/nonmyeloablative transplants have less immediate toxicity than conventional radiation therapy based transplants, they remain arduous procedures with many short- and medium-term complications.
6 That randomized controlled clinical trials remain the best way to produce definitive data as to the relative merits of treatments in blood and lymphoid malignancies.

References

1 Thomas ED, Lochte Jr HL, Lu WC & Ferrebee JW. Intravenous infusion of bone marrow in patients receiving radiation and chemotherapy. *N Engl J Med* 1957; 257: 491–496.
2 Weiden PL, Sullivan KM, Flournoy M, Storb R & Thomas ED. Antileukemic effect of chronic graft versus-host disease: contribution to improved survival after allogeneic bone marrow transplantation. *N Engl J Med* 1981; 304: 1592–1633.
3 Kolb HJ, Mittermuller J, Clemm C *et al.* Donor leucocyte transfusions for treatment of recurrent chronic myelogenous leukaemia in marrow transplant patients. *Blood* 1990; 76: 2462–2465.
4 Giralt S, Estey E, Albitar M *et al.* Engraftment of allogeneic hematopoietic progenitor cells with purine analog-containing chemotherapy: harnessing graft versus leukemia without myeloablative therapy. *Blood* 1997; 89: 4531–4536.
5 Gratwohl A, Baldomero H, Frauendorfer K *et al.* Results of the EBMT activity survey 2005 on haematopoietic stem cell transplantation: focus on increasing use of unrelated donors. *Bone Marrow Transplantation* 2007; 39: 71–87.

6 Brunstein CG, Gutman JA, Weisdorf DJ *et al.* Allogeneic hematopoietic cell transplantation for hematologic malignancy: relative risks and benefits of double umbilical cord blood. *Blood* 2010; 116: 4693–4699.

7 Sacchi N, Costeas P, Hartwell L *et al.* Haematopoietic stem cell donor registries: World Bone Marrow Donor Association recommendations for evaluation of donor health. *Bone Marrow Transplantation* 2008; 42: 1–6.

8 Gharton G. Risk assessment in haematopoietic stem cell transplantation: impact of donor-recipient sex combination in allogeneic transplantation. *Best Pract Res Clin Haematol* 2007; 20: 219–229.

9 Schmitz N, Eapen M, Horowitz MM *et al.* Long-term outcome of patients given transplants of mobilized blood or bone marrow: a report from the International Bone Marrow Transplant Registry and the European Group for Blood and Marrow Transplantation *Blood* 2006; 108: 4288–4290.

10 Eapen M, Logan BR, Confer DL *et al.* Peripheral blood grafts from unrelated donors are associated with increased acute and chronic graft versus-host disease without improved survival. *Biol Blood Marrow Transplantation* 2007; 13: 1461–1468.

11 Ljungman P, Bregni M, Brune M *et al.* Allogeneic and autologous transplantation for haematological disease, solid tumours and immune disorders: current practice in Europe 2009. *Bone Marrow Transplantation* 2010; 45: 219–234.

12 Deeg HJ & Sandmaier B. Who is fit for allogeneic transplantation? *Blood* 2010; 116: 4762–4770.

13 Sorror ML, Maris MB, Storb R *et al.* Hematopoietic cell transplantation (HCT) – specific comorbidity index: a new tool for risk assessment before allogeneic HCT. *Blood* 2005; 106: 2912–2919.

14 Mattson J, Ringden O & Storb R. Graft failure after allogeneic haematopoietic cell transplantation. *Biol Blood Marrow Transplantation* 2008; 14: 165–170.

15 Goker H, Haznedaroglu IC, Chao NJ. Acute graft-vs-host disease: Pathobiology and management. *Exp Hematol* 2001; 29: 259–77.

16 Ljungman P, Reusser P, de la Camara R *et al.* Management of CMV infections: recommendations from the infectious diseases working party of the EBMT. *Bone Marrow Transplantation* 2004; 33: 1075–1081.

17 Majhail NJ, Rizzo DJ, Lee SJ *et al.* Recommended screening and preventative practices for long-term survivors after haematopoietic cell transplantation. *Biol Blood Marrow Transplantation* 2012; 18: 348–371.

18 Liesveld JL & Rothberg PG. Mixed chimerism in SCT: conflict or peaceful coexistence? *Bone Marrow Transplantation* 2008; 42: 297–310.

19 Comoli P, Basso S, Zecca M *et al.* Preemptive therapy of EBV-related lymphoproliferative disease after pediatric haploidentical stem cell transplantation. *Am J Transplantation* 2007; 7: 1648–1655.

Further reading

Ballen KK *et al.* Selection of optimal alternative graft source: mismatched unrelated, umbilical cord blood, or haploidentical transplant. *Blood* 2012; 119: 1972–1980.

Barker JN, Byam C & Scaradavou A. How I treat the selection and acquisition of unrelated cord blood grafts. *Blood* 2011, 117; 2332–2339.

British Society of Blood and Marrow Transplantation (BSBMT) site: http://bsbmt.org/.

Centre for International Blood and Marrow Transplant Research (CIBMTR) site: http://www.cibmtr.org.

European Group for Blood and Marrow Transplantation (EBMT) site. http://www.ebmt.org/.

Slavin S. Immunotherapy of cancer with alloreactive lymphocytes. *Lancet Oncology* 2001; 2: 491–498.

Socie G *et al.* Long-term survival and late deaths after allogeneic bone marrow transplantation. *N Engl J Med* 1999; 341: 14–21.

Storek J *et al.* Immunity of patients surviving 20 to 30 years after allogeneic or syngeneic bone marrow transplantation. *Blood* 2001; 98: 3505–3512.

Thomas, ED. Does BMT confer a normal life span? *N Engl J Med* 1999; 341: 50–51.

42 Cord blood transplantation

Rachael Hough

University College London Hospital's NHS Foundation Trust, London, UK

Introduction

Over the last five decades, transplantation of haemopoietic stem cells (HSCs) from related or unrelated donors has provided curative therapy for thousands of patients with a wide range of malignant, metabolic and immunological disorders [1]. HSCs have conventionally been harvested from the donor's bone marrow or granulocyte colony-stimulating factor (GCSF) mobilized peripheral blood, with minimal risks to the donor.

The impetus to explore alternative HSC sources arose because a suitably HLA-matched donor could not be identified for a substantial proportion of patients and the time to acquisition of donor cells was too long for those requiring an urgent transplant.

The optimal HSC donor for any patient is an HLA-identical sibling. However, the chance of any brother or sister being 'matched' is 1 in 4 and, as a result, a sibling allograft is an option for only around 30% of patients. Over recent years, there has been a considerable effort and success in expanding international volunteer donor registry panels, with over 14 million donors currently registered. However, the likelihood of identifying a 'suitably matched' unrelated donor is dependent on the ethnicity of the recipient; whilst Caucasians may have at least a 50% chance of finding a donor, the likelihood falls to around 10% for certain ethnic or mixed race groups who are poorly represented on the registry panels.

In addition, the time taken from commencing an unrelated donor search to the delivery of HSCs to the patient is an average of 4 months [2]. For patients who are clinically unstable and require an urgent transplant, this can be too long and patients may succumb to their disease or toxicity of further chemotherapy in the interim.

Over the last decade, the use of more stringent molecular HLA typing methods has optimized donor selection and improved transplant survival outcomes [3]. However, it has also further prolonged the search process and reduced the likelihood of finding any HLA-matched volunteer donor.

The first umbilical cord blood transplant (UCBT) was performed in 1988 in a boy with Fanconi anaemia, using cells collected from his sibling's umbilical cord blood [4]. This successful transplant was proof of the principle that umbilical cord blood (UCB) could be harvested, cryopreserved and thawed and still contain sufficient viable stem cells to successfully repopulate the recipient's bone marrow and immune system. Further successful related donor UCBTs followed quickly and led to the establishment of public UCB banks, the first of which was the New York Cord Blood Bank in 1993. These banks have rapidly expanded internationally since, with a current

Practical Transfusion Medicine, Fourth Edition. Edited by Michael F. Murphy, Derwood H. Pamphilon and Nancy M. Heddle.
© 2013 John Wiley & Sons, Ltd. Published 2013 by John Wiley & Sons, Ltd.

worldwide repository in excess of 600 000 units, which have facilitated over 20 000 UCBT so far.

Umbilical cord blood banking

Cryopreserved UCB may be safely stored for many years without significant deleterious effect on the viability of stem cells, in either public or private cord banks.

The large public banks store UCB that has been altruistically donated for transplantation into unrelated recipients. Some countries also have national, publicly funded banks for directed donations, usually collected for siblings with known life-threatening disease. More recently, siblings have been specifically conceived using preimplantation genetic diagnosis to select HLA-matched and disease-unaffected embryos for implantation, from whom UCB can be harvested after delivery and used for transplantation of an existing sick child [5]. The practice of storing UCB, collected by either altruistic or directed donations, is now well established and has already saved many thousands of lives.

An increasing number of private UCB banks are becoming available and offer cryopreservation of UCB for the specific use of the donating family as an 'insurance policy' and source of stem cells for either:
- the conventional indications for an HSC transplant;
- the future use in the treatment of other diseases (regenerative medicine).

At the present time, the utility of private cord banking is unclear. The chances of using a privately stored unit for transplantation have been estimated to be between 1 in 1400 and 1 in 20 000 [6]. The issue is further complicated by the possibility of contamination of autologous cord blood by disease, which subsequently presents in childhood, such as acute leukaemia. There is considerable current scientific exploration into the potential of cord blood as a source of nonhaemopoietic cells that could be utilized in the treatment of many different diseases, in particular degenerative diseases. Should this potential be realized, the utility of storing autologous cord blood for subsequent use may become clearer.

Quality assurance for the collection (including maternal consent), processing and storage of UCB is

Table 42.1 Donor recruitment, selection and consent.

Donor recruitment
- Need consent to collect before delivery (EU Directive)
- Prenatal information to mothers
  - leaflets, posters, videos
- Antenatal/parents classes
- Brief medical history for obvious exclusions

Maternal interview 24–48 h postdelivery
- Informed written consent for use for CBT± R+D
- Medical, lifestyle, ethnic and travel history
- Maternal samples

Follow-up donor interview
- Telephone at 12 weeks
  - Postnatal health of mother and baby
  - Medical, genetic and family history
- Haemoglobinopathy screening results
- UK Congenital Malformation Register checked when unit is issued

Consent
- Collection and storage of CB for transplantation into unrelated individuals worldwide
- Possible risks and benefits to mother and/or infant, including medical and ethical concerns
- Maintenance of linkage for the purpose of notifying infant family of communicable or genetic diseases
- Examination of the mother's and infant's relevant medical notes and dialogue with relevant clinical professionals
- Permission for microbiological testing, including for HIV, and for the donor to be counselled in the event of results relevant to their health
- Storage of samples for future testing
- Storage of personal information
- Right of the mother to refuse without prejudice
- Research and development use if the donation is unsuitable for clinical use

NB. UK NHSBT Cord Bank Procedure.

now provided by inspection against international standards (Netcord-FACT standards).

Table 42.1 lists the key elements involved in the recruitment of expectant women who may wish to altruistically donate their baby's UCB to public banks. As the potential role of UCB becomes more widely appreciated, an increasing number of women actively seek the opportunity to donate. For others, literature or verbal information may be provided at booking

Table 42.2 Testing.

At processing/cryopreservation
Maternal
- HIV (Ab + PCR), HCV (Ab + PCR), HBV, (HBsAg + anti HBcore), HTLV 1 + 2 Ab, TPHA, CMV IgG, ±Malaria Ab

Cord sample
- HIV Ab, HCV Ab, HBsAg, TPHA, HTLV Ab
- ABO/Rh
- Bacteriology
- HLA-A, -B, -DR (DNA typing)
- FBC pre- and postprocess
- CD34/viability
- nRCC (manual)

Medical review and quality checked
At issue
Maternal
- HLA type
- HBV PCR

Cord sample
- Confirmatory HLA typing (high resolution)
- Additional microbiology
  - Anti-HBc
  - HIV, HBV & HCV PCR
  - CMV IgG + CMV PCR
  - Others as necessary
- Blood film examination
- Bleedline
  - STR analysis
  - CFU assay
  - CD34 count + viability

Congenital malformation registry
Medical review and results checked

clinics or antenatal classes. A history is taken from mothers-to-be who are interested in donation, focusing on ethnicity and the risks of transmissible infection or genetic disease. The consent process ensures that the future mother is aware that her child's UCB may be used at any time for transplantation in an unknown recipient, the need for testing for transmissible infectious or genetic diseases and the potential for discard or use in research if the unit collected does not meet key criteria for clinical grade banking (Table 42.1).

Table 42.2 lists the mandatory tests of both mother and UCB, performed at the time of banking and subsequently prior to issue. There is an increasing tendency for collection centres to appoint and train a

team of UCB harvesters who collect the placenta from the delivery room following placental delivery. This obviates the need for midwives to be involved in UCB collection, which might otherwise distract them from nursing the new mother and baby.

The exact timing of collection is currently controversial. Some centres harvest UCB whilst the placenta is still *in utero*. Although this approach optimizes the volume and stem cell yield from the collection, it potentially distracts from the birthing process and may present a risk to both mother and newborn. In fact, some midwives and obstetricians advocate delaying the clamping of the umbilical cord even after placental delivery. This recommendation is based on the observation that delayed cord clamping leads to a higher ferritin in the newborn child, which may impact favourably on their subsequent development [7]. Unfortunately, delaying cord clamping will have a significant impact on the volume and number of stem cells present in each UCB unit, which may considerably limit the usefulness of many collected. This controversial issue is currently being debated by neonatologists and obstetricians internationally.

Clinical outcomes of UCBT

Malignant disease

The efficacy of allogeneic HSC transplantation in haematological malignant diseases is achieved by the cytoreductive impact of the conditioning chemotherapy and/or radiotherapy and a later immune-mediated clearance of any residual malignant cells, called the graft-versus-malignancy (GVM) or graft-versus-leukaemia (GVL) effect.

Early experience of UCBT in malignant disease used single unit transplants from related and, subsequently, unrelated donors in children. Table 42.3 summarizes these outcome data compared to other stem cell sources. The key observations, established over time, are that UCBTs are associated with equivalent survival and relapse rates (demonstrating a preserved GVM effect) compared to bone marrow or peripheral blood stem cell transplants. Interestingly, the incidence and severity of acute and chronic graft-versus-host disease (GVHD) is less than observed with conventional HSC sources, which allows for a more permissive 'matching system' between the recipient and donor. In general, unrelated donors are only used if they are matched at

Table 42.3 Summary of studies comparing CBT with HSC sources in paediatric patients.

Author	HSC source	n	Median age (range)	Cell dose (range) ($\times 10^7$/kg)	Time to ANC >500 $\times$ 10^3/mL (days)	aGVHD II–IV (%)	Severe cGVHD (%)	Relapse (%)	Survival (%)	TRM (%)
Rocha et al. [8]	CB related	113	5 (<1–15)	4.7 (<10–36)	26	14	6		14	64*
	BM related	2052	8 (<1–15)	35 (<10–410)	18	26	16		12	66*
Rocha et al. [9]	CB unrelated	99	6 (2.5–10)	3.8 (2.4–36)	32	26	25	38		35†
	BM unrelated T-cell depleted	262	8 (5–12)	42 (14–56)	18	39	46	39		49†
	BM unrelated	180	36 (6–12)	38 (11–53)	16	30	12	47		41†

*3 years' survival.

†2 years' survival.

HSC, haemopoietic stem cell; aGVHD, acute graft-versus-host disease; cGVHD, chronic graft-versus-host disease; TRM, transplant-related mortality; BM, bone marrow; ANC, absolute neutrophil count.

9 or 10 out of 10 HLA alleles, whilst unrelated donor UCB units can be used if matched at 4 or more out of 6 alleles (with less stringent matching at class I antigens).

The key limitation of using UCB as an alternative stem cell source is that the time to and probability of 'engraftment' or recovery of the neutrophil and platelet counts are both inferior when compared to bone marrow or peripheral blood stem cell transplants. The time to neutrophil recovery is around one week longer than using bone marrow, leading to a prolonged risk of early transplant mortality, predominantly due to infection.

One of the key determinants of engraftment, transplant-related mortality and survival is the cell dose (as measure by the total nucleated cell count or CD34+ cell count) infused into the recipient [10]. Outcome improves with increasing cell dose, with an apparent pre-thaw threshold of around 2–3 $\times$ 10^7 TNC/kg or 2 $\times$ 10^5 CD34+/kg, below which toxicity is prohibitively high. Engraftment, transplant-related mortality and survival also improve with closer HLA matching, although the deleterious impact of each mismatch can be overcome to some extent by a higher cell dose [11].

Initial outcome data in adults showed a high risk of graft failure and transplant-related mortality, with UCBT tending to be restricted to patients with advanced stage disease who were heavily pretreated. However, with modified conditioning regimens (including reduced intensity regimens) and an increasing awareness of the key factors in optimizing

graft selection, adult UCBT outcomes have improved considerably (Table 42.4) and are now also considered to be standard of care, when a conventional donor is unavailable.

Metabolic disorders

The metabolic disorders are a range of diseases that result from enzyme deficiencies or transport protein defects, which lead to accumulation of toxic substrates in critical organs, leading to progressive, and often, fatal organ failure. Allogeneic HSCT has been shown to arrest disease progression in selected disorders. The mechanism of benefit is unclear, but may be due to production of continuous and sufficient enzyme by graft-derived cells and a concomitant reduction of central nervous system inflammation.

The largest experience of HSCT in a metabolic disorder is in Hurler's syndrome, an autosomal recessive deficiency of α-L-iduronidase. The key factors considered in HSC choice in this disorder are:
• the need for rapid transplant before neurological damage occurs;
• the lack of necessity for GVM (thus GVHD is less tolerable than in the context of malignancy).

UCB has the advantage of being rapidly available for transplant and, in a small series of 20 patients published to date, has a high rate of survival (85% EFS) with an incidence of grade II–IV acute GVHD of 28% – outcomes at least equivalent to that previously reported for other stem cell sources [15]. Whilst

Table 42.4 Summary of studies comparing CBT with other unrelated HSC sources in adult patients.

Author	Study period	HSC source	n	Median age (range) (×10⁷/kg)	Cell dose (range)	aGVHD II–IV (%)	Severe cGVHD (%)	Relapse (%)	TRM (%)	LFS (%)	Time to ANC >500 × 10³/mL (days)
Takahashi et al. [12]	1998–2001	CB	68	36 (16–53)	2.5 (1.1–5.3)	22	30	13	16	9	74
		BM matched	45	26 (16–50)	33 (6.6–50)	18	30	14	25	29	44
Rocha et al. [13]	1998–2002	CB	98	25 (15–55)	2.3 (0.9–6.0)	26	26	30	23	44	33
		BM matched	584	32 (15–59)	29 (<10–90)	19	39	46	23	38	38
Laughlin et al. [14]	1996–2001	CB	150	(16–60)	2.2 (1.0–6.5)	27	41	33	17	63	23
		BM matched	367	(16–60)	24 (0.2–170)	18	48	52	23	46	33
		BM mismatched	83	(16–60)	22 (0.1–58)	20	52	71	14	65	19

HSC, haemopoietic stem cell; aGVHD, acute graft-versus-host disease; cGVHD, chronic graft-versus-host disease; TRM, transplant-related mortality; BM, bone marrow; LFS, leukaemia-free survival.

Table 42.5 Advantages and disadvantages of different stem cell sources (from Warwick & Brubaker [17]).

	Autologous HSCT	HLA identical related donor HSCT	Unrelated donor HSCT	Unrelated donor UCBT	Haploidentical related donor HSCT
Available donor pool	–	–	>14 million	>600 000	–
Estimation of likelihood of suitable donor	>90%	Approx 30%	10/10 = 40% 9/10 = 70% Ethnic minority = 20%	≥5/6 = 40% ≥4/6 = 70%	>90%
Speed of access	Immediate	Immediate	3–4 months	3–4 weeks	Immediate
Cost of graft	Low	Low	High	High	Low
Ability to rearrange infusion date	Easy	Easy	May be difficult	Easy	Easy
Ability to reaccess	Impossible	Yes	Possible	No	Yes
Quality of product	Assured	Assured	Assured	Variable	Assured
Speed of engraftment	Fast	Moderate	Moderate	Slow	Fast
Risk of graft failure	Low	Low	Moderate	High	Moderate
Risk of transplant related mortality	Very low	Low	High	High	High
Risk of GVHD	None	Moderate	High	Moderate	Low
Speed of immune reconstitution	Rapid	Moderate	Moderate	Moderate	Very slow
Risk of viral transmission	None	Yes	Yes	None	Yes
Risk of transmission of congenital disease	Yes	Yes	No	Yes	No

further data are clearly required, UCB appears to be an attractive stem cell choice for some metabolic disorders.

Primary immunodeficiencies

The primary immunodeficiency syndromes are a rare group of inherited disorders in which there is a single or combined deficiency in key elements of the innate and/or adaptive immune systems. Early death due to infection may be prevented by enzyme therapy in some children and gene therapy offers the promise of disease amelioration for others in the future. However, for many, replacement of the immune system by allogeneic HSCT provides the only curative therapeutic strategy at present.

The outcome of allogeneic HSCT has improved considerably over recent years with improvements in supportive care, better prevention of GVHD and the use of reduced intensity conditioning regimens. The critical determinant of a successful transplant is for the procedure to be performed prior to the onset of significant infections or comorbidities, which may lead to death within the first year of life in some disorders such as severe combined immune deficiency syndrome (SCID). Whilst the donor of choice for such children is a sibling with overall survival rates of 70–100%, the likelihood of having an HLA-matched sibling who is unaffected by the same inherited disease is only around 10% [1].

UCB is an attractive stem cell source for children with primary immunodeficiencies, given the rapid availability and low risk of GVHD. Four small series have been published to date showing survival rates of 71–88% [1]. However, the slower engraftment rates compared to conventional transplants may increase the risk of peritransplant infections. Currently an UCBT is considered to be an acceptable alternative

469

when no sibling or unrelated donor is available [16].

Advantages and disadvantages of UCB

The wealth of experience of UCBT to date has demonstrated a number of advantages and disadvantages compared to other stem cell sources, which are summarized in Table 42.5. The reduced stringency required in 'HLA matching' between recipient and donor, due to a lower incidence of GVHD following UCBT, allows patients access to a life-saving allogeneic HSCT, when previously they would not have had a 'suitable' donor. This access is increased further by targeting collection centres in areas where the population has a broader ethic mix, which allows specific harvesting of units from a racially diverse HLA background, currently underrepresented on international volunteer donor panels. UCB can be collected with no risk to either the donor or mother. Once stored, UCB units are available immediately, thus allowing rapid access when a transplant is urgently indicated and also easy rearrangement of the transplant date when necessary. Adult volunteer donors may also become unwell or be unavailable for donation when required; there is no such 'donor attrition' with UCB. There is also a very low risk of transmission of infectious agents with transplantation of HSCs collected from a newborn baby.

The principal limitation of UCB is that it is a 'one-off' collection of a finite number of HSCs. Futher stem cells cannot be harvested in the event of graft failure and donor lymphocytes cannot be given as immunotherapy in the management of relapse, serious infection or mixed chimerism. The stem cell dose is a crucial determinant of outcome and a single UCB will generally have insufficient HSCs to transplant a larger adolescent or adult patient safely. The other potential disadvantage of UCB is that the stem cells may harbour transmissible genetic disease, not yet apparent in the baby from whom it came.

Future developments

The focus of recent and ongoing research efforts has been on improving engraftment and shortening the duration of cytopenia posttransplant, with the aim

Table 42.6 Stategies to overcome the limitations of lower cell dose.

Mechanism	Approach
Increase cell dose infused	Double unit transplant
	Coinfusion of CD34 selected haploidentical cells
	Ex vivo expansion
Improved homing	Direct intro-osseous infusion
Allow host haemopoiesis to abrogate duration of neutropenia	Reduced intensity conditioning

of reducing early mortality and improving survival (Table 42.6).

The most successful so far has been the coinfusion of two unrelated UCB units in larger children, adolescents and adults. Initial concerns that this could lead to graft failure due to an immunological reaction between the two units or to prohibitive GVHD have not been substantiated. This work, pioneered by researchers in Minneapolis, have shown that the duration of neutropenia is acceptable and the likelihood of engraftment increased, even in large adult patients [18]. Although there is an increase in GVHD compared to a single unit transplant, the impact of this on survival appears to be offset by a reduced incidence of relapse. This strategy has led to safe and efficacious UCBT in adults, with a consequent rapid increase in the number of these transplants performed internationally. Interestingly, although both infused units contribute to initial haemopoiesis, ultimately one unit will predominate and will usually eradicate the 'losing' unit by around 3 months posttransplant.

Another significant development has been the use of reduced intensity conditioning regimens. It has been shown that UCB will engraft even in this setting and importantly the duration of neutropenia is considerably reduced to around 12 days, due to a temporary contribution of haemopoiesis from nonablated recipient stem cells [19]. Again, the engrafting unit will subsequently eradicate host cells that have effectively 'bridged' the neutropenic phase. This approach has made it possible for older patients or those with significant comorbidities to safely proceed to transplant.

Other approaches, including the coinfusion of CD34-selected haploidentical stem cells [20], ex vivo expansion [21] and direct intraosseous injection of UCB [22], are also showing promising results in ongoing international clinical trials.

Conclusions

Allogeneic HSCT provides a life-saving treatment option for patients with many malignant and genetic diseases. Over the last 30 years, UCB has emerged as a safe and effective alternative stem cell source for patients lacking an HLA-matched sibling or unrelated donor, available within the required time-frame. Previously considered a waste product, UCB is abundantly and rapidly available, without risk to the donor or mother. UCB also has a lower incidence of GVHD and transmissible infection. The limitations of finite cell dose and slower engraftment are being overcome by novel approaches, thus expanding access to transplantation to older, larger recipients and those with comorbidities.

Key points

1 Over the last 30 years, UCB, previously a biological waste product of pregnancy, has been shown to be an effective and safe alternative source of HSCs for transplantation in patients with life-threatening diseases who otherwise would not have a suitable related or unrelated donor.

2 The lower stringency required for recipient and donor matching and the targeted collection of ethnic minority and mixed race UCB units has extended access to transplantation considerably, particularly for those of racial backgrounds poorly represented on volunteer donor panels.

3 UCB collection presents no risk to the mother or baby and provides a rapidly available HSC source when urgently required, with no risk of donor attrition.

4 The incidence and severity of acute and chronic GVHD is lower, following an UCBT compared to BMT, despite greater HLA disparity. Transplant-related mortality, relapse rate and overall survival are at least comparable with BM.

5 A limited cell dose, resulting in a slower and reduced probability of engraftment, remains the biggest obstacle to the wider use of UCBT.

6 Double unit UCBT has been shown to be safe and efficacious in larger adolescents and adults, in whom a single unit transplant would result in an unacceptably high risk of graft failure and early mortality.

7 Other strategies, such as *ex vivo* expansion, intraosseous injection and coinfusion of haploidentical CD34-selected stem cells all show promise and may yet expand the utility of UCBT further.

References

1 Hough R, Cooper N & Veys P. Allogeneic haemopoietic stem cell transplantation in children: what alternative donor should we choose when no matched sibling is available? *Br J Haematol* 2009, December; 147(5): 593–613. Epub 25 August 2009.

2 Barker JN, Krepski TP, DeFor TE, Davies SM, Wagner JE & Weisdorf DJ. Searching for unrelated donor hematopoietic stem cells: availability and speed of umbilical cord blood versus bone marrow. Biology of blood and marrow transplantation. *J Am Soc for Blood and Marrow Transplantation* 2002; 8(5): 257–260. PubMed PMID: 12064362.

3 Eapen M, Klein JP, Sanz GF, Spellman S, Ruggeri A, Anasetti C *et al.* Effect of donor-recipient HLA matching at HLA A, B, C, and DRB1 on outcomes after umbilical-cord blood transplantation for leukaemia and myelodysplastic syndrome: a retrospective analysis. *Lancet Oncol* 2011, December; 12(13): 1214–1221. PubMed PMID: 21982422, Pubmed Central PMCID: 3245836.

4 Gluckman E, Broxmeyer HA, Auerbach AD, Friedman HS, Douglas GW, Devergie A *et al.* Hematopoietic reconstitution in a patient with Fanconi's anemia by means of umbilical-cord blood from an HLA-identical sibling. *N Engl J Med* 1989, 26 October; 321(17): 1174–1178. PubMed PMID: 2571931.

5 Samuel GN, Strong KA, Kerridge I, Jordens CF, Ankeny RA & Shaw PJ. Establishing the role of pre-implantation genetic diagnosis with human leucocyte antigen typing: what place do 'saviour siblings' have in paediatric transplantation? *Archiv Disease in Childhood* 2009, April; 94(4): 317–320. PubMed PMID: 18684746.

6 Fisk NM, Roberts IA, Markwald R & Mironov V. Can routine commercial cord blood banking be scientifically and ethically justified? *PLoS Med* 2005, February; 2(2): e44. PubMed PMID: 15737000, Pubmed Central PMCID: 549592.

7 Mercer JS & Erickson-Owens DA. Rethinking placental transfusion and cord clamping issues. *J Perinatal and Neonatal Nursing* 2012, July; 26(3): 202–217. PubMed PMID: 22843002.

8 Rocha V, Wagner Jr JE, Sobocinski KA *et al.* Eurocord and International Bone Marrow Transplant Registry Working Committee on Alternative Donor and Stem Cell Sources. Graft-versus-host disease in children who have received a cord-blood or bone marrow transplant from an HLA-identical sibling. *N Engl J Med* 2000, June; 342(25): 1846–1854.

9 Rocha V, Cornish J, Sievers E *et al.* Comparison of outcomes of unrelated bone marrow and umbilical cord blood transplants in children with acute leukemia. *Blood* 2001; 97: 2962–2971.

10 Wagner JE, Barker JN, DeFor TE, Baker KS, Blazar BR, Eide C *et al.* Transplantation of unrelated donor umbilical cord blood in 102 patients with malignant and nonmalignant diseases: influence of CD34 cell dose and HLA disparity on treatment-related mortality and survival. *Blood* 2002, 1 September; 100(5): 1611–1618. PubMed PMID: 12176879.

11 Eapen M, Rubinstein P, Zhang MJ, Stevens C, Kurtzberg J, Scaradavou A *et al.* Outcomes of transplantation of unrelated donor umbilical cord blood and bone marrow in children with acute leukaemia: a comparison study. *Lancet* 2007, 9 June; 369(9577): 1947–1954. PubMed PMID: 17560447.

12 Takahashi S, Iseki T, Ooi J *et al.* Single-institute comparative analysis of unrelated bone marrow transplantation and cord blood transplantation for adult patients with hematologic malignancies. *Blood* 2004; 104: 3873–3820.

13 Rocha V, Labopin M, Sanz G *et al.* Acute Leukemia Working Party of European Blood and Marrow Transplant Group; Eurocord-Netcord Registry. Transplants of umbilical cord blood or bone marrow from unrelated donors in adults with acute leukemia. *N Engl J Med* 2004; 351: 2276–2285.

14 Laughlin MJ, Eapen M, Rubinstein P *et al.* Outcomes after transplantation of cord blood or bone marrow from unrelated donors in adults with leukemia. *N Engl J Med* 2004; 351: 2265–2275.

15 Staba SL, Escolar ML, Poe M, Kim Y, Martin PL, Szabolcs P *et al.* Cord-blood transplants from unrelated donors in patients with Hurler's syndrome. *N Engl J Med* 2004, 6 May; 350(19): 1960–1969. PubMed PMID: 15128896.

16 Shaw BE, Veys P, Pagliuca A, Addada J, Cook G, Craddock CF *et al.* Recommendations for a standard UK approach to incorporating umbilical cord blood into clinical transplantation practice: conditioning protocols and donor selection algorithms. *Bone Marrow Transplantation* 2009, July; 44(1): 7–12. Epub 12 January 2009.

17 Warwick RM & Brubaker SA (eds). *Tissue and Cell Clinical Use.* Oxford: Blackwell Publishing; 2012.

18 Barker JN, Weisdorf DJ, DeFor TE, Blazar BR, McGlave PB, Miller JS *et al.* Transplantation of 2 partially HLA-matched umbilical cord blood units to enhance engraftment in adults with hematologic malignancy. *Blood* 2005, 1 February; 105(3): 1343–1347. PubMed PMID: 15466923.

19 Barker JN, Weisdorf DJ, DeFor TE, Blazar BR, Miller JS & Wagner JE. Rapid and complete donor chimerism in adult recipients of unrelated donor umbilical cord blood transplantation after reduced-intensity conditioning. *Blood* 2003, 1 September; 102(5): 1915–1919. PubMed PMID: 12738676.

20 Fernandez MN, Regidor C, Cabrera R, Garcia-Marco JA, Fores R, Sanjuan I *et al.* Unrelated umbilical cord blood transplants in adults: early recovery of neutrophils by supportive co-transplantation of a low number of highly purified peripheral blood CD34+ cells from an HLA-haploidentical donor. *Expl Hematol* 2003, June; 31(6): 535–544. PubMed PMID: 12829030.

21 de Lima M, McMannis J, Gee A, Komanduri K, Couriel D, Andersson BS *et al.* Transplantation of *ex vivo* expanded cord blood cells using the copper chelator tetraethylenepentamine: a phase I/II clinical trial. *Bone Marrow Transplantation* 2008, May; 41(9): 771–778. PubMed PMID: 18209724.

22 Frassoni F, Gualandi F, Podesta M, Raiola AM, Ibatici A, Piaggio G *et al.* Direct intrabone transplant of unrelated cord-blood cells in acute leukaemia: a phase I/II study. *Lancet Oncol* 2008, September; 9(9): 831–839. PubMed PMID: 18693069.

Further reading

Boelens JJ. Trends in haematopoietic cell transplantation for inborn errors of metabolism. *J Inherit Metab Dis* 2006; 29: 413–420.

Brunstein CG, Barker KS & Wagner JE. Umbilical cord blood transplantation for myeloid malignancies. *Curr Opin Hematol* 2007; 14: 162–169.

Brunstein CG, Setubal DC & Wagner JE. Expanding the role of umbilical cord blood transplantation. *Br J Haematol* 2007; 137: 20–35.

Gluckman E & Rocha V. Donor selection for unrelated cord blood transplants. *Curr Opin Immunol* 2006; 18: 565–570.

Locatelli F, Rocha V, Reed W *et al.* Related umbilical cord blood transplantation in patients with thalassemia and sickle cell disease. *Blood* 2003; 101: 2137–2143.

Martin PL, Carter SL, Kernan NA *et al.* Results of the Cord Blood Transplantation Study (COBLT): outcomes of unrelated donor umbilical cord blood transplantation in pediatric patients with lysosomal and peroxisomal storage diseases. *Biol Blood Marrow Transplantation* 2006; 12: 184–194.

43 Recent advances in clinical cellular immunotherapy

Mark W. Lowdell[1] & Emma Morris[2]

[1]Royal Free and University College Medical School, Royal Free Hospital, London, UK
[2]Department of Immunology and Molecular Pathology, Royal Free and University College
Medical School and Department of Haematology, University College London Hospitals NHS
Trust, London, UK

Introduction

Immunotherapy in the form of vaccination has been part of medical practice since Jenner in the 18th century. This so-called 'active' immunization requires that the recipient has the capacity to mount an immune response against the antigens within the vaccine. In contrast, the infusion of antibodies or immune cells raised in other animals or individuals, in response to deliberate vaccination or prior antigen exposure, into patients at risk of infection – 'passive' immunization – allows treatment of immunodeficient or immunocompromised patients.

Until recently, infusion of pathogen-specific antisera was the only routine form of passive immunotherapy, equine antitetanus antisera being a well-known example. Successful passive cellular immunotherapy requires precise matching of donor : recipient histocompatibility antigens and thus advances in HLA-typing over the past 40 years has allowed this form of immunotherapy to move closer to routine treatment.

Cellular immunotherapy in haemopoietic progenitor cell transplantation

The antileukaemic activity of allogeneic bone marrow transplantation was first described, in murine experiments, more than 40 years ago, but was appreciated in the clinic only in the late 1970s when attempts at preventing graft-versus-host disease (GVHD) by T-cell depletion were sometimes frustrated by an increase in the risk of leukaemia recurrence. The clinical antileukaemic effect of GVHD was first reported in 1979 and confirmed later by registry data from the International Bone Marrow Transplant Registry (IBMTR) [1]. The observed benefit of GVHD was particularly evident in patients transplanted for chronic myeloid leukaemia and led to the trial of post-transplant infusions of donor leucocyte infusions (DLI). The first peer-reviewed report of DLI therapy included a single patient who achieved molecular remission with no evidence of clinical GVHD, supporting the hypothesis that graft-versus-leukaemia (GVL) could be directed at leukaemia-specific or leukaemia-restricted target antigens [2]. GVHD after DLI remained a significant clinical problem, which has been somewhat reduced by the use of incremental doses of DLI, but the search for the 'holy grail' of leukaemia-specific GVL in the complete absence of GVHD continues to be an active research theme.

Nonspecific T-cell immunotherapy

A pragmatic approach to the dissection of GVHD from GVL was the concept of removal of alloreactive T cells from donor grafts whilst retaining nonalloreactive cells that could mediate GVL and antiviral

---

Practical Transfusion Medicine, Fourth Edition. Edited by Michael F. Murphy, Derwood H. Pamphilon and Nancy M. Heddle.
© 2013 John Wiley & Sons, Ltd. Published 2013 by John Wiley & Sons, Ltd.

responses. These approaches were all based upon *ex vivo* stimulation of allogeneic donor T cells with normal haemopoietic cells from the recipient to provoke a clinical-scale mixed lymphocyte response. Reacting T cells were then identified by the expression of one or more activation antigens (e.g. CD25, CD69) and depleted by immunotoxin or immunomagnetic selection. Whilst possibly successful in the reduction of GVHD, the clinical trials of this approach showed no evidence of a GVL effect, although antiviral immune responses have been enhanced in some cases. The principal criticism of these studies was that too few allo-depleted T cells were infused to definitively test the hypothesis that GVHD was prevented. Subsequently an extremely thorough study of the nature of alloreactive T cell activation *in vitro* in a mixed lymphocyte reaction concluded that the oligoclonal T-cell response is random and hence unpredictable from day to day. These data demonstrated that not all alloreactive T-cell clones will activate in a single mixed cell reaction and thus clinically relevant minor alloreactive T cells are likely to remain and induce GVHD upon infusion.

Another nonspecific approach has been the selective depletion of CD8 T cells from DLI [3]. Based upon the fact that the target cells of GVHD mostly lack expression of HLA-class II it has been considered that infusions of allogeneic CD4 T cells induce less GVHD. Many haemopoietic malignancies express HLA-class II antigens and are potential targets for CD4 T cells. Evidence of GVL, resolution of mixed T-cell chimerism and improved antiviral immunity in the absence of GVHD have all been reported in clinical trials of CD8-depleted DLI. Trials of this form of immunotherapy are continuing and are reporting encouraging results with respect to reversal of mixed chimerism and GVL [4].

Tumour-specific or tumour-restricted T-cell immunotherapy

Unselected DLI currently remains the mainstay of anti-tumour cellular immunotherapy following haemopoietic progenitor cell (HPC) transplantation; however, tumour antigen-specific T-cell responses can be generated by vaccination or by the generation of tumour antigen-specific T cells for adoptive transfer. T-cell-recognized tumour antigens can be divided into two main categories:

• The first are known as tumour-specific antigens (TSA), and the genes encoding TSA are only present in tumour cells and not in normal tissues.
• The second group, called tumour-associated antigens (TAA), are expressed at elevated levels in tumour cells but are also present in normal cells.

The majority of T-cell-recognized tumour antigens in humans are TAAs. The significance of this is that a low level of gene expression in normal cells can lead to the inactivation of high avidity T cells by immunological tolerance mechanisms. As a consequence, low avidity T-cell responses in patients are often inadequate in providing tumour protection. Therefore, TSA are theoretically the most desirable target antigens for cellular immunotherapy (vaccination or adoptive transfer), as there is no pre-existing immunological self-tolerance and TSA-specific immune responses are unlikely to damage normal tissues. Unfortunately TSAs with specific mutations are often invisible to cytotoxic T-lymphocytes (CTL) as a result of impaired antigen presentation due to competition with normal cellular antigens for proteasomal degradation, transportation by TAP molecules and binding to MHC. To date, most tumour antigens indentified as CTL targets are TAAs.

The majority of antitumour vaccination trials in humans has been against melanoma antigens and not in the context of stem cell transplantation. In these situations, vaccination can lead to TAA or TSA-reactive CTL responses, but there has rarely been a corresponding clinical benefit.

Recently, vaccination against the Wilms' tumour antigen 1 (WT1, a leukaemia-associated antigen) has been shown to induce WT1-specific T-cell responses in patients with myeloid malignancies. In the next 5 years it is anticipated that phase I/II clinical trials will test whether vaccination against WT1 epitopes early post-transplant can augment the reconstitution of WT1-specific CTL and act as maintenance immunotherapy.

TCR gene transfer

The inability to generate antigen-specific T cells is a serious limitation of adoptive cellular therapy for cancer. As discussed above, tumour antigens are often poorly immunogenic and patients are frequently immunocompromised as a consequence of the tumour burden or as a result of previous therapies. TcCR gene transfer offers a strategy to produce T cells with a

TCR specific for a tumour antigen (antigen-specific T cells) independent of precursor frequency [5]. Over the last 5 years, TCR gene transfer has been demonstrated to redirect reliably the antigen specificity of a given population of T cells via the introduction of a cloned TCR using retroviral transduction. This allows for the rapid generation and expansion of tumour antigen-specific T cells. Both the specificity and avidity of the TCR-transduced T cells are similar to the parental CTL clone from which the TCR has been isolated. Tumour antigen-specific TCR-transduced T cells have been shown to provide tumour protection in murine models and result in re-call responses up to 3 months post adoptive transfer. Recently, the first clinical trial using TCR-transduced T cells in melanoma patients has been published, demonstrating that TCR-transduced autologous T cells can have an antitumour effect. Patient T cells were transduced with a retroviral construct encoding the alpha and beta chains of the MART-1-specific TCR to target melanoma tumour cells. This milestone study demonstrated the feasibility and potential of TCR gene therapy. However, further modifications are required to the approach in order to maximize the clinical benefit. These include:

• modifications of the TCR construct to enhance cell surface expression of the introduced TCR and reduce the incidence of mispairing with endogenous alpha and beta chains (Figure 43.1);

• optimization of the conditioning regimen used prior to adoptive transfer;

• generation of functional TCR-transduced helper T cells.

Chimeric antigen receptor (CAR) modified T cells

The inability to generate antigen-specific T cells (see above) can be overcome by inserting a B-cell receptor with an intracellular TCR domain through gene transfer – a chimeric receptor. Murine monoclonal antibodies are readily generated to human proteins, some of which may be tumour restricted or at least tumour associated. CD19 is a protein expressed on B cells from the pre-B-cell stage to the mature B cell but is absent from plasma cells. T cells transfected with a sequence encoding the F(ab) domain of an anti-CD19 and the intracellular domain of CD3ζ can bind to CD19 expressing leukaemia cells and be triggered functionally as if they received signalling through the CD3–TCR complex. This is not a new concept; CAR-T cells have been tested experimentally for many years but the clinical effects have been transient due to failure of the cells to survive *in vivo*.

Recently the first successful clinical trial of CAR-transduced T cells used in adoptive immunotherapy was reported from Pennsylvania State University [6]. This group combined the anti-CD19 CAR with the

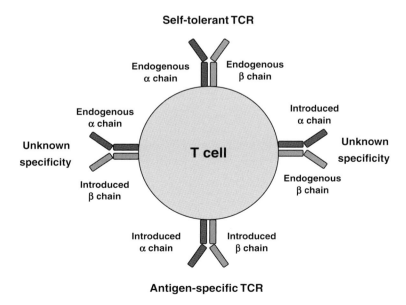

Fig 43.1 Schematic illustrating mis-pairing with endogenous TCR chains by the introduced TCR chains following retroviral TCR gene transfer.

sequence encoding human CD137, the costimulatory receptor 4-1BB, which is involved in T-cell survival. These CAR-T cells targeted CD19 expressing chronic lymphocytic leukaemia cells *in vivo* and successfully matured into memory T cells, which were detectable in recipient blood samples for prolonged periods.

Tumour-restricted natural killer cell immunotherapy

Some of the earliest trials of antitumour cellular immunotherapy were based upon infusion of NK cell activating cytokines or of *ex vivo* activated NK cells. Most of the early trials were in the autologous setting and, with the notable exception of a single report of acute myeloid leukaemia (AML) patients after autologous haemopoietic progenitor cell (HPC) transplant, were uniformly disappointing. However, these early trials were conducted before the complex mechanisms underlying NK cell function were understood.

Human NK cells are controlled by a variety of inhibitory and stimulatory signals though cell surface receptors, which allow them to distinguish between normal and malignant or infected cells. These receptors fall into one of four families:
• killer immunoglobulin-like receptor (KIR);
• C-type lectins;
• immunoglobulin-like transcript (ILT);
• natural cytotoxicity receptor (NCR).

The first two families include both inhibitory and activating receptors whilst the ILT and NCR families contain only activating receptors. All human NK cells express multiple receptors from each family and it is now apparent that functional subsets of NK cells exist.

In the 1980s Klaus Karre first demonstrated that murine NK cells preferentially lysed MHC class I negative tumours. This led him to construct his 'missing self' hypothesis, in which he proposed that NK cells are inhibited from lysis of normal cells that express MHC class I but are capable of lysing MHC class I negative tumour cells. Murine NK cells express surface receptors for MHC class I molecules and their ligation transduces inhibitory signals that prevent NK-mediated lysis. As implied above, the human NK regulatory system is more complex. Killer immunoglobulin-like receptors (KIRs) bind to HLA

class I molecules and the majority transduce inhibitory signals upon ligation by their specific HLA class I ligand. KIR molecules are classified on the basis of the number of extracellular domains and the length of the intracellular domain. For example:
• KIR2DL1 is a molecule with two extracellular domains and one long intracellular domain. This KIR binds to the family of HLA-C molecules with asparginine in position 77, the so-called 'type 2' HLA-C. The inhibitory signal is via an ITIM in the long intracellular domain.
• KIR2DL2, in contrast, binds to the remaining 'type 1' HLA-C molecules, those with a serine in position 77.
• KIR3DL1 binds to HLA-Bw4 alleles.
• KIR3DL2 binds HLA-A3 or A11 alleles.
• Other KIRs have been shown to bind HLA-G (Figure 43.2).

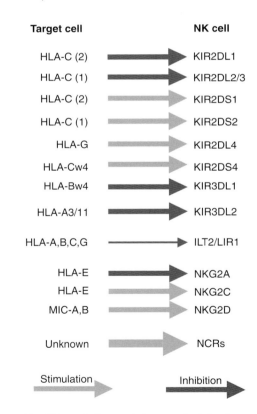

Fig 43.2 Ligands controlling NK cell activation and triggering.

In a co-culture of NK cells, autologous normal cells and HLA-class I deficient tumour cells one can demonstrate the colocalization of the KIR : HLA interaction between the NK and normal cell whilst the tumour cells show no such signalling (see Plate 43.1 in the plate section).

Given the concept that NK cells are 'kept in check' by inhibitory signals initiated through binding HLA molecules on normal somatic cells one might imagine that the KIR repertoire of any given individual is determined by their HLA type. This is not, however, the case and many healthy individuals will maintain NK cell clones that lack the appropriate inhibitory KIR molecules. However, the C-type lectin, NKG2A, which forms a heterodimer with CD94, appears to be universally expressed on human NK cells and presumably can provide the requisite inhibitory signals through its ligation to HLA-E. Most healthy individuals sustain a population of NK cells that lacks both KIR and NKG2A; these cells appear to be hyporesponsive to activating stimuli.

The clinical relevance of the understanding of NK cell inhibition is evident in haploidentical HPC transplantation where certain HLA class I mismatches generate a situation of HLA : KIR incompatibility. Highly significant reductions in relapse have been reported among AML patients receiving HLA : KIR incompatible haploidentical HPC grafts compared to patients receiving grafts in which the donor NK repertoire is matched to the HLA type of the patient.

Whilst these data stand on their own merit, much remains to be done to understand the mechanisms behind their results since the KIR effect seems to be limited to excessively T-cell-depleted haploidentical grafts and there is little or no role for CD94/NKG2A or for the activating receptors that appear so important in autologous NK cell function.

The implication from the haploidentical transplant data is that the lack of KIR-mediated NK cell inhibition is sufficient to initiate NK activation and lysis. However, since the patients with known KIR : HLA incompatibility did not experience NK-mediated GVHD one must assume that normal cells failing to inhibit NK cells were spared. NK activating signals may be provided via numerous receptors, although their ligands remain largely unknown. Recent published work has shown that, like T cells, NK cells generally require more than one signal to initiate cytokine secretion or lysis and that these signals may need to be provided sequentially to the cell.

Despite the lack of a complete understanding of human NK biology, clinical trials of allogeneic NK immunotherapy are already underway and some have been reported.

A remarkable study in which minimally conditioned patients with AML received bolus infusions of partially enriched IL2-activated NK cells from HLA-mismatched donors without concomitant HPC transplant showed engraftment of donor NK cells in the presence of recipient T, B and myeloid cells [7]. At the highest NK dose and the greatest level of preinfusion conditioning with cyclophosphamide and fludarabine, 5 of 19 patients achieved complete remission. Donor NK cells were detected in their peripheral blood and bone marrow. Despite the engraftment of haplomismatched NK cells the patients maintained normal bone marrow function and normal levels of autologous T cells, B cells and granulocytes.

The antileukaemic effect was relatively short lived in this trial but the data support the safety of such an approach and it is possible that such patients could receive multiple courses of NK cell infusions to maintain control of residual disease. The concept of repetitive passive cellular immunotherapy is novel and contrary to the design of most current approaches, which have been conceived within a mindset of 'cure by vaccination'. However, most tumour antigens elicit relatively weak immune responses and the physiological immune response to tumours may be one of control rather than eradication.

Passive cellular immunotherapy of infectious disease

Possibly the most remarkable clinical results from cellular immunotherapies have been seen in the treatment of opportunistic viral infections in immunocompromised patients. Most of these trials have been in the posttransplant setting, particularly in recipients of allogeneic HPC grafts:
• The earliest studies involved infusion of enormous numbers of cloned CMV-reactive CD8 T cells, which caused resolution of refractory CMV disease in patients postallogeneic HPCT.

• Subsequently, others elegantly demonstrated the specific resolution of posttransplant EBV-driven lymphoma following infusion of donor-derived anti-EBV CTLs.

Ex vivo generation of very large numbers of antiviral T cells is complex and expensive. However, in 2003, a phase I trial of allogeneic donor-derived CMV-reactive T cells grown for 21–28 days *ex vivo* on monocyte-derived dendritic cells that were pulsed with fixed whole CMV was reported. These expanded cells were infused into patients with molecular evidence of CMV reactivation postallogeneic HPCT and 8/16 patients resolved the reactivation without recourse to antiviral chemotherapy. No patient received a dose greater than 10^5 T cells per kilogram body weight and the average dose of CMV-specific T cells in each dose was no greater than 200–300 per kilogram. Despite this incredibly low dose of cells, virus-specific T cells were detectable in the peripheral blood of responding recipients at levels equivalent to a 35 000-fold expansion. The small numbers of cells infused in this demonstrated that the production of donor-specific cell therapies could be cost effective.

Despite the acknowledged clinical success of these trials neither led to a wide-scale adoption of cellular therapy due to the extreme technical complexity of cell therapy production. However, with recent advances in the availability of clinical-grade reagents and disposables the translation of laboratory-grade procedures to clinical application has advanced rapidly. For several years immunologists have been able to immunomagnetically select specifically activated T cells on the basis of the secretion of gamma-interferon and its capture on the cell surface with a bispecific antibody complexed to a paramagnetic nanoparticle. This approach selects both CD4 and CD8 cells [8].

An alternative approach is the use of multimeric recombinant MHC class I complexes loaded with an immunodominant viral peptide antigen restricted to the specific class I antigen [9]. These HLA-multimers can be complexed with the same sort of paramagnetic nanoparticles used in the gamma-secretion process described above and directly select antiviral-specific CD8 T cells from donor blood. These two patented technologies are now produced to clinical grade and are already central to a number of trials, including a phase III trial of allogeneic immunotherapy of CMV reactivation post-HPCT – the first multicentre randomized clinical trial of directed donation cellular immunotherapy.

There is undoubted promise in the clinical application of cellular immunity and the field has advanced very substantially in the last 5 years. However, the true potential of adoptive cellular immunotherapy remains constrained by the perceived need for directed donations (autologous or HLA-matched allogeneic) and by confusion over the regulatory framework in which the therapies fall. The first issue is the greatest barrier although some recent studies do support the feasibility of the ultimate goal of 'off the shelf' products [10]. The haploidentical NK study discussed above used NK cells from HLA-mismatched donors and demonstrated transient engraftment. A group in Edinburgh, UK, recently used 'off the shelf' HLA-mismatched T-cell lines to treat posttransplant EBV lymphoma in recipients of renal transplants [11].

Technical advances facilitating translational research in cellular immunotherapy

In Europe, since the ratification of the EU Clinical Trials Directive in member states in 2004, cellular immunotherapies have becomes susceptible to regulation as investigational medicinal products (IMPs). Whether a specific cell therapy product constitutes an IMP is determined by the relevant authority in each member state but, once a product is regulated as an IMP then production must meet Good Manufacturing Practice (GMP), and this has been difficult in the field of cellular immunotherapy. However, a number of European companies now manufacturer CE-marked reagents, consumables and devices for clinical-grade cell production. Closed and semi-closed systems are available for handling large-volume cell suspensions. Gas-permeable cell culture and expansion bags allowing closed-system culture are now widely available and the availability of clinical-grade cytokines is improving.

One of the most significant advances in the field has been the development of CE-marked clinical-grade immunomagnetic cell sorters. These are now widely used for the specific selection of subsets of haemopoietic progenitor cells and other leukocytes and can even select antigen-reactive cells on the basis of cytokine secretion, multimeric HLA-peptide reagents or expression of activation markers.

As the regulatory position becomes clearer more trials will be conducted to good clinical practice and the regulatory authorities will gather more evidence and experience of the field. In the not too distant future hospital blood banks may become more of a 'cell pharmacy' than ever before.

Key points

1 Allogeneic GVL by DLI is proof-of-principal of cellular immunotherapy.
2 Cellular immunotherapy of viral infections is becoming an alternative to antiviral chemotherapy.
3 HLA-matching may not be necessary.
4 Technical and regulatory difficulties in production of cell therapies are being overcome.

References

1 Horowitz MM, Gale RP, Sondel PM *et al.* Graft-versus-leukemia reactions after bone marrow transplantation. *Blood* 1990; 75: 555–562.
2 Kolb HJ, Mittermueller J, Clemm C *et al.* Donor leukocyte transfusion for treatment of recurrent chronic myelogenous leukemia in marrow transplant patients. *Blood* 1990; 76: 2462–2465.
3 Shimoni A, Gajewski JA, Donato M *et al.* Long-term follow up of recipients of CD8-depleted DLI for the treatment of CML relapsing after allogeneic progenitor cell transplantation. *Biol Blood Marrow Transplantation* 2001; 7: 568–575.
4 Orti G, Lowdell M, Fielding A *et al.* Phase I study of high-stringency CD8 depletion of donor leukocyte infusions after allogeneic hematopoietic stem cell transplantation. *Transplantation* 2009; 88: 1312–1318.
5 Xue SA & Stauss HJ. Enhancing immune responses for cancer therapy. *Cell Mol Immunol* 2007; 4: 173–184.
6 Kalos M, Levine BL, Porter DL *et al.* T cells with chimeric antigen receptors have potent antitumor effects and can establish memory in patients with advanced leukemia. *Sci Translational Med* 2011; 3: 95ra73.
7 Miller JS, Soignier Y, Panoskaltis-Mortari A *et al.* Successful adoptive transfer and *in vivo* expansion of human haploidentical NK cells in patients with cancer. *Blood* 2005; 105: 3051–3057.
8 Peggs K, Thomson K, Samuel E *et al.* Directly selected cytomegalovirus-reactive donor T cells confer rapid and safe systemic reconstitution of virus-specific immunity following stem cell transplantation. *Clin Infect Dis* 2011; 52: 49–57.
9 Cobbold M, Khan N, Pourgheysari B *et al.* Adoptive transfer of CMV-specific CTL to stem cell transplant patients after selection by HLA-peptide tetramers. *J Expl Med* 2005; 202: 379–386.
10 Leen AM, Myers GD, Sili U *et al.* Monoculture-derived T lymphocytes specific for multiple viruses expand and produce clinically relevant effects in immunocompromised individuals. *Nat Med* 2006; 12: 1160–1166.
11 Haque T, Wilkie GM, Jones MM *et al.* Allogeneic cytotoxic T cell therapy for EBV-positive PTLD: results of a phase II multicentre clinical trial. *Blood* 2007; 110: 1123–1131.

Further reading

Kadowaki N & Kitawaki T. Recent advance in antigen-specific immunotherapy for acute myeloid leukemia. *Clin Dev Immunol* 2011; 2011: 104926. Epub 19 October 2011. Review.
Kolb HJ, Schattenberg A, Goldman JM, Hertenstein B, Jacobsen N, Arcese W, Ljungman P, Ferrant A, Verdonck L, Niederwieser D, van Rhee F, Mittermueller J, de Witte T, Holler E, Ansari H; European Group for Blood and Marrow Transplantation Working Party. Chronic leukemia. Graft-versus-leukemia effect of donor lymphocyte transfusions in marrow grafted patients. *Blood* 1995. 1 September; 86(5): 2041–2050.
Linley AJ, Ahmad M & Rees RC. Tumour-associated antigens: considerations for their use in tumour immunotherapy. *Int J Hematol* 2011, March; 93(3): 263–273. Epub 1 March 2011. Review.
Vincent K, Roy DC & Perreault C. Next generation leukaemia immunotherapy. *Blood* 2011, 15 September; 118(11): 2951–2959. Epub 6 July 2011. Review. PMID: 21734234 [PubMed – indexed for MEDLINE].

44 Tissue banking

Akila Chandrasekar, Paul Rooney & John Kearney

NHS Blood and Transplant Tissue Services, Liverpool, UK

Regulation

The European Union Tissue and Cells Directives (EUTCD) set a benchmark for the standards that must be met when carrying out any activity involving tissues and cells for human application (patient treatment) by all member states. The EUTCD is made up of three Directives, the parent Directive (2004/23/EC), which provides the framework legislation, and two technical directives (2006/17/EC and 2006/86/EC), which provide the detailed requirements of the EUTCD.

The Human Tissue Act (2004) established the Human Tissue Authority (HTA) as the competent authority, with the responsibility for regulating tissues and cells (other than gametes and embryos) for human application within England, Wales and Northern Ireland. There is separate legislation in Scotland - the Human Tissue (Scotland) Act 2006 – with a high degree of similarity between both acts. The EU Directives were fully implemented into UK law in 2007, via the Human Tissue (Quality and Safety for Human Application) Regulations 2007. The HTA codes of practice provide guidance and lay down expected standards for the sectors regulated by the organization. The revised codes, effective since 2009, are designed to support professionals with advice and guidance based on real-life experience. More information is available at http://www.hta.gov.uk.

Tissue banks in the USA are regulated by the Food and Drug Administration (FDA) with standards set by the American Association of Tissue Banks (AATB).

Consent

Consent is the fundamental principle of the Human Tissue Act and underpins the lawful removal, storage and the use of donated tissue for any purpose. The Act provides for financial and custodial penalties for breaches of its requirements. While provisions of the Human Tissue (Scotland) Act 2006 are based on authorization rather than consent, these are essentially both expressions of the same principle. In Europe, the legal requirements for obtaining permission for retrieval of tissues after death vary from country to country [1]. However, even where 'opting out' or 'presumed consent' systems are operated, it is considered best professional practice to confirm that no relatives object to the donation proceeding.

To ensure that tissue donation for any purpose, either for clinical use or research purposes, is lawful, informed and valid consent must be obtained from an appropriate person, prior to tissue retrieval. Different consent requirements apply when dealing with tissue from deceased and living donors. With a living donor, the appropriate person is generally the donor themselves. For deceased donors, this can be the wishes of the deceased themselves expressed in life, e.g. through the organ donor register, or their nominated representative, a person who was appointed in life by the deceased to make these decisions. In the absence of either of these, the consent of a person in a 'qualifying relationship' with them immediately before they died must be sought. This may be (in

Practical Transfusion Medicine, Fourth Edition. Edited by Michael F. Murphy, Derwood H. Pamphilon and Nancy M. Heddle.
© 2013 John Wiley & Sons, Ltd. Published 2013 by John Wiley & Sons, Ltd.

order of priority) a spouse or partner, blood relation or friend.

Consent must be given voluntarily. It is also important that the person giving consent is fully informed about all aspects of the donation process and, where appropriate, what the risks are. The information should be provided on the following areas:

• the tissues donated and the intended clinical use of the donation, in general terms;
• the need for testing for transmissible infections and the implications and follow-up of positive results;
• information on how tissues are retrieved and stored;
• the possible need for a review of medical records;
• if applicable, the potential use of the tissue for research and development if it proves unsuitable for clinical use.

The duration of the consent must also be specified; this may be enduring (it remains in force unless it is specifically withdrawn) or time limited. The person giving consent may also withdraw it at any point before or after donation, providing that the tissue has not already been used, and it is important that they are informed of this right.

Consent should be taken only by those trained to do so. Seeking and obtaining consent is a sensitive issue; hence, staff seeking consent should have a good understanding of the activities they are seeking consent for. With the exception of anatomical examination or public display, where written consent is required, the Human Tissue Act does not specify the format in which consent should be recorded. Verbal consent documented either by audio recording or in the patient's notes is also valid.

Donor selection and testing

Tissue donors must be carefully selected to minimize the risk of transmitting diseases and to ensure suitable quality of grafts for transplantation. The major donor exclusion criteria described in the EU Directive is based on these two principles. The major reasons for deferral of donors include: malignancy, sepsis or significant local infection in the tissues to be donated, history or evidence of risk of transmissible viral infections such as HIV and hepatitis, risk of prion diseases and diseases of unknown aetiology [2]. Donors with a history of chronic or systemic autoimmune disease that could have a detrimental effect on the tissues

to be donated must be excluded. In the case of deceased donors, the donors must be excluded where the cause of death is not known, although the post mortem report is likely to provide this information after tissue retrieval. Detailed donor selection guidance for living and deceased tissue donors for the UK Blood and Tissue Transplantation Services is available at http://www.transfusionguidelines.org.uk.

The donor selection process includes a structured interview with the living donors to obtain a detailed medical and behavioural history. In the case of deceased donors this interview is conducted with someone who knew the donor well – usually, but not always, a relative. The reliability of a family interview depends on how well the interviewee knew their deceased relative. Family members or even partners may be unaware of some aspects of the donor's medical history or may not wish to disclose certain information or they may be in denial about some risk behaviours such as intravenous drug use. Additional sources of information can supplement the process of donor selection. Information is sought from the general practitioner and, when necessary, from the referring hospital practitioner if the donor was admitted to hospital prior to death, to obtain as accurate a medical history as possible. The result of post mortem examination is reviewed, if one was carried out.

Donor blood samples for testing of the mandatory and any additional discretionary microbiological markers (determined by the donor's medical or travel history, e.g. malaria and *Trypanosoma cruzi*) must be obtained at the time of donation or within seven days postdonation for living donors. The sample from deceased donors must be obtained just prior to death or within 24 hours after death. Fluids administered in the 48 hours prior to death must be recorded to allow an estimation of any plasma dilution effect. Tissues from donors with plasma dilution of more than 50% can be accepted only if testing procedures used for screening are validated for such plasma dilution or if a pretransfusion sample is available.

The minimum requirement for mandatory tests required by the EU Directive includes screening for hepatitis C (anti-HCV), hepatitis B (HBsAg and anti-HBc), HIV (anti-HIV I and II) and syphilis. Individual nations are permitted to set higher standards than the minimum requirements. For example, anti-HTLV testing is mandatory in UK Blood Service guidelines whereas the EU Directive requires anti-HTLV testing only for donors living in or originating from high incidence areas or if the donor's sexual partner or donor's parents originate from high incidence areas. In the USA, HTLV testing is not required for tissues that are acellular. There is a requirement in the EU Directive to quarantine living tissue donations to obtain a second blood sample from the donor after an interval of 180 days to repeat the mandatory tests; however, if the blood sample taken at the time of donation is additionally tested by the nucleic acid amplification method (NAT) for HIV, HCV and HBV, a retesting is not required after 180 days. In UK blood services, all tissue donors are screened by NAT for HIV, hepatitis C and hepatitis B, in addition to the antibody and antigen tests mentioned above. The interval between the time of infection to the onset of detectable infection on screening tests is known as the 'window period'. This window period for genome detection by NAT is much shorter than the window period for antibody detection. NAT thereby reduces the risk of transmission of infection during the early phase of the infection following exposure to the virus, before antibodies can be detected on screening. However, the serology screen may serve as an indicator of a past exposure and as an indicator of lifestyle risks. This combination of NAT and antibody test is especially important for testing of deceased tissue donors, where only a single blood sample can be taken at the time of donation. A negative NAT at the time of donation from a seronegative individual also removes the requirement for quarantining the donation from living donors, as explained above.

Tissue procurement

Tissue procurement or retrieval is a very different procedure for living and deceased donations. By necessity, living donations are retrieved during surgery by the operating team. Clear, written instructions, staff training and standard sterile kits are provided by the tissue bank for tissue collection. Regular auditing to ensure compliance with agreed procedures, detailed in a written agreement between the tissue bank and the hospital, is an integral part of a living donation programme. The critical aspect of retrieval is the identification of the donor, the donation and associated blood samples for donor testing and tissue samples for bacteriology and fungal testing. The use of barcoded donation number labels for donations,

samples and associated documentation greatly increases the security in this step (see below).

With deceased donors, it is important to ensure the quality of the tissues removed. Tissues can deteriorate post mortem due to microbial contamination and autolysis, or be contaminated during the retrieval process. The optimal time and place to procure tissues from deceased donors is in an operating theatre, immediately after death or postcessation of circulation. However, the availability of these facilities for tissue donation is limited, and is generally restricted to tissue grafts that can be obtained during routine organ procurement procedures, such as removal of the heart for valve donation. In the UK, the large majority of tissue donations are performed in hospital mortuaries or on rare occasions in funeral homes. In addition, NHSBT Tissue Services (Liverpool) has a dedicated tissue donation facility, equipped with laminar air flow, for tissue retrieval; similar donation suites can be found both in Europe and in the USA. Consent is obtained from the donor family for moving the donor to the facility for tissue donation and returning the donor to the hospital or the funeral home within specified time limits. The environment is controlled to a defined specification, which is easier to maintain and monitor. The other advantages of an on-site dedicated facility are reduction in staff travelling time and the opportunity for close supervision and training of staff as senior expertise is available on-site.

Donor identification by means of a wristband, toe-tag or by mortuary staff is a crucial step before commencing the retrieval. A minimum of three points of identification such as name, date of birth, hospital number, address and tattoos (described by the family) are required to positively identify the donor. Before the tissue retrieval, a thorough external examination of the donor body appearance is conducted and recorded as a part of donor assessment. This examination should include detection and recording of tattoos, jaundice, evidence of drug use, body piercing, open wounds or signs of infection, scars and bruises, intravenous cannula sites, operation incision sites and other significant abnormalities.

Following death, autodegradation of all tissues commences as cells die and release lytic enzymes into the tissue. The intestinal microflora begins to migrate throughout the body, contaminating other tissues. The rate of both these processes is critically dependent on temperature; therefore it is crucial that warm ischaemia time is minimized and the body is refrigerated as soon as possible after death. In general, tissues should be recovered within the shortest possible period from the time of death. Standards vary around the world from 12 to 48 hours depending on the tissue and the processing method to which it will be subjected.

Minimizing bacterial contamination is further ensured by staff wearing sterile clothing and applying an aseptic technique during the tissue recovery process. This includes cleaning the donor using surgical detergents, alcohol wipes and sterile water; shaving the incision and skin retrieval areas; and draping the donor body before commencing the retrieval. Single-use equipment is used where possible.

Generally, skin grafts (if consented for) will be retrieved first to prevent the skin becoming contaminated by internal body fluids following incisions to remove internal tissues. In the UK, skin grafts are retrieved from the back of the torso and the back and front of both legs. Other tissue grafts are located internally and must be retrieved by incision. If retrieving heart, pericardium and thoracic aorta, the chest cavity must be exposed. Many other tissue grafts are obtained from the lower limbs, including bone (femur and proximal tibia), tendons and ligaments (Patellar, Achilles and hamstrings), meniscal cartilage and femoral arteries. An important aspect of tissue recovery is the careful reconstruction of the donor body. Extendable plastic or wooden prostheses are used to replace large bones.

Tissue processing

Tissue grafts are processed to improve safety, efficacy and for long-term storage of the donated material. There are multiple ways of processing, depending on the properties of the graft that need to be retained [3]. The core methodology by which viable tissues (skin, heart valve, cardiovascular and meniscus grafts) are processed comprises dissection, decontamination by antibiotic cocktail and cryopreservation. Whilst it may be desirable to sterilize a graft to increase safety, this is not practical where retention of donor cell viability is required. For many types of tissue allograft, in particular musculoskeletal allografts, the presence of viable cells is not required and, in these cases, processing reduces the risk of disease transmission by removal

of blood and marrow and by reducing or eliminating contamination by chemical or physical means. Pooling of tissues from different donors during processing is not permitted by standards in Europe or the USA.

Each tissue bank should have a policy for acceptance or rejection of tissues if certain organisms are detected in bacterial screening during different stages of processing. The policy should be based on the pathogenicity of the organism and the validated effectiveness of any subsequent decontamination or sterilization steps.

Femoral heads from living donors removed during surgery in an operating theatre can be frozen and transplanted without further processing in the absence of bacterial or fungal contamination in validated tests.

Processing facilities

The required standard of EU tissue processing facilities is defined in Directive 2006/86/EC and is recognized as a key factor for the safety of tissues at risk of contamination. In general, the directive defines the minimum air quality in which tissues are exposed as Grade A (as defined in the European Guide to Good Manufacturing Practice, Annex 1) with a minimum background air quality of Grade D. The Directive defines a number of circumstances where lower standards must be justified and shown to give adequate protection to the tissue. Individual member states may apply more stringent criteria and may require a background of Grade B for some or all tissues exposed to the environment without terminal sterilization.

Supply and traceability of tissues

Directive 2006/86/EC requires the development of a European coding system, which will facilitate tracking of tissue from the donor to the recipient. A variety of different coding systems are currently in use, some using manually recorded codes and others using computerized systems with barcoding. The use of ISBT128 coding standard for blood is widespread in blood services in Europe and in the USA and has been further developed to include tissue product nomenclature (see www.iccbba.org).

Currently most tissue banks supply tissues direct to operating theatre departments and it is the

responsibility of the receiving hospital to track from the receipt of the tissue to the graft's ultimate fate. Many tissue banks supply the hospital with a recipient record to be completed for each graft and returned to the bank. The users should always be advised:
• to keep a log of tissue received and used;
• to record any allograft unit numbers in the patient's notes;
• to inform the tissue bank immediately of any adverse reaction that might be attributable to the tissue graft.

In many cases, tissues are supplied for specific cases and stocks are not held locally, but some units prefer to keep stocks of tissue immediately at hand for use in emergency or unexpected cases. Depending on the type of tissue, the hospital may require a licence to store tissue grafts for more than 48 hours; tissues containing donor cells such as cryopreserved skin grafts require a licence for storage, whereas acellular tissues, such as processed freeze dried bone grafts, do not.

Clinical applications

Tissue allografts are used in a variety of clinical indications in orthopaedic, spinal, cardiac, vascular, ophthalmic and plastic and reconstructive surgical procedures. Some of them are listed in Table 44.1.

Serious adverse events and reactions

Directive 2006/86/EC requires member states to have systems for reporting adverse reactions and events related to the procurement, processing, storage, testing or distribution of the tissue, which might seriously affect the recipient. The EUTCD definitions are as follows:

Adverse event:

Any untoward occurrence associated with the procurement, testing, processing, storage and distribution of tissues and cells that might lead to the transmission of communicable disease, to death or life-threatening, disabling or incapacitating conditions for patients or which might result in or prolong hospitalisation or morbidity.

Adverse reaction:

An unintended response, including a communicable disease in the donor or in the recipient associated with the procurement or human application of tissues and cells that is fatal, life-threatening, disabling, incapacitating or which results in or prolongs hospitalisation or morbidity.

Table 44.1 Indications for tissue allografts.

Types of graft	Surgical specialty	Surgical procedure (examples)
Heart valves	Cardiac	Valve replacement
Tendons and ligaments	Knee surgery	Ligament reconstruction
Meniscus	Knee surgery	Replacement of damaged meniscus (in selected cases)
Frozen femoral head, morcellized bone grafts	Orthopaedic (hip and knee)	Impaction grafting at revision joint surgery
Massive bone allograft	Orthopaedics	Post-trauma or tumour excision reconstruction
Demineralized bone	Spinal surgery, orthopaedic, oral and maxillofacial	Spinal fusion, nonunion or trauma defects, to fill cysts and tumour cavity defects
Cornea	Ophthalmology	Keratoconus, corneal ulcers, trauma, chemical burns
Skin	Burns	Burns, toxic epidermal necrolysis
Decellularized dermis	Plastic and reconstructive, breast surgery, abdominal surgery	Chronic wounds, breast reconstruction, abdominal wall repair
Blood vessels	Vascular	To replace infected prosthetic graft, lower limb ischaemia
Pericardium	Cardiac, andrology, ophthalmology	Vessel wall repair, Peyronie's disease, glaucoma surgery

In the UK, the HTA has developed an electronic reporting system for tissue and cell facilities, in line with the requirements of Directive 2006/86/EC. Each tissue bank receiving information about such a reaction or event must report it to the HTA when it comes to their attention and then again when the investigation of the event is completed. Such reactions and events can also be reported by the organization applying the graft, direct to the HTA.

Advances in tissue processing and regenerative medicine

There is still a need for traditionally banked human tissue, skin, bone, tendon, etc., but there is a recognition that, when grafted, these tissues may not provide the optimal environment for tissue regeneration; e.g. the presence of cells in the allograft (viable or dead) can give rise to an immune response and a delay or inhibition of recipient cellular infiltration or incorporation into the recipient. As such, traditionally processed and banked tissue essentially provides a replacement to damaged or diseased host tissue and some tissue, such as massive bone allografts, will never become fully incorporated into a recipient.

Regenerative medicine uses techniques of tissue engineering to remove donor cells without affecting the biological, biomechanical or biochemical parameters of the tissue [4]. Decellularized tissue, in particular decellularized dermis, has been available as an allograft since 1995 and several tissue banks now offer decellularized dermis and decellularized heart valves to surgeons. Clinical evaluation of results indicate that the decellularized tissue scaffold performs well, aids healing (if used in chronic wounds) and becomes infiltrated with recipient cells. Importantly, the infiltrating cells are not inflammatory cells resorbing the graft; instead they include progenitor and precursor cells, which can differentiate into an appropriate cell type, often influenced by factors remaining in the scaffold.

A major advantage of decellularized tissue becoming repopulated by recipient cells is that, over time, the grafted tissue becomes remodelled by the recipient cells, the donor extracellular matrix is replaced with recipient matrix and the allograft becomes part of the host. Two consequences of this are (1) a lack of the need for anti-inflammatory/antirejection drugs and (2) the ability of the grafted/remodelled tissue to grow and

be able to repair itself as part of the recipient. Recent studies on implantation of decellularized heart valves indicate that the tissue does become repopulated with recipient cells and there is a reduction in complications and the need for further operations with time when compared to conventionally cryopreserved valves [5]. The use of decellularized heart valves opens up the possibility that when used in paediatric patients, only one heart valve transplant may be required during the lifetime of the patient and the implanted valve will increase in size when required as part of the recipient's natural growth.

The ability to add cells to banked tissue allografts is a major step forward in regenerative medicine treatment. Amniotic membrane has been used as a conventional allograft to treat severe ocular surface diseases for several years due to its ability to facilitate corneal re-epithelialization and reduce scarring and inflammation; however, more recently amniotic membrane has been used as a substrate on which epithelial stem cells can be expanded prior to transplant. The epithelial stem cells are derived from biopsies of the limbal region of the corneum; the stem cells can locate to stem cell niches when transplanted and thus provide a long-term solution to limbal stem cell deficiency. Limbal stem cells can be obtained either from the patient or from a donor.

Recent advances in regenerative medicine have involved adding recipient cells to a decellularized tissue, either in advance in the laboratory or at the point of transplant, making the procedure 'personalised' regenerative medicine. In 2008, a patient in Spain received a transplant of a portion of trachea that had been decellularized and then repopulated with her own cells, within a bioreactor [6]. Cells of different lineages, epithelial from bronchus and chondrocytes from bone marrow, were added to the inside and the outside of the trachea respectively at the University of Bristol (UK) before the repopulated tissue was shipped back to Spain. The cells were cultured in the bioreactor for four days before shipping. Similar procedures have been performed in the UK in 2010 using the entire trachea and adding stem cells 2–4 hours prior to transplant [7]. The initial transplant required 42 days for decellularization, but more recent transplants have been decellularized in 10 days or less.

Regenerative medicine may not always require human tissue for generation of a graft but it does require the addition of human cells. In 2006, it was reported that seven children/youths suffering from myelomeningocele and resultant dysfunctional bladder received successful transplants of artificial bladders impregnated with smooth muscle and bladder urothelial cells [8]. The bladders had been produced by erecting a scaffold and adding the cells in the laboratory. All patients reported improvement.

More recently, in June 2011, an entire artificial trachea was produced by scientists at University College London using a polymer-based nanocomposite and shipped to the Karolinska Institute in Sweden where recipient stem cells were added in a bioreactor for two days before being transplanted into a 36-year-old patient by the same surgeon who performed the first tissue-engineered tracheal transplant in 2008 [9].

Research is currently being performed on micronizing or solubilizing decellularized extracellular matrices such that the tissue is capable of being percutaneously injected to a site of required repair rather than incision. These matrices are biphasic in that they are a viscous fluid at low temperatures but set into a solid state at physiological temperature; therefore when injected into a repair site, the fluid becomes a solid tissue-like structure. These biphasic gels could be added with either bioactive factors or host cells to stimulate more rapid repair.

Regenerative medicine opens up the possibility of replacing almost every damaged or worn-out tissue with a new tissue capable of becoming part of the patient and returning normal functionality.

Summary

The banking of tissues is increasing within blood services, where expertise in donor selection, donor testing and quality management is being applied to the banking of many tissues including bone, tendons, heart valves and skin. Living donors can donate bone, amnion and heart valves during joint replacement, delivery of an infant or heart transplant surgery, respectively. All other types of tissue donation are made after death. For deceased donors, a thorough medical and behavioural history from a number of alternative sources is recorded to compensate for the lack of a face-to-face donor interview. This additional information should be sought from the donor's family doctor and the post mortem examination report (where applicable).

Living donations are retrieved during surgery by the operating team. In the UK, the large majority of tissue donations after death are performed in hospital mortuaries. Tissues should be retrieved within the shortest possible time period after death. Delayed tissue recovery increases the risk of bacterial contamination. Minimizing bacterial cross-contamination is ensured by applying aseptic retrieval techniques.

Tissue processing is necessarily open and usually involves decontamination or terminal sterilization. As a minimum, facilities for tissue processing in the EU should be designed to achieve class C for tissues destined for terminal sterilization and class A, with class D background, for the manipulation of tissues in the absence of a terminal sterilization step, but following chemical or antibiotic decontamination. Many EU member states apply more stringent requirements.

Traceability is an essential aspect of the quality chain and should be supported by machine readable identification codes. If these are compatible with blood coding systems, traceability within the transplanting hospital can be greatly enhanced. Requirements are now in place for the reporting of serious adverse events and reactions to regulatory authorities to support the further enhancement of safety and quality in tissue banking.

Tissue banking and processing is a rapidly evolving field and is becoming more and more related to personalized regenerative medicine. Conventional tissue allografts often require replacement (with another allograft) with time, but tissue engineered allografts raise the possibility that, particularly in children, only one allograft will be required for the lifetime of the patient.

Key points

1 Tissue grafts are used in surgical procedures to replace damaged or lost tissues in patients. Most tissue allografts are donated by deceased donors and some by living donors undergoing surgery.
2 The European Union Tissue and Cells Directives (EUTCD) set out to establish a harmonized approach to the regulation of tissues and cells across Europe, requiring EC member states to have inspection and accreditation systems to ensure that all tissue banks comply with mandated technical requirements.

3 Consent should be taken only by those trained to do so and the associated discussion should include information on intended clinical use of the tissue, including research use, virological testing and the implications of positive results.

4 The primary source of donor selection information for deceased donors is the interview with someone who knew the donor well and this may not necessarily be the person who gives consent for the donation. Where a post mortem examination has been performed or is scheduled, the results should be reviewed as part of the donor selection process.

5 An external examination of the donor body should be conducted, recorded and form part of the donor selection assessment prior to the tissue recovery. After tissue recovery, it is important to carefully reconstruct the donor body. Aseptic procedures must be followed to minimize bacterial contamination.

6 Processing tissue reduces the risk of disease transmission by removing blood and marrow and by reducing or eliminating contamination by chemical and physical means. Pooling of donations during processing is not permitted by standards in Europe or the USA.

7 Tissue allografts have been used in surgical procedures for many years with great success but with known limitations. Regenerative medicine using decellularized and tissue engineered allografts may allow full incorporation of the graft into the patient such that it becomes part of the patient and is able to grow with and repair itself.

References

1 Schulz-Baldes A, Biller-Andorno N & Capron AM. International perspectives on the ethics and regulation of human cell and tissue transplantation. *Bull World Health Org* 2007; 85: 941–948.

2 Chandrasekar A, Warwick RM & Clarkson A. Exclusion of deceased donors post-procurement of tissues. *Cell Tissue Bank* 2011; 12: 191–198.

3 Galea E (ed.). *Essentials of Tissue Banking*, 1st edn. Springer; 2010, 245 pp.

4 Mirsadraee S, Wilcox H, Korossis S *et al*. Development and characterisation of an acellular human pericardial matrix for tissue engineering. *Tissue Engng* 2006; 12: 763–773.

5 da Costa FD, Santos LR, Collatusso C *et al*. Thirteen years' experience of the Ross operation. *J Heart Valve Dis* 2009; 18: 84–94.

6 Macchiarini P, Jungebluth P, Go T *et al*. Clinical transplantation of a tissue-engineered airway. *Lancet* 2008; 372: 2023–2030.

7 Baiguera S, Birchall MA & Macchiarini P. Tissue engineered tracheal transplantation. *Transplantation* 2010; 89: 485–491.

8 Atala A, Bauer SB, Soker S *et al*. Tissue engineered autologous bladder for patients needing cystoplasty. *Lancet* 2006; 367: 1241–1246.

9 Jungebluth P, Alici E, Baiguera S *et al*. Tracheobronchial transplantation with a stem-cell-seeded bioartificial nanocomposite: a proof-of-concept study. *Lancet* 2011; 378: 1997–2004.

Further reading

Barron DJ, Khan NE, Jones TJ, Willets RG & Brawn WJ. What tissue bankers should know about the use of allograft heart valves. *Cell Tissue Bank* 2010; 11: 47–55.

Eagle MJ, Rooney P, Lomas R & Kearney JN. Validation of radiation dose received by frozen unprocessed and processed bone during terminal sterilisation. *Cell Tissue Bank* 2005; 6: 221–230.

Fehily S, Warwick RM, Kearney J & Galea G. Bone banking in the UK blood services. *Organs and Tissues* 2004; 3: 177–182.

Getgood A & Bollen S. What tissue bankers should know about the use of allograft tendons and cartilage in orthopaedics. *Cell Tissue Bank* 2010; 11: 87–97.

Kearney JN. Guidelines on processing and clinical use of skin allografts. *Clinics in Dermatology* 2005; 23: 357–364.

McDermott ID. What tissue bankers should know about the use of allograft meniscus in orthopaedics. *Cell Tissue Bank* 2010; 11: 75–85.

PART SEVEN

Development of the Evidence Base for Transfusion

45 Observational and interventional trials in transfusion medicine

Alan Tinmouth[1,2], *Dean Fergusson*[2] & *Paul C. Hébert*[2]

[1]General Hematology and Transfusion Medicine, Division of Hematology, Department of Medicine, Ottawa Hospital, Ottawa, Ontario, Canada
[2]University of Ottawa Centre for Transfusion Research, Clinical Epidemiology Program, The Ottawa Health Research Institute, Ottawa, Ontario, Canada

Introduction

Randomized controlled clinical trials (RCTs) have evolved to become the 'gold standard' clinical research design used to distinguish the risks and benefits of therapeutic interventions. In 1948, for the first time a controlled clinical trial made use of random allocation, a control group and blinding. Additional principles guiding the design of RCTs were first elaborated by Sir Austin Bradford-Hill in the 1960s [1].

Many important questions regarding the use of blood components and alternatives such as blood conservation therapies have not been the subject of well-designed and executed RCTs. Consequently, clinicians frequently base their therapeutic decisions on suboptimal levels of clinical evidence, including observational studies, poorly controlled clinical trials or laboratory studies, and personal experience or observations, which are not evidence based. There are a number of plausible reasons why there are so few large clinical trials in transfusion medicine:

• transfusion medicine has historically been a laboratory-based specialty with research focused on the product;
• a relative lack of clinical epidemiologists and clinical trialists interested in transfusion medicine;
• difficulty in obtaining funding for research of a supportive as opposed to a curative therapy;

• many of the products have been in standard use for years without good evidence to define the benefits or harms, or specific indications of use; and
• few industry partners willing to invest in large clinical trials given that products are already in wide use.

It could also be postulated that unique difficulties in the field may have impeded the development of important clinical studies. In this chapter, we outline some of the methodological issues central to the development and conduct of observational and interventional trials, including RCTs, in transfusion medicine.

What is unique about transfusion medicine?

There are a number of unique difficulties in transfusion medicine that require consideration in the development of clinical research. First and foremost, transfusion medicine as a discipline is largely based upon the provision of supportive interventions in the treatment of a wide variety of acute illnesses as opposed to disciplines such as cardiology or oncology where interventions are evaluated in well-defined diseases. Furthermore, studies are conducted by trialists trained within a specific discipline (e.g. oncologists, cardiac surgeons). In comparison, blood components are indicated in response to conditions such as anaemia or coagulopathy induced by medications or disease

Practical Transfusion Medicine, Fourth Edition. Edited by Michael F. Murphy, Derwood H. Pamphilon and Nancy M. Heddle.
© 2013 John Wiley & Sons, Ltd. Published 2013 by John Wiley & Sons, Ltd.

entities. The supportive nature of transfusions leads to consideration of outcomes that may not be directly clinically relevant to the underlying disease process. In addition, most benefits and risks of care either would not be attributed to supportive interventions or the supportive intervention may not be considered the prime factor influencing the outcome(s).

Conditions that require blood components, such as anaemia and coagulopathies, occur in a broad range of diseases. This raises significant difficulties in designing studies and setting a research agenda. Evaluating a transfusion intervention in many diseases can be problematic as the frequency of the outcome(s) of interest will vary. Larger sample sizes and more robust outcomes would then be required to account for the variation within the patient population. The alternative strategy of smaller trials in targeted populations will limit the generalizability of the study as the conclusions may not be applicable to patient groups outside the studied target population.

A further concern is the complex biological nature of blood components. For instance, red cell concentrates are prepared using a variety of techniques and storage media, and intravenous immunoglobulins are manufactured by different companies using different processes. This leads investigators to consider whether studies evaluating a transfusion intervention should only be done with one product or preparation, or with many different preparations. Indeed, there may be unforeseen or unexpected clinical consequences due to different approaches to the preparation of blood components. In the planning of studies, one must carefully consider whether products are sufficiently similar to consider including in the same study. Regulatory concerns within or between jurisdictions may also impact on the choice of products included in the study.

As discussed in subsequent sections, regulations may not permit the conduct of randomized trials for studies assessing the clinical consequences of different products or testing procedures. Under such constraints, quasi-experimental designs such as before-and-after studies or time-series analyses should be considered.

One of the remaining unique aspects of conducting clinical research in transfusion medicine is that transfusions are often incorporated into complex care paths or within therapeutic algorithms of care. The evaluation of transfusions with many other interventions and diagnostic tests increases the complexity of any clinical evaluation.

Types of studies

To ascertain the effectiveness of an intervention, the RCT remains the preferred study design as it should minimize the most important biases if properly conceived and executed. Despite being the 'gold standard', there are often practical, legal, financial and ethical limitations to the use of clinical trials. For instance, exposing subjects to undesirable and dangerous interventions such as cigarettes and toxins would not be permitted in an RCT. While many of these limitations have been well described, one unique obstacle encountered in transfusion medicine is the conduct of an RCT when an intervention is universally implemented, such as a new processing method or testing procedure for the entire blood supply. By implementing an intervention such as universal pre-storage leucocyte reduction or universal polymerase chain reaction (PCR) testing for hepatitis C, an RCT becomes impossible within that population. If an RCT is not possible, other study designs including quasi-experimental and observational designs should be considered.

Observational studies

Two types of observational designs are often considered in clinical research, case–control studies and cohort or prognostic studies (Figure 45.1). In all observational studies, the first step is to define (a) the research hypothesis, (b) the population, (c) the exposure(s), (d) the outcome(s) and (e) the covariates (factors other than the exposure that may influence the occurrence of the outcomes). A case–control study refers to a study where one identifies a group of individuals with an outcome and another group of individuals who would be considered at risk of developing the outcome. Once both groups have been identified, investigators usually seek to identify potential risk factors in both the group with the outcome and the controls. This classic epidemiological design is ideally suited to the investigation of rare diseases and the identification of potential aetiological or risk factors, particulary if there is a long latency period [2]. In transfusion medicine, case–control studies would be

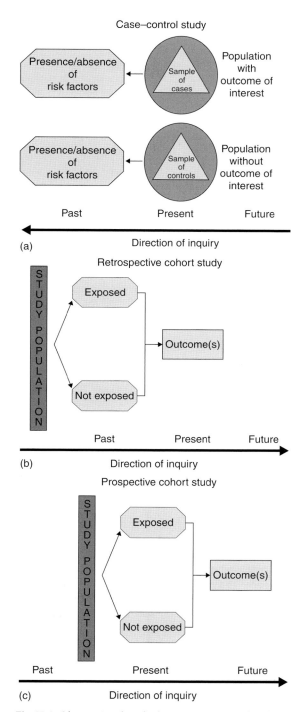

Case–control study

Prospective cohort study

Fig 45.1 Observational study designs: case–control and cohort studies. Adapted from Tay and Tinmouth [26].

ideally suited for the initial study of rare conditions such as transfusion-related acute lung injury (TRALI) and the association between blood transfusion and variant Creutzfeldt–Jakob disease (vCJD). By definition, this study design is always retrospective in nature. Cases, controls and potential risk factors are identified from historical records or past events. By comparing 46 cases of patients with TRALI (cases) and 225 randomly selected transfusion recipients without TRALI (controls), Silliman *et al.* [3] were able to identify that certain diagnoses (haematological malignancies and cardiac disease) and the age of the platelets were associated with TRALI. In a smaller subset of cases and controls, the implicated units also had greater neutrophil priming activity as compared with controls. While these results demonstrate an association between neutrophil priming activity, which increases in older platelets, and TRALI reactions, the case–control design does not allow causation to be determined.

Despite some of the potential advantages of this study design, it is difficult to do well and is fraught with potential biases. A systematic review of case–control studies attempting to establish the association between blood transfusion and vCJD demonstrated that blood transfusion had a protective effect [4]. Such a protective effect makes little sense and is probably the result of some biased approach to the sampling of controls.

The second observational design choice is a cohort study. In this type of study, individuals are identified well in advance of developing a disease and followed forward in time. Ideally, information on potential risk factors would be gathered from patients throughout the period of observation until the occurrence of an outcome or the end of the study. If subjects are identified well in advance of the development of a disease, then comparing individuals who have a given risk factor with individuals who do not may provide important clues to the aetiology of a disease or health state. It may also lead to a better understanding of the course of the disease and its incidence. If patients are identified and followed once a disease has developed, then this design may also provide invaluable prognostic information.

Cohort studies follow patients forward in time and evaluate outcomes based on a known exposure, risk factor or treatment. This design is most powerful when all eligible individuals are identified early,

493

followed prospectively and without any losses to follow-up. A number of cohort studies have examined the relationship between anaemia, red cell transfusion and outcomes such as hospital mortality. These studies illustrate both positive and negative attributes of cohort studies. A retrospective study conducted by Carson and colleagues evaluated the relationship between increasing degrees of anaemia, the presence of ischaemic heart disease and mortality rates [5]. In 1958 for Jehovah's Witness patients, the adjusted odds of death increased from 2.3 (95% confidence interval (CI) 1.4–4.0) to 12.3 (95% CI 2.5–62.1), as preoperative haemoglobin concentrations declined from 10.0–10.9 g/dL to 6.0–6.9 g/dL in patients with cardiac disease as compared with patients without cardiac disease. This study shows a clear relationship between increasing anaemia and death.

In comparison, the risks of anaemia or transfusing older red blood cells and benefits of transfusions may be quite complex. This interdependence is often referred to as confounding by indication. Confounding is the mixing or blurring of effects where an outcome is related to an exposure but the effect is due to a third factor [6]. Observational studies in transfusion medicine have attempted to compare clinical outcomes in patients receiving red blood cells with varied storage times. These studies have major limitations including confounding by indication [7]. Koch *et al.* [8] retrospectively studied the records of Medicare of 8366 patients who received a red blood cell transfusion during cardiac surgery at a single institution over an 8-year period. Patients were arbitrarily divided into groups that received only red cells stored 14 days or less (newer) or red cells stored for greater than 14 days (older). Patients who received mixed aged red cells ($n = 2364$) were excluded from the analysis. Transfusion of newer red cells was associated with reductions in a composite outcome of serious adverse events including MI, stroke, sepsis, organ failure and death (adjusted odds ratio 1.16; 95% confidence interval, 1.01 to 1.33; $p = 0.03$) and a reduction in-hospital mortality (2.8% versus 1.7%, $p = 0.004$) and 1-year mortality (7.4% versus 11.0%, $p < 0.001$). Even though the study was published in a prestigious journal, there were several major limitations, making it difficult to draw useful conclusions:

- association between increased number of units transfused and older red cell units;
- confounding by indication;
- dichotomization by a single age point introduces artificial cut-off;
- a primary composite outcome including 17 items;
- the timing of the transfusions were unknown;
- inability to adjust for important but unmeasured variables; and
- a prolonged observation period that may include changes in transfusion and/or medical practice.

One of the positive aspects of the study by Koch and colleagues was their approach to analysis. They did not include patients who received both newer and older red cells, and they used propensity scoring to match patients in the newer and older red cell transfusion groups. However, as most seen with observational studies, the potential biases and limitations of the analysis do not allow for any definitive inclusions.

The use of cohort studies can be of particular value in the evaluation of a universally implemented intervention such as pre-storage leucocyte reduction. In such a case, subjects must either be sampled over a period of time prior to and after the implementation of the programme (a 'before-and-after' or interrupted time-series study) or sampling must occur among subjects who received leucocyte-reduced blood components and another population that did not receive such products (standardized incidence study).

In a before-and-after study design, the frequency of an outcome in a specified population is measured during a period of time when the exposure is absent, followed by a measurement in the same population during a period of time where exposure is present. Consecutive periods before and after the implementation of a treatment are often compared. When a single measurement in both the pre- and postintervention periods are compared, there is the risk that changes occurring as a result of other ongoing factors may be attributed to the intervention. To limit this temporal bias, the changes in the experimental group may be compared to a control group not exposed to the intervention (controlled before-and-after study). Alternatively, an interrupted time-series design (a before-and-after study that makes determinations of an outcome at multiple time points before and after the implementation of an intervention) may be used to account for any temporal changes occurring during the period observation.

In a standardized incidence study, a standardized incidence ratio is calculated by comparing (standardizing) the incidence of an outcome in a defined exposed population with that of a nonexposed population. In the standardization procedure, care is taken to adjust for important confounders. Using universal leucocyte reduction as an example, the incidence of nosocomial infection in Canadian patients receiving a transfusion could be compared to a US population of transfused patients receiving non-leucocyte-reduced blood components.

Well-executed case–control studies may provide clues about the aetiology or risk factors associated with the development of a disease or a complication. A cohort study may provide the best estimate of incidence, prognosis and risks associated with the development of a disease or its complications. Both designs provide weak inferences regarding specific therapeutic interventions because many forms of bias and confounding remain even after complex multivariable analysis. Before-and-after studies and time-series analysis, both quasi-experimental designs, may provide some inferences regarding clinical consequences attributed to the implementation of a universal programme when a randomized trial is not possible [9]. Inherent in both case–control and cohort studies is the inability to determine causality between a risk factor or treatment and a specific outcome.

Randomized controlled trials

Overall design approaches for RCTs

Clinicians, hospital administrators and policymakers should always seek to identify the best evidence for decision making. Researchers should aspire to conduct the highest quality studies. For therapeutic interventions, there is little debate that this should be an RCT. However, there should be an awareness that randomized trials may be complex. The question being addressed, the many choices and compromises made by the investigators pertaining to different study manoeuvres, such as the selection of patients and centres, may affect inferences made from the results of the trial. In this section, a conceptual framework is provided for randomized trials that should assist providers and consumers of clinical research.

The ideal RCT establishes whether therapeutic interventions work and determines the overall benefits and risks of each alternative in predefined patient populations. This is accomplished by minimizing the influence of chance, bias and confounding through appropriate methodology. In addition, the ideal RCT should attempt to fulfil its objectives with the fewest patients possible (often termed 'statistical efficiency'). Unfortunately, these objectives are often in direct conflict rather than complementary. More importantly, economic considerations often limit our ability to fulfil all these objectives. For instance, by maximizing the efficiency of a study, investigators might sacrifice their ability to draw conclusions in clinically important subgroups because of an inadequate sample size.

The most important consequence of these conflicting objectives is that choices made in the design of RCTs must focus on whether an intervention works or whether it results in more good than harm for patients [10]. Trials that attempt to determine therapeutic *efficacy* address the question 'Will the therapy work under ideal conditions?' Trials attempting to determine therapeutic *effectiveness* address the question 'Will the therapy do more good than harm under usual practice conditions in all patients who are offered the intervention?' Clearly, both questions will yield useful information for health practitioners. Efficacy is often established first and then the intervention may be evaluated for its effectiveness. In pivotal RCTs used in the final phase of obtaining regulatory approval (phase III trials), pharmaceutical companies primarily wish to demonstrate that their product has proven efficacy; rarely are attempts made to demonstrate therapeutic effectiveness.

The design characteristics of efficacy and effectiveness trials tend to differ considerably (Table 45.1). As a consequence of design choices, inferences and threats to the validity of effectiveness and efficacy trials are different. Therefore, one of the first steps in planning an RCT is to determine which of these two design approaches will best reflect the primary study question. Efficacy trials often opt for restricted eligibility, rigorous treatment protocols and disease-specific outcomes responsive to the potential benefits of the experimental intervention. By using this approach efficacy studies attempt to maximize internal validity, defined as the extent to which the experimental findings represent the true effect in study participants. As a consequence, this design approach will often lack the ability to maximize external validity, defined as the extent to which the experimental findings in the study represent the true effect in the target. Hence, there is often a trade-off between the two forms of validity in any one study.

Table 45.1 Comparison of study characteristics using either an efficacy or an effectiveness approach when designing a study.

Study characteristics	Efficacy trial	Effectiveness trial
Research question	Will the intervention work under ideal conditions?	Will the intervention result in more good than harm under usual practice conditions?
Setting	Restricted to specialized centres	Open to all institutions
Patient selection	Selected, well-defined patients	A wider range of patients identified using broad eligibility criteria
Study design	Smaller RCT using stringent rules	Larger multicentre RCT using simpler rules
Baseline assessment	Elaborate and detailed	Simple and clinician friendly
Intervention	Tightly controlled	Less controlled
	Optimal therapy under optimal study conditions	Therapy administered by investigators using accepted approaches
Treatment protocols	Rigorous and detailed.	Very general.
Compliance		Non compliance tolerated.
Endpoints	Disease-related	Patient-related such as all-cause mortality or quality of life
	Related to biologic effect	
	Surrogate endpoints	
Analysis	By treatment received	Intention-to-treat
	Noncompliers removed	All patients included
Data management		
Data collection	Elaborate	Minimal and simple
Data monitoring*	Detailed and rigorous.	Minimal

*Data monitoring refers to the review of source documents and adjudication/verification of outcomes.

As an example of an efficacy trial, Rivers and colleagues undertook an RCT in which they randomly allocated 263 patients with early sepsis and septic shock to receive either goal-directed therapy using a monitor of continuous central venous saturation in one group versus standard care in the other arm of the trial [11]. Both groups received fluids, vasopressors such as noradrenaline (norepinephrine), inotropic agents such as dobutamine and red cell transfusions according to a strict clinical algorithm. In addition to the clinical algorithm, the goal-directed therapy arm was required to maintain mixed venous saturation greater than 70%. Saturations below 70% suggest an ongoing oxygen debt and shock. In the first 6 hours of care in the emergency department, the experimental group received more fluids (4981 mL versus 3499 mL, $p < 0.001$), more inotropic agents (13.7% versus 0.8% of patients, $p < 0.001$) and more red cell transfusions (64.1% versus 18.5% of patients, $p < 0.001$). As a result of the multiple interventions including red cells, in-hospital mortality was decreased from 46.5 to 30.5% ($p < 0.009$). In this efficacy study, many of the study manoeuvres were tightly controlled. Specifically, the trial was conducted in a single tertiary centre, by a small number of experts, in a well-defined patient population using elaborate treatment algorithms in both the experimental and standard of care groups. This efficacy approach may be contrasted with large cardiovascular trials such as the International Study of Infarct Survival trials in acute myocardial infarction, which enrolled thousands of patients [12]. One of the major shortcomings of effectiveness trials is the limited data collection and the limited control imposed on most aspects of the study design, thereby increasing biological variability, minimizing information on biological mechanisms and curtailing the possibility of understanding negative results, or the influence of cointerventions and confounding on study outcomes. One of the few examples of a large simple trial design in transfusion medicine is the saline-versus-albumin fluid evaluation (SAFE) study, which randomized 7000 critically ill with a wide variety of illnesses to 4% albumin or saline as a resuscitation fluid [13]. This trial found that mortality did not differ between the two groups. The lack of benefit of albumin makes its use, which is expensive, hard to justify in this group of patients. However, as a downside of the broad inclusion criteria, questions remain about the benefits of albumin in subgroups such as septic patients where a biologic rationale supporting its use exist.

Many trials opted for a hybrid approach between large simple trials and tightly controlled clinical studies. The Transfusion Requirements in Critical Care (TRICC) trial [14] or the Platelet Dose (PLADO) trial [15] provide examples. The former was an 838-patient trial that randomly allocated patients to either a restrictive or a liberal transfusion strategy. The study was conducted in 25 clinical centres, enrolled patients using broad eligibility criteria, followed simple treatment strategies for the administration of red cells and ascertained mortality rates and rates of organ failure [14]. The latter randomized 1272 patients in 26 sites with hypoproliferative thrombocytopenia to receive low, medium or high dose prophylactic platelet transfusions, and assessed the bleeding complications and platelet utilization in recipients [15].

RCT design alternatives

Once investigators have chosen whether an efficacy, effectiveness or a hybrid approach will best answer the research question, there are several design options that may be considered (Table 45.2). A two-group parallel design is the most common of RCT design choices (Figure 45.2a). In this design, patients are randomly allocated to one of two therapeutic interventions and followed forward in time. It is the simplest to plan, implement, analyse and, most importantly, interpret. Therefore, a parallel group design is the most frequently adopted choice of RCT design. Parallel group designs may also be used to independently compare three or more treatments [16].

The use of factorial designs may also be considered when a number of therapies are being evaluated in combination. For instance, in a two-by-two (2×2) factorial design, two interventions are tested both alone and in combination, and compared with a control group (usually a placebo) (Figure 45.2b) [17]. This means that investigators can efficiently test two interventions with only marginal increases in sample

Table 45.2 Types of randomized clinical trial (RCT) designs.

Type of RCT	Description	Advantage	Disadvantage
Two group parallel	Patients randomized to one of two groups	Simplest approach widely used and accepted	Limited to simple comparisons
Factorial (2×2)	Patients randomized to one of four groups; therapy a, therapy b, therapy a + b or control	Combinations of therapy may be compared	Larger sample size required More complex design
Sequential study	Pairs of outcomes continuously compared in patients randomized to one of two therapies	Ongoing evaluations of therapy	Limited uses (efficacy only) Not a well-accepted approach Sample size unpredictable
Two-period crossover	Patients allocated to one of two therapies and then receive other therapy in second treatment period	Smaller sample required	Limited to reversible outcomes Major concern with carryover effect
N-of-1 trials	Single patient sequentially and repeatedly receives a therapy and a placebo	Optimal method of determining if a therapy is beneficial to a given patients	Results not generalizable Difficult in unstable patients Very labour intensive
Cluster design	Groups of patients are randomized	Ideal for programme or guideline evaluation	Less well accepted in clinical practice Difficult to implement when large variability between clusters

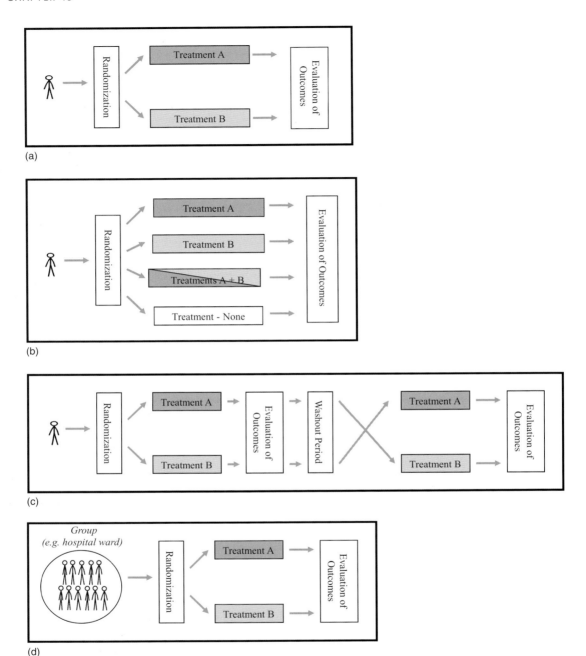

Fig 45.2 Design approaches for randomized controlled trials. Adapted from Tinmouth and Hébert [27]. (a) Randomized two-group parallel design: subjects randomly assigned to treatment A or B. (b) Factorial design: all subjects randomly assigned to treatment A, treatment B, treatment A + B or no treatment. (c) Randomized crossover design: subjects randomly assigned to treatment A followed by treatment B (after washout period) or treatment B followed by treatment A. (d) Randomized cluster design: all subjects in one group/area (e.g. by physician, by hospital, by ward) are assigned to treatment A or B.

size. In addition, the benefits of treatment combinations can be evaluated in a controlled manner. This design is most useful when interactions are either very strong or nonexistent. Thus, before embarking on a large, more complex factorial study, investigators should expect either strong additive or synergistic effects from combined therapy or none at all [17]. Prospective investigators should realize that detecting interactions is also more difficult and requires a much larger sample size as compared with comparison of either therapy with a placebo. Factorial designs have been used very successfully to evaluate thrombolytic therapy in combination with an antiplatelet agent in acute myocardial infarction and unstable angina [18].

Factorial designs imply concurrent comparisons between at least two therapies. It is also possible to implement a design that compares interventions sequentially. For example, two therapies in the early treatment of a disease could be compared, followed by the evaluation of a second intervention in the late phase of care several days later. The authors are not aware of any clinical studies in transfusion medicine that have made use of a factorial design. An example of a factorial trial would be to randomize patients to an algorithm of care versus standard care in addition to either a conservative or liberal transfusion threshold. Traditionally, the factorial design is used to answer two separate study questions.

Both the simple parallel group design and a factorial design are designed using classical or frequentist statistical approaches, where the sample size is fixed according to pre-established assumptions (anticipated outcomes in treatment and control group, power and significance levels) prior to the commencement of enrolment. There are other experimental designs that are more responsive to patient outcomes as the study progresses. Sequential designs use frequentist statistical methods to set boundaries for significance levels that consider the increasing number of comparisons and sample size throughout the study. True sequential studies randomly allocate patients to receive one of two therapies. Pairs of patients are then sequentially compared. The study is terminated as soon as one of the significance boundaries is crossed. One of the major concerns with this design may be its inability to conceal the randomization process and the uncertainty of not knowing the exact sample size in advance. From this methodology, several biostatisticians have developed methods of performing interim analyses in large clinical trials, referred to as group sequential methods [19]. A Bayesian statistical approach offers an alternative methodology. In a Bayesian analysis, previous beliefs about the effectiveness of a therapy are combined with the observed data from the trial to provide a new revised set of likely values for the effectiveness of the therapy. This approach allows for repeated or continuous monitoring of study results as patients accrue. As a result, predetermined sample sizes are not required and enrolment continues until the results meet predetermined significance levels. This can allow for increased trial efficiency as studies will not enrol additional patients unnecessarily or terminate the study prematurely. A Bayesian approach has also been advocated for interim analyses of large clinical trials [20].

Another RCT design option particularly amenable to an efficacy evaluation is a two-period crossover study in which patients are used as their own controls. In a two-period crossover trial, patients are randomized to one of two therapies for a fixed period of time and then proceed to receive the other therapy in a second comparable interval (Figure 45.2c). Minimizing 'between-subject' variability in this manner makes significant gains in efficiency. Crossover studies are therefore best suited to relatively stable conditions (stability is required during the study), interventions with rapid onset of action and a very short half-life (the biological effect must disappear prior to the second treatment period), and rapidly modifiable endpoints such as haemodynamic and respiratory measures [17]. An example of a crossover trial in transfusion medicine would be the evaluation of a modified red cell product (e.g. bacterially inactivated or pegylated red cells) in patients with transfusion-dependent congenital anaemias. The time to next transfusion or red cell survival could be measured in patients who receive, in a random order, standard red cell transfusions and modified red cell transfusions for fixed periods of time. An appropriate washout time between the two interventions is required to ensure there is no contamination of the modified red cells during the period of standard transfusions.

All designs discussed so far have described the evaluation of interventions for individual patients. However, it is sometimes necessary to evaluate therapies, protocols, guidelines or treatment programmes for groups of individuals. Using this design, groups or 'clusters' such as ICUs, wards, hospitals and physician practice are randomized to receive an intervention or control (Figure 45.2d). Cluster design may be the most appropriate design for evaluating complex or multidimensional interventions such as the implementation of care paths, educational interventions, transfusion audits or other interventions to change transfusion practice. For these evaluations, the cluster is a more natural method of allocation than the individual [9]. Cluster trials are advantageous when there is a real risk that the intervention will be implemented in all patients rather than only the patients assigned to receive the therapy. When individuals in the control group receive the intervention or elements of the intervention, this contamination biases the results of the study. This may easily occur when one is evaluating guidelines, educational interventions, interventions designed to modify health provider behaviour and administrative changes to systems. However, the allocation of interventions to groups rather than individuals comes at a cost. The sample size is usually larger as a result of the nonindependence within the group and it is often difficult to infer what happened at an individual level [21]. As a result, this design has many detractors. An additional concern in cluster trials is the possibility of large variations between clusters that may make it difficult to detect actual differences between therapies [21].

In a cluster randomized trial, Murphy *et al.* [22] randomized wards at different hospitals to receive units of red cells with labels reminding nurses to check the patient and component identification. The randomization by wards was important to ensure that transfusions given without the reminder were not given by nurses who had been previously exposed to the intervention (reminders tags). In this study, the reminder tags did not result in an improvement in the bedside check for transfusion.

Selecting a study population

In transfusion medicine, most blood components are currently used in a wide variety of diseases and conditions. The choice of study population will invariably depend on the study question, the underlying hypothesis and on a number of other factors. The choice of a hypothesis that will address either therapeutic efficacy or effectiveness will have a substantial impact on the selection of the study population [10]. Specifically, in choosing an efficacy approach, investigators usually perform the study in a well-defined patient population where the intervention has the highest probability of demonstrating an effect. This may be done by narrowly defining the patient population through the use of restrictive eligibility criteria and disease definitions, as well as selecting specialized centres with clinical expertise in the field. Choosing a narrowly defined study population will decrease overall variability attributed to patient selection but may have adverse consequences such as hampering patient recruitment and jeopardizing the generalizability of study results. When defining the eligibility criteria for an effectiveness trial, investigators should consider utilizing more liberal criteria in a wide range of clinical settings (e.g. medical or surgical critically ill patients with a broad range of primary diagnoses or underlying conditions from a range of tertiary care centres).

On the spectrum between highly selected patients (efficacy) and a large patient population (effectiveness), investigators should consider a number of factors in making the decision (Table 45.3). The spectrum of biological activity of the intervention is an important consideration. For instance, a narrow spectrum of biological activity should translate into restricted eligibility while a broad spectrum of biological activity should yield more liberal eligibility criteria. Eligibility may also be restricted through the selection of

Table 45.3 Considerations in determining which design approach to implement in transfusion trials.

Criteria to consider	Choice of design	
	Favouring efficacy	Favouring effectiveness
Evidence	Limited evidence	Efficacy well documented
Importance of the question	Rare and less serious	Common and serious problem
Feasibility	Not demonstrated	Adequate accrual and confirmed feasibility
Risks	Unknown or significant consequences	Minimal or acceptable risks given benefits
Benefits	Limited or unknown benefits	Significant benefits anticipated

study centres. In efficacy trials, highly specialized units should be sought while studies evaluating the effectiveness of an intervention would require the inclusion of a large number of nonspecialized centres. In practice, investigators should first focus on therapeutic efficacy and study the intervention in high risk and/or well-defined patient populations.

Selecting outcomes (Table 45.4)

In most clinical trials, the clinical investigative team should consider a number of potential outcomes, both fatal and nonfatal. An outcome is defined as a measurement (e.g. haematocrit) or an event (e.g. death) potentially modified following the implementation of an intervention. If all are given equal consideration, concerns arise about multiple comparisons and interpretation of a study with heterogeneous findings. Thus it is important to choose a primary outcome that will determine an intervention's therapeutic success or failure. Secondary outcomes will provide supportive evidence in secondary analyses and assess potential adverse outcomes. As a corollary, a predefined hierarchy implies that the investigators believe that clinically or statistically important differences in secondary outcomes, in the absence of important changes in the primary outcome, will not be interpreted as strong evidence of therapeutic benefit. The primary outcome is also essential in determining the sample size requirements in a clinical trial. Thus, once a decision has been made to determine either therapeutic efficacy or

Table 45.4 Guides to the choice of outcome measure in an RCT.

1 Is the outcome causally related to the consequences of the disease?
2 Is the outcome clinically relevant to the healthcare providers and/or patients?
3 Has the validity of the outcome (for complex outcomes such as scoring systems or composite outcomes) been established?
4 Is the outcome easily and accurately determined?
5 Is the outcome responsive to changes in a patient's condition?
6 Is the outcome measure potentially able to discriminate between patients who benefit from a therapy from patients in the control group?

effectiveness (or possibly a combined approach), the second task facing investigators is determining and ranking outcomes as primary and secondary.

The choice of study outcome is one of the most important design considerations to be made by investigators. However, there are a number of factors that should be considered prior to selection of an outcome. The primary outcomes should be considered clinically important and easily ascertained. By fulfilling these two criteria, the investigator will have a much greater chance of influencing clinical practice once a study has been completed and published. Outcomes should also measure what they are supposed to measure (validity) and be precise and reproducible. An outcome must be able to detect a clinically important true positive or negative change in the patient's condition following a therapy.

The sample size in a clinical trial comparing two therapies is based on the baseline event rate, the expected incremental benefit or difference, the level of significance (α) and the power to detect differences ($1 - \beta$). Establishing the incremental benefit of a new therapy is vitally important because of the enormous sample size repercussions. A sample size calculation for an RCT requires that the investigators establish the minimum therapeutic effect detectable within the trial. This difference in outcomes between interventions is referred to as the minimally important difference (MID) or minimal clinically important difference (MCID) [10]. The MID is essentially establishing the level of discrimination in the study population who are exposed to the interventions given acceptable levels of type I (finding a difference when one does not truly exist) and type II (not finding a difference when one truly exists) errors and the baseline event rate. Too often, investigators calculate a sample size based on very large and unrealistic expected differences in outcomes. To determine a plausible effect size, investigators should ask themselves the following questions:

• What difference or incremental benefit can be realistically expected of the experimental therapy? (Anticipated biological effect of therapy.)
• Are the required number of patients available to participate in the clinical trial? (Feasibility.)
• How much of a benefit, given the added costs and expected adverse effects of therapy, would be required for clinicians, patients and administrators to adopt a new therapy? (Overall benefit of therapy.)

As a concrete example, assuming that a given study population has an expected mortality rate of 25% in the standard therapy group while the experimental therapy is expected to decrease mortality by an absolute difference of 12.5% (a 50% relative risk reduction), the total number of patients required would be approximately 250. Most therapies used in the ICU would not be expected to decrease mortality so dramatically. More realistic expectations may be in the range of a 5% absolute decrease (a 20% relative risk reduction), which would require a total sample size of 2200 patients respectively if the baseline mortality was 25%. Investigators need to consider whether an absolute incremental benefit in the range of 5–10% is attainable using the experimental therapy. If not, another more discriminating outcome should be sought.

Frequently, the treatment effect or difference in the desired outcome is small. As a result, a surrogate or composite outcome may be chosen as the primary outcome for a trial to reduce the sample size. A surrogate outcome is defined as a laboratory or physical measure that accurately reflects a clinically meaningful outcome and, therefore, can act as a substitute outcome with the goal of reducing the sample size [23, 24]. A composite outcome combines more than one individual outcome. The latter may increase statistical efficiency and can combine multiple endpoints that are equally important [24]. Both approaches must be used judiciously and results interpreted with caution [24, 25]. Surrogate endpoints should clearly predict the clinical outcome, which may not be the case (e.g. corrected count increment and bleeding in platelet transfusion trials) [23, 25]. Composite outcomes must be related, equally important, biologically plausible and clinically relevant [23, 24].

Conclusion

In this chapter on interventional studies in transfusion medicine, several major observational and interventional design characteristics have been discussed. Study design issues of special interest to health professionals interested in transfusion medicine have been outlined. Suggestions when planning a RCT in transfusion medicine are provided in Table 45.5. Observational and quasi-experimental studies may provide invaluable information in transfusion medicine.

Table 45.5 Suggestions when planning an RCT in transfusion medicine.

1 Explicitly determine whether you are primarily interested in establishing therapeutic efficacy or effectiveness.
2 Whenever possible, undertake an RCT as part of a broader research programme.
3 If the study intervention is complex (or risky) or if other aspects of study feasibility are questionable, a pilot study should be considered.
4 Whenever possible, investigators should use simple rather than complex designs (two groups parallel design versus factorial design).
5 The study population should be tailored to the intervention.
6 Ideally, the study intervention and treatment protocols should not aim to substantially modify or affect usual clinical practice.
7 Given the complexity of RCTs, data collection should aim to clearly describe the study population, describe cointerventions and all major study outcomes.
8 In choosing primary study endpoints investigators should focus on patient-oriented outcomes rather than surrogate or biological markers.
9 If you are planning a seminal RCT, you may only have one chance to get it right. When making compromises, always opt to answer questions that most clinicians consider most important.
10 In establishing the minimally important difference, select a potentially achievable benefit.

Although RCTs provide the most unbiased and accurate assessment of the efficacy and effectiveness of therapeutic and preventive interventions, they remain challenging and expensive to conduct. As more research groups form to address unanswered therapeutic questions in transfusion medicine, investigators will invariably better understand the strengths and limitations of different RCT design characteristics.

Key points

1 Properly conducted RCTs are the best means to evaluate the risk and benefits of therapeutic interventions.
2 Observational studies can be useful when RCTs are not feasible: case–control studies are particularly

useful to evaluate rare outcomes and cohort studies can examine outcomes following known exposures, risk factors or therapies; however, all observational studies are prone to biases and cannot show causation.

3 The design of an RCT depends on whether the investigators wish to evaluate the *efficacy* or the *effectiveness* of an intervention.

4 A two-group parallel group design is the simplest RCT to design, execute and evaluate, but alternative designs can be useful in specific circumstances.

5 Selecting the appropriate study population and the outcomes are critical to ensure both the feasibility of completing the RCT and the generalizability and clinical relevance of the study results.

Acknowledgement

The authors wish to thank our students, teachers and colleagues who contributed many of the ideas outlined in this manuscript.

References

1 Hill AB. The clinical trial. *N Engl J Med* 1952; 247(4): 113–119.

2 Kelsey RA, Whittemore AS, Evans AS & Thompson WD. *Case Control Studies: I. Planning and Execution*. Oxford: Oxford University Press; 1996, pp. 188–213.

3 Silliman CC, Boshkov LK, Mehdizadehkashi Z, Elzi DJ, Dickey WO, Podlosky L et al. Transfusion-related acute lung injury: epidemiology and a prospective analysis of etiologic factors. *Blood* 2003; 101(2): 454–462.

4 Wilson K, Code C & Ricketts MN. Risk of acquiring Creutzfeldt–Jakob disease from blood transfusions: systematic review of case–control studies. *Br Med J* 2000; 321(7252): 17–19.

5 Carson JL, Duff A, Berlin JA, Lawrence VA, Poses RM, Huber EC et al. Perioperative blood transfusion and postoperative mortality. *J Am Med Assoc* 1998; 279(3): 199–205.

6 Grimes DA & Schulz KF. Bias and causal associations in observational research. *Lancet* 2002; 359(9302): 248–252.

7 van de Watering L, for the Biomedical Excellence for Safer Transfusion (BEST) Collaborative. Pitfalls in the current published observational literature on the effects of red blood cell storage. *Transfusion* 2011; 51(8): 1847–1854.

8 Koch CG, Li L, Sessler DI, Figueroa P, Hoeltge GA, Mihaljevic T et al. Duration of red-cell storage and complications after cardiac surgery. *N Engl J Med* 2008; 358(12): 1229–1239.

9 Grimshaw J, Campbell M, Eccles M & Steen N. Experimental and quasi-experimental designs for evaluating guideline implementation strategies. *Fam Pract* 2000; 17 (Suppl. 1): S11–S16.

10 Sackett D. The principles behind the tactic of performing clinical trials. In: RB Haynes, D Sackett, G Guyatt & P Tugwell (eds). *Clinical Epidemiology: How to Do Clinical Practice Research*. Lippincott Williams and Wilkins; 2009, pp. 173–243.

11 Walker ID, Walker JJ, Colvin BT, Letsky EA, Rivers R & Stevens R. Investigation and management of haemorrhagic disorders in pregnancy. Haemostasis and Thrombosis Task Force. *J Clin Pathol* 1994; 47(2): 100–108.

12 Randomised trial of intravenous atenolol among 16 027 cases of suspected acute myocardial infarction: ISIS-1. First International Study of Infarct Survival Collaborative Group. *Lancet* 1986; 2(8498): 57–66.

13 Finfer S, Bellomo R, Boyce N, French J, Myburgh J & Norton R. A comparison of albumin and saline for fluid resuscitation in the intensive care unit. *N Engl J Med* 2004; 350(22): 2247–2256.

14 Hebert PC, Wells G, Blajchman MA, Marshall J, Martin C, Pagliarello G et al. A multicenter, randomized, controlled clinical trial of transfusion requirements in critical care. Transfusion Requirements in Critical Care Investigators, Canadian Critical Care Trials Group. *N Engl J Med* 1999; 340(6): 409–417.

15 Slichter SJ, Kaufman RM, Assmann SF, McCullough J, Triulzi DJ, Strauss RG et al. Dose of prophylactic platelet transfusions and prevention of hemorrhage. *N Engl J Med* 2010; 362(7): 600–613.

16 Fergusson DA, Hebert PC, Mazer CD, Fremes S, MacAdams C, Murkin JM et al. A comparison of aprotinin and lysine analogues in high-risk cardiac surgery. *N Engl J Med* 2008; 358(22): 2319–2331.

17 Friedman LM, Furberg CD & DeMets DL. *Fundamentals of Clinical Trials*, 3rd edn. New York: Springer-Verlag; 1998.

18 ISIS-3: a randomised comparison of streptokinase vs tissue plasminogen activator vsanistreplase and of aspirin plus heparin vs aspirin alone among 41,299 cases of suspected acute myocardial infarction. ISIS-3 (Third International Study of Infarct Survival) Collaborative Group. *Lancet* 1992; 339(8796): 753–770.

19 Spiegelhalter DJ, Myles JP, Jones DR & Abrams KR. Bayesian methods in health technology assessment: a review. *Health Technol Assess* 2000; 4(38): 1–130.

20 Freedman LS, Spiegelhalter DJ & Parmar MK. The what, why and how of Bayesian clinical trials monitoring. *Stat Med* 1994; 13(13–14): 1371–1383.

21 Donner A Klar N. *Design and Analysis of Cluster Randomization Trials in Health Research*. London: Arnold; 2000.

22 Murphy MF, Casbard AC, Ballard S, Shulman IA, Heddle N, AuBuchon JP *et al*. Prevention of bedside errors in transfusion medicine (PROBE-TM) study: a cluster-randomized, matched-paired clinical areas trial of a simple intervention to reduce errors in the pretransfusion bedside check. *Transfusion* 2007; 47(5): 771–780.

23 Heddle NM, Arnold DM & Webert KE. Time to rethink clinically important outcomes in platelet transfusion trials. *Transfusion* 2011; 51(2): 430–434.

24 Heddle NM & Cook RJ. Composite outcomes in clinical trials: what are they and when should they be used? *Transfusion* 2011; 51(1): 11–13.

25 Arnold DM & Lim W. The use and abuse of surrogate endpoints in clinical research in transfusion medicine. *Transfusion* 2008; 48(8): 1547–1549.

26 Tay J & Tinmouth A. Observational studies: what is a cohort study? *Transfusion* 2007; 47(7): 1115–1117.

27 Tinmouth A & Hébert P. Interventional trials: an overview of design alternatives. *Transfusion* 2007; 47(4): 565–567.

Further reading

Campbell DT, Stanley JC. *Experimental and Quasi-experimental Designs for Research*. Chicago, IL: Rand McNally College Publishing Company; 1966.

Carson JL, Duff A, Poses RM *et al*. Effects of anaemia and cardiovascular disease on surgical mortality and morbidity. *Lancet* 1996; 348: 1055–1060.

Friedman LM, Furberg CD & Demets DL. *Fundamentals of Clinical Trials*, 3rd edn. St Louis, MI: Mosby Year Book; 1996.

Grimes DA & Schulz KF. Bias and causal associations in observational research. *Lancet* 2002; 359(9302): 248–252.

Guyatt GH, Sackett DL & Cook DJ. Users' guides to the medical literature II. How to use an article about therapy or prevention. Are the results of the study valid? *J Am Med Assoc* 1993; 270: 2598–2601.

Haynes RB, Sackett DL, Guyatt GH & Tugwell P. *Clinical Epidemiology: A Basic Science for Clinical Medicine*, 3rd edn. Philadelphia, PA: Lippincott Williams and Wilkins, 2006.

Hébert PC, Wells G, Blajchman MA *et al*. and the Transfusion Requirements in Critical Care investigators for the Canadian Critical Care Trials Group. Transfusion Requirements in Critical Care: a multicentre randomized controlled clinical trial. *N Engl J Med* 1999; 340: 409–417.

Sackett DL. Bias in analytic research. *J Chron Dis* 1979; 32: 51–63.

Sackett DL. The competing objectives of randomized trials. *N Engl J Med* 1980; 303: 1059–1060.

Sackett DL & Gent M. Controversy in counting and attributing events in clinical trials. *N Engl J Med* 1979; 301: 1410–1412.

The SAFE Study Investigators. A comparison of albumin and saline for fluid resuscitation. *New Engl J Med* 2004; 350: 2247–2256.

46 Getting the most out of the evidence for transfusion medicine

Simon J. Stanworth[1], Susan J. Brunskill[2], Carolyn Doree[2], Sally Hopewell[3] & Donald M. Arnold[4]

[1]University of Oxford and NHS Blood and Transplant and Department of Haematology, John Radcliffe Hospital, Oxford, UK

[2]NHS Blood and Transplant, Systematic Review Initiative, Oxford, UK

[3]UK Cochrane Centre, Oxford, UK

[4]Department of Medicine, McMaster University and Canadian Blood Services, Hamilton, Ontario, Canada

What is meant by evidence-based medicine?

Evidence-based medicine (EBM) has been described by Sackett as 'the integration of best research evidence with clinical expertise and patient values' [1]. Proponents of EBM have particularly highlighted the nature of the evidence that is used to make clinical decisions, i.e. where is it from, how believable is it, how relevant is it to my patient and can it be supported by other data? However, evidence is only one of the factors driving clinical decision making, and clinicians will also need to consider the available resources and opportunities, individual patients' values and needs (physical, psychological and social), local clinical expertise and cost. In some situations, clinical judgement will determine that the available evidence for a specific problem is not applicable.

EBM is not just about obtaining and evaluating clinical research evidence; it is also a means by which effective strategies for self-learning can be applied, aimed at continuously improving clinical performance. The focus of this chapter will be to discuss core elements of EBM with particular reference to clinical research in transfusion medicine and to provide a practical approach to critical appraisal and study design.

Hierarchies of clinical evidence

Health research studies are designed to ultimately show evidence of causality. While causality is extremely difficult (or impossible) to prove, hierarchical levels of evidence provide increasing support for such association. Optimal evidence is the best evidence available to answer a question. Data derived from randomized controlled trials (RCTs) have generally been regarded as the strongest support for evidence of efficacy or effectiveness.

In 1948, the first modern RCT in medicine was published comparing streptomycin and bedrest for patients with pulmonary tuberculosis [2]. The authors chose to perform a controlled trial because 'the natural course of pulmonary tuberculosis is in fact so variable and unpredictable that evidence of improvement or cure following the use of a new drug in a few cases cannot be accepted as proof of the effect of that drug'. In that trial, assignment of patients to streptomycin or bedrest was done by 'reference to a statistical series based on random sampling numbers drawn up for each sex at each centre'. There were fewer deaths in the patients assigned to streptomycin (4 out of 55 patients) compared to bedrest alone (14 out of 52 patients) [2]. If the process of randomization is done correctly, differences in outcome(s) between groups should be attributable to the intervention and

Practical Transfusion Medicine, Fourth Edition. Edited by Michael F. Murphy, Derwood H. Pamphilon and Nancy M. Heddle.
© 2013 John Wiley & Sons, Ltd. Published 2013 by John Wiley & Sons, Ltd.

not to other confounding factors related to the patients demography, study setting or quality of care.

The most common (and simple) design for an RCT is a parallel design, in which participants are randomly allocated to one of two groups. However, the RCT design comes with inherent challenges:
• RCTs are costly and logistic problems can arise if these studies are conducted at multiple centres (which is necessary for large trials).
• Small RCTs may overestimate the effect of the intervention and may place too much emphasis on those outcomes with more striking results.
• Small RCTs may be designed to detect unreasonably large treatment effects (which they will never be able to show because of their small size).
• RCTs with nonsignificant results may never be fully reported or only found in abstract form – a phenomenon known as publication bias.
• Effects of interventions may be overgeneralized and inappropriately applied to different patient populations.
• RCTs are not suited to investigating low frequency rare adverse effects, prevalence rates or diagnostic criteria.

In contrast to RCTs, observational studies, such as cohort or case–control studies, whether prospective or retrospective, may demonstrate an association between intervention and outcome; however, it is often difficult to be sure that this association does not reflect the effects of unknown confounding factors. The influence of confounding factors and biased participant selection can dramatically distort the accuracy of the study findings in observational studies. This does not mean that findings from well-designed observational studies should be disregarded; such study designs can be very effective in establishing or confirming effects of large size. Interpretation is more difficult when the observed effects are small. Clinical questions addressing possible aetiology or monitoring adverse effects may be more suited to observational studies.

The above points have highlighted some of the limitations with both RCTs and observational studies. In order to identify any limitations in a study and understand the possible impact of such limitations, it is important for readers, and investigators gearing up to design their own studies, to know how to appraise the methodological quality of the research. Critical appraisal and evaluation will be discussed next.

Appraisal of primary research evidence for its validity and usefulness

One component of EBM is the critical appraisal of evidence generated from a study. Published RCTs should report sufficient detail pertaining to the study design, population, condition, intervention and outcome to allow the reader to make an independent assessment of the trial's strengths and weaknesses. Guidelines and checklists have been designed to help with the reporting and assessment of RCTs, such as those based on the CONSORT statement [3, 4]. As shown in Table 46.1, key components of the critical appraisal process for clinical trials relate to the methodology of the study (the participants, interventions and comparators, the outcomes, the sample size, the methods used for the randomization process, and whether research staff were blinded to treatment allocation) and the reporting of the results (the numbers randomized and the numbers analysed/evaluated, the numbers not available for analysis with reasons and the role of chance, i.e. confidence intervals). Inadequate methodology and poor reporting of the study methods and its findings does not provide the needed reassurance to readers that patient selection, study group

Table 46.1 Key components of the critical appraisal process for clinical trials. Reproduced from The Critical Appraisal Skills Programme worksheets, Milton Keynes Primary Care Trust, 2002.

Did the study ask a focused question?
Was the allocation of participants to the study arms appropriate?
Were the study staff and participants unaware (blind) to the treatment allocation?
Were all the participants who entered the study accounted for within the results?
Were all the participants followed up and data collected in the same way?
Was the study sample size big enough to minimize any play of chance that may occur?
How are the results presented and what is the main result?
How precise are the results?
Were all the important outcomes for this patient population considered?
Can the results be applied to practice/different populations?

assignment and outcome detection were not prone to bias, which may result in inaccurate inferences drawn from the data. Critical appraisal guidelines are also useful for authors of primary research because they define the information that should be included in their published reports.

One aspect of trial appraisal concerns the understanding of chance variation and sample size calculation. One needs to distinguish between 'no evidence of effect' and 'evidence of no effect': the former may be derived from results that are either underpowered or nonsignificant, whereas the latter implies a sufficient sample size to show superiority, equivalency or noninferiority. Information about sample size calculations should therefore be provided in the published report of clinical trials.

Comparable standards can be applied to the critique of observational studies using a framework called STROBE (Strengthening the Reporting of Observational Studies in Epidemiology) [5, 6].

Reviews: narrative and systematic

Reviews have long been used to provide summary statements of the evidence for clinical practice. Reviews can be narrative or systematic. Often written by experts in the field, narrative reviews provide an overview of the relevant findings, as well as being educational and informative. However, narrative reviews summarize the evidence based on what the authors feel is important. On the other hand, systematic reviews gather the totality of the evidence on a subject and summarize it in an objective way using prespecfied methods for study identification, selection, quality assessment and analysis that limits bias.

Systematic reviews aim to be more explicit and less biased in their approach to reviewing a subject than traditional (narrative) literature reviews and they can provide a synthesis of results of primary studies, making them more accessible to clinicians and policy makers. Systematic reviews also form the background for clinical trial design by establishing what is currently known, what methods were used to achieve that knowledge and what gaps remain. Systematic reviews are not substitutes for adequately powered clinical trials, but should be considered as complementary methods of clinical research.

There are generally accepted 'rules' about how to undertake a systematic review, which include:
• developing a focused review question;
• comprehensively searching for all material relevant to this question (Table 46.2 provides some practical suggestions when developing a more comprehensive search strategy);
• using explicit criteria to assess eligibility and methodological quality of identified studies;
• reporting and explaining why studies were excluded; and
• using explicit methods for combining data from primary studies including, where appropriate, meta-analysis of the study data.

Meta-analysis, strictly speaking, refers to mathematically pooling data from primary studies. This method is acceptable for a systematic review when primary studies are sufficiently homogeneous in their design and quality to show any difference in treatment effect between the two treatment groups.

Results from each study within a systematic review are typically presented in the form of a graphical display, called a 'forest plot'. A hypothetical example is shown in Figure 46.1. The result for the outcome point estimate in each trial is represented by a square, together with a horizontal line that corresponds to the 95% confidence intervals (CIs). For summary statistics of binary or dichotomous data, effect measures are typically summarized as either a relative risk or an odds ratio (for definitions, see Figure 46.1). The 95% CI provides a very useful measure of effect, in that it represents the range of values that will contain the true size of treatment effect 95% of the time, should the study be repeated again and again. The solid vertical line corresponds to no effect of treatment (or a relative risk of 1.0 for the analysis of dichotomous data, see Figure 46.1). Forest plots, therefore, are a visual representation of the size of treatment effects between different trials and allow the reader to assess:
• the effect of treatment by examining whether the bounds of the confidence interval exceed or overlap the minimal clinically important benefit;
• the consistency of the direction of the treatment effects across multiple studies; and
• outlying results from some studies relative to others.

Figure 46.2 provides an overall guide for assessing the validity of evidence for treatment decisions for the different types of studies, trials and reviews mentioned in this section. Although sometimes criticized for their

Table 46.2 List of selected sources that can be searched to identify reports of trials and clinical evidence.

PRINCIPLES OF EFFECTIVE LITERATURE SEARCHING

A. WRITING THE RESEARCH QUESTION & SELECTING SEARCH TERMS

Construct your question as simply as possible by combining (ideally) any two of the four parts of the PICO formula below. Then add any relevant synonyms and/or alternative spellings, while keeping the search as simple as possible. For example, the question "Is Factor VIIa effective for the prevention of bleeding in patients without haemophilia" is best searched for as intervention AND outcome – "Factor VIIa" **AND** "the prevention of bleeding":

PATIENT/CONDITION	INTERVENTION	COMPARISON	OUTCOME
Nonhaemophiliacs [too large a group to search for – exclude from search)	**(factor VIIa OR activated factor vii OR activated factor seven OR recombinant factor vii OR recombinant factor seven OR rfviia OR fviia OR novoseven)**	Other methods of bleeding prevention (again, too large a group to search for–exclude)	**(bleeding OR bloodloss OR blood loss OR hemorrhage OR haemorrhage OR hemorrhaging OR haemorrhaging)**

B. TIPS FOR SEARCHING IN PUBMED

1) Use Boolean operators "AND" and "OR" to combine groups of search terms, but use "NOT" with care
2) Use truncation to reduce the number of search terms: e.g. bleed* or haemorrhag* OR hemorrhag*
3) Make use of the MeSH (Medical Subject Headings) indexing system, exploding terms if a broader (more sensitive) search is required [mh], or restricting to major MeSH headings if a more targeted search is needed [majr]
4) For a narrow, targeted search, try by title alone – e.g. factor viia[ti] OR fviia[ti] OR rfviia[ti]
5) Quick therapy search: (systematic[sb] OR randomized controlled trial[pt] AND search terms)

C. CHOOSING A STUDY DESIGN(S)

Search for information from the highest level evidence, working down this list if there is little or no relevant evidence at higher levels:
Levels of evidence
1) Evidence from at least one **systematic review**
2) Evidence from at least one **randomised controlled trial (RCT)**
3) Evidence from a well-designed **observational study** (i.e. **cohort or case control studies**)
4) Evidence from well-designed nonexperimental studies (e.g. **case series and case reports**)
5) Expert opinion (e.g. overviews, narrative reviews)

D. SOURCES TO SEARCH

i) For **Therapeutic studies** – Start by searching for systematic reviews and randomised controlled trials (RCTs), thereafter ongoing RCTs (to source current research) and lastly observational studies.

Systematic Reviews:	**Randomised Controlled Trials:**
• Transfusion Evidence Library – www.transfusionevidencelibrary.com • PubMed Clinical Queries (NLM) – www.ncbi.nlm.nih.gov/pubmed/clinical • TRIP database – www.tripdatabase.com • Cochrane Database of Systematic Reviews (CDSR) & Database of Abstracts of Reviews of Effects (DARE), *The Cochrane Library* (Wiley) – www.thecochranelibrary.com	• CENTRAL, *The Cochrane Library* (Wiley) – www.thecochranelibrary.com • PubMed Clinical Queries (NLM) – www.ncbi.nlm.nih.gov/pubmed/clinical • MEDLINE (Ovid/EBSCO) – enter "Randomized Controlled Trial.pt" AND (search terms) • EMBASE (Ovid/ESBSCO) – enter search terms + Additional Limits – Clinical Queries – Therapy • CINAHL (EBSCO) – enter (search terms) AND randomi*.ti,ab
Ongoing Trials:	**Observational Studies:**
• WHO International Clinical Trials Registry Platform - http://apps.who.int/trialsearch/	• MEDLINE, EMBASE and CINAHL, using 'Expert Searches'

ii) For **Diagnostic studies** – PubMed Clinical Queries – select 'Diagnosis', either broad or narrow (see above)
iii) For **Prognostic studies** – PubMed Clinical Queries – select 'Prognosis', either broad or narrow (see above)
iv) For **Cost effectiveness studies** – NHS EED in *The Cochrane Library* (www.thecochranelibrary.com)
v) For **Uncertainties about Treatment Effects** – DUETS (www.library.nhs.uk/duets/).

E. FURTHER SUGGESTIONS

• If time is at a premium, look first at sources that synthesise the evidence (e.g. Transfusion Evidence Library, PubMed, TRIP, NHS Evidence)
• Manage multiple searches by downloading results into bibliographic software – e.g. EndNote or Reference Manager
• If searching for a research project or paper, always record the search terms used and databases and dates searched
• Stay up-to-date by saving your searches and setting up regular autoalerts in PubMed and/or other databases
• For further help, or to perform more extensive, systematic searches, make a friend of your hospital librarian!

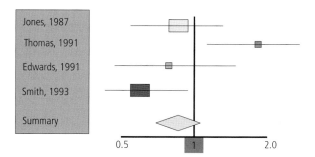

- The figure shows a forest plot display for four hypothetical studies.
- The point estimates for each trial have been presented as a relative risk for an outcome with discrete data. The blocks for the point estimates are different sizes, in proportion to the weight that each study takes in the analysis. Weighting is used in order to draw the reader's eye to the more precise studies.
- The relative risk (RR) is the ratio of risk in the intervention group to the risk in the control group. A RR of one (RR = 1.0) indicates no difference between comparison groups. For undesirable outcomes an RR that is less than 1 indicates that the intervention was effective in reducing the risk of that outcome.
- The diamond shape represents a summary point estimate for all trials. The vertical line corresponds to no effect of treatment. Thus if the 95% confidence interval crosses the vertical line, this indicates that the difference in effect of intervention therapy compared to control is not statistically significant at the level of $p > 0.05$ (please note there will be a 1 in 20 chance that the confidence interval does not include the true value). Such is the case in this example.
- Perhaps, the most important aspect of displaying the results graphically in this way is that it helps the reader look at the overall effects for each trial. Therefore, in this example, it should prompt the reader to ask why the results for one trial seem to be so different from the others (Thomas, 1991)?

Fig 46.1 A hypothetical forest plot.

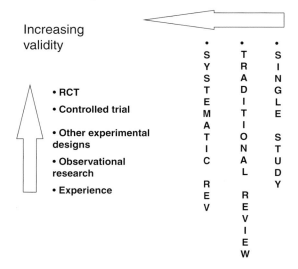

Fig 46.2 A guide for judging the validity of evidence for treatment decisions from different types of studies and reviews.

overemphasis on methodology at the expense of clinical relevance, and the inappropriate use of meta-analysis, systematic reviews have an important place in clinical practice as a means of transparently summarizing evidence from multiple sources. As for RCTs, guidelines for the reporting of systematic reviews have been developed including PRISMA (preferred reporting items for systematic reviews and meta-analyses) for the reporting of systematic reviews of RCTs and MOOSE (meta-analysis of observational studies in epidemiology) for the reporting of systematic reviews of observational studies [7, 8]. Quality assessment tools have also been development for critical appraisal of systematic reviews (the Critical Appraisal Skills Programme) (Table 46.3).

Evaluating systematic reviews and guidelines

The GRADE (Grading of Recommendations Assessment, Development and Evaluation) evaluation tool has been devised as a system for rating the quality of evidence in systematic reviews and grading the strength of recommendations in guidelines. The system is designed for reviews and guidelines that examine alternative management strategies or interventions, which may include no intervention or current best management. An example relevant to transfusion medicine is the recent guidelines on immune thrombocytopenia from the American Society of Hematology, which utilized GRADE methodology to evaluate the strength of recommendations [9, 10].

Comparative effectiveness research

Comparative effectiveness research (CER) is gaining support from both researchers and funding agencies, particularly in the USA and Canada. CER is defined as the conduct and synthesis of systematic research comparing different interventions and strategies to prevent, diagnose, treat and monitor health conditions. While experimental study designs like RCTs are highly valued methods of CER, they are costly, resource-intensive and their results may not be easily generalizable to nonstudy patients. Nonexperimental approaches using observational data are also useful tools for CER; however, they are inherently limited by heterogeneous methodologies, diverse designs and susceptibility to bias. As methods of observational studies continue to be refined, the data they derive may become more widely applicable, e.g. advances in the design of clinical registries and the use of encounter-generated data from sources such as electronic medical records.

The informing fresh-versus-old red cell management (INFORM) pilot trial is an example of CER in transfusion medicine [11]. The design was pragmatic; patients were randomized to receive one of two treatments that are already routinely used, thus obviating the need for individual informed consent; data were collected in real time from existing electronic databases, thereby reducing costs; and study procedures were streamlined, enabling randomization of more than 900 patients from a single centre in six months at very low cost. A larger pragmatic RCT with a similar design is planned to answer the question of the risk of mortality with fresh-versus-older blood. These data will inform policy decision around the maximum storage threshold that would optimize the balance between adequate supply and acceptable risk.

Table 46.3 Key components of the critical appraisal process for systematic reviews. Reproduced from The Critical Appraisal Skills Programme worksheets, Milton Keynes Primary Care Trust, 2002 and Systematic Review Initiative NBS in-house worksheets.

Did the review ask a clearly focused question?
Did the reviewers try to identify all relevant studies?
Were the eligibility criteria of the included studies detailed in the review?
Did the reviewers assess the quality of the included studies?
Have the results of the studies been combined and was it reasonable to do so?
How many studies were included in the review?
What is the main result for each outcome?
How precise are the results?
Were all the important outcomes for the review question considered?
How applicable are these results to clinical practice?

Evidence base for transfusion medicine

So, how good is the evidence base for transfusion medicine? As a first step, identification of all relevant RCTs in transfusion medicine would be essential. The Cochrane Collaboration's database of RCTs, the Cochrane Central Register of Controlled Trials (CENTRAL) (updated quarterly) is a good starting point. This database uses sensitive literature search filters that aim to identify all RCTs that have been catalogued on MEDLINE from 1966 and on the European medical bibliographic database, EMBASE, from 1980. High level evidence can be derived not only from methodologically sound RCTs but also from systematic reviews of RCTs. An excellent database of systematic reviews pertaining to transfusion medicine is the NHS Blood and Transplant's Systematic Review Initiative's Transfusion Evidence Library (www.transfusionevidencelibrary.com), a comprehensive online library of systematic reviews (updated monthly). The Transfusion Evidence Library will also, by 2013, include all RCTs relevant to transfusion medicine.

In addition, other databases of reviews for clinical evidence exist for clinicians, e.g. Bandolier (a print and Internet journal about healthcare using EBM techniques) and DARE (www.crd.york.ac.uk/crdweb). Table 46.2 presents a list of sources that can be searched to identify relevant reports of clinical trials and reviews.

The total number of published systematic reviews relevant to the broad theme of transfusion medicine was approximately 650 as of November 2011. These identified reviews cover topics ranging from the effective use of blood components including red cell thresholds [12] and fractionated blood components to alternatives to blood components and methods to minimize the need for blood in a surgical setting, and to blood safety. It should be noted that the searching filters for this exercise included stem cell and tissue transplantation and that the boundaries between transfusion medicine and other areas of medicine overlap (e.g. a systematic review of resuscitation fluids is relevant to transfusion medicine, critical care and anaesthesia). The search strategy also identified a number of areas of transfusion practice where few published systematic reviews exist, especially donation screening and blood donor selection. In paediatric transfusion practice, there is a paucity of evidence from RCTs or systematic reviews on which to base clinical decisions; notable recent examples of trials include a study of liberal and restrictive red cell transfusion thresholds and the treatment of neonatal sepsis with intravenous immune globulin trial [13–15]. For other clinical settings, even when systematic reviews were identified, many were only able to draw upon information from a very limited number of relevant randomized trials.

Evidence base for transfusion medicine: individual examples

Frozen plasma

Two recent relevant systematic reviews have attempted to address evidence relevant to the clinical use of FFP. The first asked the question about the evidence for whether abnormalities in coagulation tests predict an increased risk of clinical bleeding, as such abnormalities are important drivers for decisions to transfuse FFP. All relevant publications describing bleeding outcomes in patients with abnormalities in coagulation tests prior to invasive procedures were assessed. Overall, the published studies did not support evidence for a predictive value of PT/INR for bleeding [16].

The second systematic review was undertaken to identify and analyse all RCTs examining the clinical effectiveness of FFP (the first review published in 2005 has now been updated) [17, 18]. Comprehensive searching of the databases MEDLINE (1966–2002), Embase (1980–2002) and the Cochrane Library (2002, Issue 4) and detailed eligibility criteria, identified 80 RCTs as relevant for inclusion and analysis.

The analysis focused on:
• Studies of interventions comparing FFP with no FFP/plasma. These studies would be expected to provide the clearest evidence for a direct effect of FFP.
• Studies of interventions comparing FFP with a non-blood component (e.g. solutions of colloids and/or crystalloids).
• Studies of interventions comparing FFP with a different blood component or different formulations of FFP, e.g. solvent–detergent and methylene-blue treated.

Few of the identified studies included details of the study methodology (method of randomization, blinding of particicpants and study personnel). The sample size of many included studies was small (mean range 8–78 patients per arm). Few studies took adequate account of the extent to which adverse events might negate the clinical benefits of treatment with FFP. Taken together, many of the identified trials in groups such as cardiac, neonatal and other clinical conditions evaluated a prophylactic transfusion strategy. When these trials evaluating prophylactic usage were more closely assessed as a group in the systematic review, irrespective of clinical setting, it appeared that there was evidence (including from larger trials) for a *lack of effect* of prophylactic FFP. The overall finding of the review was that, for most clinical situations, RCTs examining the clinical use of FFP are limited.

Platelets

A number of different systematic reviews have been published that have more critically evaluated the evidence underpinning the following questions [19–21]:
• What is the appropriate threshold platelet count to trigger prophylactic platelet transfusions?
• What is the optimal dose for platelet transfusions?
• What is the evidence that a strategy of prophylactic platelet transfusions is superior to the use of platelet transfusions only in the event of bleeding (therapeutic use)?

The results from the four identified trials in the updated Cochrane Systematic Review evaluating different thresholds do not provide assurance that a 10×10^9/L threshold is as safe and effective as 20×10^9/L for all clinical outcomes, and indeed raise the critical question as to whether the combined studies have sufficient power to demonstrate equivalence in terms of the safety of the lower prophylactic threshold. This is because the combined results of the quantitative meta-analysis have confidence intervals that include both detrimental and beneficial effects. In contrast, the forest plots for summarizing the effect sizes in identified trials evaluating different platelet doses for transfusion clearly demonstrate no effect by dose, with much narrower confidence intervals.

The more fundamental question about whether a prophylactic platelet transfusion policy is any better than a therapeutic policy based on the aggressive use of platelet transfusions to treat the onset of clinical bleeding is unproven. The older age of the published identified randomized studies addressing this question raises questions of their applicability to current clinical practice, since the trials were conducted at a time when product specifications and quality control were very different, when supportive care for chemotherapy patients was less advanced and when antipyretics with antiplatelet activity, such as aspirin, were in common use. In addition to the small number of patients randomized in the trials, there was also considerable heterogeneity in the study population in relation to the indications for platelet transfusion, the definition of clinically significant bleeding, the threshold in the prophylaxis arm and in the dose of platelets given. Taken together, these analyses cast doubt on the validity of the data from published trials aimed at evaluating evidence for the effectiveness of prophylactic platelet transfusions.

Alternatives to transfusion

Many patients without haemophilia have now been treated, off-licence, with activated recombinant factor VII (rFVIIa). The patients settings are very diverse, including surgery (especially cardiac), gastrointestinal bleeding, liver dysfunction, intarcranial haemorrhage and trauma, for example. Data from 25 RCTs enrolling around 3500 patients have now evaluated the use of rFVIIa as both prophylaxis to prevent bleeding (14 trials) or therapeutically to treat major bleeding (11 trials), in patients without haemophilia [22]. This literature provides the more robust means

of assessing the effectivenss and safety of rFVIIa, and formed the basis of a recent updated Cochrane Review. When combined in meta-analysis, the trials showed modest reductions in total blood loss or red cell transfusion requirements (equivalent to less than one unit of red cell transfusion). However, the reductions were likely to be overestimated due to the limitations of the data. For other endpoints, including clinically relevant outcomes, there were no consistent indications of benefit and almost all of the findings in support of and against the effectiveness of recombinant factor VIIa could be due to chance. The one, and important, exception was thromboembolic events. In both groups of trials, there was an overall trend to increased thromboembolic events in patients receiving rFVIIa. The forest plots for total arterial thromboembolic events are shown in Figure 46.3 and reach statististical significance.

Common practices of transfusion and interventions to improve transfusion practice

Systematic reviews may also be applied to important questions about the evidence base for common or well-established practices in transfusion [23]. For example, some recent reviews based on observational, nonrandomized studies have addressed:

• What is the maximum time that one unit of RBCs can be out of the fridge before it becomes unsafe?
• How often should blood administration sets be changed while a patient is being transfused?
• Which blood transfusion administration method – one-person or two-person checks – is safest?

It is surprising and salutary to realize that some of these common recommendations appear to have little firm evidence base, yet are commonly reproduced in guidelines and protocols.

Are there limitations to evidence-based practice?

It is important to acknowledge some of the limitations of EBM that have been discussed by critics and supporters alike. EBM alone cannot provide a clinical decision; instead the findings generated from EBM are one strand of input driving decision-making in clinical practice. Each clinician will also need to consider the available resources and opportunities, the values

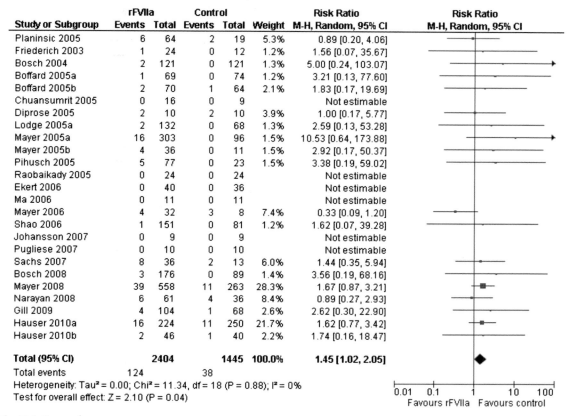

Study or Subgroup	rFVIIa Events	Total	Control Events	Total	Weight	Risk Ratio M-H, Random, 95% CI
Planinsic 2005	6	64	2	19	5.3%	0.89 [0.20, 4.06]
Friederich 2003	1	24	0	12	1.2%	1.56 [0.07, 35.67]
Bosch 2004	2	121	0	121	1.3%	5.00 [0.24, 103.07]
Boffard 2005a	1	69	0	74	1.2%	3.21 [0.13, 77.60]
Boffard 2005b	2	70	1	64	2.1%	1.83 [0.17, 19.69]
Chuansumrit 2005	0	16	0	9		Not estimable
Diprose 2005	2	10	2	10	3.9%	1.00 [0.17, 5.77]
Lodge 2005a	2	132	0	68	1.3%	2.59 [0.13, 53.28]
Mayer 2005a	16	303	0	96	1.5%	10.53 [0.64, 173.88]
Mayer 2005b	4	36	0	11	1.5%	2.92 [0.17, 50.37]
Pihusch 2005	5	77	0	23	1.5%	3.38 [0.19, 59.02]
Raobaikady 2005	0	24	0	24		Not estimable
Ekert 2006	0	40	0	36		Not estimable
Ma 2006	0	11	0	11		Not estimable
Mayer 2006	4	32	3	8	7.4%	0.33 [0.09, 1.20]
Shao 2006	1	151	0	81	1.2%	1.62 [0.07, 39.28]
Johansson 2007	0	9	0	9		Not estimable
Pugliese 2007	0	10	0	10		Not estimable
Sachs 2007	8	36	2	13	6.0%	1.44 [0.35, 5.94]
Bosch 2008	3	176	0	89	1.4%	3.56 [0.19, 68.16]
Mayer 2008	39	558	11	263	28.3%	1.67 [0.87, 3.21]
Narayan 2008	6	61	4	36	8.4%	0.89 [0.27, 2.93]
Gill 2009	4	104	1	68	2.6%	2.62 [0.30, 22.90]
Hauser 2010a	16	224	11	250	21.7%	1.62 [0.77, 3.42]
Hauser 2010b	2	46	1	40	2.2%	1.74 [0.16, 18.47]
Total (95% CI)		**2404**		**1445**	**100.0%**	**1.45 [1.02, 2.05]**
Total events	124		38			

Heterogeneity: Tau² = 0.00; Chi² = 11.34, df = 18 (P = 0.88); I² = 0%
Test for overall effect: Z = 2.10 (P = 0.04)

Favours rFVIIa Favours control

Fig 46.3 Forest plot.

and needs (physical, psychological and social) of the patient, the local clinical expertise and the costs of the intervention. Patients enrolled in clinical trials are not always the same as the individual patients requiring treatment, and generalizing to different clinical settings may not be appropriate. It has also been said that within EBM there is an overemphasis on methodology at the expense of clinical relevance, with the risks of generating conclusions that are either overly pessimistic or inappropriate for the clinical question. Perhaps we need to get away from the mentality that 'there is no good RCT evidence available to answer this clinical question' to thinking more about why this should be so, what can be learned from those studies that have already been completed, and what design of trial would answer the main area of uncertainty in this transfusion setting.

This chapter has attempted to explain why it is essential to assess the quality of primary clinical research and consider the risks of evidence being misleading, e.g. in the case of few trials or a failure to identify appropriate clinical research questions. Systematic reviews and the statistical method of meta-analysis are useful tools to achieve this, but, like trials themselves, can become outdated and must be carefully scrutinized to ensure unbiased results. Transfusion medicine is no different from many other branches of medicine, and the evidence base that informs much of the practice has not developed to the point that it can be universally applied with confidence. There is a need to recognize these uncertainties and to identify those transfusion issues that require high priority for clinical research.

Finally, appraising the evidence base for transfusion medicine is one part of improving practice; another is the effective dissemination of the evidence to clinicians. For example, clinicians may not have the time to search and evaluate the evidence themselves given the increasing numbers of publications and journals. As many of the sources are web-based, access at any one moment may be easier but the skills of appraisal need to be regularly maintained. Chapter 48 discusses aspects of changing practice in more detail.

Summary

There has been growing recognition that research, especially empirical research (based on observing what has happened), has been underutilized in making healthcare decisions at all levels. This appears to be as true for transfusion medicine as much as other clinical areas. EBM is an approach to developing and improving skills to identify and apply research evidence to clinical decisions. Even the most ardent proponents of EBM have never claimed it is a panacea, and there is recognition that it should amplify rather than replace clinical skills and knowledge, and be a driver for keeping healthcare practices up-to-date.

Systematic reviews can help bring together relevant literature on a particular problem and assess its strengths, weaknesses and overall meaning. Such reviews can be used in different ways including improving the precision of estimates of effect, generating hypotheses, providing background to new primary research or informing policy. Progress is being made to ensure that most areas in transfusion medicine are being systematically reviewed and some of these have encouraged plans for new RCTs.

Key points

1 The process of EBM consists of question formulation, searching for literature, critically appraising studies (identifying strengths and weaknesses) and decisions around applicability to one's patients.
2 It is essential to assess the quality of primary clinical research and consider the risks of evidence being misleading, e.g. in the case of few trials or a failure to identify appropriate clinical research questions.
3 Systematic reviews of RCTs combine evidence most likely to provide valid (truthful) answers on particular questions of effectiveness, and form an important component to the evaluation of evidence-based practice in transfusion medicine.

4 There is a common perception that much of transfusion medicine practice is based on limited evidence, but this is changing and systematic reviews are an important tool to collate, analyse and update the evidence base.

Acknowledgement

D. Arnold is funded by a New Investigator Award from the Canadian Institutes of Health Research in partnership with Hoffmann-LaRoche.

References

1 Sackett DL, Strauss SE, Richardson WS, Rosenberg W & Haynes RB. *Evidence Based Medicine: How to Practice and Teach EBM*, 2nd edn. Edinburgh: Churchill Livingstone; 2000.
2 Streptomycin treatment of pulmonary tuberculosis [no authors listed]. *Br Med J* 1948, 30 October; 2(4582): 769–782. PMID: 18890300.
3 Moher DF, Schulz KF & Altman DG. The CONSORT statement: revised recommendations for improving the quality of reports of parallel-group randomised trials. *Clin Oral Investig* 2003; 7(1): 2–7.
4 Schulz KF, Altman DG & Moher D, for the CONSORT Group. CONSORT 2010 Statement: Updated Guidelines for Reporting Parallel Group Randomised Trials. *PLoS Med* 2010; 7(3): e1000251. DOI: 10.1371/journal.pmed.100025; *Ann Intern Med* 2010. 1 June; 152(11): 726–732.
5 von Elm E, Altman DG, Egger M, Pocock SJ, Gøtzsche PC & Vandenbroucke JP, for the STROBE Initiative. The Strengthening the Reporting of Observational Studies in Epidemiology (STROBE) statement: guidelines for reporting observational studies. *Ann Intern Med* 2007; 147(8): 573–577.
6 von Elm E, Altman DG, Egger M, Pocock SJ, Gøtzsche PC & Vandenbroucke JP, for the STROBE Initiative. The Strengthening the Reporting of Observational Studies in Epidemiology (STROBE) statement: guidelines for reporting observational studies. *Lancet* 2007, 20 October; 370(9596): 1453–1457. PMID: 18064739.
7 Moher D, Liberati A, Tetzlaff J & Altman DG. The PRISMA Group (2009) Preferred Reporting Items for Systematic Reviews and Meta-Analyses: The PRISMA Statement. *PLoS Med* 6(7): e1000097. doi:10.1371/journal.pmed.1000097.
8 Stroup DF, Berlin JA, Morton SC, Olkin I, Williamson GD, Rennie D, Moher D, Becker BJ, Sipe TA &

Thacker SB, for the MOOSE (Meta-analysis of Observational Studies in Epidemiology) Group. Meta-analysis of observational studies in epidemiology: a proposal for reporting. *J Am Med Assoc* 2000, 19 April; 283(15): 2008–2012.

9 Guyatt GH, Oxman AD, Schünemann HJ, Tugwell P & Knotterus A. GRADE guidelines: a new series of articles in the *Journal of Clinical Epidemiology*. *J Clin Epidemiol* 2010, 23 December. Epub ahead of print.

10 Neunert C, Lim W, Crowther M, Cohen A, Solberg Jr L & Crowther MA, American Society of Hematology. The American Society of Hematology 2011 evidence-based practice guideline for immune thrombocytopenia. *Blood* 2011, 21 April; 117(16): 4190–4207.

11 Heddle NM, Cook RJ, Arnold DM, Crowther MA, Warkentin TE, Webert KE, Hirsh J, Barty RL, Liu Y, Lester C & Eikelboom JW. The effect of blood storage duration on in-hospital mortality: a randomized controlled pilot feasibility trial. *Transfusion* 2012, 18 January. DOI: 10.1111/j.1537-2995.2011.03521.x. Epub ahead of print.

12 Doree C, Stanworth S, Brunskill SJ, Hopewell S, Hyde CJ & Murphy MF. Where are the systematic reviews in transfusion medicine? A study of the transfusion evidence base. *Transfus Med Rev* 2010, 24(4): 286–294.

13 Carson JL, Hill S, Carless P, Hébert P & Henry D. Transfusion triggers: a systematic review of the literature. *Transfus Med Rev* 2002; 16(3): 187–199.

14 Lacroix J, Hébert PC, Hutchison JS, Hume HA, Tucci M, Ducruet T, Gauvin F, Collet JP, Toledano BJ, Robillard P, Joffe A, Biarent D, Meert K & Peters MJ; TRIPICU Investigators, Canadian Critical Care Trials Group, Pediatric Acute Lung Injury and Sepsis Investigators Network. Transfusion strategies for patients in pediatric intensive care units *N Engl J Med* 2007; 19 April; 356(16): 1609–1619.

15 INIS Collaborative Group; Brocklehurst P, Farrell B, King A, Juszczak E, Darlow B, Haque K, Salt A, Stenson B & Tarnow-Mordi W. *N Engl J Med* 2011, 29 September; 365(13): 1201–1211. PMID: 21962214.

16 Segal JB & Dzik WH. Paucity of studies to support that abnormal coagulation test results predict bleeding in the setting of invasive procedures: an evidence-based review. *Transfusion* 2005; 45: 1413–1425.

17 Stanworth SJ, Brunskill SJ, Hyde CJ, McLelland DBL & Murphy MF. Is fresh frozen plasma clinically effective? A systematic review of randomized controlled trials. *Br J Haematol* 2004; 126: 139–152.

18 Yang L, Stanworth SJ, Hopewell S, Doree C & Murphy M. Is fresh frozen plasma clinically effective? An update of a systematic review of randomized controlled trials. *Transfusion* 2011 (in press).

19 Cid J & Lozano M. Lower or higher doses for prophylactic platelet transfusions: results of a meta-analysis of randomized controlled trials. *Transfusion* 2007; 47(3): 464–470.

20 Estcourt L, Stanworth SJ, Hopewell S, Heddle N, Tinmouth A & Murphy MF. Prophylactic platelet transfusion for haemorrhage after chemotherapy and stem cell transplantation. *Cochrane Database Syst Rev* 2004/2011 (update), Issue 4. DOI: 10.1002/14651858. CD004269.pub2.

21 Tinmouth AT & Freedman J. Prophylactic platelet transfusions: which dose is the best dose? A review of the literature. *Transfus Med Rev* 2003; 17(3): 181–193.

22 Simpson E, Lin Y, Stanworth S, Birchall J, Doree C & Hyde C. Recombinant factor VIIa for the prevention and treatment of bleeding in patients without haemophilia. *Cochrane Database Syst Rev* 2011, Issue 2, Article No.: CD005011. DOI: 10.1002/14651858.CD005011. pub3.

23 Watson D, Murdock J, Doree C *et al.* Blood transfusion administration – 1 or 2 person checks, which is the safest method? *Transfusion* 2008; 48(4): 783–789.

Further reading

Centre for Reviews and Dissemination. Systematic Reviews CRD's guidance for undertaking reviews in healthcare. CRD, University of York; 2009.

Egger M, Davey Smith G & Altman DG. *Systematic Reviews in Health Care. Meta-analysis in Context*, 2nd edn. London: BMJ Publishing Group; 2001.

Guyatt GH & Rennie D. *Users' Guide to the Medical Literature: Essentials of Evidence-Based Clinical Practice*. Chicago, IL: American Medical Association; 2002.

Heddle NM. Evidence-based clinical reporting: a need for improvement. *Transfusion* 2002; 42: 1106–1110.

Higgins JPT & Green S (eds). Cochrane Handbook for Systematic Reviews of Interventions Version 5.1.0 [updated March 2011]. The Cochrane Collaboration, 2011. Available from: www.cochrane-handbook.org.

Hyde CJ, Stanworth SJ & Murphy MF. Can you see the wood for the trees! Making sense of the forest plot. 1. Presentation of the data from the included studies. *Transfusion* 2008; 48(2): 218–220.

Hyde CJ, Stanworth SJ & Murphy MF. Can you see the wood for the trees! Making sense of the forest plot. 2. Analysis of the combined results from the included studies. *Transfusion* 2008; 48(4): 580–583.

The Equator Network: Enhancing the Quality and Transparency of Health Research. Available at: http://www .equator-network.org/.

47 Variation in transfusion practice and how to influence clinicians' use of blood in hospitals

Simon J. Stanworth[1], *J.J. Francis*[2], *Michael F. Murphy*[1] *&*
Alan T. Tinmouth[3]

[1]University of Oxford and NHS Blood and Transplant and Department of Haematology, John Radcliffe Hospital, Oxford, UK
[2]Health Services Research Unit, University of Aberdeen, Aberdeen, Scotland
[3]General Hematology and Transfusion Medicine, Division of Hematology, Ottawa Hospital and University of Ottawa Centre for Transfusion Research, Clinical Epidemiology Program, The Ottawa Health Research Institute, Ottawa, Ontario, Canada

Background

Changing established patterns of transfusion practice is not easy. As the evidence base for transfusion medicine advances, there is an increasing need to ensure that important new research is rapidly implemented and that practice which is shown to be less effective (or cost-inefficient) is discontinued. Many of the methods used to facilitate change in clinical behaviour are familiar to hospital healthcare workers in the field of transfusion medicine. They include:

- guideline adoption and dissemination;
- educational materials or teaching sessions;
- the use of audits with feedback; and
- reminders.

But which is best or, put another way, which intervention delivers more effective and sustained change in transfusion prescribing behaviour in a cost-effective manner? Answers to these questions may help address comments frequently expressed at meetings, such as 'What is the point of doing yet another audit?' The wider volume of literature relevant to promoting clinical effectiveness and the uptake of effective practice is increasing substantially and this chapter will look at these issues with regard to reducing inappropriate transfusion practice.

Interventions to change practice

The different means of achieving changes in practice have been reviewed by many groups and cover a wide range of candidate 'strategies'. One (empirically based) general taxonomy of interventions developed and used by the Cochrane Collaboration Effective Practice and Organization of Care (EPOC) Group is reproduced below, to illustrate the breadth of different interventions.

(a) Professional
 - audit and feedback;
 - reminders;
 - educational – groups, meetings, outreach visits;
 - patient-mediated interventions; and
 - local opinion leaders.
(b) Financial
 - fee-for-service and
 - provider incentives.
(c) Organizational
 - clinical multidisciplinary teams and
 - changes to the setting/site of service delivery.
(d) Regulatory
 - changes in medical liability and
 - peer review.

Professional interventions represent the main group of 'strategies' with which healthcare workers in transfusion are familiar. Audit and feedback is defined by EPOC as 'any summary of clinical performance of health care over a specified period of time. The summary may also have included recommendations for clinical action.' Audit and feedback is a very well-established tool for evaluation and improvement of the quality of clinical care and quality assurance in hospitals with the objective to improve patient care

Practical Transfusion Medicine, Fourth Edition. Edited by Michael F. Murphy, Derwood H. Pamphilon and Nancy M. Heddle.
© 2013 John Wiley & Sons, Ltd. Published 2013 by John Wiley & Sons, Ltd.

and outcomes through careful review of care provided against explicit standards. Where indicated, changes are then implemented at an individual, team or service level. Further monitoring is used to confirm improvement in healthcare delivery. Audit and feedback is widely used across the National Health Service (NHS) in the UK as a quality improvement method and is used by transfusion services worldwide to monitor parameters such as the number of units transfused/patient for a given procedure or condition and/or the proportion of patients receiving any blood. The proportion of transfusions deemed to be appropriate is sometimes assessed (also see Chapter 23). However, as currently used, audit and feedback does not work consistently and the effects are generally considered small to moderate. The method of feedback (e.g. at the individual or team level) is acknowledged as critical to delivering change, and will be discussed again later.

Educational outreach involves the 'use of a trained person who meets with providers in their practice settings to give information with the intent of changing the provider's practice'. Educational meetings are defined by EPOC as 'participation of healthcare providers in conferences, lectures, workshops or traineeships'. Other examples of interventions include the use of local opinion leaders who are 'providers nominated by their colleagues as educationally influential'. Reminders are 'patient- or encounter-specific information, provided verbally, on paper or on a computer screen, which is designed or intended to prompt a health professional to recall information'. Computer-aided decision supports would also be examples of reminders. In transfusion practice, reminders have been incorporated into transfusion request forms or computer order entry.

Changes in practice may also be instigated by combinations of these interventions and multifaceted interventions include 'any intervention including two or more components'. Multifaceted interventions are likely to be more costly than single-component interventions. A recent example by Rothschild et al. of a combined approach to changing and improving transfusion decisions was a report of a study examining transfusion practices before and after a conventional educational intervention followed by a randomized controlled trial of a decision support intervention based on computerized physician order entry [1]. Education and computerized decision

support both decreased the percentage of inappropriate transfusions, although, the residual amount of inappropriate transfusions remained high.

Organizational interventions are also widely used to deliver change in some areas of transfusion practice. In contrast to professional interventions looking at usage of blood, organizational interventions have been designed to deliver safer transfusion practice. Examples might include: the introduction of two-person pretransfusion bedside checking or patient identification using barcoding. Aspects of wider quality assurance systems for delivering safer transfusion practice might also be considered as organizational interventions for change, but these categories will not be considered further in this chapter.

Comparing and enhancing interventions to change practice

Different forms of behavioural interventions are undertaken by hospitals and blood transfusion services worldwide with the aim of changing transfusion practice, but there are few data on their relative or absolute effectiveness. The broad principles of clinical research appraisal should be applied to evaluate all studies of interventions, as for any pharmaceutical intervention in medical care. Randomized controlled trials would be expected to provide the highest level of evidence. For example, a controlled trial by Soumerai et al. of an intensive educational outreach programme (based around printed materials, presentations and face-to-face visits by transfusion medicine specialists) indicated good evidence for improved appropriateness of blood component use [2, 3]. What this trial did not perhaps address were questions regarding the sustainability of changes and overall cost effectiveness.

An update of two previous systematic reviews [4, 5] has identified and appraised all relevant publications evaluating different interventions in transfusion. The identification of the eligible literature in the field of practice improvement was challenging because of the wider numbers of potentially relevant journals and the lack of specific indexing to trials trying to change transfusion practice. In addition, many of the identified studies reported multiple and different endpoints or defined appropriateness of transfusion in different ways. In total, 43 studies (17 published since 2001) were identified and, taken as a whole, the reported results indicated variable effectiveness of guidelines, audit and feedback, and other interventions such as the implementation of a new transfusion request form or various education initiatives.

In general, interventions for the reduction of transfusion studied in clinical trials seemed to be effective. For red cell transfusions, the reported absolute reductions of inappropriate transfusions were −31% to +4%, an absolute reduction of 0.55 to −0.01 in the number of units transfused per patient and a relative reduction of −75% to +1% for the total number of units transfused (Table 47.1). Due to the lack of emphasis placed on detailing the interventions and use of a multifaceted intervention in most of the studies, determining the relative effectiveness of different types of interventions to change transfusion practice is difficult. However, no specific type of intervention appeared to be clearly more effective than others and there was no clear benefit of multifaceted interventions [4, 5]. There were significant limitations to the quality of the evidence. Most of the studies were not controlled trials, but 'before-and-after' studies with no concurrent controls. This type of study design cannot account for changes that may occur over time for other reasons, and are also more prone to bias in favour of the intervention. Most were single-centre studies and many were performed more than 10 years ago. The reported successes in these published studies also raise the possibility of a 'Hawthorne effect', which

describes an initial improvement in performance due to the simple act of observing the performance. These concerns about the true effectiveness and the durability of the effect of these interventions were raised in one study that reported a return to the baseline rate of transfusions three months after the completion of the intervention, and were also reported in a follow-up assessment from another study that also found a return to previous transfusion practice. None of the studies formally reported cost-effectiveness comparisons, and it is also likely that these publications will be susceptible to 'publication bias' in that studies with negative results may not have been submitted for publication.

The results of the systematic review support the concept that interventions can be successful in changing physicians' transfusion practices. These findings are similar to other studies that have examined the effects of interventions to change physician practice in other settings. However, given the limitations of the studies, there is uncertainty as to the nature of the 'active ingredients' of interventions (or combinations of ingredients) that have the maximum effectiveness in delivering sustained (and cost-effective) changes in transfusion practice. For example, considerable scope exists to improve the impact of audit and feedback on patient care and outcomes; as described later, the effectiveness and consistency of audit and feedback may be considerably enhanced by ensuring that the feedback is behaviourally specific and

Table 47.1 Changes in red blood cell utilization following introduction of behavioural interventions to change transfusion practice.

Outcome	Number of studies with reduction	Mean absolute reduction (relative reduction)	Range of absolute reduction* (relative reduction)
Randomized controlled trials			
No. of units/patient	1/1	−0.02 (−8%)	–
Inappropriate transfusions (%)	4/4	− 9%	−20% to +2%
Before and after studies			
No. of units	8/9	– (−27%)	– (−75% to 1%)
No. of units/patient	13/13	−0.2 (−14%)	−0.55 to −0.01 (−29% to −5%)
Patients transfused (%)	8/10	−8%	−50% to +30%
Inappropriate transfusions (%)	7/7	−19%	−31% to +4%

*Range is lowest and highest reductions reported in individual studies.

accompanied by a behavioural target and a targeted action plan.

Variation in practice

The variability in transfusion practice should not be a surprise to any healthcare professional involved in this area of medicine. Indeed, in a wider context, all healthcare systems experience inappropriate variation in treatments and treatment rates that suggest there is considerable inappropriate practice. Alongside the public and political anxiety surrounding blood transfusion, this variation in practice has arguably been more comprehensively documented over a longer period of time for transfusion medicine than many other areas of healthcare, and is frequently reported as a key driver for the need for, and use of, interventions to change practice. One of the first and more commonly quoted studies on this topic was reported by the Sanguis Study Group [6]. They evaluated the use of blood components for elective surgery at multiple European hospitals and reported large differences between hospitals and clinical teams in the use of red cell transfusion for the same surgical procedures, with no clear explanation based on patient and clinical factors such as age, preoperative haemoglobin or perioperative blood loss.

Variation in usage has also been reported for other blood components. In a comparison of plasma use in a number of countries, the ratio of frozen plasma (FP) units to red blood cell units transfused varied from 1:3.6 in the USA to 1:8.5 in France [7]. Other studies have reported wide variation in the use of plasma and platelets among centres within the same country, including patients undergoing cardiac surgery and critical care patients. Other studies have suggested that FFP may be associated with the highest rate of inappropriate transfusion, with some studies indicating a rate of inappropriate transfusions as high as 50%.

However, the reasons for variation in transfusion practice are complex. Arguably some of this variation may be expected given the complicated nature of healthcare and wide differences between patients and their responses to intensive medical or surgical treatments, which are frequently the setting for transfusion. Although some variation is to be expected in any healthcare setting, it is variation against an explicit set of criteria or guidelines based on good evidence that is the key issue. When there is good scientific evidence that supports evidence-based transfusions guidelines, then practice variation that continues and deviates from these guidelines is a concern that requires scrutiny.

An increasing number of transfusion trials are being undertaken and reported using clinically relevant outcomes and are providing worthwhile additions to the evidence base for transfusion practice. Interestingly, these trials are beginning to challenge some of the preconceived notions of the clinical benefits of transfusion. For example, in the topic of red cell transfusions, a number of threshold studies are now published [8, 9]. The transfusion requirements in critical care (TRICC) trial compared two transfusion thresholds for adult patients admitted to Canadian intensive care units; the results of a subgroup analysis showed a trend towards lower 30-day mortality in the restrictive transfusion group. In the paediatric intensive care unit setting, a similar restrictive transfusion strategy was found not to be inferior to a more liberal strategy. Comparable trials evaluating red cell transfusion strategies in neonates and recently for hip fracture surgery have also been published [9–11]. As a broad generalization, the combined weight of evidence from these trials of red cell transfusion does not support unrestricted use of red cell transfusions in many patient groups and therefore appears to argue against the intuitive desire to raise haemoglobin levels.

In the UK, national comparative audits of transfusion practice provide baseline information on compliance with standards and are undertaken through a collaboration between NHS Blood and Transplant and the Royal College of Physicians. These audits continue to demonstrate that approximately 20% of red cell transfusions, and an even higher proportion of transfusions of plasma and platelets, are not compliant with national guidelines, particularly in medical settings, and suggest that blood usage can be reduced [12, 13].

Models of behaviour and change

It is important to study systematically the wider influences on decisions to transfuse in the context of the considerable variation in practice. At one level, inappropriate variation in blood usage may reflect poor knowledge by physicians. However, there are likely to be many other influences on clinical practice and a number of ways to improve and optimize transfusion practice that may not focus solely around knowledge (or the lack of it).

It has been suggested that the clinical actions of healthcare professionals are influenced by the same factors that influence human behaviour in general. Assuming that this is correct, models of change can then be used to understand the behaviour of health professionals better and to inform the development of interventions to change behaviour [14–16]. Some models propose that the ways in which people think about and manage changes in practice, and not just their knowledge, will influence their behaviour. For example, one synthesis of evidence proposes 11 'theoretical domains' or factors that influence behaviour change in practice (Figure 47.1).

These domains could be explored using the following questions:

1 Do I (or my staff) have the necessary skills (e.g. communication skills, technical skills) to implement the recommended change? (Skills)
2 Is the recommended change in practice consistent with my professional training? Do I see it as my professional responsibility? (Professional role and identity)

3 Am I confident that we can do this effectively? (Beliefs about capabilities)
4 Do we have the necessary resources (e.g. time, staff, equipment, space)? (Environmental context and resources)
5 What protocols, procedures, monitoring or prompts will be needed to ensure that our policies are implemented? (Behavioural regulation)
6 Does the proposed new practice create unpleasantness, discomfort or work stress? (Emotion)
7 What are the views of other important or relevant people? Are my senior colleagues in favour of a change in practice? What will be the views of staff coming on to the ward on the next shift? Do the patients' relatives have strong views? (Social influence)
8 Is the new practice something that I may forget to do? Am I clear which patients should receive care differently? (Memory, attention and decision processes)
9 Where does the new practice fall on my list of clinical priorities? How important is it? (Motivation and goals)
10 Is it good practice? What is my understanding of the evidence about effectiveness versus risk? How do I weigh up the pros and cons? What might be the consequences of the action (for the patient, for other patients in the unit, for me or for the clinical team)? (Beliefs about consequences).

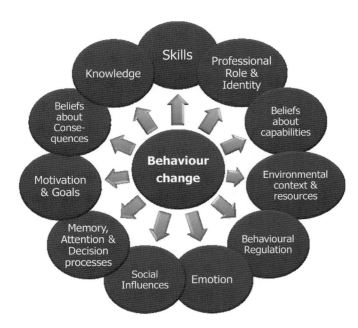

Fig 47.1 Depiction of 11 theoretical domains that may explain behaviour change in clinical practice. Reproduced from Michie *et al.* [16].

A behavioural perspective on enhancing the uptake of evidence-based transfusion practice may not only help unravel the complexities of decisions to transfuse but lead to new strategies for influencing clinicians' use of blood. For example, different domains influencing behaviour change can be elaborated further in ways that could identify the major drivers of decisions about whether or not to transfuse in a specific situation. These drivers focus on how individual clinicians might weigh up the relative importance of various factors to do with transfusion. Attitudes arise not only from the perceived advantages and disadvantages of transfusing, but also on how individuals balance them up against one another. It might be understandable if immediate adverse events were weighed more heavily than delayed adverse events, even though the likelihood of the delayed event may be greater. Similarly, the influences of other people with different views (say, the patient's family) is likely to be greater when those people are present in the ward than when they are distant. Further, factors influencing the clinician's control over the behaviour may exert different amounts of influence. For example, time constraints will have a more powerful influence when other critically ill patients are in greater need of attention. Published research has identified consistent patterns of influences on transfusion behaviour, encompassing theoretical domains of knowledge, social influences, beliefs about capabilities, beliefs about consequences and behavioural regulation. Of note, behavioural regulation (including techniques such as goal setting and providing feedback) was identified as a key domain influencing transfusion practice [17, 18].

Implementation research

There is increasing recognition that the findings from clinical research will not change population health outcomes unless healthcare systems and professionals adopt them in practice. However, a consistent finding from many groups and organizations is that this transfer of research findings into practice is unpredictable and in many cases slow and inconsistent. This gap between evidence and practice is a strategically important problem for policy makers, healthcare systems and research funders because it limits the health, social and economic impacts of clinical research. There is no reason to believe that this is any different for

transfusion medicine and the problem of slow uptake will become more important as new primary research is published. Recognition of this quality gap in practice has led to much more interest in active quality improvement strategies over the last 10 years, and a body of implementation research has developed in many different healthcare areas [19–21]. As a generalization, this again demonstrates that interventions can be effective, although providing less information to guide the choice or to optimize the interventions in actual practice.

The starting position for implementation research is the recognition that identifying factors predictive of clinicians' behaviour that are amenable to change may guide the design and choice of interventions with the highest chance of success. However, our understanding of potential barriers and enablers to quality improvement is largely limited in transfusion and hindered by a lack of a 'basic science' relating to determinants of professional and organizational behaviour and potential targets for intervention. A systematic investigation of the beliefs associated with inappropriate transfusion practice and barriers to change could therefore point to potentially effective ways to optimize practice.

As an example, audit and feedback is widely used and embedded within the NHS, providing an existing vehicle for quality improvement that can be optimized for transfusion. Systematic reviews indicate small to medium effects of 6–16% on clinical practice and patient outcomes, although effects are often variable [19, 20]. Clearly, there is potential to improve the practice of audit and feedback. However, there is little rigorous evidence on how to optimize its content or delivery, target key health professionals and parts of the organization necessary for conducting it or reliably maximize its effectiveness. Research is beginning to provide data on how to enhance its effects and understand the key mechanisms for its effectiveness. Feedback can be enhanced by reviewing the written content to deliver direct responses better or by targeting its delivery to the relevant staff with discussion and agreement of action plans. Enhanced delivery might include practical guidance for clinical teams on how best to implement the process of delivering feedback, including the development of materials for clinical teams to facilitate discussion and agreement of contextually appropriate goals and action plans.

Conclusions

Many healthcare professionals are becoming more aware of the need to practise evidence-based transfusion medicine. However, there remains considerable variation in transfusion practice in spite of explicit criteria and guidelines. Some surgical teams carry out major procedures without blood transfusion by attention to patient care throughout the perioperative period. For example, a combination of educational support for algorithms for blood management and restrictive transfusion thresholds may offer a more effective approach to blood conservation than the implementation of more complex (or costly) single interventions, but better evidence on the relative effectiveness of these (or other) strategies is required. While interventions to change transfusion practice can be aimed at a number of levels (individual health care professionals, healthcare groups or teams, organizations providing healthcare, the larger healthcare system or environment), the majority of interventions have been aimed at individual practitioners, as ultimately it is the individual clinician who dictates much of the decision-making around patient care. More resources need to be devoted towards a better understanding of the promotion of clinical effectiveness and the uptake of clinically effective transfusion practice (*evidence-based implementation*). Evidence of 'what to do' is one thing, but learning 'how to implement' is another.

Key points

1 The evidence base for transfusion practice is poorly developed but is improving. As it increases, changes in transfusion behaviour will need to be enacted more frequently.
2 Transfusion practice is also characterized by variation in spite of explicit criteria and guidelines.
3 The decision to transfuse is a complex process and knowledge is unlikely to be the only influence; research into these factors is generally sparse.
4 A better understanding of the determinants of transfusion behaviour should guide the design and choice of interventions better in order to deliver changes and improvements in transfusion practice. These need to be evaluated in rigorous clinical studies.

References

1 Rothschild JM, McGurk S, Honour M *et al.* Assessment of education and computerised decision support interventions for improving transfusion practice. *Transfusion* 2007; 47: 228–239.
2 Salem-Schatz SR, Avorn J & Soumerai SB. Influence of clinical knowledge, organisational context and practice style on transfusion decision making: implications for practice change strategies. *J Am Med Assoc* 1990; 264: 476–483.
3 Soumerai SB, Salem-Schatz SR, Avorn J *et al.* A controlled trial of education outreach to improve blood transfusion practice. *J Am Med Assoc* 1993; 270: 961–966.
4 Tinmouth A, MacDougall L, Fergusson D *et al.* Reducing the amount of blood transfused. *Arch Intern Med* 2005; 165: 845–852.
5 Wilson K, MacDougall L, Fergusson D, Graham L, Tinmouth A & Hebert, PC. The effectiveness of interventions to reduce physician's levels of inappropriate transfusion: what can be learned from a systematic review of the literature. *Transfusion* 2002; 42(9): 1224–1229.
6 Sanguis Study Group. Use of blood products for elective surgery in 43 European hospitals. *Transfus Med* 1994; 4: 251–268.
7 Stanworth S & Tinmouth A. Plasma transfusion and use of albumin. In: TL Simon, EL Snyder, CP Stowell, RG Strauss, BG Solheim & M Petrides (eds), *Rossi's Textbook of Transfusion Medicine*, 4th edn. Wiley-Blackwell andAABB Press; 2012 (in press).
8 Carless PA, Henry DA, Carson JL, Hebert PP, McClelland B & Ker K. Transfusion thresholds and other strategies for guiding allogeneic red blood cell transfusion. *Cochrane Database Syst Rev* 2010, Issue 10, Article No.: CD002042. DOI: 10.1002/14651858.CD002042.pub2.
9 Lacroix J, Hébert PC, Hutchison JS, Hume HA, Tucci M, Ducruet T, Gauvin F, Collet JP, Toledano BJ, Robillard P, Joffe A, Biarent D, Meert K & Peters MJ; TRIPICU Investigators; Canadian Critical Care Trials Group; Pediatric Acute Lung Injury and Sepsis Investigators Network. Transfusion strategies for patients in pediatric intensive care units N Engl J Med 2007, 19 April; 356(16):1609–1619.
10 Kirplani H, Whyte RK & Anderson C. The premature infants in need of transfusion (PINT) study: a randomised controlled trial of a restrictive (low) versus liberal (high) transfusion threshold for extremely low birthweight infants. *J Pediatr* 2006; 149: 301–307.
11 Carson JL, Terrin ML, Noveck H, Sanders DW, Chaitman BR, Rhoads GG, Nemo G, Dragert K, Beaupre L,

Hildebrand K, Macaulay W, Lewis C, Cook DR, Dobbin G, Zakriya KJ, Apple FS, Horney RA & Magaziner J; FOCUS Investigators. Liberal or restrictive transfusion in high-risk patients after hip surgery. *N Engl J Med* 2011, 29 December; 365(26): 2453–2462. Epub 14 December 2011.

12 Stanworth SJ, Grant-Casey J, Lowe D, Laffan M, New H, Murphy MF & Allard S. The use of fresh frozen plasma in England: high levels of inappropriate use in adults and children. *Transfusion* 2010; 51(1): 62–70.

13 Estcourt L. National comparative audit of platelet transfusions, 2010. Key findings of the audit with regard to the inappropriate use of platelet transfusions. http://hospital.blood.co.uk/library/pdf/PlateletRe-audit-Key_Findings_2010.pdf.

14 Carver CS & Scheier MF. Control theory: a useful conceptual framework for personality-social, clinical and health psychology. *Psycholog Bull* 1998; 92, 111e135.

15 Ajzen I. The theory of planned behaviour. *Organ Behav Hum Decis Process* 1991; 50: 179–211.

16 Michie S, Johnson A, Abraham C, Lawton R, Parker D & Walker A. Making psychological theory useful for implementing evidence based practice: a consensus approach. *Qual Safety Health Care* 2005; 14: 26–33.

17 Francis JJ, Stockton C, Eccles MP, Johnston M, Cuthbertson BH, Grimshaw JM, Hyde C, Tinmouth A & Stanworth SJ. Evidence-based selection of theories for designing behaviour change interventions: using methods based on theoretical construct domains to understand clinicians' blood transfusion behaviour. *Br J Health Psychol* 2009; 14: 625–646.

18 Francis JJ, Tinmouth A, Stanworth SJ, Grimshaw JM, Johnston M, Hyde C, Stockton C, Brehaut JC, Fergusson D & Eccles MP. Using theories of behaviour to understand transfusion prescribing in three clinical contexts in two countries: Development work for an implementation trial. *Implement Sci* 2009, 24 October; 4: 70. PMID: 19852832.

19 Grimshaw JM, Thomas RE, MacLennan G, Fraser C, Ramsay CR, Vale L, Whitty P, Eccles MP, Matowe L, Shirran L *et al.* Effectiveness and efficiency of guideline dissemination and implementation strategies. *Health Technol Assess* 2004, Report, p. 8.

20 Jamtvedt G, Young JM, Kristoffersen DT, O'Brien MA & Oxman AD. Audit and feedback: effects on professional practice and health care outcomes. *Cochrane Database Syst Rev* 2006; Issue 2, Article No.: CD000259. DOI: 10.1002/14651858.CD000259.pub2.

21 Craig P, Dieppe P, Macintyre S, Michie S, Nazareth I & Petticrew M. Developing and evaluating complex interventions: the new Medical Research Council guidance. *Br Med J* 2008; 337: a1655.

Further reading

Cooksey R. *A Review of UK Health Research Funding.* Norwich: HMSO; 2006.

Effective Health Care. Bulletin on the effectiveness of health service interventions for decision makers. Centre for Reviews and Dissemination, The Royal Society of Medicine. Available at: www.york.ac.uk.

Eisenstaedt RS. Modifying physicians' transfusion practice. *Transfus Med Rev* 1997; 11: 27–37.

Glasziou P, Chalmers I, Altman D, Bastian H, Boutron I, Brice A, Jamtvedt G, Farmer A, Ghersi D, Groves T *et al.* Taking healthcare interventions from trial to practice. *Br Med J* 2010; 341: c3852.

Grol R. Implementation of changes in practice. In: R Grol, M Wensing & M Eccles (eds), *Improving Patient Care: Implementing Change in Clinical Practice.* Oxford: Elsevier; 2004.

48 Scanning the future of transfusion medicine

Dana V. Devine[1], Walter H. Dzik[2] & Zbigniew M. Szczepiorkowski[3]

[1]Canadian Blood Services, Ottawa, Ontario and Centre for Blood Research, University of British Columbia, Vancouver, British Columbia, Canada

[2]Blood Transfusion Service, Massachusetts General Hospital and Harvard Medical School, Boston, Massachusetts, USA

[3]Transfusion Medicine Service, Cellular Therapy Center, Dartmouth-Hitchcock Medical Center and Geisel School of Medicine at Dartmouth, Hanover, New Hampshire, USA

Transfusion medicine is a technology-based discipline. The early years of the 21st century have witnessed exciting innovation and discovery throughout the biological sciences including transfusion medicine. New technology is being introduced that is changing the way blood is collected, processed and used for therapeutic benefit. Beginning from the vantage point of recent changes to our profession, this chapter attempts to summarize developments anticipated to occur before the year 2018 as well as innovations that may lie further in the future. Considerations of blood collection and component preparation, hospital-based transfusion practice and cellular therapies are considered in turn (see Table 48.1). The authors recognize that the actual pace of change is often slower than the pace of innovation and acknowledge that some predictions may be influenced by optimism. Indeed, significant advances in healthcare and transfusion are expensive and the appetite of modern society to create new technology will need to be tempered by the wisdom of its application.

Blood collection and component production

Over the past two decades, blood organizations have become increasingly focused on the use of good manufacturing practices (GMPs) adapted from pharmaceutical manufacturing to bring increased standardization to the production of blood components. At the same time, technological advances have brought an increasing level of automation with new approaches on the horizon. These developments have taken place against a backdrop of blood management practices that have actually slowed or reduced the demand for red cells in many developed countries, while platelet concentrate demand continues to increase. These trends keep donor recruitment professionals hard at work and cause us to maintain our heightened emphasis on blood component safety.

Donors

Recent: are we doing donors harm?

Despite considerable effort to create artificial blood components over the last decades, the maintenance of a blood supply remains completely dependent on the goodwill of our fellow citizens. Having created donation practices that optimize an individual's opportunity to donate whole blood or apheresis products, we have now begun to ask whether these practices are actually causing inadvertent harm to some groups of donors. Our attention has been drawn to this area by recent work on quantification, analysis and amelioration of adverse donor events, particularly in our youngest donors [1]. The development of more sophisticated deferral criteria based on estimated blood volume should make donation safer [2]. Recent studies addressing donor iron metabolism have highlighted

Practical Transfusion Medicine, Fourth Edition. Edited by Michael F. Murphy, Derwood H. Pamphilon and Nancy M. Heddle.
© 2013 John Wiley & Sons, Ltd. Published 2013 by John Wiley & Sons, Ltd.

Table 48.1 Transfusion medicine horizon scanning.

	Recent trends	Before 2018	Beyond 2018
Donor considerations	Focus on iron status and minimizing adverse donation events	Identification of donor factors that determine stored product quality	Donor management based on individual genetic characteristics
Bloodborne infectious diseases	Concern over untested pathogens; PRT use increases	PRT applied to red cells; technology to preserve quality in PRT-treated products	Widespread use of PRT internationally. New PRT technology applied to whole blood
Risk management for blood safety	Recognition of inconsistent decision making	Development of risk-based decision-making frameworks	International harmonization of risk management for blood safety
Blood component manufacturing – quality perspective	Widespread use of leucocyte reduction; increased use of automation	Continued shift to high volume component processing centres	Near walk-away production of components; real-time quality control
Blood storage	DEHP scrutinized; focus on product storage	New storage technologies to improve quality	New quality standards focus on product efficacy
Haemovigilance	Collection of hospital data	Policy driven by outcomes	Shared databases among hospitals
Machine-readable patient identification	Early adopters: bar code at the bedside	Commercialization of platforms	A new standard of care in patient identification
Clinical indications for components	RCTs destroy old dogma	Do stored red cells deliver oxygen?	Indications for FFP finally defined
RBC genotyping	Two assays become available	Increasing use in clinical practice	Recurrent donors routinely typed
Bedside diagnostics	Viscoelasticity rediscovered	Noninvasive haemoglobin measure	Tissue oxygen sensors
Immune manipulation	Rituximab and eculizumab	Improved agents for B cell suppression	Antigen-specific tolerance
Haemostasis	PCC use increases	New oral anticoagulants	Reversible anticoagulants
HSCT	RCT to identify best graft sources	Better GVHD control	HSCT becomes a low risk procedure
Cancer immunotherapy	Early methods approved	New products available	Individualized immunotherapy
Cellular therapy in nonmalignant diseases	Trials in different disorders begin	Phase 3 trials to determine efficacy	Cellular therapy competes with small molecules
Blood components	Red cells and platelets *in vitro*	Large-scale production	Economically viable products

PRT, pathogen reduction technology; DEHP, diethyl hexyl phthalate, PCC, prothrombin complex concentrates; RCT, randomized controlled trial; HSCT, haemopoietic stem cell transplantation; GVHD, graft-versus-host disease.

the differences in managing donor iron stores across various jurisdictions and the vulnerability of some donors to chronic disruption of iron stores [3]. The challenge, as always, will be to ensure that blood system operators attend to the responsibility of their advocacy and stewardship, not only of the blood supply but of those who create it.

Looking ahead: optimizing the donor's impact on product quality

Donors represent the 'raw material' for the manufacture of blood components. In almost all other manufacturing processes, the raw materials are qualified to increase the probability of making a high quality product. In blood transfusion we have been, and remain, appropriately focused on qualifying our donors with respect to their behaviours that may influence product safety from the standpoint of transmissible diseases. In addition, to avoid causing bodily harm to donors, we also focus on their suitability to undergo the process of donation. In the next decade, our focus will be not only on increasing the donor base to offset any increase in demand due to shifting demographics or increased accessibility of health care but will be on improving our understanding of donor characteristics as they relate to product quality. As the tools of proteomics, genomics and metabolomics are beginning to be applied to understanding the characteristics of stored blood components, the role of the variability of donor characteristics becomes increasingly apparent [4]. Armed with this information, we will manage donors with tailored strategies for donation and produce those products that are most likely to have the highest product quality. This will lead to much more sophisticated donor information utilization, clinic design and donor relationship management.

Blood component manufacturing – safety

Recent: safer but unaffordable?

We remain frozen in the headlights of blood safety risk. Good work has been accomplished in lowering the risk of known transfusion transmissible diseases through the development of sophisticated tests. However, these come with significant cost and it is clear that we are reaching the breaking point with respect to how much additional safety even wealthy nations can afford. For the developing world, there are even greater challenges. Yet despite massive financial investment, we know that fatal complications from bloodborne pathogens still occur due to lack of testing (e.g. *Babesia*), highlighting the pitfall of our current risk reduction strategy: we cannot afford to test for everything. The development of the first generation of pathogen reduction treatments for platelets and plasma has brought an opportunity to rethink the blood safety paradigm. We must find a more cost-effective way to deal with known and emerging threats to blood safety than our current reactive approach of incremental test addition (also see Chapter 16). An important part of this discussion is the generation of a more uniform process for risk-based decision making in the area of blood safety that can be used by blood operators and regulatory authorities alike [5].

Future: make it simple, make it safe

Pathogen reduction technology (PRT) will become more widely used and applied to a broader range of blood components. Newer developments in PRT will include strategies to protect therapeutic elements in components from the damage caused by pathogen inactivation. Blood systems in the developed world will continue to mature after learning the lessons of HIV and hepatitis, moving from reactionary fear of any risk to blood safety to the recognition that risk must be balanced against other factors, including the security of the blood supply, cost and social justice.

Blood component manufacturing – quality

Recent: get the white out

In addition to the widespread application of GMP and quality management, two specific developments have led to a significant improvement in product quality in the last decade. The first is the wider use of pre-storage leucocyte reduction of blood components, resulting in the minimization of leucocyte-derived biological response modifiers in cellular blood components as well as the direct detrimental effects of passenger leucocytes themselves. The second is the increasing drive towards automation and standardization in blood component production. Whether this occurs through the use of apheresis equipment or the use of instrumentation to assist in the production of components from whole blood donations, it has fundamentally altered the way that blood services operate. Investment in such equipment and the quality systems required to operate GMP production facilities have in turn led to manufacturing consolidation with the creation of high throughput component production laboratories and mergers among smaller blood centres. Other recent developments in component manufacture will drive change in the future, including the spreading renewed concern over the use of diethyl hexyl phthalate (DEHP) as a plasticizer in storage sets [6] and renewed appreciation of the impact of component outdating on the cost of transfusion products, particularly platelets.

Future: the next major steps in the quality journey

The world of the blood operator will continue to be one of significant change. We will see newer generations of automated component equipment to process whole blood donations that do not have the high cost and large footprint of the current generation machinery; these will feed the increasing demand in developing countries for alternative strategies to improve technology and increase quality and consistency.

Storage as we know it will change dramatically. Products may be frozen or freeze-dried, allowing prolonged storage. Liquid cellular products are likely to be found in containers that have much improved preservation characteristics, readily addressing the concerns about the age of stored red cells or the short shelf life of platelets. Containers will have 'smarts', including the ability to self-interrogate and report their status to the blood bank throughout the storage period without breaking sterility of the system. This will permit the removal of products from the inventory that have an unacceptable loss of quality prior to their expected outdate.

However, before these new storage systems become available, concerns over possible harm caused by older red cell concentrates may force the development of new inventory management strategies focused on demand for red cells with a shorter shelf life. Unfortunately, this demand is likely to exist even if current randomized controlled trials fail to demonstrate any significant advantage to shorter shelf life red cells.

New quality parameters focused on product efficacy will be developed. For example, platelet count can only partially predict product efficacy and an improved understanding of the physiology of stored platelets will lead to the development of quality standards that more accurately reflect product efficacy. Similarly, the factors that affect the efficacy of red cells during storage will be identified. These will make strong candidates for better markers to monitor the quality of blood components produced by all methods.

Hospital blood transfusion practice

Improving hospital transfusion care

Hospital biovigilance lights the path to improved care

Recent trends: haemovigilance extends to the hospitals Led by programmes in the UK, Quebec and France, haemovigilance has spread worldwide and has become an expected standard of blood transfusion systems in economically advantaged nations (see Chapter 18). Recent efforts have focused on the root causes of patient harm. In 2010, the USA launched the haemovigilance module of the National Healthcare Safety Network, a programme run under the overall direction of the Centers for Disease Control. This programme is expected to gather information systematically on the frequency of *reported* adverse events among transfusion recipients. Nevertheless, even better data would be useful. We still do not understand well the reason why physicians request blood components, the clinical benefits of transfusion, nor the true frequency of adverse events. Data need not be collected from all hospitals in order to draw meaningful conclusions. A system that prospectively collects detailed data from a group of sentinel hospitals – whose size and complexity is representative of all hospitals – would serve to provide much needed data on blood transfusion therapies.

Looking ahead: policy driven by data Changes in transfusion medicine policy and regulation can be connected to haemovigilance data resulting in evidence-based prioritization and metrics for assessment. For example, recognition of rates of platelet bacterial contamination led to diversion of the initial portion of donor blood and screening for bacterial overgrowth. Haemovigilance data on the frequency of transfusion-associated acute lung injury led to policies that reduced high plasma volume products donated by female donors with HLA antibodies. As haemovigilance draws closer to the bedside to determine toxicities of blood transfusion accurately, policies and technologies can be rationally applied based on the reality of harm rather than the perception of threat.

Beyond 2018, shared databases will improve patient outcomes. The Quebec haemovigilance programme documented a statistically significant reduction in the frequency of haemolytic transfusion reactions as a result of sharing patient data among hospital transfusion services. For example, patients whose current antibody screen is negative but who previously had a red cell alloantibody identified at another hospital can avoid delayed haemolytic reactions. More importantly, ABO results on a first-time patient sample tested at one hospital can be instantly compared to prior ABO results obtained at other hospitals (see Chapter 23). Given the truly prodigious capacity of shared information systems in an Internet world, and given the technology for secure digital transactions upon which the world economy and legal systems already operate, there is no reason not to share data related to vital aspects of transfusion safety.

Machine-readable technology for patient identification

Early adopters show the way The use of bar codes to improve patient identification at the bedside was begun by a few early adopters in the first decade of the 21st century. The transfusion medicine programmes at the John Radcliffe Hospital in Oxford (UK) and the University of Iowa hospitals (USA) (among others) demonstrated that barcode-based systems could be used for the bedside clerical check. Despite these early steps, most hospitals continue to use eye-readable technology for the bedside identification check with poor performance. Surveys by the American College of Pathology document that all aspects of the pretransfusion bedside patient identification were performed in only 25% of transfusions [7].

Looking ahead to a new standard of care We anticipate that commercially available systems will be increasingly deployed in the next few years. Advances in point-of-care diagnostics (e.g. glucometry) that use barcode inputs for patient information and the increasing use of the electronic medical record will make machine-readable bedside technology for blood transfusion naturally integrated with other bedside nursing activities. In addition to bar codes, inexpensive radiofrequency chips embedded in wristbands and in bag labels will carry more information and are expected to make machine-readable technology even more user-friendly [8].

Beyond 2018, it is difficult to imagine that machine-readable patient identification will *not* become the standard of care. In all other areas of society, transactions are increasingly done using digital (not handwritten) technology. We look forward to the day when the current process – whereby healthcare workers in distracted environments attempt to check eye-readable information found on printed labels and on printed wristbands – will be a thing of the past.

Clinical indications for standard blood components

Recent trends: randomized controlled trials destroy old dogma Recent years have witnessed multiple examples of transfusion dogma overturned by higher quality evidence obtained from randomized clinical trials. Examples include the PLADO study, which found no benefit to the use of >3 platelet units when transfused as prophylaxis against bleeding among patients with haematologic malignancy [9]. The FOCUS trial demonstrated that elderly patients undergoing orthopedic surgery do not fair better if maintained at a haemoglobin >10 g/dL [10]. The TRACS trial underscored the wisdom of a conservative policy for red cell transfusion for patients undergoing cardiac surgery [11]. Studies such as these breathe fresh air into the profession and become the bedrock for future advances.

Looking ahead: do stored red cells deliver oxygen? A central question in the profession is whether or not stored red cells adequately deliver oxygen to tissues. Four large prospective trials are currently underway to examine clinical outcomes among recipients randomized to short storage-versus-prolonged storage red cells. In the next five years the results of these trials are likely to have long-term implications for the management of worldwide RBC inventories [12].

Beyond 2018, we can anticipate that indications for FFP will finally be clarified. Despite the current excitement over the use of increasing amounts of FFP in the resuscitation of trauma patients, we should require randomized trials that will measure the benefit and the toxicity of large volumes of FFP. Of even greater value would be randomized trials among intensive care patients that identify the threshold INR values at which benefit from FFP occurs, when used for prophylaxis or for treatment of bleeding. As the number of critical care patients continues to grow, transfusion medicine will need high quality data to identify an appropriate trigger for FFP transfusion.

Diagnostics

Genotyping applied to transfusion care

Recent: commercial assays become available While many laboratories have developed in-house methods for analysis of DNA polymorphisms corresponding to red cell antigens, the field has been advanced by the development of commercially available assays for use in clinical transfusion medicine. BLOODchip™ (Progenika, Cambridge, MA) is a DNA-based system that uses a prepared solid support coated with probes for red cell antigen single nucleotide polymorphisms. Sample DNA is amplified with fluorescent nucleotides, hybridized with the probes, unbound DNA is washed away and the solid support examined for fluorescence. In the BeadChip™ (Bioarray Solutions, Warren, NJ) assay, coloured polystyrene beads are each coated with a different probe. The beads are hybridized with the test DNA and, after washing, the hybridized DNA is elongated with fluorescent nucleotides. A photograph determines which coloured beads acquired fluorescence. The Luminex™ platform is also being used for analysis of RBC DNA polymorphisms [13].

Looking ahead: increasing use of DNA methods for transfusion care Developments in DNA-based diagnostics should find increasing application in several areas of clinical transfusion care. For multitransfused patients or patients with strongly reactive autoantibodies, DNA-based methods provide a fast and reliable method of determining the probable phenotype. The method will prove valuable for antigens for which reliable antisera are in short supply. DNA assays are also well suited to determining fetal blood types and for resolution of variant D antigens [14].

Beyond 2018, with increasing throughput of DNA technology, DNA-based typing may be applied to recurrent group O blood donors. Genotyping, done once, could be reported on the bag label for each subsequent donation, creating an enormous pool of donors with extensive characterization of their red cell expected phenotype. This resource could be used not only for patients with alloantibodies but also in programmes of deliberate antigen matching to prevent sensitization [15].

Bedside diagnostics influence decision to transfuse

Recent: rediscovery of viscoelasticity Invented in 1948, measurement of clot viscoelasticity was largely a curiosity confined to liver transplant surgery complicated by fibrinolysis. In recent years two commercial systems have resurfaced: TEG® (thromboelastograph, Haemonetics, USA) and ROTEM® (rotation thromboelastometry, TEM International, Germany) (also see Chapter 25). Both systems employ a sensor placed in blood during rotational movement. The change in torque is detected electronically

in TEG® and optically in ROTEM®. Both systems assess time to initial clot formation, speed and strength of clot, and time to clot lysis. There is widespread interest in whether or not either of these systems can improve upon traditional coagulation testing as methods not only to diagnose defects in haemostasis but also to guide transfusion therapy. Good parallel studies with clinical outcomes will be needed and welcome [16].

Looking ahead: noninvasive monitoring may guide transfusion A recently developed clip-on finger oximeter offers a continuous readout of the patient's haemoglobin concentration. This technology, if validated in clinical practice, may change transfusion decisions for critically ill patients, especially during surgery. The technology, coupled with bedside cardiac echo imaging, could provide the three measures needed to calculate systemic oxygen delivery: haemoglobin concentration, percent saturation and cardiac output. Transfusions based on better physiologic measurements should be the shared clinical goal.

In the future, noninvasive measurement of tissue oxygen utilization will be the ultimate guide to red cell transfusion. Two devices represent early steps in this direction [17]. The Fore-Sight® (CAS Medical Systems, USA) system shines near infrared laser light on the scalp and measures reflected light from the surface and from the deeper (2.5–3 cm) underlying brain tissue. After subtracting the surface light component, the amount and wavelength of reflected deeper penetration light is used to estimate cerebral O_2 saturation. The In-spectra® device (Hutchinson Technology Inc., USA) measures real-time changes in tissue oxygen saturation of the thenar muscle, calculating the ratio of oxygenated-to-total haemoglobin at 0–14 mm beneath the skin. Whether or not devices such as these may one day serve to guide transfusion awaits research to be done.

Therapeutics

Advances in immune manipulation

Recent: rituximab and eculizumab Antibody-directed and complement-mediated cell destruction is central to the pathophysiology of haemolysis, humoral allograft rejection, platelet refractoriness, autoimmune neurologic disorders, certain varieties of vasculitis and other immune disorders. In recent years, anti-CD20 (rituximab) has been increasingly used for treatment of autoimmune blood disorders [18]. Eculizumab, a recombinant humanized murine monoclonal that inhibits cleavage of complement protein C5, effectively reduces complement-mediated membrane lysis in paroxysmal nocturnal haemoglobinuria and may be of benefit in the treatment of autoimmune haemolytic anaemia and atypical haemolytic uremic syndrome [19]. Eculizumab may have potential benefit in humoral allograft rejection, haemolytic transfusion reactions, hyperhaemolysis syndrome and certain varieties of vasculitis, including cryoglobulinemia. More research is needed to evaluate this agent either used singly or in combination with other immune inhibitors.

Looking ahead: increasing options for B-cell suppression and parallel further decline of plasma exchange New drugs directed at B-cell activity are emerging. These include B-cell depleting agents such as rituximab, alemtuzumab, ofatumumab and anti-CD19; B-cell activation inhibitors including epratuzumab (anti-CD22), belimumab and atacicept; and drugs directed at plasma cells, including the proteosome inhibitor bortezomib. In addition, recombinant factor H and factor I in the complement system would represent attractive infusion molecules for patients with immune-mediated tissue damage. The introduction of these and other drugs over the next decade should gradually replace plasma exchange as a treatment for immune-mediated disorders [20].

Beyond 2018, improved pharmacologic agents that act directly upon plasma cells or that induce antigen-specific immune suppression would be welcome. For example, in a patient who has made anticellano antibodies, one can imagine specific targeting of B-cell surface immunoglobulin resulting in clonal deletion of those cells generating anticellano. The human polyclonal immune response to blood group antigens represents an excellent model for the investigation of antigen-specific immune suppression. Application to HLA antibodies would have an immediate benefit for solid organ transplant patients.

New strategies for haemostasis

Recent: rise of prothrombin complex concentrates (PCCs) PCCs are pooled plasma-derived factor concentrates initially developed and licensed for the treatment of haemophilia B. Three-factor PCCs have qualified levels of factor IX, variable levels of factors II and X, and low levels of factor VII. Four-factor PCCs, in contrast, have therapeutic levels of factors II, VII, IX, X, C and S. Although four-factor PCCs are widely available in Canada, the UK and Europe, three-factor PCCs are the only currently licensed products available in the USA and Australia. Because four-factor PCCs offer ease of administration and small volume, they have recently been combined with vitamin K for emergency reversal of coumadin. Despite lack of evidence, enthusiasm for four-factor PCCs has led some to use them as an alternative to FFP in other clinical settings, such as liver disease, surgical bleeding and trauma [21]. The manufacturer of one four-factor PCC (Beriplex®) has applied to the US Food and Drug Administration for approval to market their product in the USA. If approved, the availability of this product will increase the options in the USA for emergency reversal of coumadin.

Looking ahead: alternatives to coumadin become widespread Two classes of oral medications serving as alternatives to coumadin were introduced in 2011: the direct thrombin inhibitor dabigatran and direct inhibitors of the factor Xa complex (rivaroxaban, apixaban and endoxaban). These drugs offer the convenience of fixed dosing without the need for blood test monitoring and a level of efficacy that is not inferior to coumadin. However, their anticoagulant effect is prolonged by renal insufficiency and the drugs all suffer the disadvantage of not having an agent proven to reverse their anticoagulant effect. Transfusion medicine specialists will certainly contribute to the challenging management of bleeding in the setting of these nonreversible anticoagulants [22].

As experience with the difficulties of managing bleeding among patients taking nonreversible anticoagulants grows, there will be pressure to develop reversible anticoagulants. In some ways, this advance will be a return to features originally offered by unfractionated heparin and coumadin, but with newer drugs that shed the disadvantages of blood monitoring, heparin-induced thrombocytopenia or vitamin K and drug interactions. Already, agents to reverse factor Xa inhibitors are under development and include recombinant Xa molecules where the active procoagulant site is blocked and where glutamic acid domains are depleted, resulting in a decoy substrate for direct Xa inhibitor medications.

Cellular therapy

Chronic, incurable or devastating conditions are often portrayed as the best targets for miraculous treatments with novel cellular therapies, including, among others, mesenchymal stem cells (MSCs), embryonic stem cells (ESCs) or induced pluripotent stem cells (iPSCs). It seems as if any human tissue contains cells that can be coaxed into pluri- or multipotent stem cells, which in turn can be used to alleviate, if not cure, any human condition. This is, of course, if one relies exclusively on headlines intended for the general public. Scientists including transfusion medicine specialists will need to manage societal expectations, otherwise cellular therapy may come to resemble the bloodletting of the 17th century or hydrotherapy of the 19th century. Cellular therapy, gene therapy and regenerative medicine have great promise, but only if clinical trials are well designed and research endeavours and achievements are honestly presented. In this section we will focus on a few examples of cell-based therapies and their potential impact on the future of healthcare.

Haematopoietic stem cell transplantation

Recent developments

Progress in haemopoietic stem cell transplantation (HSCT), the cell-based therapy recently celebrating its 50th anniversary, has been extremely encouraging. Since its inception, HSCT had to deal with several challenges, including optimal matching of the donor with recipient, the choice of the graft source assuring prompt engraftment with minimal complications and long-term complications including acute and chronic graft-versus-host disease (GVHD), delayed immune reconstitution and posttransplant lymphoproliferative disorders (PTLDs). Graft selection has been enhanced by the availability of cord blood units and new strategies for cellular expansion. The first randomized controlled study comparing apheresis versus marrow sources of haemopoietic stem cells (HSCs) was very recently reported. The study confirmed more rapid engraftment with apheresis HSC, but found a significantly increased incidence of chronic GVHD with apheresis HSC compared with HSC obtained from marrow (53% versus 40%) [23]. A new cellular therapy modality utilizing small molecules interacting with modified components of the human intrinsic apoptotic pathway (e.g. caspase 9) has been shown to be a powerful tool in the induction of cell death in patients receiving cell therapy [24]. This approach seems to be much more efficient than previous attempts to insert thymidine kinase-dependent suicide genes, which were activated in the presence of ganciclovir. Furthermore, manipulation of lymphocytes to generate cytotoxic T cells against adenovirus, cytomegalovirus and Epstein–Barr virus (EBV) has shown promise in the treatment of infections with these viruses and with EBV-associated PTLD. These virus-specific T-cell lines also showed efficacy against infections with all three viruses in partially HLA-matched third party recipients. Thus, they may become an 'off the shelf' treatment for many more patients [25].

Looking ahead

We should see an increased demand for marrow-derived HPC as the source for HSCT with a corresponding decrease in demand for apheresis collections. The impact is most likely to be moderate and transient as apheresis-derived HPC will still remain the first choice for the growing number of older patients and for those with aggressive malignant conditions. Advances in personalized medicine may further increase options in ameliorating GVHD without compromising graft versus tumour/leukaemia effect or increasing posttransplant infections. The survival rate of HSCT recipients with better selected donors and personalized graft processing should continue to improve. We should also see increased utilization of HSCT in nonmalignant conditions, such as HIV-infected patients with cells from CCR5 negative donors, once transplant related mortality and morbidity decrease further.

Immunotherapy in cancer treatment

Recent developments

The last two decades have seen numerous trials evaluating manipulation of the immune system in patients with cancer. One of the major issues facing the field is identification of appropriate endpoints, which range from the generation of antitumour lymphocytes to measurements of tumour burden, up to patient survival. The Cancer Immunotherapy Consortium established three novel endpoint recommendations: harmonization of assays of the immune response, definition of new immune-related response criteria and use of hazard ratios as a function of time to address delayed separation of survival curves [26]. Additional efforts to standardize the design and evaluation of so many heterogeneous immunotherapy trials should help to identify true biologic effects. Studies with only a few patients who respond well to immunotherapy, often hailed as final solutions, should be correctly interpreted as a proof-of-principle endeavour. Thus far, the biggest recognition in cancer immunotherapy was given to Sipuleucel-T (Provenge®; Dendreon), which was licensed in the USA in April 2010 for patients with metastatic prostate cancer. The logistics of this autologous therapy are very complex and the median increased survival of approximately four months is limited. Nevertheless, the demand for this therapy appears to be growing.

Looking ahead
Cancer immunotherapy is likely to continue to grow, despite the expense of treatments based on exclusively autologous therapies. New approaches to creating an immune response in the cancer patients will be tried and some of the new products will reach the market within the next 5 to 10 years. However, these therapies will continue to be challenged by small molecules and other directed therapies, which are generally easier to generate, test and bring to the market.

Cellular therapy in nonmalignant diseases

Recent developments
Cell-based therapies are being extensively studied in the cardiovascular area, especially in the treatment of acute and chronic heart failure and peripheral vascular disease. There are multiple approaches to identify the appropriate cell source (e.g. bone marrow, cord blood, peripheral blood, cardiomyocytes, pluripotent stem cells), cell manipulation (e.g. buffy coat enrichment, immunomagnetic selection) and form of administration (e.g. location, catheter, cell dose). All these variables make it difficult to assess which type of cells will be most successful in providing a long-lasting effect. Other medical specialties are also involved in a growing number of clinical trials. Examples include allogeneic mesenchymal stem cells in inflammatory bowel disease, pluripotent stem cells in spinal cord injury or growth of islet cells for patients with diabetes.

Looking ahead
This is the area of cellular therapy where the most will happen over the next few years. There will be

increased interest in identifying the best cellular therapy products for these chronic conditions with a very large market and potentially long-lasting impact on the health of many affected individuals. We should see first-generation products available for patients prior to 2018 and most likely in the area of cardiology, gastroenterology and metabolic disorders.

Ex vivo generation of blood components

Recent developments
Transfusion medicine specialists have both hoped and feared that one day all blood components would be generated *ex vivo*. Although initial efforts focused only on the expansion of HSCs *in vitro*, a growing knowledge of haemopoiesis allowed both expansion and maturation in culture. The first reports of *ex vivo* generation of fully mature human erythrocytes have been published in the last decade [27–29]. Different sources of stem cells were used, including CD34 positive HSCs from peripheral blood, bone marrow or cord blood, embryonic stem cells and human iPSCs. The process is time consuming and labour intensive but the final product is not different from adult red cells, at least in the initial studies. Recent studies showed that as few as 15 iPSC clones would be sufficient to cover all the needs of the French National Registry of People with a rare blood phenotype/genotype for individuals of Caucasian ancestry [29]. The reports of *ex vivo* generation of platelets have been also published.

Looking ahead
There is a dose of healthy scepticism regarding *ex vivo* production of blood components. The challenges of GMP and scale-up make these products prohibitively expensive for the immediate future. However, there are some products (e.g. red cells lacking high frequency antigens) that may be first to see a positive return on investment. While the developments remain exciting, it may be several decades before *ex vivo* generated blood components replace healthy volunteers for routine transfusions.

Economics of cellular therapy

Recent developments
The financial support for the vast majority of phase I and phase II cellular therapy trials comes from not-for-profit foundations and/or governmental grants. Small

for-profit companies, with only a few exceptions, have been able to bring their products to pivotal trials where they required additional capital to complete phase III trials. Only recently have large pharmaceutical companies showed interest in cell-based therapies in their earlier phases. Funding is also complicated by a very lengthy and primarily uncharted regulatory pathway for approval. The licensure of Provenge® by Dendreon in 2010 was the first example of successful navigation of a cellular therapy product from phase I through approval. Although the cost of a full treatment stands at $93 000 per patient, the company was able to navigate the complex private and public insurance market to have its product approved for reimbursement. Even with such success it is said that the investment costs may never be recouped. Other publicly traded companies involved in cellular therapy products have also experienced financial volatility. Recently, the widely publicized exit of Geron Corporation from the stem cell market illustrates the complexity of the economic environment of cellular therapy.

Looking ahead

Funding for cellular therapies will be an important component of the success or demise of the cell-based therapies. Continuous growth of public expectations of miraculous treatments could be met by many years of only incremental success. It is quite possible that current leading companies will not survive due to lack of financial support. Although we anticipate that some of the promised therapies will reach patients, the cost of development may disillusion many. Combination therapies, nanotechnology and small engineered molecules may prove to be a more dynamic therapeutic strategy leading to a shift in resources away from classical cellular therapy.

Conclusion: resetting priorities of health and healthcare

World economic recession

December 2007 marked the beginning of a prolonged economic recession in the USA, resulting from failings in the financial and mortgage markets and lack of oversight of banking and lending practices. Japan had already been in prolonged recession following the burst of an overinflated domestic real estate market in the 1990s. By 2011, sovereign debt among southern European nations resulted in a crisis of confidence in the euro. Worldwide unemployment reached record levels in wealthy nations, reduced tax revenues and placed greater strains on the delivery of national healthcare. There is no reason to believe that the recession now straining North America and Europe will resolve any faster than that which struck Japan a decade earlier. Thus, any expectations for advances in transfusion care and healthcare over the next decade should be set in the context of global worldwide economic constraints.

Cost of new technology collides with world demographics

In 2011, the world's population for the first time reached 7 billion and is expected to exceed 10 billion before mid-century. Most population growth has occurred in low income nations with impoverished healthcare. Meanwhile, in wealthy nations, population has increased but average per capita expenditure on healthcare has increased even more, fuelling substantial profits for suppliers to the healthcare industry. For example, in the USA the proportion of the gross domestic product spent on healthcare has risen steadily and in 2011 approached 18%. The effect of these two forces – the rising cost of healthcare technology and the rising world's population in low income nations – has increased the disparity in the per capita wealth devoted to human health (see Figure 48.1). For example, in 2007, the United States spent over $6000 per person on healthcare, while each of the nations of sub-Saharan Africa spent approximately one-hundredth as much ($60 per person per year) [30].

Changing how we use technology

While better products and technology account for some of the spiralling costs of healthcare, much healthcare expenditure is wasteful, redundant and unnecessary. Wasteful transfusion decisions, for example, may be fuelled by a combination of lack of knowledge on the part of the requesting clinician, fear of being 'wrong', pharmaceutical marketing and a professional ethos that fosters clinical extravagance over parsimony. If we are to use healthcare services in general and transfusion services in particular, more wisely and with greater *value*, then healthcare professionals

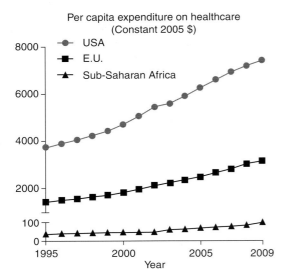

Per capita expenditure on healthcare
(Constant 2005 $)

Fig 48.1 Per capita expenditure on healthcare in the USA, Europe and sub-Saharan Africa. Note the split scale of the y axis. *Source:* World Bank, 2011.

will need to improve decision making under circumstances of risk. Patient management based on conservative use of healthcare resources is far more difficult than that based on unbridled use, involves the assumption of risk and requires a commitment to address the likely outcomes rather than all possible outcomes. Healthcare expenditures in wealthy nations are also fuelled by an unwarranted sense of entitlement by both doctor and patient. The expectations of both will need to become more realistic in a world where healthcare is no longer an enterprise characterized by extravagance.

Deciding who we are: healthcare priorities in a global context

How we choose to advance human health in the 21st century will ultimately reflect who we are. Some choices will reflect both our appetite for and our celebration of a level of technological achievement considered unreachable to earlier generations. Those advances will, however, not be affordable by or available to all who need them and will highlight the concentration of wealth and privilege among an ever smaller subset of the world's population. Other choices will serve to distribute basic healthcare

more broadly to the billions of humans who share the planet. Those advances will, however, require a redirection of energy and resources away from the spectacular achievements of organ transplantation, designer drugs and ultrahigh technology critical care. While many who enjoy the benefits of wealthy nations would argue that both paths are possible, the evidence – most clearly reflected by the growing worldwide disparity of per capita wealth devoted to healthcare – argues otherwise. It is entirely possible that we cannot have it both ways – that a choice is to be made between advancing healthcare technology or advancing world health. That choice is beyond the confines of the medical profession alone and will involve politicians, economists, religious groups, governments – each of us. Ultimately, how we chose to care for one another will define who we are.

Key points

1 Blood component processing continues to become more automated with strong quality systems in place driving consolidation of production activity.
2 Emphasis on blood component safety from transfusion-transmitted infections must be done from a perspective of cost effectiveness and informed risk-based decision making.
3 Management of blood donors is evolving to be better aligned with the needs of the hospital blood bank and to optimize the individual characteristics of each donor that impacts the quality of stored blood components.
4 Haemovigilance programmes focused on the hospital transfusion service can provide a data-driven method to improve patient outcomes.
5 Noninvasive measures of haemoglobin concentration and tissue oxygenation may improve clinical decision making for transfusion of red cells.
6 Reversible oral and intravenous anticoagulants and antigen-specific immune suppression would represent substantial therapeutic advances.
7 Haemopoietic stem cell transplantation will continue to evolve into a safer modality with more sophisticated approaches to minimize graft-versus-host disease and other complications.
8 Cell-based cancer immunotherapy will provide for better and more efficient individualized therapies, though at a significant cost.

9 Cell-based solutions affect many specialties (e.g. neurology, cardiology) and may also lead to an *ex vivo* generation of blood components for clinical use in the future.

References

1 Eder AF, Hillyer CD, Dy BA, Notari EP & Benjamin RJ. Adverse reactions to allogeneic whole blood donation by 16- and 17-year-olds. *J Am Med Assoc* 2008, 21 May; 299(19): 2279–2286.

2 Wiltbank TB, Giordano GF, Kamel H, Tomasulo P & Custer B Faint and prefaint reactions in whole-blood donors: an analysis of predonation measurements and their predictive value. *Transfusion* 2008, September; 48(9): 1799–1808.

3 Cable RG, Glynn SA, Kiss JE, Mast AE, Steele WR, Murphy EL *et al*. Iron deficiency in blood donors: the REDS-II Donor Iron Status Evaluation (RISE) study. *Transfusion* 2011; 51: 511–522.

4 Devine DV & Schubert P. Proteomic applications in blood transfusion: working the jigsaw puzzle. *Vox Sanguinis* 2011, January; 100(1): 84–91.

5 Stein J, Besley J, Brook C, Hamill M, Klein E, Krewski D *et al*. Risk-based decision-making for blood safety: preliminary report of a consensus conference. *Vox Sanguinis* 2011, November; 101(4): 277–281.

6 Shaz BH, Grima K & Hillyer CD. 2-(Diethylhexyl) phthalate in blood bags: is this a public health issue? *Transfusion* 2011, November; 51(11): 2510–2517.

7 Novis DA, Miller KA, Howanitz PJ, Renner SW & Walsh MK. Audit of transfusion procedures in 660 hospitals. A College of American Pathologists Q-Probes study of patient identification and vital sign monitoring frequencies in 16494 transfusions. *Arch Pathol Lab Med* 2003, May; 127(5): 541–548.

8 Murphy MF, Stanworth SJ & Yazer M. Transfusion practice and safety: current status and possibilities for improvement. *Vox Sanguinis* 2011, January; 100(1): 46–59.

9 Slichter SJ, Kaufman RM, Assmann SF, McCullough J, Triulzi DJ, Strauss RG *et al*. Dose of prophylactic platelet transfusions and prevention of hemorrhage. *N Engl J Med* 2010, 18 February; 362(7): 600–613.

10 Carson JL, Terrin ML, Noveck H, Sanders DW, Chaitman BR, Rhoads GG *et al*. Liberal or restrictive transfusion in high-risk patients after hip surgery. *N Engl J Med* 2011, 14 December; 365: 2453–2462.

11 Hajjar LA, Vincent JL, Galas FR, Nakamura RE, Silva CM, Santos MH *et al*. Transfusion requirements after cardiac surgery: the TRACS randomized controlled trial.

J Am Med Assoc 2010, 13 October; 304(14): 1559–1567.

12 Triulzi DJ & Yazer MH. Clinical studies of the effect of blood storage on patient outcomes. *Transfus Apher Sci* 2010, August; 43(1): 95–106.

13 Moulds JM, Sloan SR & Ness PM (eds). *BeadChip Molecular Immunohematology: Toward Routine Donor and Patient Antigen Profiling by DNA Analysis*. New York: Springer; 2011, pp. 1–152.

14 Anstee DJ. Red cell genotyping and the future of pretransfusion testing. *Blood* 2009, 9 July; 114(2): 248–256.

15 Denomme GA, Johnson ST & Pietz BC. Mass-scale red cell genotyping of blood donors. *Transfus Apher Sci* 2011, February; 44(1): 93–99.

16 Bolliger D, Seeberger MD, Tanaka KA *et al*. Principles and practice of thromboelastography in clinical coagulation management and transfusion practice *Transfus Med Rev* 2012; 26: 1–13.

17 Sakr Y. Techniques to assess tissue oxygenation in the clinical setting. *Transfus Apher Sci* 2010, August; 43(1): 79–94.

18 Stasi R. Rituximab in autoimmune hematologic diseases: not just a matter of B cells. *Semin Hematol* 2010, April; 47(2): 170–179.

19 Kavanagh D & Goodship TH. Atypical hemolytic uremic syndrome, genetic basis, and clinical manifestations. *Hematol Am Soc Hematol Educ Program* 2011; 2011: 15–20.

20 Clatworthy MR. Targeting B cells and antibody in transplantation. *Am J Transplant* 2011, July; 11(7): 1359–1367.

21 Patanwala AE, Acquisto NM & Erstad BL. Prothrombin complex concentrate for critical bleeding. *Ann Pharmacother* 2011, July; 45(7–8): 990–999.

22 Bauer KA. Recent progress in anticoagulant therapy: oral direct inhibitors of thrombin and factor Xa. *J Thromb Haemost* 2011, July; 9 (Suppl. 1): 12–19.

23 Anasetti C, Logan BR, Lee SJ, Waller EK, Weisdorf DJ, Wingard JR *et. al*. Peripheral-blood stem cells versus bone marrow from unrelated donors. *N Engl J Med* 2012, 18 October; 367(16): 1487–1496.

24 Di Stasi A, Tey SK, Dotti G, Fujita Y, Kennedy-Nasser A, Martinez C *et al*. Inducible apoptosis as a safety switch for adoptive cell therapy. *N Engl J Med* [Clinical Trial Research Support, NIH, Extramural] 2011, 3 November; 365(18): 1673–1683.

25 Sili U, Leen AM, Vera JF, Gee AP, Huls H, Heslop HE *et al*. Production of good manufacturing practice-grade cytotoxic T lymphocytes specific for Epstein–Barr virus, cytomegalovirus and adenovirus to prevent or treat viral infections post-allogeneic hematopoietic stem cell transplant. *Cytotherapy* 2012, January; 14(1): 7–11.

26 Hoos A, Eggermont AM, Janetzki S, Hodi FS, Ibrahim R, Anderson A *et al*. Improved endpoints for cancer immunotherapy trials. *J Natl Cancer Inst* [Research Support, Non-US Government Review] 2010, 22 September; 102(18): 1388–1397.

27 Anstee DJ. Production of erythroid cells from human embryonic stem cells (hESC) and human induced pluripotent stem cells (hiPSC). Transfusion clinique et biologique. *J Societé Francaise de Transfusion Sanguine* [Research Support, Non-US Government Review] 2010, September; 17(3): 104–109.

28 Mountford JC & Turner M. *In vitro* production of red blood cells. *Transfus Apher Sci* 2011, August; 45(1): 85–89.

29 Peyrard T, Bardiaux L, Krause C, Kobari L, Lapillonne H, Andreu G *et al*. Banking of pluripotent adult stem cells as an unlimited source for red blood cell production: potential applications for alloimmunized patients and rare blood challenges. *Transfus Med Rev* [Research Support, Non-US Government Review] 2011, July; 25(3): 206–216.

30 *Human Development Report*, 2007, United Nations. Available at: web: hdr.undp.org.

Further reading

Blajchman MA. The clinical benefits of the leukoreduction of blood products. *J Trauma* 2006, June; 60(6 Suppl.): S83–90.

Daley GQ & Scadden DT. Prospects for stem cell-based therapy. *Cell* 2008; 132: 544–548.

Gelderman MP & Vostal JG. Current and future cellular transfusion products. *Clin Lab Med* 2010, June; 30(2): 443–452.

Klein HG, Glynn SA, Ness PM & Blajchman MA; NHLBI Working Group on Research Opportunities for the Pathogen Reduction/Inactivation of Blood Components. Research opportunities for pathogen reduction/inactivation of blood components: summary of an NHLBI workshop. *Transfusion* 2009, June; 49(6): 1262–1268.

Mohsin S, Siddiqi S, Collins B & Sussman MA. Empowering adult stem cells for myocardial regeneration. *Circ Res* 2011, 9 December; 109(12): 1415–1428.

Riviere I, Dunbar CE & Sadelain M. Hematopoietic stem cell engineering at a crossroads. *Blood* 2011. Epub 2011/11/19.

Index

Page numbers in **bold** represent tables, those in *italics* represent figures.

Practical Transfusion Medicine, Fourth Edition. Edited by Michael F. Murphy, Derwood H. Pamphilon and Nancy M. Heddle.
© 2013 John Wiley & Sons, Ltd. Published 2013 by John Wiley & Sons, Ltd.